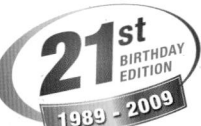

21st BIRTHDAY EDITION

1989 - 2009

THE CALORIEKING®
Calorie, F...

W9-ARQ-680

Weight Control Tips

✔ Eat Sensibly

- Avoid fad diets. Eat 3 sensible meals daily with adequate fruit and vegetables.
- Limit portion size. Limit fats and high-fat foods, sugar, soda and alcohol. *(Sample Meal Plan ~ Page 11)*

✔ Exercise Daily

- Get active and exercise every day!
- Include muscle-strengthening exercises. You'll lose more fat and keep it off. You'll also feel and look better, and you can eat a little more! *(Exercise Guide ~ Page 12)*

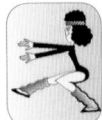

✔ Reshape Eating Behaviors

- Be aware of eating habits and behaviors that lead to overeating.
- Also focus on social and emotional situations that lead you to snack compulsively. *(Extra Notes ~ Page 14)*

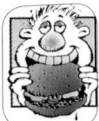

✔ Keep a Food & Exercise Journal

- A journal helps you see exactly what you eat and drink, and how much you exercise. *(Extra Notes ~ Page 15)*
- An excellent motivator and proven weight loss aid. Keeps you honest!

✔ Arrange Moral Support

Gain the support of family and friends. Get extra professional help if required, from your doctor, dietitian, psychologist, exercise trainer, or diet club. Beware of family saboteurs who discourage you from adopting a healthier lifestyle!

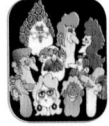

DOCTOR CHECK-UP

Ask your doctor to check your blood pressure, blood sugar and blood cholesterol levels.

HEALTHY WEIGHTS
~ MEN & WOMEN ~
(Over 18 Years)

Based on weights with least risk of disease or death from heart disease, diabetes, stroke and cancer.

Based on Body Mass Index of 20-25

BMI calculated as: $\dfrac{\text{Weight (kg)}}{\text{Height (m)}^2}$

Height (No Shoes) Ft Ins		Healthy Weight Range (Pounds)
4'7"	~	86-108
4'8"	~	88-110
4'9"	~	92-114
4'10"	~	97-121
4'11"	~	99-123
5'0"	~	101-127
5'1"	~	105-132
5'2"	~	110-136
5'3"	~	112-140
5'4"	~	114-145
5'5"	~	119-149
5'6"	~	123-156
5'7"	~	127-158
5'8"	~	129-162
5'9"	~	134-167
5'10"	~	138-173
5'11"	~	143-178
6'0"	~	145-182
6'1"	~	149-187
6'2"	~	156-193
6'3"	~	158-198
6'4"	~	162-202
6'5"	~	170-211
6'6"	~	172-215
6'7"	~	175-220

Body Fat Distribution & Health

Moderate amounts of body fat do not compromise health. However, excess fat above the hips carries a far greater health risk than fat on or below the hips - better to be a 'pear-shape' than an 'apple-shape'.

Abdominal obesity greatly increases the risk of developing diabetes, heart disease, high blood fats, hypertension, stroke, sleep apnea, arthritis and some cancers. So-called **'cellulite'** carries no extra health risk.

Waist Circumference directly reflects the increased health risk of abdominal obesity. Waist size associated with a high health risk:
Men ~ Over 40 inches **Women** ~ Over 35 inches

Body Mass Index (BMI)

BMI is a general (but not specific) indicator of body fatness. Although BMI alone is not diagnostic, the higher the BMI, the greater the health risk of developing diabetes, high blood pressure and heart disease. BMI does not apply to heavily muscled persons. BMI is used in a different way for children.

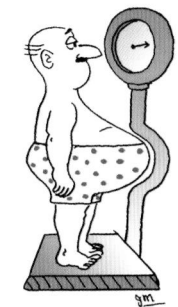

Abdominal obesity greatly increases the risk of ill-health and earlier death.

Check Your BMI: Find your height (no shoes) - look across the row to the weight nearest your own. Then track down to BMI.

Ht	WEIGHT (LBS) ~ ADULTS													
5'1"	100	106	111	116	122	127	132	137	143	148	153	158	185	211
5'2"	104	109	115	120	126	131	136	142	147	153	158	164	191	218
5'3"	107	113	118	124	130	135	141	146	152	158	163	169	197	225
5'4"	110	116	122	128	134	140	145	151	157	163	169	174	204	232
5'5"	114	120	126	132	138	144	150	156	162	168	174	180	210	240
5'6"	118	124	130	136	142	148	155	161	167	173	179	186	216	247
5'7"	121	127	134	140	146	153	159	166	172	178	185	191	223	255
5'8"	125	131	138	144	151	158	164	171	177	184	190	197	230	262
5'9"	128	135	142	149	155	162	169	176	182	189	196	206	236	270
5'10"	132	139	146	153	160	167	174	181	188	195	202	207	243	278
5'11"	136	143	150	157	165	172	179	186	193	200	208	215	250	286
6'0"	140	147	154	162	169	177	184	191	199	206	213	221	258	294
6'1"	144	151	159	166	174	182	189	197	204	212	219	227	265	302
6'2"	148	155	163	171	179	186	194	202	210	218	225	233	272	311
6'3"	152	160	168	176	184	192	200	208	216	224	232	240	279	319
6'4"	156	164	172	180	189	197	205	213	221	230	238	246	287	328
BMI	19	20	21	22	23	24	25	26	27	28	29	30	35	40

BMI Classification:

BMI Below 19
Underweight

BMI 19-24.9
Healthy Weight
(Low Health Risk)

BMI 25-29.9
Overweight
(Moderate Health Risk)

BMI 30-40
Obese (High Health Risk)

BMI Over 40
Morbid Obesity
(Very High Risk)

Interactive BMI Calculator
www.calorieking.com

3

Calories in Food

Calories in food are derived from protein, fat and carbohydrate. Alcohol also provides calories. Vitamins, minerals and water provide no calories.

Calorie Values Per Gram

Fat/Oil	~ 9 Calories
Carbohydrate	~ 4 Calories
Protein	~ 4 Calories
Alcohol	~ 7 Calories

Note that fats have over double the calories of protein and carbohydrate. The higher the fat content of food, the higher the calories.

Sample Calculation

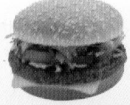

QUARTER POUNDER® WITH CHEESE has 510 calories derived from:

26g Fat (x 9 cals/gram)	= 234
40g Carbohyd.(x 4 cals/gram)	= 160
29g Protein (x 4 cals/gram)	= 116
Total Calories	= 510

Calorie Levels for Weight Loss

Start with a calorie-controlled diet that allows a moderate weight loss of ½ - 1 pound per week. Weight loss is usually much greater in the first few weeks due to extra fluid losses.

Note: It is better to increase exercise rather than lessen food calories too drastically.

Suggested Calories for Weight Loss

Women:	Non-active	1000 - 1200
	Active	1200 - 1500
Men:	Non-active	1200 - 1500
	Active	1500 - 1800
Teenagers:		1200 - 1800

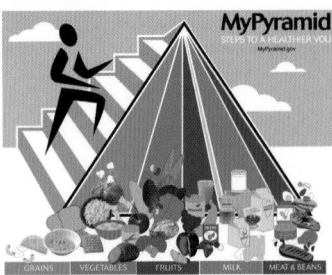

The MyPyramid symbol represents the recommended proportion of foods from each food group and focuses on the importance of making smart food choices in every food group, every day. Daily physical activity is also important. *(More info: www.MyPyramid.gov)*

Examples of Single Serving Sizes

Grains (Eat 6 servings per day):
- 1 slice whole-grain bread (1 oz)
- ½ bun, small bagel or English muffin
- 4 small crackers or 1 tortilla
- 1 oz ready-to-eat whole-grain cereal
- ½ cup cooked cereal, rice or pasta

Vegetable (Eat 3-5 servings per day):
- 1 cup raw leafy vegetables
- 1½ cups raw chopped vegetables
- ½ cup cooked vegetables
- ½ - ¾ cup vegetable juice

Fruits (Eat 3-5 servings per day):
- 1 medium apple, orange, banana
- ½ cup canned fruit (in own juice)
- ¼ cup dried fruit
- ¾ cup fruit juice (unsweetened)
- ¼ medium avocado

Milk (2-3 servings per day):
- 1 cup (8 fl.oz) milk/soy (enriched)/yogurt
- 1½ oz cheese or ½ cup cottage cheese

Meat & Beans (Eat 2-3 servings per day):
- 2-3 oz (cooked) lean meat/poultry/fish
- 2 eggs or 7 oz tofu or ¼ cup nuts
- 1 cup (cooked) dried beans or chickpeas
- 4 Tbsp peanut butter or ½ cup nuts/seeds

Portion Size Counts!

Food portion size is critical to controlling calorie intake for weight control.

Super-sized food servings have become more common when eating out and in the home. This can mean a day's worth of calories being consumed in one meal; or a snack being equivalent to a full meal.

It is easy to underestimate portion size of foods and drinks, and unwittingly consume excess calories – even if the fat content is low or even zero!

To more accurately estimate portion size of different foods, weigh and measure your food with food scales, measuring spoons and cups. Better control of calories will result.

For a visual idea of portion sizes, visit www.CalorieKing.com. See examples (fries and cola) on this page.

Allow for Extra Calories in Packaged Food

The actual weight of packaged foods is usually 5-10% more than the label net weight (the minimum legal weight) - and in some cases up to 50% more. However, manufacturers calculate the calories based on the net weight. For actual calories, weigh the product and calculate the extra calories.

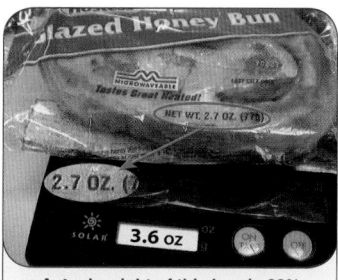

Actual weight of this bun is 33% more than the stated net weight.

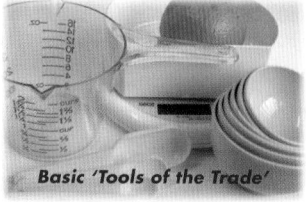

Basic 'Tools of the Trade'

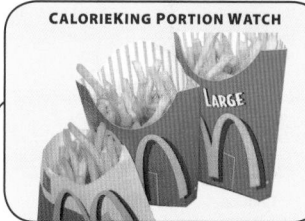

CALORIEKING PORTION WATCH

Fries	Cal	Fat	Carb
Small	250	13	30
Medium	380	20	47
Large	570	30	70

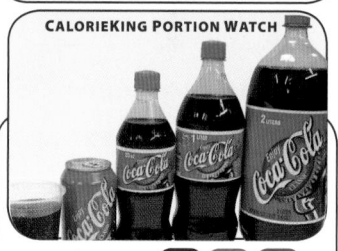

CALORIEKING PORTION WATCH

Cola	Cal	Fat	Carb
8 fl.oz Cup	100	0	25
12 fl.oz Can	150	0	37
20 fl.oz Bottle	250	0	63
1 Liter Bottle	400	0	100
2 Liter Bottle	800	0	200

Recommended Fat Intake

Americans consume too much fat with many getting over 40% of total daily calories from fat – either as fat or oil, or as fat in foods and drinks. A range of 20-30% is healthier.

Fat Intake - Healthy Ranges

Children	~	30-60g
Teenagers (Active)	~	40-80g
Women	~	30-60g
Men: Active	~	40-80g
Heavy Activity/Athlete	~	80-120g

MAXIMUM DESIRABLE FAT INTAKE (Daily)

Calories	Fat	% Fat Cals
1200 cals	30g fat	23%
1500 cals	40g fat	24%
1800 cals	50g fat	25%
2000 cals	60g fat	27%
2200 cals	70g fat	28%
2500 cals	80g fat	29%
3000 cals	100g fat	30%
4000 cals	135g fat	30%

Percentage Fat Calories Formula:

$$\frac{\text{Grams of Fat Per Serving} \times (900)}{\text{Total Calories Per Serving}}$$

Fat Percent Content

(Grams of fat per 100 grams of food)

Don't be fooled by promotion of foods claiming to have a low percentage of fat. **It's serving size and total grams of fat that count.**

Examples: Whole Milk with 3.5% fat sounds low (3.5g fat/100ml) but an 8 fl.oz cup contains 8g fat; and 2 cups contain 16g fat.

Ice cream with 10% fat seems high, yet a regular scoop (3 fl.oz) has only 5g fat.

(Low-fat ice cream has less than 2g fat/serving.)

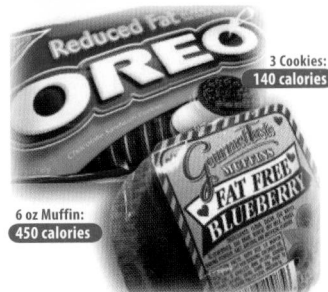

3 Cookies: 140 calories

6 oz Muffin: 450 calories

Reduced fat & fat-free foods are not necessarily low calorie. Portion size is still important.

It is a mistake to think that eating low-fat or fat-free foods allows you to eat double the quantity. You can end up with even more calories than eating smaller amounts of regular fat products.

Also fat-free but high in calories are soda drinks, fruit juices, beer, alcoholic spirits, sugar and candy. Bread, rice and pasta also have negligible fat.

Total Calories Count!

Ultimately, it is food portion size and total calories that count whether from fat, carbohydrate or protein. Remember, cows get fat on grass!

FOOD LABEL MEANINGS

FDA Nutrition Claim Definitions
(All are on a Per Serving Basis)

Low Calorie: 40 Calories or less

Light or Lite: One third fewer calories or, 50% or less fat than regular product

Fat-Free: Less than half a gram of fat

Low-Fat: 3 grams or less of fat

Reduced Fat: 25% less fat than regular product

Fewer or Less Calories: At least 25% fewer calories than regular product

Meats, Poultry, Fish

- Choose **lean cuts** of meat with little marbling. **Trim all visible fat** from meat and remove the skin from poultry. Removal of fat after cooking, is okay (to prevent dryness). Choose 'extra lean' ground beef.
- **Avoid high-fat meat products** such as salami, bacon, sausage and franks.
- **Broil or bake. Avoid frying in oil.** Allow casseroles to cool and skim off surface fat.
- **Avoid fried fish**, frozen fish in batter and canned fish in oil.

Fats & Oils

- **Use minimal amounts** of all types of fat and oil. All are high in calories.
- **Choose** 'light' and 'reduced fat' spreads but still use sparingly.
- Use minimal amounts of oil when stir-frying. Use no-stick sprays like Pam.

Salad Dressings & Sauces

- **Avoid regular mayonnaise and oil dressings.** Choose 'light', 'reduced fat' or 'fat-free' brands.
- **Choose** low-fat or fat-free sauces (mainly tomato-based). Avoid 'pesto', 'alfredo', 'cheese' and 'creamy' sauces.

Milk, Cheese

- **Choose** low-fat or nonfat milks and yogurts. **Avoid** full-cream milk, cream, Half & Half.
- **Cheese:** Choose fat-free, and low-fat cheese. Part-skim ricotta is still high in fat. Low-fat cottage cheese is a good choice. Cheese substitutes can still be high in fat.

Snacks, Cookies, Candy

- **Avoid** high-fat snacks such as potato chips, corn/tortilla chips, cheese puffs, buttered popcorn, chocolate and carob bars.

Desserts/Sweets

- **Avoid high-fat desserts**, such as cake, pie, pastries, cheesecake, full-fat puddings.
- **Choose** fresh fruits, fresh fruit salad, canned fruit in water pack, low-fat ice cream. Use low-fat yogurt in place of cream.

Fast-Foods & Take-Out

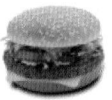

Check the Fast-Foods Section of this book for actual fat and calorie counts.

- **Avoid deep-fried chicken**, french fries, and onion rings.
- **Pizzas:** Avoid sausage/pepperoni. Choose vegetarian topping and modest quantity of cheese. Eat a moderate serving. Eat extra salad and fresh fruit.
- **Hamburgers:** Choose medium size, lower fat burgers. Avoid bacon. Have a side salad (with fat-free dressing).
- **Delis:** Choose sandwiches/bread rolls, pitas with low-fat fillings and plain salad. Limit meat/cheese to small portions.
- **Coffees:** Avoid large sizes of latte and frappuccino. Request nonfat milk and no whipped cream. Avoid cookies and pastries.

Extra Information: www.CalorieKing.com

FRYING ADDS FAT!

The greater the surface area of potato exposed to fat or oil, the higher the fat content and calories.

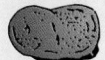

Whole Potato (3 oz)
 0g Fat, 65 Cals

Roast Potato (3 oz)
 5g Fat, 155 Cals

Fries (Large cut, 3 oz)
 12g Fat, 220 Cals

Fries (Small, 3 oz)
 15g Fat, 265 Cals

Potato Chips (3 oz)
 30g Fat, 450 Cals

Carbohydrates ~ Friend or Foe?

Naturally-Friendly Carbs

- **Carbohydrate foods in their more natural forms** (not overly processed) are essential to good health. They are the main source of fuel for the body, and also provide important vitamins, minerals, antioxidants and fiber – all of which help protect against heart disease, diabetes, hypertension, constipation-related ailments and many other diseases.

- Carbohydrates even help the body produce serotonin, the 'feel good' brain chemical that helps control appetite and overeating. Too little serotonin can lead to mood swings and depression.

Carbohydrates are found in different forms in food as:

- Sugars in fruit, sugar cane, milk
- Starches in whole grains, legumes, nuts, seeds and vegetables
- Dietary fiber (See Fiber Guide ~ Page 276)
Glycemic Index & Diabetes ~ Page 20

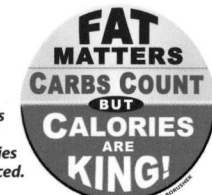

Low-carb diets only work if total calories are reduced.

FAT MATTERS
CARBS COUNT
BUT
CALORIES ARE KING!
©ALLAN BORUSHEK

RECOMMENDED CARBOHYDRATE INTAKE		
Calories (Daily)	Carbohydrate (Grams)	Percent Carbohydrate Calories
1200 cals	120g	40%
1500 cals	170g	45%
1800 cals	210g	47%
2000 cals	250g	50%
2500 cals	345g	55%
3000 cals	450g	60%

How Much Do We Need?

- As shown in the chart, well-balanced diets above 2000 calories contain 50-60% of total calories from carbohydrates.
- At lower calorie levels used for weight control (1200-1500 calories), carbohydrates account for as little as 40% of total calories. This is because protein calories have nutritional priority.
- Carbohydrates & Diabetes ~ *See Page 20*

Low-Carbohydrate Diets

- Popular low-carbohydrate diets are extreme in their recommendations to initially cut carb intake to as little as 20 grams per day – the amount in 1 thick slice of bread, or 1 medium apple, or 1 small potato. This greatly increases the risk of nutritional deficiencies and compromises health, particularly if fat intake is excessive through fatty meats, high-fat dairy products, and fried foods.

- While overweight Americans do need to reduce carbohydrate intake, it should be done **sensibly as part of reducing portion size and total calories.**

- Simply eating 'low-carb' food products without regard to portion size, calories or fats, will do little to promote weight loss or good health.

- **Low-carb diets (and indeed any diet) only work if total calories are reduced.**

- Refined sugars should be one of the first targets in moderating carb intake.
Extra Info ~ www.CalorieKing.com

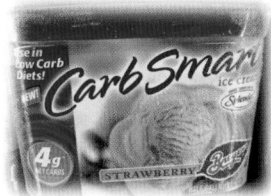

Lower carbohydrate products may still be high in calories and fat.

- Many overweight, inactive people consume over 500 calories of refined sugars per day, either self-added or as part of food products. This is equivalent to over 30 level teaspoons – a significant amount in weight control terms. Halving this amount would be reasonable and worthwhile.

  Note: Naturally occurring sugars in fruits, vegetables and milk are fine when consumed in normal recommended amounts. These foods are also rich in other nutrients.

  Refined sugar is referred to as having 'empty calories' because it supplies calories but negligible nutrients and no fiber.

- **Most sugar in our diet is 'hidden'** in processed foods such as soft drinks, fruit drinks, candy, cookies, cake, jam, sauces, ice cream, desserts, canned foods, and breakfast cereals.

  Certainly enjoy moderate quantities of these foods, but for serious weight control, look for 'low calorie', 'diet' or 'sugar-free'.

  However, be careful not to substitute sugar-rich foods with high-fat foods which might boost calories even more!

- Be aware that sugar comes in different forms such as sucrose, glucose, fructose, malt, high-fructose corn syrup, molasses, honey and maple syrup. Check the label.

- **Sugar alcohols such as sorbitol,** mannitol and maltitol are carb-based and have $1/2$ - $3/4$ the calories of regular sugar. While not counted as sugar on food labels, they do add to the carb count. Excess amounts can cause bloating, gas and diarrhea.

- **Sugar-free sweeteners** such as *Equal, DiabetiSweet, NutraSweet, Splenda, Sweet'n Low* and *Stevia* make it easy to reduce sugar in drinks and recipes. Use only in moderation.

  Note: Most recipes can be adapted to contain less sugar with little effect on taste or quality.

Extra Info ~ www.CalorieKing.com

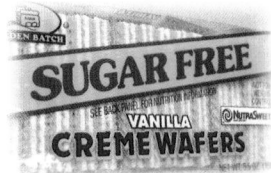

Sugar-free snacks and foods may be higher in fat and calories than the regular product.

Example ~ Creme Wafers (3):
Regular ~ 115 cals, 6g fat
Sugar-Free ~ 160 cals, 10g fat

SUGAR CONTENT OF SOME COMMON FOODS

	Teaspoons of Sugar
Coca Cola or *Pepsi*, 12 fl.oz	10
20 fl.oz size	17
Iced Tea, sweetened, 12 fl.oz	8
Chocolate Milk, 12 fl.oz	6
Honey Smacks Cereal, 1 oz	4
Popcorn, caramel, 1 cup	3.5
Chocolate Bar, 1.5 oz	6
M&M's 1.7 oz pkg	7
Muffin, large, 4 oz	6
Choc Chip Cookie, 1 oz	2
Donut, iced	6
Apple Pie, 1 piece	7
Jell-O, $1/2$ cup	4.5
Jam, 1 Tbsp, 20g	2.5
Syrup, maple, 1 Tbsp	3

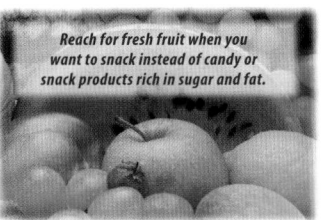

Reach for fresh fruit when you want to snack instead of candy or snack products rich in sugar and fat.

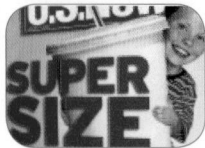

The XL Generation

Some 15% of American kids and adolescents are overweight; and childhood obesity has doubled over the last 20 years. Diabetes, high blood pressure and high cholesterol are major problem areas for overweight children and adolescents, as are depression, low self-esteem, sleep apnea and bone joint problems.

To address this problem, cooperation is required between kids, parents, schools and government. Weight control is a family and community affair.

Five Simple Tips To Get Started:

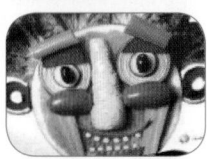

❶ Watch Soda Intake

Limit soda and sugary drinks to one serving on the weekends. Soda should not be an everyday beverage – water should be. When at restaurants or using a soda fountain, choose small servings with ice or choose diet soda instead. Schools should provide water and restrict access to soda as should parents when eating out or in the home!

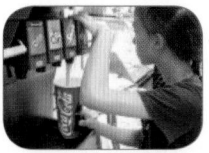

❷ Cut back on Fast-Foods and Eating Out

Many more calories are consumed when you eat out. Healthy meals prepared at home are best for the whole family.

❸ Say "No" to Super-Sizing

When meals are upsized, loads more calories are consumed. Choose sensible portion sizes when eating out and at home. Use smaller plates and choose smaller packages.

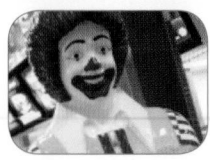

❹ Limit Between-Meal Snacking

Watch out for high-fat and high-calorie snacks – they can have more calories than a meal! Keep your eye on portion sizes and limit salty snack foods and candy to parties and special occasions. Choose fresh fruit, vegetables, nuts and low-fat milk instead.

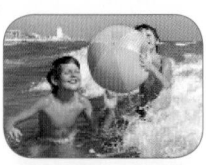

❺ Get Moving ~ Watch Less TV

Kids need at least 60 minutes of physical activity every day. It's critical for their fitness, and greatly lessens the risk of obesity.

Encourage kids to be active out of school hours. Wearing a pedometer can be highly motivational for kids to move more – as can playing dance video games such as *Dance Dance Revolution*. *Wii Fit* (Nintendo) is also useful as a fitness motivator.

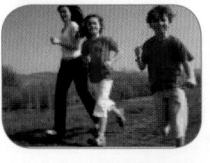

Limit TV and non-active computer games to just one hour per day. Also limit the accompanying snacks! Include exercise in family activities.

Extra information and tips ~ www.CalorieKing.com

Sample Meal Plan - 1400 Calories

For Healthy, Overweight Persons ~ Not for Persons With Any Medical Condition
~ Please Check With Your Doctor & Dietitian ~

 Breakfast (approx. 300 cal)

	1 Small Fruit or ½ oz Dried Fruit
Plus	Cereal: 1½ Dry (high fiber)
	or 1 cup cooked Oatmeal
Plus	½ oz Almonds/Seeds
Plus	Milk (from daily allowance) or Yogurt (low-fat)

Breakfast ~ Choice 2

	1 Small Fruit
Plus	2 Eggs (no added fat)
	or 2 oz Cheese (low-fat)
	or 4 oz Cottage Cheese (low-fat)
	or 2 oz Lean/Canadian Bacon
Plus	1 Tomato
Plus	1 Slice Whole-Grain Toast

Daily Milk Allowance (approx. 160 calories)
2 cups Non-Fat Milk or 1½ cups Low-fat (1%) Milk
or equivalent Soy Drink, Yogurt, Cheese, Tofu

Fat Allowance (140 calories; 15g Fat)
4 tsp Fat or 6-8 tsp Diet Margarine or 3 tsp Oil
or 1½ Tbsp Mayonnaise or ½ medium Avocado
or 1½ Tbsp Peanut Butter or 30g Nuts/Seeds

 Lunch (approx. 440 calories)

	2 slices Whole-Grain Bread (2 oz)
	or 4 Crispbreads/Crackers or 6" Pita
Plus	2 oz lean Meat, Chicken or Turkey
	or 3½oz Tuna (in water) or 2½ oz Salmon
	or 1 oz Cheese or ½ cup (4 oz) Cottage Cheese
	or ½ cup (4 oz) Ricotta Cheese (low-fat)
	or ½ cup (4 oz) Fruit Yogurt (low-fat)
	or ½ cup (4 oz) Bean Salad
Plus	Large Salad (Oil-free dressing)
Plus	1 small Fruit or ½ oz Dried Fruit

 Dinner (approx. 360 calories)

	Soup (fat-free)
Plus	3 oz lean Meat (cooked weight)
	or 4 oz Chicken Breast (no skin)
	or 3 oz Chicken Thigh/Leg (no skin)
	or 5 oz Fish (grilled, no fat)
	or ¾ cup (6 oz) Beans (Soy, Kidney, Pinto etc)/Lentils
	or Low-fat Entree (e.g. Lean Cuisine)
Plus	1 small Potato or ½ cup Rice/Pasta/Sweet Corn
	or 1 slice Whole-Grain Bread
Plus	2-3 servings Vegetables/Salad
Plus	1 small Fruit + Diet Gelatin Dessert

 Between Meals Water, Coffee, Tea, Diet drinks,
Fruit from main meals; Raw vegetable pieces, Milk from Daily Allowance

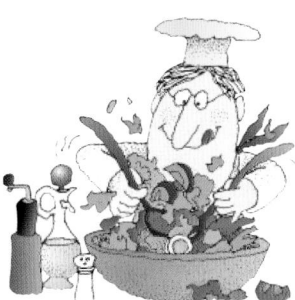

Exercise & Weight Control

- Persons who exercise regularly lose more weight and keep it off longer than non-exercisers.

- Exercise also improves general health and well-being. Mood, confidence and self-esteem are enhanced by a sense of control and accomplishment.

- **Exercise increases the metabolic rate** of the body even for hours after exercise - a good way to 'wake up' a sluggish metabolism and burn extra fat. Exercise compensates for any decrease in metabolic rate with increasing age and also in some heavy smokers who stop smoking.

- **Strength training** further builds muscle and aids body reshaping. You can also eat a little more food! Note: Each extra pound of muscle burns an extra 50 calories daily ~ even while you sleep! Weight from exercised muscles is okay. It is surplus fat (particularly abdominal fat) that is potentially harmful to health.

- **Avoid injury** by beginning with walking, low impact aerobics, or weight-supported exercise (e.g. swimming, cycling). Avoid competitive sports.

- **How Much?** Start with 10 - 20 minutes/day and progress to 30 - 60 minutes/day.
  Also walk up stairs instead of using elevators. Take a brisk walk at lunch. Use an exercise bike, treadmill or stair machine while watching TV. Walk the dog.

- **How Often?** While aerobic fitness requires only 3 - 4 sessions weekly, **weight control is a daily event which requires daily exercise.**

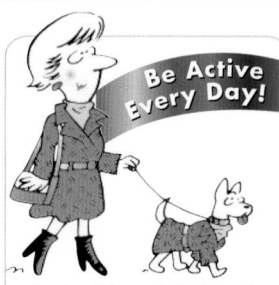

Brisk walking each day is a safe and effective way to keep trim and fit. Try it – you'll like it!
Strength-training with light weights helps to retain or rebuild muscle tissue. It enhances weight control.

FATNESS VS FITNESS

An overweight but fit person can be healthier than a thin, unfit person.

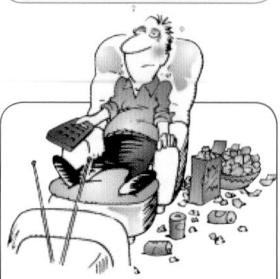

Too little exercise and too much food are the main contributors to middle-age spread.
Daily exercise and sensible eating can minimize middle-age spread. Include some strength-training to retain or build muscle.

TV CAN BE FATTENING!

- Many adults and children spend over 20 hours per week watching TV or at the computer (playing games or 'surfing') – at the same time as eating high-calorie snacks and drinks.

- Are you a TV couch potato or computer addict? Limit your TV and computer hours and plan healthy physical activities.

- At home, limit kids to just one hour daily for TV and computers. Kids need at least 60 minutes of physical activity every day.

Calories Used in Exercise

LIGHT	MODERATE	HEAVY
130 lbs ~ 3 Cals/Min	130 lbs ~ 5 Cals/Min	130 lbs ~ 8 Cals/Min
170 lbs ~ 4 Cals/Min	170 lbs ~ 6 Cals/Min	170 lbs ~ 10 Cals/Min
220 lbs ~ 5 Cals/Min	220 lbs ~ 7 Cals/Min	220 lbs ~ 12 Cals/Min

LIGHT	MODERATE	HEAVY
Walking, slow	Walking, brisk	Walking (power), Jogging
Cycling, light	Cycling, moderate	Cycling (vigorous), Spinning
Gardening light	Swimming, crawl	Swimming, strenuous
Golf, social	Weight-training, light	Weight-training, heavy
Tennis, doubles	Tennis, moderate	Wrestling/Judo, advanced
Housework, cleaning	Racquetball, beginners	Racquetball, advanced
Calisthenics, Yoga	Aerobics, light	Tae Bo, Kick Boxing
Bowling	Football, touch	Football, training
Ping-pong, social	Basketball, Baseball	Basketball (Pro)
Ice Skating	Walking Downstairs	Climbing Stairs
Aquarobics, light	Snow Skiing (downhill)	Skipping Rope
Skate Boarding	Shovelling snow	Skiing (cross country)
Line/Square Dancing	Dancing (ballroom)	Aquarobics, advanced
		Dancing (strenuous), Zumba

Note: Only those sports or activities that are sustained over a period of time (e.g running)
qualify for heavy exercise. Stop-start sports such as tennis are considered 'moderate'.

Interactive Calculations ~ www.CalorieKing.com/tools

WALKING PROGRAM

USE DISTANCE, STEPS OR TIME

Weeks	Distance	Steps Pedometer	Time
1-2	1 mile	2000	20 mins
3-5	1.5 miles	3000	18 mins
6-8	2 miles	3500	35 mins
9-10	2.5 miles	4500	45 mins
11+	3.5 miles	6000	60 mins

10,000 STEPS PER DAY

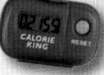

A pedometer can motivate you to be more active. It clips to your belt or waist band and registers each step.

Aim for 8,000 - 10,000 steps per day, instead of an average of only 3,000 - 4,000 steps.

For Extra Information:
www.CalorieKing.com

Reshaping Eating Behaviors

- Eating is a behavior that is largely controlled by people with whom we live or socialize, places in which we carry out our lives, and our emotions. Become aware of those situations that commonly lead to extra food being eaten.

- We may also be unaware of 'bad' eating habits that can lead to excess calorie intake; e.g. eating quickly, large mouthfuls, eating when tense or bored, finishing a large serving of food when not hungry.

Tips to help uncover and correct those 'bad' eating habits:

- **Don't eat while engaged in other activities;** for example, watching TV, reading. Eat only at the table, not at the fridge or while standing.

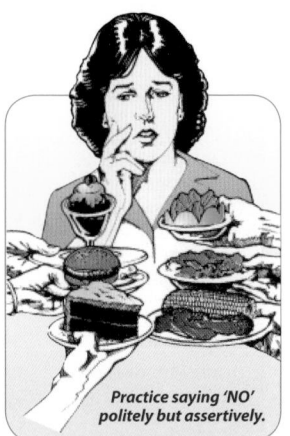

Practice saying 'NO' politely but assertively.

- **Don't eat quickly.** Chewing slowly allows time to register a feeling of fullness. Don't use fingers, only utensils. Cut food into smaller pieces. Don't load your fork until the previous mouthful is finished.

- **Don't purchase problem high calorie foods.** Shop from a set list to prevent impulse buying. Avoid shopping with children.

- **Buy snack foods** in the smallest package. The larger the serving size or package, the more you are likely to eat or drink.

- **Plan meals in advance. Stick to a set menu.**

- **Plan a strategy to avoid uncontrolled eating** and drinking at social events, or when your emotions urge you to binge.

  Rehearse repeatedly in your mind exactly what you will do in such situations. Remind yourself several times each day that you are in charge of your actions and that you can be strong-willed. Seek counseling or coaching on various strategies.

- **Promise yourself** that when you feel the urge to snack, you will engage in some activity that will distract you away from food (e.g. go for a walk, brush your teeth, phone a friend.)

  If you eat out of boredom, find some new hobby or interest that gets you out of the house. Even enroll in an adult education class.

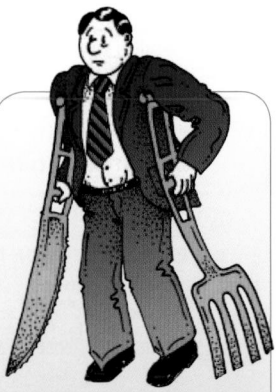

Do you use food as an emotional crutch? If so, professional counseling may be helpful.

The food journal is the most powerful proven aid for dieters. Persons who keep a food and exercise journal not only lose more weight, they also keep it off. Here are some of the reasons:

- **Recording your eating and exercise habits** jolts you into realizing just what you do eat and drink each day; and also whether you exercise sufficiently.

- **Helps you identify problem foods** and drinks with excessive calories and fat.

- **Helps identify moods**, situations and events that lead to excessive eating of unwanted calories. You can then plan to overcome or avoid them.

- **Prevents 'calorie amnesia'**, the forgetfulness that leads to rebound weight gain after successful weight loss. Recording puts you back on the right track.

- **Helps you develop greater self-discipline.** You will think twice about overindulging if you have to record it - especially if someone checks your journal regularly. It certainly keeps you honest!

- **Motivates you** to carefully plan your meals and to exercise each day.

- **Serves as a check system** for your doctor, dietitian or counselor to assess your progress and make recommendations.

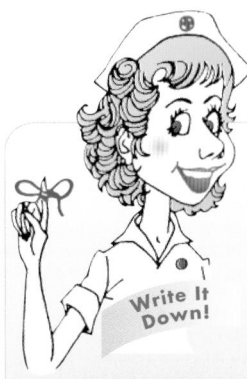

"Keeping a journal gives me feedback on exactly what I eat and drink each day.

It helps prevent 'calorie amnesia' and reminds me to exercise each day.

It's a 'must' for successful weight control!"

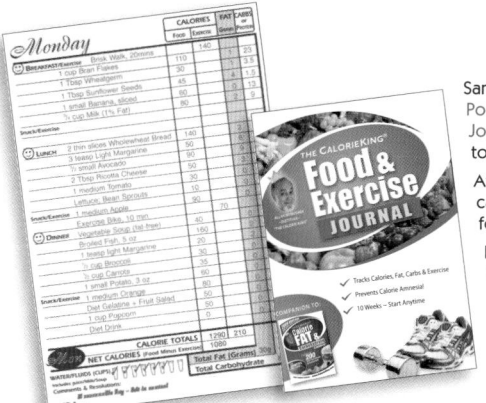

Sample Page from The Pocket Food & Exercise Journal, a 10-week journal to record food and exercise.

At day's end, exercise calories are deducted from food calories.

Includes Weekly Summary Page & Progress Checklist.

EXTRA DETAILS

~ SEE PAGE 302

What is Diabetes?

Diabetes is a disorder whereby the body cannot use carbohydrates (sugar and starches) properly.

- **After digestion**, sugar and starches are changed into **glucose** – the simplest form of sugar vital for body energy and growth.
- **Insulin** is the hormone which acts like a key that opens the door to body cells and allows glucose to enter.
- **Without enough insulin**, glucose builds up in the blood and passes into the urine. High blood glucose levels lead to frequent urination, extreme thirst, and tiredness.
- **Untreated diabetes** increases the risk of damage to nerves and blood vessels. This, in turn, increases the risk of heart disease, stroke, blindness, kidney damage, foot ulcers and gangrene (with amputation), impotence and other complications.

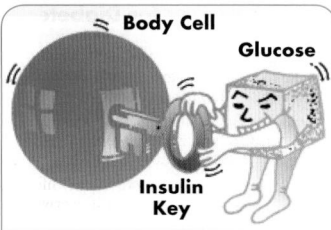

Insulin acts like a key. It opens the door to body cells and allows glucose to enter.

People with type 1 diabetes and some with type 2 have too few or no keys and require insulin injections.

Others (primarily type 2) make enough insulin but the body doesn't use it as well as it should – particularly if obese and inactive.

SYMPTOMS OF DIABETES

- Frequent urination
- Extreme thirst
- Unusual hunger
- Rapid weight loss
- Extreme fatigue
- Blurred vision
- Skin infections that are slow to heal
- Tingling/numbness in feet

DON'T IGNORE DIABETES

Note: Diabetes can be present even with no symptoms.

TYPE 2 DIABETES

- Occurs in 90% of diabetes cases
- Occurs mainly in adults - particularly in overweight and inactive persons
- Insulin is produced but body cells resist its action and glucose cannot enter cells
- Usually treated with meal planning and physical activity. Sometimes requires medication (pills or insulin)

TYPE 1 DIABETES

- Occurs in 10% of diabetes cases
- Usually in children and young adults
- Pancreas produces little or no insulin. Daily insulin injections (or use of an insulin pump or inhaled insulin) are necessary, as well as:
  - Matching pre-meal insulin to the amount of carbohydrate eaten
  - Weight control and regular physical activity

GESTATIONAL DIABETES

- Occurs in some women during pregnancy
- Usually disappears after the baby's birth
- Women who have had gestational diabetes still have a high risk of developing type 2 diabetes within 5 to 10 years
- Requires weight control, a healthy lifestyle and regular medical checks

Are You At Risk for Diabetes?
Pre-Diabetes ~ An Early Warning!

Pre-diabetes means that your blood glucose levels are higher than normal, but not high enough to be called diabetes.

If you have pre-diabetes, you have a higher risk for getting diabetes later on.

The good news is that you can start taking steps to prevent diabetes by making healthy lifestyle changes – such as losing weight if overweight, and being more physically active.

WHAT'S YOUR RISK?
Find out if you're at risk for diabetes by answering the following questions:

- ☐ I have been told I have pre-diabetes
- ☐ I have a family history of diabetes
- ☐ I am African American, Latino American, Asian American, Native American or a Pacific Islander
- ☐ I have had gestational diabetes (diabetes during pregnancy)
- ☐ I am over age 65
- ☐ I am overweight
- ☐ I get little or no physical activity
- ☐ My waist is larger than: 35 inches (for a woman) or 40 inches (for a man)
- ☐ My blood pressure is higher than 130 over 85
- ☐ My HDL (good cholesterol) is too low
- ☐ My triglycerides (blood fats) are too high

 CHECK YOUR RESULT

- If you've put a check mark in two or more of the boxes, you may be more likely to develop type 2 diabetes.
- Talk with your healthcare provider to see if you should have a blood test for diabetes.

BLOOD GLUCOSE CLASSIFICATION OF DIABETES

Normal:	Below 100 mg/dl*
Pre-Diabetes:	100-125 mg/dl*
Diabetes:	Over 125 mg/dl*

(*Fasting Blood Glucose)

KNOW YOUR BGL
(Blood Glucose Level)
Everyone over the age of 45 should have a blood glucose test every three years

Importance of Weight Control

- **Type 2 diabetes** is more common in people who are overweight.
- **Being overweight** means that your insulin doesn't work as well to control blood glucose levels.
- **Losing just 10 to 20 pounds** can help you better manage your diabetes and lower your risk for heart disease.
- Keys to weight control include:
  - Following a healthy eating plan
  - Controlling food portions
  - Being physically active most days of the week
  - Keeping food records
  - Setting realistic goals
- **Work with a registered dietitian** who can help you reach a weight that's good for you.

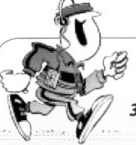

KEEP MOVING!
Every day, do at least 30 minutes of moderate intensity exercise.
(even in 5-minute sets)

It's the key to improving insulin action. Add muscle strength training 3-4 times a week to double the benefits.

Managing Diabetes

Don't battle diabetes alone. Establish a partnership with your doctor, dietitian, certified diabetes educator, and pharmacist.

Extra Support: • *Joslin Diabetes Center*
  • *American Diabetes Association*
  • *American Association of Diabetes Educators*
  • *Juvenile Diabetes Research Foundation*
  • *National Diabetes Education Program*

Hints to keep blood glucose within safe limits:

• **Control your food intake.** Know what and when you will eat. Seek referral to a dietitian for expert advice.

• **Exercise regularly.** It assists weight control and can improve sensitivity of body cells to insulin. Plan physical activity into your daily routine.

• **Monitor your blood glucose** at home and work with a blood glucose meter. It will help you become familiar with your blood glucose patterns, and the effects of food, activity and medication.

• **Take insulin or oral medication as prescribed.** If on insulin, know what action to take if hypoglycemia (low blood glucose) occurs. Also educate your family and friends.
  More Info: www.joslin.org

Be Heart Smart ~ Know Your ABC's

If you have diabetes, you are at a higher risk for heart attack and stroke than someone without diabetes. But you can fight back!

Be smart about your heart!
Take control of the ABC's of diabetes and live a long and healthy life. Talk to your healthcare provider about your ABC targets.

Be Smart About Your **Heart**
Control the ABCs of **Diabetes**
— A1C
— Blood Pressure
— Cholesterol

National Diabetes Education Program

Ⓐ is for A1C
The A1C (A-one-C) test – short for hemoglobin A1C – measures your average blood glucose (sugar) over the last 3 months.
Suggested target: below 7%

Ⓑ is for Blood Pressure
High blood pressure makes your heart work too hard. **Suggested target: below 130/80**

Ⓒ is for Cholesterol
Bad cholesterol, or LDL, can build up and clog your arteries. **Suggested target: below 100**

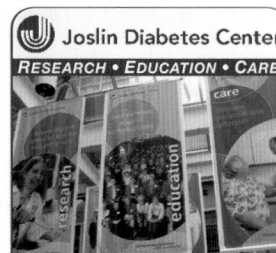

Joslin Diabetes Center, an affiliate of Harvard Medical School, is the world's largest diabetes research center, diabetes clinic and provider of diabetes education.

MORE INFORMATION
www.joslin.org or call 800-344-4501

Blood glucose meters and insulin pumps can greatly improve control of diabetes

BLOOD GLUCOSE METERS (EXAMPLES)

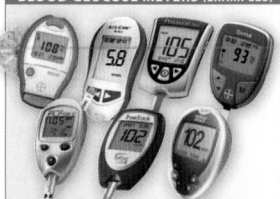

INSULIN PUMPS (EXAMPLES)

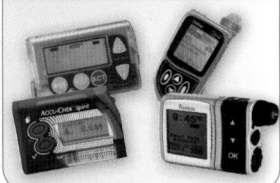

Guidelines for choosing a healthy diet apply equally to people with or without diabetes. Eating a wide variety of foods that are mainly low in fat, low in refined sugars, and high in fiber, is recommended.

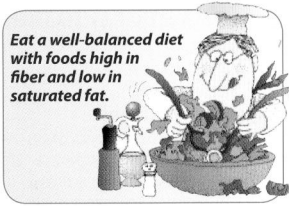

Eat a well-balanced diet with foods high in fiber and low in saturated fat.

However, actual food quantities, as well as when you eat, will also influence control of blood glucose. Your dietitian will individualize a meal plan to suit your food preferences, lifestyle and medical status. Here are a few tips:

- **Maintain a healthy weight.** If overweight, even a modest weight loss plus daily physical activity can help manage blood glucose in type 2 diabetes.

- **Don't skip meals.** If you take insulin or an oral hypoglycemic agent, regular meals are important.

The Plate Method is an easy way to eat healthfully. (See next page)

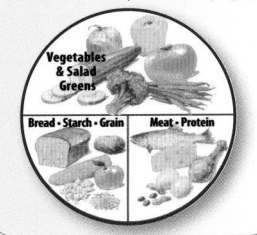

- **If on insulin,** eat meals at the same time each day. Eat a similar amount of food at each meal. Eating about the same amount of carbohydrate over the day will make best use of insulin and prevent wide variations in blood glucose levels.

- **Know how much carbohydrate you should eat** at your meals and snacks each day.

- **Choose whole-grain breads, cereals and pasta.** Eat fresh fruits, vegetables and legumes. These foods contain more fiber and slow the release of glucose into your blood after a meal.

- **Limit foods high in saturated fat, trans fat and cholesterol.** Enjoy fish, soy foods, and other foods rich in omega-3 fats. *(Extra Notes: Page 271)*

- **Limit sugars and foods high in added sugar** particularly if overweight. Small amounts of sugar as part of a meal may occasionally be okay. Check with your dietitian. *(Extra Notes: Page 9)*

- **Read the Nutrition Facts label** on foods. Check the serving size, total fat and total carbohydrate.

ALCOHOL TIPS

- **If you drink alcohol, have only moderate amounts:**
  Men ~ 1-2 drinks/day
  Women ~ 1 drink/day
  For some people, safe drinking will mean no alcoholic drinks at all.
  (Also see Alcohol Guide ~ Page 25)

- **Drink along with your food** – especially if you use insulin or diabetes pills.

- **Do not omit any carb food** in exchange for an alcoholic drink. However, non-alcoholic beers (12 fl oz) count as one carb exchange.

- **Alcohol increases the risk of hypoglycemia** (low blood sugar) and drug interactions if you take insulin and certain types of diabetes pills.

- **Check with your doctor and dietitian.**
  Extra Info: www.joslin.org

The Plate Method — An Easy Way to Eat Healthfully

The plate method is a helpful tool to guide your food choices until you see a dietitian for your own meal plan.

For a healthy meal:

- **Fill half of your plate** with non-starchy vegetables (broccoli, green beans, carrots).
- **Fill a quarter of your plate** with carbohydrate (whole-grain bread, pasta, potato, brown rice).
- **Fill the other quarter of your plate** with 3-4 ounces of lean meat, poultry, or fish.
- **Use 1-2 teaspoons of tub margarine** or a heart-healthy vegetable oil.
- **Add** a small piece of fruit or 8 ounces of skim/low-fat milk or yogurt.

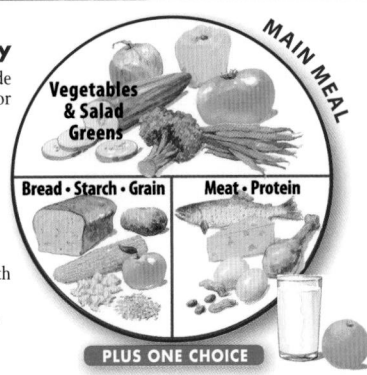

MAIN MEAL

Vegetables & Salad Greens

Bread · Starch · Grain

Meat · Protein

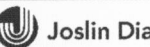

PLUS ONE CHOICE

Milk, Fruit, Dessert or other Carb Food

How Much Carbohydrate Should You Eat?

A dietitian can best determine how much carbohydrate you need at each of your meals, based on your lifestyle, food preferences, and overall diabetes control.

Until you see a dietitian, aim to keep the amount of carbohydrate you eat the same at each of your meals.

CARB CHOICES MEAL PLAN
One Carb Choice = 15 Grams of Carb

The amount in: 1 slice Bread **or** ¾ cup Cereal (unsweetened) **or** 1 small Potato **or** 1 small Fruit

🍽 **Breakfast**
- Eat 2-3 carb choices (30-45 grams)
- Include a low-fat protein source such as egg whites or skim milk.

🍽 **Lunch and Dinner**
- Eat 3-4 carb choices (45-60 grams carb)
- Include fruit and non-starchy vegetables. Choose small portions of low-fat protein foods.

🍽 **Snacks:** If needed, eat 1-2 carb choices (15-30 grams carb).

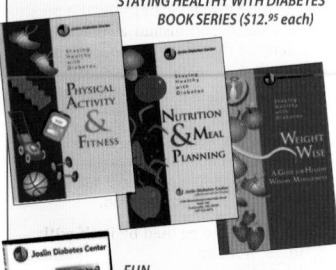
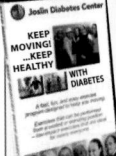

Carb Type Affects Blood Glucose

The various forms of carbohydrate affect blood glucose levels in different ways. It is difficult to predict the effect of particular foods, sugars, or meals, simply by their carbohydrate content.

Thus the same amount of carbohydrate from different foods may affect blood sugar levels very differently. Many factors affect the rate of digestion and absorption – particularly the type of sugar, starch, and fiber; the degree of processing and cooking (which increases digestion rate); and the amount of protein and fat (which slow stomach emptying and digestion).

Glycemic Index (GI)

The GI is a method of ranking carbohydrate foods on a scale (0-100) according to how they affect blood glucose levels. (See next column). The higher the GI value, the greater the food's ability to rapidly raise blood glucose levels, and the more insulin needed by the body (not desirable).

Eating low-GI foods may lead to better control of blood glucose and insulin levels (which in turn lowers the risk of damage to blood vessels and nerves). The slower digestion of low-GI foods may also help to delay hunger pangs and benefit weight control.

Note: Choosing low-GI foods is not a license to eat unlimited amounts. Calorie restriction and portion control for weight control is of prime importance.

- GI is not meant to be used by itself without regard to **portion size**, and other dietary recommendations for healthy eating. Foods are not good or bad on the basis of their GI.

- While GI may be a helpful tool for some people with diabetes, what is most important is to control the total amount of carbohydrate that you eat.

Extra Info: *www.joslin.org*
www.glycemicindex.com

LOWER-GLYCEMIC FOODS

Slower-Acting Carbohydrates

These foods are more slowly digested and absorbed. They help maintain more even blood glucose levels, as long as excessive amounts are not eaten. Use these foods regularly but still limit portion size for weight control.

Examples:
- Dried beans, peas, lentils
- Nuts and seeds
- Whole-grain breads
- Bran cereals, oats
- Sweet corn, barley, buckwheat
- Whole-grain pasta, basmati rice
- Fresh fruit: apples, avocados, bananas (firm), cherries, grapefruit, grapes, olives, oranges, peaches, pears, plums. Fresh juices.
- Vegetables: broccoli, yam, sweet potatoes, salad greens
- Milk, yogurt, soy drinks
- Dark chocolate
- Sugar alcohols (sorbitol, maltitol)

HIGHER-GLYCEMIC FOODS

Quicker-Acting Carbohydrates

These foods more rapidly raise blood glucose levels. Eat only in moderation.

- White bread, rice cakes, bagels, croissants, doughnuts
- Low-fiber cereals: Cornflakes, *Rice Krispies, Froot Loops*
- White potatoes, white rice
- Watermelon, ripe bananas, cantaloupe, pineapple
- Soda, sugar-sweetened sports and energy drinks
- Sugar, candy, popcorn (plain)
- Ice cream (low-fat), frozen yogurt

High-GI fruits and potatoes are still healthy choices when eaten in moderate amounts.

Calcium & Osteoporosis Guide

Calcium's Role in the Body

Calcium plays a vital role in nerve and muscle function, clotting of blood, enzyme regulation, insulin secretion and overall bone strength. Bones and teeth store 99% of the body's calcium.

The calcium level in blood is kept at a steady level by the continual exchange of calcium between blood and bone. When insufficient calcium is obtained from food the body draws calcium out of the bones.

This bone loss over a period of years may lead to **osteoporosis** – thinning of the bones (porous bones).

The bones become weak, brittle and easy to fracture, particularly the bones of the wrist, hips and spine. Loss of height and curvature of the spine may also result, as may periodontal disease - the deterioration of the jaw bones that support the teeth.

Common in Women & Men

While osteoporosis also occurs in men, women are particularly vulnerable (1 in 4 by age 60). They have about 30% less bone than men, and a greater bone loss at menopause when oestrogen levels drop. Slender framed women are at greater risk. (A woman in her eighties can have lost up to two thirds of her skeleton.)

Insufficient dietary calcium during pregnancy and breastfeeding will see bone reserves drawn upon, increasing the risk of osteoporosis in later years.

Hip fractures account for 300,000 hospitalizations each year. One in 5 older Americans with hip fracture die within a year – and 1 in 5 end up in a nursing home.

Causes of Osteoporosis

The major factors associated with the bone loss of osteoporosis appear to be:

- hormone changes of menopause
- inadequate dietary intake of calcium and other bone nutrients such as magnesium, vitamin D, zinc and protein
- insufficient exercise (weight bearing - such as walking, cycling ~ 30-60 minutes daily)
- family history of osteoporosis

Other contributing factors may include:

- excessive cola (regular or diet) and alcohol intake
- cigarette smoking
- some drug medications (e.g. steroids, thyroid)

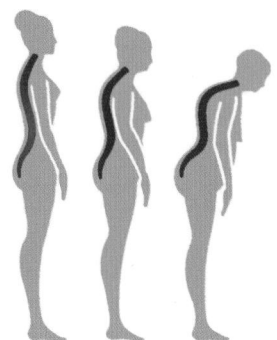

As osteoporosis progresses after menopause, vertebrae may collapse causing the spine to curve and shoulders to hunch.

RECOMMENDED DAILY INTAKE OF CALCIUM		
Children:	1-3 yrs ~	500mg
	4-8 yrs ~	800mg
	9-12 yrs ~	1300mg
Teenagers:		
	13-18 yrs ~	1300mg
Adults:	19-50 yrs ~	1000mg
	51+ yrs ~	1200mg
Women:		
Pre-menopausal		~ 1000mg
Menopausal (beginning)		~ 1200mg
Post-menopausal		~ 1500mg
Pregnant & Breast-feeding		
	14-18 yrs ~	1300mg
	19+ yrs ~	1000mg

Early Prevention Important

Gradual loss of bone begins in the thirties after maximum bone mass is reached. The stronger the bones at that time, the less trouble is likely to occur later. The earlier that prevention or treatment begins the greater the benefit. **The key to prevention is to build strong, dense bones early in life. By age 16, some 80% of peak bone mass is already reached.**

Young women may lessen the risk by:

- eating high-calcium foods as well as adequate fruits, vegetables, whole grains and nuts
- drinking less soda, and more milk
- not engaging in extreme dieting that results in menstrual period cessation (via less estrogen)
- taking regular exercise and not smoking

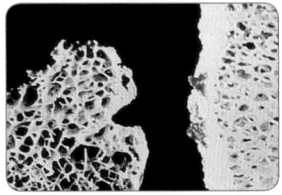

▲ Osteoporotic Fragile Bone ▲ Healthy Dense Bone

Good Dietary Sources of Calcium
(Eat 3-4 servings a day of calcium-rich foods)

- Milk, Yogurt, Cheese
- Flavored Milk Drinks & Fruit Smoothies
- Ice Cream (low-fat), Frozen Yogurt (low-fat)
- Soy Drinks (calcium-enriched)
- Orange Juice (calcium-fortified)
- Tofu (with calcium coagulant), Miso, Tempeh
- Canned Salmon or Sardines (with edible bones)
- Breakfast Cereals (calcium-enriched): *Total, Wheaties*
- Broccoli, Dried Beans, Baked Beans
- Almonds, Brazil nuts, Hazelnuts, Seeds

Calculating Calcium From Food Labels

The calcium content of packaged foods and drinks is shown in the Nutrition Facts label as a percentage of the DRI (dietary reference intake) of 1000 mg calcium.

To convert this percentage into milligrams of calcium, simply multiply the percent figure by 10 (or add a zero). Examples: 5% = 50 mg calcium; 35% = 350 mg calcium.

Food Calcium Counter ~ www.CalorieKing.com

Calcium Supplements

Because absorption of dietary calcium decreases with age, prescribed high doses of calcium (1500-2000mg/day) may benefit persons with osteoporosis - as well as vitamin D (preferably in D3 form, not D2), vitamin K, magnesium and zinc. Check with your doctor.

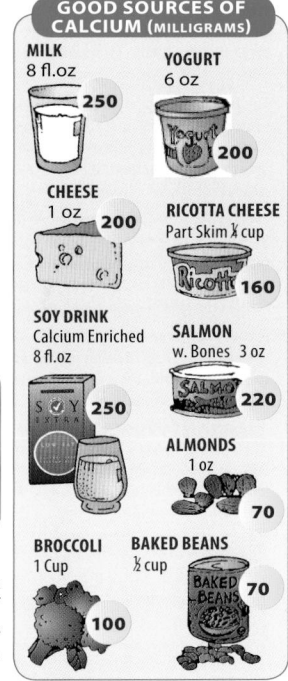

GOOD SOURCES OF CALCIUM (MILLIGRAMS)

MILK
8 fl.oz — 250

YOGURT
6 oz — 200

CHEESE
1 oz — 200

RICOTTA CHEESE
Part Skim ¼ cup — 160

SOY DRINK
Calcium Enriched
8 fl.oz — 250

SALMON
w. Bones 3 oz — 220

ALMONDS
1 oz — 70

BROCCOLI
1 Cup — 100

BAKED BEANS
½ cup — 70

Notes ◆ Abbreviations ◆ Disclaimer

≫ **Calorie and fat values have been rounded off.**
Calories ~ to the nearest 5 or 10 calories.
Fat ~ to nearest half gram. **Note:** Trace amounts of
fat (less than 0.3 grams) have been treated as zero.

≫ **Carbohydrate figures** in this book are for total
carbohydrate, and not **Net Carbs** (which deducts fiber,
polydextrose and sugar alcohols from total carbs).

≫ Because manufacturers' figures on labels are rounded
off, figures in this book may differ slightly from the
label. Serving sizes may also vary.

IMPORTANT DISCLAIMER

* The authors and publishers of this book are not physicians
and are not licensed to give medical advice. This book is not a
substitute for professional advice. Users should consult their
medical professional before making any health, medical or
other decisions based on the material contained herein.

* This book is a compilation of original material from other
sources intended for educational purposes only. Because
food manufacturers constantly change their products,
only they are the authoritative source for food's most
current nutritional information.

* Persons using the information herein for any medical
purposes, such as matching insulin dosage to carbohydrate
intake, should not rely solely on the accuracy of figures
herein and should independently check food labels or
contact the food manufacturer for the latest data.

* Because nutrition data for food products is subject to
change, users should consult the most recent edition of
this book, and the author's website www.calorieking.com
for the most up-to-date information.

* **WARRANTY DISCLAIMER:**
THE AUTHOR AND PUBLISHER DISCLAIM ANY LIABILITY
ARISING DIRECTLY OR INDIRECTLY FROM THE USE OF THIS
BOOK. THE INFORMATION HEREIN IS PROVIDED "AS IS" AND
WITHOUT ANY WARRANTY EXPRESSED OR IMPLIED. ALL
DIRECT, INDIRECT, SPECIAL, INCIDENTAL, CONSEQUENTIAL
OR PUNITIVE DAMAGES ARISING FROM ANY USE OF THIS
INFORMATION IS DISCLAIMED AND EXCLUDED.

This information is also provided subject to Family Health
Publications' Terms and Conditions found at the website,
www.calorieking.com/terms and incorporated herein.

C ~ **Calories**
F ~ **Fat (grams)**
Cb ~ **Carbohydrate (grams)**

Abbreviations

tsp	= teaspoon
Tbsp or T	= Tablespoon
oz	= ounce(s)
c	= cup
fl.oz	= fluid ounce(s)
g	= gram(s)
avg	= average
pkg	= package

Volume Measures

(All measures are level)

3 tsp	=	1 Tbsp
2 Tbsp	=	1 fl.oz
½ cup	=	4 fl.oz
1 cup	=	8 fl.oz
2 cups	=	1 Pint
2 Pints	=	1 Quart

Note: 8 oz weight is not the same
as 8 fl oz volume (space occupied).
Dense foods weigh more per set
volume. Examples:

1 cup popcorn weighs ½ oz
1 cup milk weighs 8½ oz
1 cup pudding weighs 10 oz

Metric Conversion

½ oz	=	14 grams
1 oz	=	28.4 grams
2 oz	=	57 grams
3½ oz	=	100 grams
1 fl.oz	=	30 mls
1 cup (8 fl.oz)	=	240 mls
33 fl.oz	=	1 liter (volume)

INFORMATION SOURCES
• U.S. Dept. of Agriculture
• Food Manufacturers
• Food Industry Boards & Councils
• Author extrapolations

FEEDBACK WELCOME!
Please contact the author with
your queries and suggestions.
feedback@calorieking.com

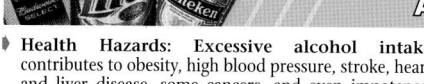

Alcohol Guide A

- **Health Hazards: Excessive alcohol intake** contributes to obesity, high blood pressure, stroke, heart and liver disease, some cancers, and even impotence. **Concentration and short-term memory** are reduced as well as athletic performance.

  Other alcohol hazards include fetal alcohol syndrome, stomach upsets, menstrual problems, depression, snoring, sleep problems, work absenteeism, impaired judgement, and social/family problems.

- **Alcohol contributes to obesity** through its high calories and by lessening the body's ability to burn fat. Fat storage is promoted, particularly in the belly - a health danger zone. Alcohol can also stimulate the appetite.

- **Alcohol is potentially more harmful while dieting.** Blood sugar levels may drop with resultant fatigue and further impairment of concentration, reflexes and driving skills - and maybe even the dieter's resolve!

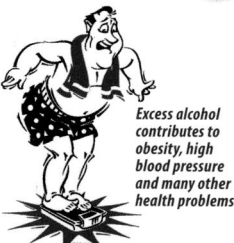

Excess alcohol contributes to obesity, high blood pressure and many other health problems

LOWER RISK ALCOHOL LIMITS

 WOMEN: No more than **1 drink** per day

 MEN: No more than **2 drinks** per day (Over 65 ~ 1 drink)

(At least 2 days a week should be alcohol-free)

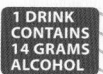 **1 DRINK CONTAINS 14 GRAMS ALCOHOL** →
- 12 fl.oz Regular Beer (5% Alc.)
- OR 14 fl.oz Light Beer (4.2% Alc.)
- OR 5 fl.oz Wine (12% Alc.)
- OR 1½ fl.oz Spirits (80 Proof)

Note: You cannot save daily drinks for one occasion. Binge drinking is particularly harmful ~ 4 drinks for males or 3 drinks for females (within 2 hours).

For some people, **safe drinking** means no alcohol at all. Even one drink may impair driving skills, particularly if tired. For women who drink frequently, breast cancer risk is increased by 9% for each drink after the first drink.

- **It is advisable not to drink at all if you are:**
- pregnant, trying to conceive or breastfeeding
- taking medication or have liver or heart disease (unless approved by your doctor or pharmacist)
- planning to drive, use machinery or play sports
- studying or needing to concentrate
- a child or adolescent

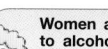 Women and adolescents are more prone to alcohol's ill-effects due to their lower body weight, smaller livers and lesser capacity to metabolize alcohol. As we age, our ability to handle alcohol decreases.

HOW TO CALCULATE ALCOHOL CONTENT

Percent alcohol on label refers to alcohol volume (ml alcohol/100ml). Note: 100ml = 3½ fl.oz

To convert to grams (weight) of alcohol, multiply the percent volume by 0.8 – since 1 ml of alcohol weighs only 0.8 grams.

EXAMPLE:
12 fl.oz Can Beer (5% alcohol)
5% alc. volume
= 5% of 12 fl.oz = 0.6 fl.oz
= 18ml alcohol (Note: 1 fl.oz = 30ml)
Weight (18ml x 0.8) = 14.4g alcohol

GOVERNMENT WARNINGS!

(1) According to the Surgeon General, women should not drink alcoholic beverages during pregnancy because of the risk of birth defects.

(2) Consumption of alcoholic beverages impairs your ability to drive a car or operate machinery, and may cause health problems.

EXTRA INFORMATION
Alcohol & Diabetes ~ See Page 19
Alcohol & The Heart ~ See Page 274
Tips to Avoid Harmful Drinking ~ p. 31

25

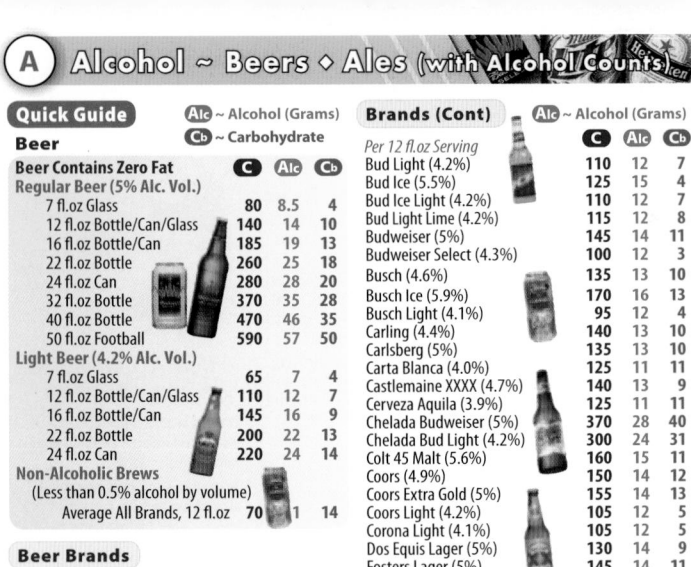

A — Alcohol ~ Beers ◆ Ales (with Alcohol Counts)

Quick Guide

Alc ~ Alcohol (Grams)
Cb ~ Carbohydrate

Beer

Beer Contains Zero Fat	C	Alc	Cb
Regular Beer (5% Alc. Vol.)			
7 fl.oz Glass	80	8.5	4
12 fl.oz Bottle/Can/Glass	140	14	10
16 fl.oz Bottle/Can	185	19	13
22 fl.oz Bottle	260	25	18
24 fl.oz Can	280	28	20
32 fl.oz Bottle	370	35	28
40 fl.oz Bottle	470	46	35
50 fl.oz Football	590	57	50
Light Beer (4.2% Alc. Vol.)			
7 fl.oz Glass	65	7	4
12 fl.oz Bottle/Can/Glass	110	12	7
16 fl.oz Bottle/Can	145	16	9
22 fl.oz Bottle	200	22	13
24 fl.oz Bottle	220	24	14
Non-Alcoholic Brews			
(Less than 0.5% alcohol by volume)			
Average All Brands, 12 fl.oz	70	1	14

Beer Brands

Per 12 fl.oz Serving
Percentage alcohol listed is by volume - not by weight.

Alc ~ Alcohol (Grams)

	C	Alc	Cb
Amber Ice (5.3% alcohol)	130	15	6
Amstel Light (3.5%)	100	10	5
Anheuser World Select (5%)	165	15	15
Anchor Steam (4.6%)	155	13	16
Artic Ice (5.3%)	150	15	8
Artic Ice Light (3.9%)	100	11	6
Asahi Super Dry (5.2%)	150	15	11
Aspen Edge Low Carb (4.1%)	95	12	3
Augsburger Bock (4.9%)	170	14	17
Bass (5.51%)	140	16	13
Beck's (5%)	145	14	12
Beck's Premier Light (2.3%)	65	6.5	4
Big Sky (4.8%)	150	14	12
Big Sky Light (4.5%)	105	13	5
Black Label (5.6%)	155	15	11
Blackhook Porter (4.9%)	160	14	14
Blatz (4.6%)	145	13	13
Blatz LA (2.3%)	75	7	6
Blatz (3.9%)	110	11	8
Blonde (4.3%)	140	12	10
Blue Moon, Belgian (5.4%)	170	15	14
Bud Dry (5%)	130	14	8

Brands (Cont)

Per 12 fl.oz Serving

Alc ~ Alcohol (Grams)

	C	Alc	Cb
Bud Light (4.2%)	110	12	7
Bud Ice (5.5%)	125	15	4
Bud Ice Light (4.2%)	110	12	7
Bud Light Lime (4.2%)	115	12	8
Budweiser (5%)	145	14	11
Budweiser Select (4.3%)	100	12	3
Busch (4.6%)	135	13	10
Busch Ice (5.9%)	170	16	13
Busch Light (4.1%)	95	12	4
Carling (4.4%)	140	13	10
Carlsberg (5%)	135	13	10
Carta Blanca (4.0%)	125	11	11
Castlemaine XXXX (4.7%)	140	13	9
Cerveza Aquila (3.9%)	125	11	11
Chelada Budweiser (5%)	370	28	40
Chelada Bud Light (4.2%)	300	24	31
Colt 45 Malt (5.6%)	160	15	11
Coors (4.9%)	150	14	12
Coors Extra Gold (5%)	155	14	13
Coors Light (4.2%)	105	12	5
Corona Light (4.1%)	105	12	5
Dos Equis Lager (5%)	130	14	9
Fosters Lager (5%)	145	14	11
Genesse: Regular (4.5%)	150	12	14
Genny Light (3.6%)	95	10	6
George Killian's: Irish Brown	185	15	15
Irish Red (5%)	160	14	13
Goebel (4.1%)	130	11	11
Goebel Light (3.9%)	110	11	8
Grolsch Premium (5%)	140	14	10
Guinness Draught (4.2%)	125	12	10
Guinness Extra Stout (5.8%)	175	17	14
Hamm's (4.7%)	145	13	12
Special Light (3.9%)	110	12	8
Harp (4.5%)	150	12	13
Heineken (5%)	150	14	12
Heineken Special Dark (5.2%)	175	16	14
Heineken Premium Light (3.5%)	100	10	7
Hurricane (5.9%)	135	16	5
Icehouse (5.0%)	135	14	9
Icehouse Light (5%)	125	14	7
Jacob Best Ice (5.8%)	160	16	11
Keystone: Ice (5.9%)	145	16	6
Light (4.2%)	105	12	6
Premium (4.4%)	110	12	6
Killarney's Red Larger (5%)	200	14	23
Killian's Irish Red (4.9%)	165	14	14
King Cobra (5.6%)	135	16	5
Kirin Ichiban (5%)	150	14	12
Kirin Light (3.2%)	95	9	8

Brands (Cont)

Beer Contains Zero Fat
Per 12 fl.oz Serving

C ~ **Alc** ~ Alcohol (Grams)
Cb ~ Carbohydrate

	C	Alc	Cb
Labatt: Blue (5%)	155	14	10
Blue Light (4%)	110	11	8
Leinenkugel's: Original (4.7%)	150	13	14
Light (4.2%)	105	11	6
Lone Star: Regular (4.7%)	135	14	12
Light (3.9%)	110	11	9
Lowenbrau Dark/Special (4.9%)	160	14	15
Magic Hat #9 (4.6% alc)	155	13	14
Magnum Malt Liquor (5.6%)	160	16	11
Meister Brau (4.5%)	130	13	12
Memphis Brown (4.6%)	120	13	6
Michelob: Larger (5%)	165	14	15
Light (4.3%)	125	12	9
Ultra (4.2%)	85	12	2.5
Ultra, fruit flavors	110	12	6
Amber (5%)	115	14	3.5
AmberBock (5.2%)	155	15	14
Honey Lager (4.9%)	180	14	19
Porter (5.9%)	195	16	18
Mickey's Malt Liquor (5.6%)	160	16	11
Miller Chill Chelada (4.2%)	110	13	7
Miller Genuine Draft (4.7%)	145	14	13
Miller High Life (4.7%)	145	14	13
Miller High Life Light (4.2%)	110	13	7
Miller Lite (4.2%)	95	13	3
Milwaukee's Best (4.3%)	130	13	12
Milwaukee's Best Ice (5.9%)	145	16	7
Milwaukee's Best Light (4.2%)	100	13	4
Minnesota's Best (4.9%)	140	14	10
Molson Canadian (5%)	150	14	12
Molson Ice (5.6%)	160	16	14
Molson Special Dry (5%)	145	14	10
Moosehead (5%)	125	14	14
Natural Ice (5.9%)	160	17	9
Natural Light (4.2%)	95	12	3
Negra Modela (5%)	155	14	14
Newcastle Brown Ale (4.5%)	140	12	13
Northstone Amber Ale (4.9%)	150	14	8
Olde English "800" (5.9%)	160	16	11
Old Milwaukee (4.6%)	145	13	13
Light (3.9%)	110	11	8
Ice (5.9%)	180	16	15
Old Style (4.7%)	145	14	12
Old Style Light (4.2%)	115	12	7
Old Style LA (2.2%)	70	6	6
Olympia Gold Light (2.2 %)	70	6	6

	C	Alc	Cb
Pabst (4.3%)	145	13	12
Pabst Blue Ribbon (4.7%)	145	14	12
Pabst Light (3.9%)	110	11	8
Pabst Extra Light (2.2%)	70	6	6
Pearl Light (2.2%)	70	6	6
Pete's Wicked Ale (5.3%)	175	15	17
Piels (4.3%)	125	12	9
Pilsner (5% alc)	140	14	9
Red Dog (5%)	150	14	14
Red Hook ESB (5.7%)	180	17	16
Red Hook India Pale Ale (4.7%)	180	13	19
Red Stripe Jamaican Ale (5.0%)	155	14	14
Rolling Rock (4.5%)	130	13	10
Samuel Adams: Lager (4.9%)	180	13	19
Summer Ale (5.3%)	160	15	12
Sam Adams Light (4.6%)	120	11	10
Sapporo Draft (3.9%)	135	11	14
Schaefer (4.6%)	145	13	12
Schaefer Light (3.9%)	110	11	8
Schlitz (4.6%)	145	13	12
Schlitz Light (3.9%)	110	11	8
Schmidt's (4.6%)	145	13	13
Schmidt's Light (3.9%)	110	11	8
Sheaf Stout, 5.7%	180	16	17
Sierra Nevada: Pale Ale (5.6%)	200	16	12
Big Foot (9.6%)	295	28	25
Porter (5.6%)	200	16	16
Wheat Beer (4.4%)	150	12	12
Silver Thunder (5.9%)	165	17	11
Skyy Sport (4.%)	160	14	15
Sol Cerveza Especial (4%)	125	11	11
Southpaw Light (5%)	125	14	7
St Pauli Girl (4.9%)	135	14	9
Stella Artois (5.2%)	155	15	12
Stroh's (4.6%)	145	13	12
Stroh's Light (3.9%)	115	11	7
Tecate (4.7%)	155	13	16
Tequiza (4.5%)	130	13	9
Tsingtao (4.7%)	155	13	16
Warsteiner Verum/Dunkel (5%)	155	14	13
Weinhard's: Pale Ale (4/6%)	155	13	13
Hefeweizen (4.9%)	155	14	12
Wheat Hook (4.8%)	150	14	12
Widmer: Hefeweizen (4.9%)	155	13	16
Zeigenbock Amber (4.4%)	145	12	13

Home-Brewed Beer: Similar to regular beers, according to alcohol content.

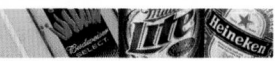

Alc ~ Alcohol (Grams)   **Cb** ~ Carbohydrate

Non-Alcoholic Brews

Less Than 0.5% Alcohol
Average All Brands
(Busch NA, Coors NA, Haake Beck, Kaliber, Kingsbury, O'Douls, Old Milwaukee NA, Pabst NA, Stroh's NA, Texas Select)

	C	Alc	Cb
12 fl.oz Can/Bottle	70	1	14
O'Doul's Amber, 12 fl.oz	90	1	18
Sharp's 12 fl.oz	60	1	12

Cider (Alcoholic)

	C	Alc	Cb
Hardcore Crisp Hard Cider (6%)	190	17	19
Hornsby's: Draft Cider (6%)	170	17	16
Hard Apple Cider (5.5%)	200	16	27
Woodchuck (5%) Amber, 12 fl.oz	200	15	21
Dark & Dry, 12 fl.oz	180	15	11
Granny Smith, 12 fl.oz	165	15	11
Wyder's: *Per 11.5 fl.oz Bottle*			
Apple (4%)	155	11	12
Peach (5%)	175	12	16
Pear (5%)	130	12	15
Raspberry (4%)	140	11	16

Quick Guide

Table Wines
Average All Varieties (11.5% Alc.)
(Wine Contains Zero Fat)

	C	Alc	Cb
4 fl.oz 1 small wine glass			
OR ½ large wine glass	90	11	3
6 fl.oz (¾ large wine glass)	135	16	4
8 fl.oz (1 large wine glass)	180	22	6
½ Carafe/Bottle, 375ml	290	34	10
1 Bottle, 750ml	580	68	20

Table Wines

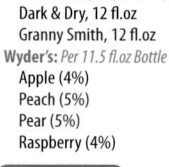

	C	Alc	Cb
Red: Claret/Burgundy/Chianti, 4 fl.oz	80	11	2
Sparkling Reds, 4 fl.oz	90	11	3
Rose: Medium, 4 fl.oz	80	11	2
White: *Per 4 fl.oz*			
Dry (Chablis/Hock/Riesling)	75	11	1
Zinfandel Sweet			
(Moselle/Sauterne), 4 fl.oz	85	11	2
Sparkling, 4 fl.oz	95	11	4

Table Wines (Cont)

	C	Alc	Cb
Champagne: *Per 4 fl.oz Serving*			
Average 1 glass, 4 fl.oz	85	11	2
w. Orange Jce (3:1 orange)	75	8	4
w. Orange Jce (1:1 orange)	65	5	7
Cold Duck 4 fl oz	108	11	8
Mulled Wine *(Gluhwein)*, 4 fl.oz	180	14	20
Non-Alcoholic Wine, avg., 4 fl.oz	50	0	12
Reduced Alcohol Wine (6%):			
Average all types, 4 fl.oz	50	0	12
Sake: Rice Wine (16% alc.), 4 oz	125	15	5

Flavored Wines

Average All Brands (6% alcohol)
(Examples: Arbor Mist, Wild Vines, Boones)

	C	Alc	Cb
1 small wine glass, 4 fl.oz	80	6	10
1 large wine glass, 8 fl.oz	160	11	20
1 bottle, 750 ml (25.4 fl.oz)	510	36	64

Dessert Wines

	C	Alc	Cb
Madeira (18% alc), 2 oz	85	9	5
Marsala (18%), 2 oz	110	9	11
Port, Muscatel (18%), 2 oz	85	9	5
Sherry (18%), 2 oz			
Dry, 1 Sherry glass	65	9	0.5
Sweet/Cream, average	85	9	5
Vermouth: Dry (18%), 2 oz	65	9	0.5
Sweet (15%), 2 oz	85	7	8

Cooking Wines

	C	Alc	Cb
Average All Brands			
Red/White: 2 Tbsp, 1 oz	20	3	1
1 cup, 8 fl.oz	160	22	12
Marsala, 2 Tbsp, 1 oz	35	4	2
Sherry, 2 Tbsp, 1 oz	40	4	2

COOKING WITH WINE

For alcohol to evaporate, sufficient heat and cooking time (at least 30 minutes) is required.
Red and white table wines would then contain negligible residual calories.
Sweetened wines (marsala/sherry) would contain 10 calories per 1 fl.oz.
Flambé Desserts: Only surface alcohol is burned off, so negligible reduction in alcohol or calories.

Quick Guide — Alc ~ Alcohol (Grams)

Spirits/Liquors

Includes Bourbon, Brandy, Gin, Rum, Scotch, Tequila, Vodka, Whiskey.
Note: All spirits with same alcohol proof have similar calories and zero fat.

Average All Brands

	C	Alc	Cb
80 Proof (40% Alcohol by Volume):			
1 fl.oz	65	9.5	0
1½ fl.oz (1 shot)	100	14	0
3 fl.oz (Double shot)	200	29	0
½ Bottle, 350 ml	810	120	0
1 Bottle, 700 ml (24 fl.oz)	1620	240	0
86 Proof (43% Alc): 1 fl.oz	70	10	0
1½ fl.oz (1 shot)	105	15	0
1 Bottle, 700 ml (24 fl.oz)	1750	250	0
100 Proof (50% Alc): 1½ fl.oz	120	18	0

Flavored Spirits ~ Average All Brands

Includes Malibu Rum; Captain Morgan (Original)

	C	Alc	Cb
70 Proof (35% Alc): 1½ fl.oz	105	13	1
3 fl.oz (Double shot)	210	26	3
Parrot Bay (21%), avg., 1½ fl.oz	100	8	12
Southern Comfort (35%), 1½ fl.oz	100	13	3

Shochu (Soju) ~ Izakaya Lounges

Average all types (20% alc), 2 fl.oz — 65 — 9 — 0

Hard Lemonade & Sodas

	C	Alc	Cb
Henry's Hard L'ade (5%), 12 fl.oz	285	14	46
Mike's Hard Lemonade (5.2%):			
11.2 fl.oz bottle	240	13	38
16 fl.oz bottle	345	19	54
Light (4%), 11.2 fl.oz	100	10	6
Mike's Hard Iced Tea (5%), 11.2 fl.oz	195	13	27
Rick's Spiked (5.2%), 12 fl.oz	250	14	39
Twisted Tea: Half & Half (5%) 12 fl.oz	250	14	30
Hard Iced (5%): All flavors	220	14	37
Light (4%), 12 fl.oz	115	11	9
Original (5%):, 12 fl.oz bottle	220	14	30
24 fl.oz can	440	28	60
Zima (4.9%), avg. all flav., 12 fl.oz	185	14	22

Alcoholic Energy Drinks (with Caffeine)

	C	Alc	Cb
Sparks: *Per 16 fl.oz Can*			
Sparks (6%)	340	23	47
Sparks Light (6%)	180	23	5
Sparks Plus (7%)	385	26	49
Tilt Green (8%), 16 fl.oz	460	30	64
Tilt Orange (6.6%), 16 fl.oz	410	25	46

Coolers & Premix Cocktails

Ready-To-Drink
Zero Fat Unless Indicated

	C	Alc	Cb
Arbor Mist: Blenders, all flavors (12.5%), 4 fl.oz	100	11	14
Bacardi Silver: *Per 12 fl.oz*			
Fruit Flavors (5%)	240	14	36
Silver O³/Raz (5%)	240	14	36
Silver Mojito (5%)	230	14	33
Ready to Pour, *(1.75 liter bottle)*			
Bahama Mama (10%), 4 fl.oz	130	13	16
Hurricane (12.5%), 4 fl.oz	144	12	16
Rum Island Ice Tea (12.5%), 4 fl.oz	150	12	16
Bartles & Jaymes			
Malt Based Coolers (3.9% alc.): *Per 12 fl.oz*			
Classic Original; Blue Hawaiian	190	11	29
Black Cherry; Berry; Peach	220	11	33
Raspb./Strawb. Daquiri	215	11	36
Margarita/Pina Colada	260	11	47
Other flavors, avg.	230	11	39
Wine Cooler (5% alc.): *12 fl.oz*			
Classic Original	200	14	29
Blue Hawaiian; Exotic Berry, avg.	230	14	33
Other flavors, average	240	14	38
Captain Morgan Parrot Bay (5% Alc), Average all flavors, 12 fl.oz	250	14	37
Daily's *(Ready-to-Drink):*			
Bag-In-Box Cocktails (6.9%), Bloody Mary, ½ cup, 4 fl.oz	70	6	6
Other flavors, 4 fl.oz	110	6	15
Frozen Pouches (5%), 10 fl.oz	280	11	44
Jack Daniels Country Cocktails:			
Average all flavors, 6.8 fl.oz	170	10	25
Jack Daniels Hard Cola (5%) 12 oz	234	14	34
Jose Cuervo Margaritas (5.9% alc)			
Premix (9.95%), Strawb./Lime, 1½ oz	50	3.5	7
Minis (5.9%), 200ml bottle	180	10	27
Sauza Diablo (5%), 12 fl.oz	260	14	40
Seagram's Coolers (5%)			
Average all flavors	240	14	35
Skyy Blue (5%), 12 fl.oz	280	14	45
Stolichnaya Citr. (5%), 12 fl.oz	240	14	36
Smirnoff Ice (5%), 330ml	220	13	33
Black Ice (5.5%), 12 fl.oz	240	19	36
TGI Friday's: *Per 3 fl.oz*			
On The Rocks: Margarita (7.5%)	90	6	14
Long Island Ice Tea (15%)	130	11	14
Mudslide (10%)	200	8	18
Blenders (12.5% alc): *Per 3 fl.oz*			
Mudslide (12.5%)	120	8.5	15
Orange Dream (12.5%)	120	8.5	15
Strawberry Shortcake (12.5%)	115	8.5	12

Coolers & Premix Cocktails (Cont)

Ready-To-Drink   **C**   **Alc**   **Cb**

The Club Premix Cocktails (8 oz Can):
Per 4 oz Serving (½ can)

	C	Alc	Cb
Long Island Ice Tea; Manhattan	220	16	30
Margar.; Screwdriver; Vodka Martini	210	7	40
Mudslide (9g fat)	270	12	41
Pina Colada; Or. Craze; Whisk. Sour	260	10	40
Zima (5.9%), 12 fl.oz	235	15	20

Shooters   **Alc** ~ Alcohol (Grams)

	C	Alc	Cb
Alabama Slammer	110	14	2
Amaretto Sour	120	6	19
B52	145	14	11
Beam Me Up Scotty	145	13	13
Blue Tequila	160	18	6
Jager Bomb	205	8	30
Jager Bomb (w. Sugar-Free Red Bull)	155	8	18
Jell-O Shot, 3 oz (w.1½ oz Vodka)	175	14	14
w. Diet Jell-O, 3 oz	110	14	0
Kamikaze	75	8	3
Kool-Aid	160	15	14
Liquid Cocaine	135	9	9
M & M	150	11	20
Orgasm	100	12	6
Peppermint Patty	200	8	11
Stinger	170	18	12
Vodka or Tequila Shot, 1½ oz	105	14	0

Cocktail Mixers

Non Alcoholic ~ No Alcohol Added
Bacardi: *Frozen Concentrate*
(Made Up from 2 fl.oz concentrate)

	C	Alc	Cb
Margarita, 8 fl.oz	90	0	25
Pina Colada, 8 fl.oz	170	0	35
Strawberry, 8 fl.oz	120	0	35
Baja Bob's (Sugar Free),			
Cocktail/Martini Mix, 4 oz	10	0	2
Daily's Pina Colada, 3 fl.oz	160	0	37
J.Cuervo Margarita, 4 fl.oz	100	0	24
Malibu Beach, all flavors, 8 fl.oz	10	0	3
Mr T's: Mai Tai, 4.5 fl.oz	140	0	33
Bloody Mary, 8 fl.oz	40	0	9
Margarita, 4 fl.oz	100	0	26
Pina Colada, 4.5 fl.oz	180	0	43
Strawberry Daiquiri, 4 fl.oz	200	0	50
Sweet 'n' Sour, 4 fl.oz	90	0	23
Sauza Margarita, 3 fl.oz	70	0	18
Skyy Cosmo, 4 fl.oz	140	0	36
TGI Fridays: Hurricane, 2.3 fl.oz	60	0	15
Long Island Ice Tea, 3.3 fl.oz	55	0	14
Mudslide, 2.3 fl.oz	120	0	24

Cocktails   **Alc** ~ Alcohol (Grams)

Made to Standard Recipes (Standard Size)
(Main Reference: The New American Bartender's Guide)

Zero Fat Unless Indicated   **C**   **Alc**   **Cb**

	C	Alc	Cb
Bacardi & Coke (w. 1½ oz Bacardi)	160	14	17
Bloody Mary (w. 1½ oz Vodka)	125	10	7
Blue Lady	220	15	17
Blushin' Russian (20g fat)	405	14	23
Bourbon & Soda (w. 2 oz Bourbon)	130	19	0
Brandy Alexander (10g fat)	300	20	15
Chi Chi's: Long Island Iced Tea, 4 fl.oz	145	12	17
Mexican Mudslide, 4 fl.oz (8g fat)	240	1.5	42
Mojito, 4 fl.oz	160	11	21
Pina Colada 4 fl.oz (6g fat)	240	4	42
White Russian 4 fl.oz (7g fat)	245	1.5	43
Chupa Naranjas (w. 1½ oz Tequila)	150	16	8
Cosmopolitan	215	12	12
Daiquiri (w. 2 oz Rum) avg. all types	140	19	4
Frozen Daiquiri (w. 2 oz Rum):			
no fruit	155	19	6
with fruit (w. 1½ oz Rum)	145	14	11
Gin Martini (w. 2 oz alcohol)	140	19	0
Grasshopper	260	17	28
Harvey Wallbanger (2 oz Alc.)	290	19	17
Highball (1½ oz Whiskey)	100	14	0
Irish Coffee (contains 10g fat)	205	14	2
Kahlua Mudslide: w.milk (3g fat)	145	11	12
w. cream (12g fat)	230	11	10
L.A. Sunrise (w. 1½ oz Vodka)	220	14	17
Long Island Iced Tea (w. 3 oz Cola)	270	19	32
with Diet Cola (w. 3 oz Cola)	235	19	22
Mai Tai (with 2 oz Rum)	290	24	33
Manhattan	130	17	5
Margarita	160	18	7
Mint Julep (w.2½ oz Bourbon)	180	24	4
Moscow Mule	185	14	24
Pina Colada (contains 10g fat)	325	19	26
Red Bull & Vodka	210	14	28
with Sugar Free Red Bull	105	14	3
Screwdriver	160	14	15
Sex On The Beach	235	19	25
Spritzer (with 3 oz Wine)	65	8	2
Tequila Sunrise	200	14	25
Tom Collins (w. 2 oz Gin)	210	19	18
Vodka Soda (w. 1½ oz Vodka)	100	14	0
Vodka Tonic (w. 1½ oz Vodka)	165	14	18
Whiskey Sour (w. 2 oz Whiskey)	155	19	7
White Russian (w. 10g fat)	240	19	7
Non-Alcoholic:			
Cinderella	45	0	11
Shirley Temple (w. 6 oz Ginger Ale)	140	0	34

Liqueurs/Cordials

	C	**Alc**	**Cb**
Per 1 fl.oz			
Advocaat (36 Proof; 2g fat)	85	4	9
Alizé: Cognac	70	11	2
Gold/Red Passion	105	4.5	11
Amaretto (56 Proof)	110	6	17
Baileys Irish Cream (34 Proof; 5g fat)	95	4	6
Lite (30 Proof; 2g fat)	75	4	7
Benedictine (80 Proof)	90	10	5
Chambord (33 Proof)	105	5	11
Chartreuse (80 Proof)	100	10	7
Cherry Brandy (48 Proof)	80	6	9
Coffee Liqueur (53 Proof)	90	6	11
Cointreau (80 Proof)	100	10	7
Creme de Cacao (54 Proof)	100	6	15
Creme de Menthe (60 Proof)	120	7	14
Curacao (70 Proof)	95	8	6
Drambuie (80 Proof)	105	10	9
Frangelico (48 Proof)	80	6	9
Galliano (80 Proof)	100	10	8
Grand Marnier (80 Proof)	100	10	7
Kahlua (53 Proof)	90	6	11
Kirsch (68 Proof)	80	8	4
Midori (42 Proof)	80	5	11
Ouzo (80 Proof)	105	11	11
Pernod (80 Proof)	75	10	2
Sambuca (84 Proof)	100	10	7
Schnapps (80 Proof)	100	10	7
Southern Comfort (70 Proof)	80	10	3
Starbucks Coffee Liqueur (40 Proof)	80	4	13
Tia Maria (64 Proof)	90	8	9
Triple Sec (60 Proof)	80	7	4

Liqueur Coffee & Hot Drinks

Per Standard Drink

Liqueur Coffee, avg. all types	200	10	10
Egg Nog	270	10	25
Hot Toddy, w. 2 oz liquor	200	19	17
Irish Coffee, w. 2 Tbsp whip. crm	80	7	4
Mulled Wine (Glühwein), 5 oz	175	14	6

Flavorings/Syrups

Angostura Bitters, ¼ tsp	3	0	0
Ginger Ale, 8 fl.oz	80	0	22
Grenadine/Cassis, 2 Tbsp, 1 oz	70	0	17
Lime/Lemon Juice, 2 Tbsp, 1 oz	10	0	2
Maraschino Cherry, 1 small	8	0	2
Pure Lemon Extract (70%) avg., 1 oz	145	20	0
Sugar Syrup, 2 Tbsp, 1 oz	70	0	17
Sour Mix, 2 Tbsp, 1 oz	10	0	2
Tonic Water, 8 fl.oz	90	0	22
Vanilla Extract, (35%), avg., 1 oz	80	10	3.5

TEN HINTS TO AVOID HARMFUL DRINKING

1. **Add up the alcohol** you typically drink each day and on social occasions. How does this compare with 'low risk' amounts?

2. **Compare the alcohol content** of different drinks and select the lowest. Request half ounces of alcohol in cocktails and mixed drinks. Dilute them and keep topping off with non-alcoholic drinks.

3. **Go easy on 'Light' beers.** At 4% alcohol, on average, they are still high in alcohol compared to regular beer (5% alcohol).

4. **Try low alcohol or non-alcohol** alternatives such as fruit juices and mineral water. Take your own to parties.

5. **Before drinking alcohol,** quench your thirst with water and non-alcoholic drinks – particularly after vigorous exercise or sports.

6. **Slow the rate of drinking.** Chugging or drinking fast is the major cause of illness and death from alcohol poisoning.

7. **Avoid drinking in 'rounds'.**

8. **Have a non-alcoholic 'spacer'** between drinks (e.g. mineral water, orange juice).

9. **Don't drink on an empty stomach.** Food slows the rate of alcohol absorption.

10. **Keep track of the number of drinks** and know when to stop. Stick to a set limit.

Note: • Alcohol can be very dangerous when taken with prescription or street drugs or when you are very tired.

Extra Info: www.CalorieKing.com

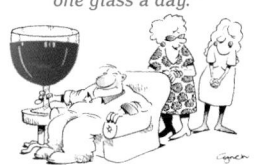

"The doctor told him to cut down to just one glass a day."

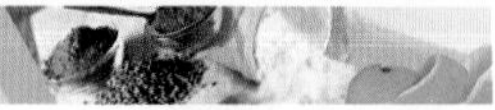

Baking Ingredients

	C	F	Cb
Almond Paste:			
(Marzipan), 2 Tbsp	170	7	24
Apple Pie Filling,			
Sweetened, 1 cup	270	0	66
Also See Page 136			
Baking Powder: Regular, 1 tsp	5	0	2
Cream of Tartar, 1 tsp	10	0	2
Baking Mix *(Bisquick)*:			
Original, ⅓ cup, 1½ oz	160	5	26
Heart Smart, ⅓ cup, 1½ oz	140	2.5	27
Blueberries, 1 cup, 5 oz	80	0.5	20
Butter/Margarine, ½ c., 4 oz	815	92	1
Stick, *Land O' Lakes*, ½ oz	100	11	0
Carob Flour, ½ cup	115	0.5	46
Chocolate Baking Bars: *Average all Brands*			
Sweet *(Baker's)*:			
1 oz portion	130	9	17
4 oz bar	520	35	65
Semi-sweet, 1 oz	140	9	16
Bittersweet, 1 oz	140	10	14
White Baking 1 oz	230	14	26
Unsweetened, 1 oz	140	14	8
Grated, 1 cup, 4½ oz	660	69	39
Chocolate Baking Chips: *Average all Brands*			
Milk Choc./Semi Sweet 1 oz	140	8	18
½ cup, 3 oz	420	24	54
1 cup, 6 oz	840	48	108
Mini Kisses *(Hershey)*, 1 pce	5	0.5	1
Cocoa Powder, Baking: *Nestle*, 1 T.	15	1	3
⅓ cup, 1 oz	80	4	12
Hershey's, 1 Tbsp	20	0.5	3
⅓ cup, 1 oz	115	3.5	21
Coconut, dried:			
Unsweet., 1 oz	195	20	6
Sweetened/flaked, 1 oz	130	8	15
½ cup, 1.3 oz	195	12	22
Toasted *(Baker's)*, 1 oz	170	13	13
Coconut Cream/Milk: *See Page 91*			
Cornstarch, 1 Tbsp	30	0	7
Eggs: Large (1)	75	4.5	0
Jumbo (1)	90	5	0
Egg White: 1 Egg White	15	0	0
½ cup (4 egg whites), 4 oz	60	0	0
Flour, white:			
1 Tbsp, 0.6 oz	55	0	12
1 cup, 4.4 oz	455	1	95
Whole Wheat, 1 cup, 4.2 oz	410	2	87

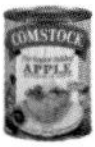

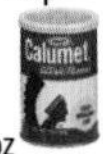

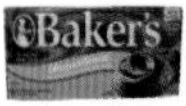

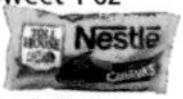

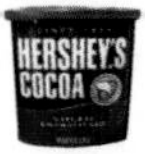

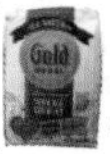

	C	F	Cb
Flavor Extracts: *Average all Brands*			
Imitation, 1 tsp	10	0	2
Pure Extract, 1 tsp	10	0	0.5
Almond, Vanilla, 1 tsp	10	0	0.5
Fruit Pectin: Swtnd, ¼ tsp	5	0	1
Unsweetened, ¼ tsp	0	0	0
Gelatin, dry, ¼ oz pkg	25	0	0
Honey, ½ cup, 6 oz	515	0	135
Lemon/Orange Peel, ¼ cup	25	0	6
Lighter Bake *(Sunsweet)*			
(Butter & Oil replacement)			
1 Tbsp, ½ oz	35	0	9
¼ Cup, 2.7 oz	140	0	36
Fat-Free, 1 1 cup, 8 fl.oz	90	0.5	13
Milk: Whole, 1 cup, 8 fl.oz	150	8	12
2%, 1 cup, 8 fl.oz	120	5	12
1%, 1 cup, 8 fl.oz	100	2.5	12
Pastry ~ *See Page 136*			
Pie Crusts ~ *See Page 136*			
Pie Fillings:			
Fruits ~ *See page 136*			
Lemon Creme, ⅓ cup	130	1	31
Mincemeat, 3½ oz	190	5	45
Pumpkin, 1 cup, 9½ oz	280	0	70
Prune Puree, ¼ cup, 3 oz	220	0	55
Raisins, ½ cup, 2.8 oz	220	0.5	56
Rennin, 1 pkg (11g)	10	0	2
Soy Milk ~ *See Pages 48-49*			
Sprinkles, all types, 1 tsp	20	1	3
Sugar: 1 Tbsp, ½ oz	50	0	12
1 oz	110	0	20
1 cup, 7 oz	770	0	192
1 lb, 16 oz	1760	0	464
Sweeteners & Sugar Substitutes ~ *See Page 164*			
Vinegar, avg. all types, 1 oz	5	0	1
Whey, sweet, dry, 1 oz	100	0.5	21
Yeast: Active, dry, ¼ oz pkg	21	0	3
Bakers, compressed, 1 oz	30	0.5	5
Fleischmann's, 0.6 oz pkg	0	0	0

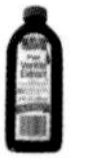

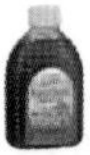

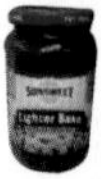

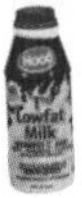

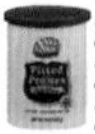

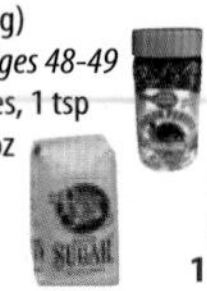

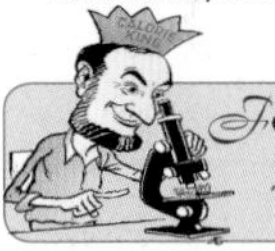

For Full Nutritional Data
& Product Updates
~ See Author's Website
www.CalorieKing.com

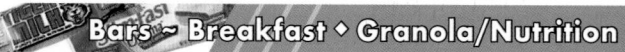

Note: Actual weight of bars is usually 5-10% more than label Net Wt. Weigh bar and allow extra calories.

Breakfast Bars

	C	F	Cb
Apex, Breakfast Squares, 2 oz	210	7	23
Atkins: Advantage Morning Bars,			
Crisp, avg., 1.3 oz bar	170	9	14
Cinnamon Bun, 1.4 oz bar	150	7	15
Barbara's Bakery: Nature's Choice	150	2	28
Fruit & Yogurt Bar, 1.1 oz	150	3	29
Full Circle, average, 1.3oz	135	2	26
General Mills: Milk'n Cereal Bars,			
Cinnamon Toast Crunch, 1.6 oz	180	4	33
Other varieties, average, 1.6 oz	160	4	28
Health Valley: Bar, avg., 1.3 oz	130	2	27
Cereal Tarts, all flav. 1 bar, 1.4oz	130	2	28
Kellogg's			
All-Bran Cereal Bar, avg., 1.2 oz	130	3	26
Crunch Cereal Bar, avg., 1 oz	110	2	22
Smart Start Bars, 1.4 oz	150	2.5	30
Pop Tarts: French Toast (1)	220	8	35
Fruit/Frosted, avg., 1.8 oz	200	5	37
Low-Fat, all flavors, 1.8 oz	190	3	39
Go Tarts, avg., 1.2 oz	140	4.5	24
Splitz: Chocolate Vanilla, 1.7 oz	200	6	35
Strawberry Blueberry, 1.7 oz	200	5	36
Market Pantry (Target), Bar, 1.4 oz	140	3	26
Nature's Path: Crispy Rice, avg.	110	3	24
Toaster Pastries, 1.8 oz	210	5	37
New England Natural Bakers			
Save the Forest Bars (1), 1 oz	120	4.5	19
Nutri-Grain Bars			
Cereal Bars, avg., 1.3 oz	140	3	26
Fruit & Nut Bar, 1.1 oz	120	3.5	22
Yogurt Bars, avg., 1.3 oz	140	3	26
Post, Honey Bunches of Oats Bar	140	4	24
Quaker			
Breakfast Cookies, 1 pce, 1.7 oz	170	4.5	33
Fruit Flavor Crisp Bar, 1.3 oz	130	2.5	26
Fruit Flavor Crisp Bites, 1 pouch	130	2.5	28
Muffin Bars, 1.3 oz	130	3.5	26
Granola Bars: *See Page 36*			
Russell Stover, Bar, 1.1 oz	100	5	13
Slim-Fast: Fruit Crisp, 1.3 oz	180	4.5	29
Muffin Bar, 1.2 oz	140	5	20
South Beach Diet *(Kraft)*			
High Protein Cereal Bars (1), 1.3 oz	140	5	15
Special K Cereal Bars, avg., 0.8 oz	90	1.5	18
Trader Joe's: Fig, 1.3 oz	120	2	24
Apple, Blueberry/Strawb., avg.	140	2.5	28

Sports & Diet Bars C F Cb

Per Bar

	C	F	Cb
ABB: Extreme XXL Bar, 4.9 oz	530	11	68
Steel Bar, 2 oz	250	4	36
AdvantEdge			
Carb Control			
Crisp Bar, 2.1 oz	240	8	27
Nutrition Bar, 2.1 oz	220	7	28
Complete Nutrition Bar, 2.1 oz	240	8	27
All-Bran Fiber Bars, avg., 1.4 oz	130	2.5	30
Alpen Cereal Bars: *Per 3.5 oz Bar*			
Alpen Light (1), 0.74 oz	285	4	56
Fruit & Nut (1), 1 oz	110	3	20
Fruit & Nut w. Chocolate (1), 1 oz	125	4	20
Groove, 1.1 oz	140	5	21
Raspberry & Yogurt (1), 1.03 oz	120	3	21
Apex: Fix Crisp Bar, 1.4 oz	160	4	21
Fix Fruit Fuel Bar	210	3.5	36
Atkins: Original Bar, average, 2.1 oz	220	9	22
Caramel Bar, average, 1.6 oz	180	6	17
Granola Bar, average, 1.7 oz	220	8	18
Back to Nature			
Bakery Squares, avg., 1.07 oz	125	4.5	20
Chewy Trail Mix Bar, avg., 1 oz	120	4.5	19
Fruit & Grain Bar, 1.07 oz	110	2	20
Balance: Balance Bars, 1.7 oz	200	6	23
Balance Bar Bare:			
Sweet & Salty, average, 1.8 oz	210	9	23
Trail Mix, average, 1.8 oz	210	7	23
Carb Well: Caramel 'n Choc., 1.7 oz	190	7	23
Chocolate Fudge, 1.7 oz	190	6	23
Chocolate Peanut Butter, 1.7 oz	200	8	22
100 Calorie Bar, 1.7 oz	100	4	14
Gold/Crunch Bars, avg., 1.7 oz	210	6	23
Barbara's Bakery: Granola, ¾ oz	80	2	14
Crunchy Granola, 1.5 oz	190	8	27
Fruit & Yogurt Bar, 1.1 oz	150	3	39
Bariatrix Proti-Bar: (15g Protein)			
Caramel Nut, 1.42 oz	150	4.5	15
Bear Valley, Meal Pack, 3.75 oz	420	13	59
Biochem: Strive, avg., 2.1 oz	190	9	4
Greens & Whey Bar, 2.1 oz	280	12	26
Raw Foods & Whey Bar, 2.1 oz	200	4	37
Bumble Bar: Original/w. Nuts1.6 oz	230	15	20
Chocolate crisp, 1.6 oz	200	11	25
Lushus Lemon, 1.6 oz	210	12	21
CarbRite Diet *(Doctor's)*, avg., 2 oz	190	4	32
Caribou Coffee, Snack Bar, avg.	140	3.5	26

Note: Actual weight of bars is usually 5-10% more than label Net Wt. Weigh bar and allow extra calories.

Bars (Cont)

Per Bar	C	F	Cb
Cascadian Farms (General Mills)			
Chewy Granola Bar, 1.3 oz	135	3	25
Champion Nutrition, SnacBar	180	3	24
Clif Bars: Regular, avg., 2.4 oz	250	5	44
Clif Minis, avg., 1 oz	100	2	18
Builders, avg., 2.4 oz	270	8	30
Luna Bar, average, 1.7 oz	180	4.5	27
Mojo Bar: Avg., 1.5 oz	200	9	21
Dipped, avg., 1.6 oz	210	10	22
Nectar Bar, average, 1.6 oz	165	6	28
Z Bar, P'nut Butter, 1.27 oz	139	3	22
Curves			
Chewy Granola Bar, avg., 25g bar	100	3	18
Chocolate Peanut, 25g bar	100	3.5	17
Designer Whey			
Big Whey Bar, 3.57 oz	420	16	38
Gourmet Bars, avg. all flav., 2.7 oz	260	7	7
Detour (Next Proteins): 2.8 oz bar	320	9	32
Core Strength, average, 1.78 oz	205	6	22
Go, 1.93 oz	210	3	34
Biker Bars, average, 1.78 oz	210	5	29
Runner Bar, 1.78 oz	200	3.5	29
Buzz Bars, 3 oz	330	10	30
Oatmeal Whole Grain, 4.28 oz	460	12	58
Lower Sugar, 3 oz	340	10	33
Disney Magic, Chewy Granola, 1 oz	115	3	21
Dr Soy: Protein Bar, Lemon, 1.76 oz	170	4	26
Chocolate/Peanut, 1.76 oz	190	5	25
Healthy Snacker, avg., 1.7 oz bar	180	6	28
EAS Advantage Edge			
Carb Control, average, 2.12 oz	230	8	27
Complete Nutrition, 2.12 oz avg.	240	8	28
EAS: Champions Energy Bar	160	4.5	26
EAS Myoplex			
Deluxe Bar, avg., 3.2 oz	350	10	36
Lite , P'nut Caramel, 1.9 oz	190	6	25
Carb Control, 2.5 oz	260	8	25
Elevate Me!: All Fruit Blend, 2.3 oz	210	3	32
Blueberry Cranberry/Goji, 2.3 oz	230	3.5	36
Expresso Cocoa Crunch, 2.3 oz	230	3	36
Other Bars, avg., 2.3 oz	240	4	36
Extend Bar, 1.4 oz	150	3	21
Fi-Bar Nectar Granola Bars, 1 oz	120	2	26
Chewy & Nutty Bar, 1.2 oz	140	4.5	23
First Endurance, EFS Bar, 2.32 oz	250	6	40
General Mills, Fiber One Granola, avg.	145	4	28

Per Bar	C	F	Cb
GeniSoy: Genisoy Bars, 2.2 oz	240	4.5	35
Natural Choice, 1.6 oz	170	4.5	20
Protein Crunch	150	5	18
Ultra Bar, 1.6 oz	160	2	27
Glenny's: Light n' Crispy, ½ oz	60	2.5	9
Slim Carb: Double Fudge, 1.3 oz	130	2.5	19
Slim 1, 1.06 oz	100	3	21
Glucerna: Meal Replacement, 2 oz	220	7	34
Snack Bar, 1.3 oz	150	4	25
Mini Snack Bar (1)	80	2.5	12
GNC ProCrunch:			
Choc Crisp	250	4.5	36
Cookies n' Cream	250	4	37
Peanut Butter Crunch, 2.3 oz	260	7	34
Pro Crunch Lite, 1.2 oz	140	1.5	19
Gnu Foods:			
Banana Walnut	130	3	30
Cinn. Raisin; Orange Cranberry	130	3	32
Choc. Brownie; P'nut Butter, avg.	150	3	32
Greens + Bar: + Energy, avg., 2 oz	245	10	33
+ High Protein, avg., 1.6 oz	255	12	22
Health Valley Fruit/Granola, avg.	190	5	29
Herbalife: Protein Deluxe!, 1.23 oz	140	4	15
Shapeworks Protein Bar, 1.41 oz	150	6	16
Hershey's Smart Zone, avg, 50g	200	7	21
Jenny Craig: Oat & Honey,1.78 oz	170	4.5	32
Cookies & Crm/Peanut Butter, 1 oz	110	3	12
Choc Chip Snack Bar, 1.21 oz	140	3	23
Joy Ride Bars, avg., 2.8 oz	34	12	17
Kashi GOLEAN: Bars, avg., 2.7 oz	290	6	48
Crunchy!, avg., 1.76 oz bar	170	4.5	30
GOLEAN Roll, avg., 1.9 oz	190	5	28
TLC: Crunchy Granola Bar, 1.42 oz	180	6	26
Chewy Granola Bar, 1.3 oz	140	5	19
Kellogg's Cereal Bars ~ See Page 33			
Kind Fruit & Nut Bars			
Almond & Apricot	170	11	16
In Yogurt	210	13	19
Almond & Coconut	190	14	14
Banana & Oatbran	160	7	23
Fruit & Nut in Yogurt	210	13	20
Macadamia & Apricot	190	14	15
Nut Delight	200	15	12
Sesame & Peanuts in Choc.	230	15	19
Walnut & Date	150	7	22
Kind Plus:			
Antioxidants: Cranb. & Almond	190	12	19
B-complex: PassionFruit Macad.	190	13	20
Calcium: Mango Macadamia	190	12	20
Omega-3: Almond & Cashew	150	9	18
Protein: Almond, Waln./Macad.	210	15	11

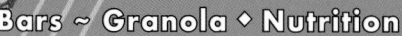

Bars (Cont)

Per Bar — **C** · **F** · **Cb**

	C	F	Cb
Kudos: Chocolate Chip, 1 oz	120	3.5	20
Peanut Butter, 1 oz	130	6	18
M&M's; Snickers, average, 0.84 oz	100	3	17
Larabar: Apple/Cherry Pie, 1.6 oz	180	10	23
Banana Cookie Dough, 1.8 oz	220	11	28
Lean Body: Cookie Bar, 3.25 oz	360	30	13
Gold, 3 oz	330	7	36
Hi Pro Granola Bar, 2.85 oz	340	11	39
Rockin' Roll, 2.5 oz	290	16	25
Lindora: Chocolate Chip	140	3	15
Other varieties, average	150	5	16
Live Active (Kraft), Granola Bars			
Avg. all flavors, 1¼ oz	140	4	26
Luna: Bars, avg., 1.69 oz	180	4.5	27
Sport, Moons Chews, avg., 1.1 oz	100	0	24
Sunrise, avg., 1.69 oz	180	4.5	27
Tea Cakes, avg., 1.4 oz	140	2	28
Marathon (Snickers): Energy, 2 oz	220	7	29
Low Carb, average, 1.7 oz	170	7	19
Protein, average, 2.8 oz	290	9	40
Market Pantry (Target)			
Chewy Granola, 1 oz, average	120	12.5	22
Sweet & Salty Bar, 1.3 oz, avg.	150	6	23
Medifast: Fit! Bar, 1.5 oz	160	5	23
Plus for Diabetics, avg., 1.5 oz	140	5	22
Met-Rx: "Big 100", 3.5 oz	360	5	53
Protein Plus, avg., 3 oz	320	9	32
MLO Bio Protein: 2.85 oz	320	7	43
Extreme, 3.2 oz	370	8	43
Mojo Bars: See Clif			
MRM Response, 2.1 oz	210	8	20
Muscle Milk, 2.57 oz	300	11	28
Muscle Tech: Nitro-Tech, average	280	7	30
Complete Cookie Bar, 2.7 oz	310	12	25
Complete Oat Bar, 3.4 oz	350	11	40
Myoplex: See EAS			
Nabisco: HoneyMaid Bars, 1.32 oz	150	6	24
100 Calorie Granola Bars:			
Chips Ahoy, 1 bar	100	1.5	22
Nutter Butter, 1 bar	100	1.5	21
Oreo, 1 bar	100	2	21
Nature Valley Granola Bars			
Chewy w. Yogurt coating, 1.4 oz	140	3.5	26
Crunchy, average, 1.5 oz	180	6	29
Heart Healthy: Honey Nut, 1.4 oz	160	4	28
Oatmeal Raisin, 1.4 oz	150	2	30
Trail Mix, average, 1.3 oz	140	4	25

Per Bar — **C** · **F** · **Cb**

	C	F	Cb
Nature's Path			
Flax Plus; Hemp Plus	140	3	27
Goji Moji (Weil), 1.6 oz	170	4.5	29
Optimum Energy, avg., 1.97 oz	230	8	33
Rebound, 2 oz	190	4	33
Granola Bars, average, 1.2 oz	160	5	26
NiteBite (Time-release Glucose Bar)			
Choc. Fudge; P'nut Butter, 0.89 oz	100	3.5	15
Nutiva: Hempseed, 1.4 oz	210	14	11
Flax Chocolate, 1.4 oz	200	12	19
NutriSystem Nourish, avg., 1.44 oz	125	3	20
Dessert Bar	160	4	28
Granola Bars: P'but Butter	170	6	18
Apple; Choc. Chip, Cranberry	150	2.5	27
Nutrilite (Quixtar):			
Butter Pretzel	200	7	22
Chocolate Nut Roll, 1.6 oz	190	6	19
Fruji Fruits Veg, 1.4 oz	130	0	30
Sport Cookie, 1.6 oz	160	5	24
Vanilla Pretzel, 1.6 oz	200	7	22
Energy Bars: Lemon, 1.6 oz	160	5	24
Sport Cookie,, 1.6 oz	160	5	24
Simply Nutrilite: Cherry Almond	180	5	26
Chocolate Crisp, 1.6 oz	170	5	32
Tropical, 1.6 oz	170	5	30
Trim Advantage Protein, 2.1 oz	260	8	25
Odwalla Energy Bars			
Choc. Chip Peanut/Crunch, avg.	245	7	38
Super Protein, 2.2 oz	230	4.5	31
Other varieties, average, 2.2 oz	240	6	41
Oh Yeah! (ISS), 3 oz	370	18	30
One Way, avg, 3 oz	340	15	29
Optifast: P'nut Butter,			
45g (1.59 oz) bar	160	4	23
Performance, 65g	230	2.5	43
Planters CarbWell			
Peanut Butter Crunch, 1.25 oz	160	12	16
Caramel Choc Crunch, 1.35 oz	180	13	17
Power Bar: Energize,	210	3.5	42
Harvest: WholeGrain	240	4.5	42
Dip'd, avg., 2.3 oz	250	5	42
Nut Naturals,			
average, 1.6 oz	210	10	24
Pria: 110 Plus, avg., 1.7 oz	110	3	16
Protein Plus: Avg., 2.75 oz	300	6	48
Reduced Sugar, avg.	265	8	31
Triple Threat, avg., 2 oz	230	8	30
Power Crunch, average, 1.3 oz	220	12	10
PR Bar average, 1.78 oz	200	6	22

Bars (Cont)

	C	F	Cb
Premier: Protein Eight, 2.4 oz	260	7	23
Premier Protein Bar, 2.5 oz	290	9	23
Odyssey Bar, avg., 2.8 oz	320	11	30
Twisted Bar, avg., 1.6 oz	190	6	21
Promax: Avg., 2.7 oz bar	290	6	40
Triple Layer, 2.5 oz	290	8	36
Protein Complete, avg., 1.97 oz	180	2.5	19
Proti 15, Choc P'nut, 1.48 oz	160	5	16
Pure Protein:			
Blueberry Crumb Cake, 2¾ oz	300	10	29
Chewy Chocolate Chip, 2¾ oz	310	8	29
Chocolate Deluxe, 2¾ oz	280	7	26
Chocolate Peanut Butter, 2¾ oz	300	10	26
Country Blueberry Pie, 2¾ oz	295	8	30
Peanut Marshmallow Eclipse, 2¾ oz	290	9	29
S'mores, 2¾ oz	280	8	31
Strawberry Shortcake, 2¾ oz	280	6	29
Pure Fit, average, 2 oz bar	235	6	27
Quaker Chewy Granola Bars			
Chewy (Regular): Avg. 0.86 oz	100	2.5	19
Peanut Butter/Chocolate	100	3	17
Chewy Dipps:			
Choc Chip	140	5	22
Peanut Butter	150	7	19
Granola Bites, 1 pouch, 0.71 oz	90	3.5	14
Snack Bars:			
Chewy Granola 25% Less Sugar	100	3.5	17
Chewy 90 Cal Granola, 0.86 oz	90	1.5	19
Rebar: Energy, 1.75 oz	180	8	29
Greens, 1.75 oz	160	0	38
Supplement, 1.75 oz	200	8	21
Resource, OptiSource Mini Bar	90	2.5	10
Revival Soy Bars *(Direct):* Per Bar			
Chocolate Temptation	270	7	32
Apple Cinnamon; Marshm. Krunch	220	3	30
Peanut Butter/Choc Pal, avg.	240	6	28
Low Carb, average all flavors	235	8	31
Slim-Fast Bars			
High Protein Meal	195	6.5	20
Cookie Bar, avg, 1 oz	120	3.5	20
Muffin Bar, average, 1.2 oz	140	5	20
Lower Carb: Average	180	6	18
Snacks, average, 1 oz	120	5	18
Optima: Fruit Crisp Bars, avg.	180	4.5	29

Per Bar

	C	F	Cb
Slim-Fast Bars (Cont)			
Meal Bars, avg., 2 oz	220	5	35
Snack Bars, avg., 1 oz	120	4	20
Granola Bars, average	220	6	35
Original: Brkfst & Lunch Bars, avg.	140	5	20
Meal-On-The-Go, average, 2 oz	220	5	35
Protein Snack Chews: Caramel, 1 pk	100	3.5	13
Peanut Butter, 1 pack	100	3.5	12
Smart Start *(Kellogg's)*			
Healthy Heart, all flavors, 1 bar, 40g	150	2.5	30
Snickers Marathon	220	7	29
SoyJoy, Bar, avg., 1.07 oz	135	6	15
Solo GI, average, 1.78 oz	200	7	26
South Beach Diet Meal Replacement			
Avg. all flavors, 2.11oz	220	7	26
Special K: Granola Snack Bites	90	2	14
Meal Bars, avg., 1½ oz	190	6	25
Protein Snack Bars, avg., 1 oz	110	3	16
Spiru-tein *(Nature's Plus),* 1.4 oz	150	5	19
Supreme, 1.8 oz	170	4.5	21
Steel Bar *(ABB),* 2 oz	250	4	36
Strive *(Biochem),* avg., 2.1 oz	230	9	24
The Sports Club/LAV:			
Caramel Cr./Choc P'nut (16g prot.)	200	5	22
P'nut Butter Fudge (13g prot.)	185	9	13
Think 5, Choc RedBerry, 2.8 oz	300	13	55
Think Organic, Cherry Nut, 1.4 oz	150	5	22
Chocolate Coconut, 1.4 oz	160	9	21
Tiger's Milk: Protein Rich, 1.25 oz	140	5	18
Peanut Butter, 1.25 oz	150	6	18
King Size Bars, 1.96 oz	230	10	28
Trader Joe's: Granola, avg.	160	7	22
Trail Mix Bars, avg., 1¼ oz	140	4	25
Tri-O-Plex: avg., 4.2 oz	430	16	45
Duo Bar, average	380	11	33
U-Turn Protein, 2.8 oz	300	8	26
Usana: Fibergy Bar, 1 oz	100	1.5	23
Nutrition Bar: Oatmeal Raisin, 1.96 oz	190	3	22
Peanut Butter Crunch, 1.46 oz	150	4	20
Vyo-Pro *(AST)* Chocolate, 2.2 oz	200	7	24
Xyience, X Smart Bar, 1.78 oz	270	7	33
Zoe Flax & Soy, Choc., 1.8 oz	190	7	19
Zone Perfect			
Dark Chocolate: Almond, 1.6 oz	190	6	22
Strawberry, 1.6 oz	180	5	22
Fruitified: Apple Cinnamon, 1.8 oz	180	2	27
Banana Nut, 1.8 oz	200	6	24
Blueberry, 1.8 oz	190	4	25
Snack Size, avg., all varieties, 0.7 oz	80	2.5	9

Cocoa & Hot Chocolate

	C	F	Cb
Cocoa (8 fl.oz cup):			
w. Whole Milk	205	8.5	22
w. Nonfat Milk	145	1	23
Tall (12 fl.oz): w. Whole Milk	280	12	26
w. Nonfat Milk	185	1	28
Hot Chocolate:			
8 fl.oz cup: w. Whole Milk	180	7	26
w. Nonfat Milk	140	2	17
Tall (12 fl.oz): w. Whole Milk	260	10	36
w. Nonfat Milk	190	2	37
Cinnabon, Mochalatta Chill, 16 oz	360	13	55
Swiss Miss Mixes, avg., 1 packet	120	2.5	22

Cocoa - Chocolate Mixes

Add extra cals/fat/carbohydrate for milk

	C	F	Cb
Carnation Breakfast Drinks: *See Page 50*			
CocoaVia, 1 pouch	25	0.5	6
Ghirardelli			
Choc Mocha, 4 Tbsp, 1.4 oz	130	1.5	33
Double Chocolate, 4 Tbsp, 1.4 oz	140	0.5	34
White Mocha, 2 Tbsp, 0.8 oz	90	0	23
Hershey's			
Choc. Milk Mix, 3 T., 24g	90	0	23
Cocoa, unsweetened, 1 T, 5g	20	0.5	3
Horlicks, Malt Extract, 1 oz	90	1	18
Land O' Lakes: *Per 1¼ oz Pkg*			
Choc.Mint/Raspb./Supreme	140	3.5	26
Nestle: *Per Single Serve Pkg*			
French Vanilla, 1 envelope	120	3	22
Milk Chocolate, 2 Tbsp	80	2.5	15
Fat-Free Hot Cocoa	25	0	1
w. Marshmallows	35	0	8
Rich Chocolate	80	3	15
No Sugar Added	50	0	10
Dble Choc Meltdown	140	3.5	28
Nesquik Powder *(Nestle): Per 2 Tbsp*			
Choc.; Dble Choc; Strawberry	60	0	15
Chocolate, No Added Sugar	40	1	7
Ovaltine Cocoa Mixes, avg., 4 tsp	80	0	20
Swiss Miss: *Per Single Serve Pkg*			
Milk Chocolate	120	2.5	23
w. Marshmallows	120	2	24
Choc. Sensation,	150	3.5	28
Hot Cocoa Diet	25	0	4
Fat-Free	50	0	10
Marshmallow Lovers	140	2.5	29
Mocha Cappuccino	110	1.5	24

Instant Coffee

	C	F	Cb
Powder/Granules: Regular or Decaffeinated			
1 level tsp	2	0	0.5
1 rounded tsp	4	0	1
Ground, 3 tsp	7	0	1
Brewed/Percolated, 1 cup, 8 fl.oz	4	0	1
Coffee With Milk/Cream/Creamers:			
Per Cup Coffee (8 fl.oz):			
Black	4	0	1
w. Whole Milk: Dash, 1 T.	15	0.5	2
2 Tbsp, 1 fl.oz	25	1	2
w. 2% Milk, 2 Tbsp	20	0.5	2
w. 1% Milk, 2 Tbsp	20	0.3	3.5
w. Fat Free Milk, 2 Tbsp	15	0	3
w. Half & Half, 2 Tbsp	50	3	2
w. ¼ cup, 2 fl.oz	90	6	3
w. Cream (light coffee), 2 Tbsp	65	6	2
w. *Coffee Mate:* Liquid, reg., 1T.	20	1	2
Liquid Fat Free, 1 Tbsp	25	0	5
Powder, 1 heaping tsp	15	1	2
Sugar ~ Add Extra: 1 heaping tsp	25	0	6
Single portion, 1 package	25	0	6
Sweeteners: *Equal/Splenda/Sweet N Low*			
Powder, pkg	0	0	0

Flavored Coffee Mixes

	C	F	Cb
Chicory: Instant Coffee, 1 tsp	5	0	1
Coffee Essence, 1 tsp	15	0	4
Caffé D'Vita: Mixes, 3 tsp	60	1.5	11
Sugar Free Mixes, 2 tsp	35	2	3
General Foods Int'l:			
Average, ½ oz	60	3	10
Sugar-free, avg, 1 tsp	30	2.5	2
Cappuccino Coolers, ½ oz	60	0	15
Hills Bros:			
Cappuccino, Fr. Vanilla			
3 Tbsp, 1 oz	120	4.5	19
Jakada *(Folgers):*			
Cappuccino, 3 tsp	80	2	16
Mocha Latte, 3 Tbsp	90	2.5	15
Maxwell House:			
Cappuccino, 1 pkt	100	1.5	19
Van., Irish Cream, 1 envelope	90	1	20
Nescafé: Average all flavors	80	0	19

Coffee Shops/Restaurants

Per 8 fl.oz Cup (Unless Indicated)

	C	F	Cb
Coffee (Regular/Percolated/Filtered)	5	0	0
Americano Drip Coffee, 1 cup	7.5	0	1
Cafe Au Lait: 1 cup, 8 fl.oz	60	3.5	5
Nonfat Milk, 1 cup, 8 fl.oz	35	0	5
Caffe Latté:			
8 fl.oz cup: w. Whole Milk	110	6	9
w. 2% Milk	100	3.5	9
w. Nonfat Milk	70	0	10
12 fl.oz: w. Whole Milk	180	9	14
w. Nonfat Milk	100	0	15
16 fl.oz: w. Whole Milk	220	11	18
w. Nonfat Milk	130	0	19
Cafe Mocha (Mochaccino): 1 cup	150	6	20
12 fl.oz	230	9	31
16 fl.oz	290	12	41
Cappuccino:			
8 fl.oz cup: w. Whole Milk	90	3.5	7
w. 2% Milk	80	3	8
w. Nonfat Milk	50	0	8
12 fl.oz: w. Whole Milk	110	6	9
w. 2% Milk	90	3.5	9
w. Nonfat Milk	60	0	9
16 fl.oz: w. Whole Milk	140	7	11
w. 2% Milk	120	3.5	11
w. Nonfat Milk	80	0	12
Mocha (with cream):			
8 fl.oz: w. Whole Milk	200	11	22
w. Nonfat Milk	160	6	22
12 fl.oz: w. Whole Milk	290	15	33
w. Non-fat Milk	230	8	34
Iced Mocha (no cream):			
12 fl.oz: w. Whole Milk	170	6	26
w. Nonfat Milk	130	2	27
Espresso: Single (Solo)	5	0	1
Doppio (Double)	10	0	2
Espresso con Panna,			
(w. dollop whipped cream), solo	30	2.5	2
Espresso Macchiato, solo	10	0	1
Frappuccino: Tall, 12 fl.oz	180	2.5	37
Grande, 16 fl.oz	240	3	48
Frappuccino Mocha			
(w. Cream): Tall, 12 fl.oz	280	11	43
Grande, 16 fl.oz	380	15	57
Iced Latte: *Similar to Caffe Latte*			
Starbucks: *See Fast-Foods Section*			

Coffee Substitute Mixes

	C	F	Cb
Roasted Cereal Beverages: (No Caffeine)			
Cafix Instant Beverage, 1 tsp	5	0	1
Kaffree Roma (*Natural Touch*) , 1 tsp	10	0	2
Postum, Instant Hot Beverage, 1 tsp	10	0	3
Revival Soy "Coffee", 1 Tbsp	0	0	0
Teeccino Caffe, 1 tsp	10	0	2

Irish & Liqueur Coffees

	C	F	Cb
Irish Coffee (no sugar)	175	10	0
Liqueur Coffee, average 1 fl.oz	100	5	7

Coffee Extras

	C	F	Cb
Chocolate (Cocoa) Topping, ½ tsp	5	0	1
Flavored Syrups: Regular, 2 Tbsp	80	0	20
Sugar-free, 2 Tbsp	0	0	0
Half & Half Cream, 2 Tbsp	40	3.5	1
Single Serve Cup, ⅜ fl.oz	15	1.5	0.5
Light Whipped Cream, 2 T.	15	1.5	1
Marshmallows, miniature (2)	5	0	1
Sugar: 1 pkg, 5 g	20	0	5
1 level tsp, 4g	15	0	4
1 heaping tsp, 6g	25	0	6
Equal/Splenda/Sweet 'N Low, pkt	0	0	0

Coffee Shop ~ Cakes, Cookies

	C	F	Cb
Cookies:			
Biscotti, 1 oz	140	6.5	18
Chocolate Chip, 3 oz	350	15	54
Oatmeal Raisin, 3 oz	350	12	56
Peanut Butter, 3 oz	410	25	39
White Choc. Macadamia, 3⅓ oz	420	20	55
Cakes/Pastries:			
Almond Croissant, 5 oz	620	35	67
Apple Danish, 5 oz	450	18	67
Banana Walnut, 4½ oz	410	17	60
Brownie, 3 oz	390	24	42
Bundt, Chocolate, 4 o	440	21	61
Carrot Cake, 4 oz	400	22	45
Chocolate Cake, 5 oz	530	28	65
Crumble Coffee Cake, 4½ oz	500	25	65
Cupcake, 3 oz	330	16	43
Pound Cake, 3 oz	330	17	40
Cinnamon Roll, 6 oz	500	15	83
Doughnuts: Sugared, 1¾ oz	220	11	27
Glazed, 2 oz	250	12	34
Pretzel, large, 4 oz	290	5	52

Bottled Coffee (Chilled)

Ready-To-Drink: Per Bottle

Caribou: Espresso, 12 fl.oz	100	0.5	22
Regular; Vanilla, 12 fl.oz	120	1.5	24

Deerfield Farms: Per 11 oz Bottle

Chai Latte, Reg./Vanilla, average	230	6	39
Mocha Cappuccino	190	3	38

Full Throttle Coffee & Energy ~ *See Page 50*

Java Monster Energy ~ *See Page 51*

Kahlúa Cappuccino Shake 8.25 fl.oz	195	3	35

Lightfull: *Satiety Smoothie*

Cafe Latte, 8.25 fl.oz	90	0.5	37
(Note: Carbs include Erythritol natural sweetener)			

Main St Cafe

French Vanilla Ice Latte, 12 fl.oz	190	3	31
Shock Coffee: Latte, 8 fl.oz bottle	150	2.5	28
Triple Latte, 8 fl.oz can	125	2	27
Triple Mocha, 8 fl.oz can	125	2	27

Starbucks: *Per Bottle*

Frappuccino: Caramel, 9.5 fl.oz	200	3	36
Coffee; Hazelnut, 9.5 fl.oz	200	3	37
Mocha: 9.5 fl.oz bottle	180	3	33
13.7 fl.oz bottle	260	4	48
Vanilla, 9.5 fl.oz	200	3	37
DoubleShot, 6.5 fl.oz can	140	6	18
Iced Coffee, 11 fl.oz can	100	1	23
Shock: Triple Latte, 8 fl.oz	125	2	27
Triple Mocha, 8 fl.oz	125	2	27
Tully's, Bellaccino, all flav., 9.5 fl.oz	210	4	36

CALORIE KING TIP!

Reduce the calories in your coffee:

- Request non-fat milk in place of whole or 2% milk
- Downsize to 8 fl.oz or 12 fl.oz
- Avoid cream on frappuccinos
- Replace sugar with *Equal*, *Splenda* or *Sweet 'N Low*
- Avoid syrup add-ons

CAFFEINE COUNTER

Moderate caffeine intake is not harmful to healthy adults. However, frequent large amounts (over 350mg/day) may cause dependency ('caffeinism') and adversely affect health. To be safe, limit caffeine to 200mg/day. Avoid if pregnant; breast feeding; a child under 8; have sleep problems or heart arrhythmia.

Caffeine (mg)

Coffee: Instant, Weak, 1 level teaspoon	30
Medium, 1 rounded teaspoon	60
Strong, 1 heaping teaspoon	100
Decaffeinated, 1 round teaspoon	2
Bags *(Folgers)*, 1 bag (6-8 fl.oz)	115
Ground, 1 Tbsp, 6g	60
Bottled (Ready-To-Drink), 9.5 fl.oz	70
Coffee Shop: Brewed, 8 fl.oz	110-150
Cappuccino: 1 cup, 8 fl.oz	75
Tall, 12 fl.oz	110
Large, 16 fl.oz	150
Decappuccino (decaffeinated)	5
Espresso: Regular/Solo	75
Double (Doppio) Espresso	150
Iced Coffee, 12 fl.oz	140
Latte, 1 cup, 8 fl.oz	75
Mocha, 1 cup, 8 fl.oz	90
Hot Chocolate, 8 fl.oz	15
Tea (Black/Green): Weak, 1 cup	20
Medium Strong, 1 cup	40
Strong, 1 cup	70
Decaffeinated Tea	0-5
Herbal Tea	0
Iced Tea, Tall Glass/Can, 12 fl.oz	25-30
Soft Drinks: *Per 12 fl.oz Can*	
Coca-Cola, Pepsi (Reg./Diet)	35
Diet Coke; TAB; RC Cola (Regular)	45
Dr. Pepper (Reg./Diet) Sunkist Orange	40
Pepsi One; Mtn Dew; Mellow Yellow; Surge	55
Pepsi Max (Reg./Diet) Sun Drop (Reg./Diet)	70
7-Up, Fanta, Sprite, Fresca, Diet Rite Cola	0
Energy Drinks (with added caffeine):	
(AMP, Adrenaline Rush, Full Throttle Monster, No Fear, Red Bull, Rockstar)	
Average all brands: 8 fl.oz	80
16 fl.oz	160
Chocolate Bars: Milk Chocolate, 2 oz	20
Dark Chocolate, 2 oz	30
Cocoa/Hot Choc. Mix, 1 oz pkt	5
Chocolate Milk, 1 cup, 8 fl.oz	2
Choc Chip Cookies, 2 medium, 2 oz	6
Chocolate Syrup, 2 Tbsp, 1.4 oz	5
Medicinals: *Excedrin,* Extra Strength (2)	130
NoDoz Maximum, 1 tablet	200

Extensive Caffeine Counter ~ www.CalorieKing.com

Quick Guide | C | F | Cb

Orange Juice
Average ~ Fresh or Sweetened:

	C	F	Cb
½ Cup, 4 fl.oz	55	0	13
Small Glass, 6 fl.oz	85	0	19
Regular Glass, 8 fl.oz	110	0.5	26
8¾ fl.oz Box	120	0.5	28
10 fl.oz Bottle	140	0.5	32
11½ fl.oz Can	160	0.5	37
16 fl.oz Bottle	225	0.5	52
20 fl.oz Bottle	280	1	64
64 fl.oz/½ Gallon	895	4	206

Juices ~ Generic

Average All Brands: Per 8 fl.oz Unless Indicated

	C	F	Cb
Aloe Vera Juice, unsweet., 2 oz	10	0	0
Apple Juice: 8 fl.oz	120	0	29
10 fl.oz Bottle	145	0.5	36
16 fl.oz	235	0.5	58
Carrot Juice: Fresh, 6 fl.oz	35	0	8
Sweetened, 6 fl.oz	75	0	17
Cranberry Juice, Cocktail/Blend	140	0	34
Fruit Blends, average, 8 fl.oz	110	0	27
Fruit Nectars, average, 8 fl.oz	140	0	36
Grape Juice, 8 fl.oz	155	0	38
Grapefruit Juice, 8 fl.oz	95	0	22
Lemon/Lime Juice: 1 Tbsp	3	0	1
1 cup, 8 fl.oz	50	0.5	16
Concentrate, 1 tsp	0	0	0
Noni Juice: *Tahitian,* 2 Tbsp, 1 fl.oz	5	0	1
Tahiti Traders, 1 fl.oz	20	0	5
Passion Fruit Juice (Fresh):			
Purple, 1 cup, 8 fl.oz	125	0	34
Yellow, 1 cup, 8 fl.oz	80	1.5	14
Papaya/Peach Nectar, avg., 8 fl.oz	140	0	36
Pear Nectar, 8 fl.oz	150	0	40
Pineapple Juice, 8 fl.oz	130	0	32
Pomegranate Juice, 8 fl.oz	160	0	40
Prune Juice, 8 fl.oz	180	0	45
Strawb./Raspberry Juice, 8 fl.oz	100	0	24
Tangerine Juice, 8 fl.oz	105	0.5	25
Tomato Juice, 8 fl.oz	40	0	10
Vegetable Juice, 8 fl.oz	45	0	11
Wheat Grass Juice: 1 fl.oz 'Shot'	5	0	1
2 fl.oz 'Shot'	15	0	2

Quick Guide | C | F | Cb

Fruit Smoothies (Jamba Juice; Smoothie King)
Average All Brands

	C	F	Cb
Fruit Only: 8 fl.oz	115	0.5	29
12 fl.oz	175	1	43
16 fl.oz	230	1	58
24 fl.oz	350	1	78
Fruit + Non-Fat Milk/Soy:			
12 fl.oz	135	0	29
16 fl.oz	155	0	37
24 fl.oz	265	1	59
Fruit + Non-Fat Frozen Yogurt/Sherbet:			
12 fl.oz	200	0	47
16 fl.oz	265	0	63
24 fl.oz	395	0	95

Juice Brands | C | F | Cb

Per 8 fl.oz Unless Indicated

	C	F	Cb
Apple & Eve			
Naturally Cranberry	130	0	32
Cranberry/Raspberry Apple	120	0	26
Cranberry Grape	140	0	34
Bolthouse			
100% Juices: Carrot, 8 fl.oz	70	0	14
Valencia Orange	110	0	24
Vedge	60	0	12
Lemonade: Cranberry	130	0	33
Mango	120	0	30
Prickly Pear	140	0	34
Fruit Smoothies:			
Berry Boost	110	0	30
Blue Goodness	170	0	41
C-Boost	150	0	36
Green Goodness	140	0	33
Strawberry Banana	120	0	29
Bossa Nova Acai Juice Blends:			
Original, 8 fl.oz	95	0	23
Blueb.; Mango/Pass./Raspb., 8 fl.oz	90	0	22
Bright & Early *(Minute Maid)*			
Orange Juice (Chilled/Frozen)	110	0	29
Campbell's			
Tomato Juice: 5.5 fl.oz can	30	0	6
11.5 fl.oz	60	0	13
Capri Sun			
Juice Drinks: *Per 6.75 fl.oz Pouch*			
Coastal Cooler	100	0	25
Mountain Cooler	90	0	22
25% Less Sugar, all flav.	70	0	18
100% Juice, avg., 6.75 fl.oz	100	0	24

Juice Brands (Cont)

	C	F	Cb
Clamato			
Tomato Cocktails, average, 8 fl.oz	60	0	11
Crystal Geyser			
Juice Squeeze: *Per Bottle (12 fl.oz)*			
Blackberry Pomegranate	170	0	43
Ruby Grapefruit	150	0	36
Average other flavors	140	0	32
Dannon			
Frusion Smoothie, avg., 10 fl.oz	260	3.5	50
Light & Fit, 7 fl.oz bottle	60	0	10
Dole			
100% Juice, Pineapple, 8 fl.oz	130	0	30
100% Fruit Juice Blends: *Per 6 fl.oz*			
Pine-Orange Banana	100	0	25
Pineapple Orange	90	0	22
Chilled, 100%: *Per 8 fl.oz*			
Berry Blend	140	0	35
Pineapple Juice	130	0	30
Pineapple Orange Banana	130	0	30
Average other flavors	120	0	29
Frozen Concentrates 100%:			
Average all flavors, ¼ cup	130	0	32
Single Serve, 100%: *Per Bottle (15.2 fl.oz)*			
100% Apple, no sugar added	210	0	49
100% Blends: Cranberry	150	0	36
Grape, no sugar added	290	0	72
Orange, no sugar added	200	0	47
Pineapple Peach Mango	130	0	31
Strawberry Kiwi	120	0	31
Five Alive *(Minute Maid):*			
Frozen Concentrate,			
Prepared, 8 fl.oz	110	0	29
Florida's Natural			
Cranb. Apple; Or. Jce	110	0	27
Ruby Red Grapefruit Juice	90	0	22
Frützzo: *Per 12 fl.oz*			
(No Added Sugar)			
Pomegranate 100%	210	0	52
with Acai, Blueberries,			
Cherry, Raspberry, avg.	195	0	49
Yumberry 100%			
Natural	150	0	33
Organic	120	0	25
with Other Juices, avg.	165	0	39

	C	F	Cb
Fuze: *Per 16 fl.oz*			
Refresh, avg. all flavors	180	0	48
Slenderize, avg.	15	0	3
Vitalize, all flavors	200	0	50
Vitamin Tea	120	0	30
Goya Nectar			
Apricot/Pear Nectar, 12 fl.oz	220	0	53
Guanabana (5% Juice), 16 fl.oz	200	0	50
Passion & Pineaple (5% Juice), 16 fl.oz	220	0	55
Hansen's			
Juice Slam: *Per 6.75 fl.oz Box*			
Awesome Apple	90	0	23
Other flavors	120	0	29
Organic, 1 Pouch	100	0	24
Junior Juice, 4.23 oz box	60	0	15
Natural (64 fl.oz Bottles): *Per 8 fl.oz*			
Apple, Strawberry	120	0	28
Grape, Pomegranate Cocktail	160	0	39
White Grape	140	0	36
Organic Juices, avg.	110	0	27
Fruit Smoothies, avg., 12 fl.oz	180	0	44
Low-Carb, avg., 12 fl.oz	40	0	9
Light Juice Cocktails, avg., 8 fl.oz	40	0	9
Hawaii's Own			
Frozen Concentrate: *Per 8 fl.oz, Prepared*			
Average all varieties	110	0	28
Hi-C Juice Drinks: Average, 8 fl.oz	120	0	32
6.75 fl.oz box, average	100	0	27
Blast, 6 fl.oz pouch	100	0	26
Hood: Apple, 8 fl.oz	120	0	31
Fruit Punch; Orange	120	0	30
Jamba Juice: *See Fast-Foods Section*			
Juicy Juice (Nestle): *Per 6.75 fl.oz Box*			
Grape	100	0	25
Average other flavors	100	0	24
4.23 fl.oz box, average	70	0	16
Kerns All Nectars			
Canned Juice: *Per 11.5 fl.oz Can*			
Pear	220	0	54
Pineapple Coconut	280	8	53
Other flavors, average	210	0	52
Kool Aid			
Jammers: Sugar Jammers	10	0	2
Kroger Smoothies, avg., 10 fl.oz	280	3.5	53
L & A: Black Cherry, 8 fl.oz	180	0	45
Grape Juice Plus	160	0	40
Mixed Berry	120	0	30
Prune Juice	180	0	41
Average other varieties	140	0	32

Juice Brands (Cont)

	C	F	Cb
Lakewood Organic: *Per 8 fl.oz*			
Acai: Berry; Coconut P'apple, avg.	130	0	25
Banana-Mango	165	0	33
Blueberry Blend	120	0	30
cranberry Lemonade	80	0	20
Fruit Garden: Summer/Green, avg.	100	0	20
Blue/Purple/Red Pomegr., avg.	110	0	24
Goji	90	0	20
Lemonade; Limeade	85	0	21
Pomegranate Blends, avg.	135	0	32
Pure: Apple	140	0	35
Blueberry; Orange	130	0	31
Carrot	95	0	23
Pink Grapefruit	90	0	22
Prune	215	0	53
Super Veggie	80	0	18
Light: Lemonade	40	0	15
Other flavors, avg.	60	0	21
(Note: Carbs include Erythritol natural sweetener)			
Langers: *Per 8 fl.oz*			
100% Juice (No Sugar Added):			
All Pomegranate	140	0	34
Apple Cider	120	0	28
Apple Juice	120	0	38
Mixed Berry	120	0	30
Red Grape Juice	160	0	40
White Grape Juice	160	0	40
Diet Low-Carb (25-50% Juice):			
Diet Apple Juice Cocktail	60	0	14
Diet Cranberry	30	0	8
Diet Pomegranate	40	0	9
Juice Cocktails (27% Juice)			
Cranberry Juice Cocktail	140	0	35
Pomegranate	140	0	34
Pomegranate Blueberry/Cranberry	140	0	34
Strawberry Peach (20% Juice)	120	0	30
White Cranberry	120	0	28
Lightfull			
Satiety Smoothies			
(Contain 5g Protein)			
Mango Oasis, 8.25 oz	90	0	38
Peachy Cream, 8.25 oz	90	0	37
Strawberry Bliss, 8.25 oz	90	0	37
(Note: Carbs include Erythritol natural sweetener)			

	C	F	Cb
Minute Maid			
Orange Juice, 100%, 8 fl.oz	110	0	27
16 fl.oz bottle	220	0	54
Light Orange Juice	50	0	13
Heart Wise; Kids Plus	110	0	27
Lemonade, all flav., avg.	120	0	28
Pomegranate: Blueberry	120	0	30
Lemonade/Flavored Tea	110	0	27
Premium Blends, avg. all flavors	120	0	28
Tropical Punches	100	0	28
Juices to Go, average, 11.5 fl.oz	155	0	45
Boxed Juices, average, 6.75 fl.oz	90	0	22
Soft Frozen Lemonade, 12 fl.oz	300	0	75
Frozen Concentrates, *8 fl.oz Prepared*			
Average all varieties	120	0	29
MonaVie Acai Blends			
Original/Active, 1 fl.oz	20	0	4
Mott's			
100% Apple Juice: *Per 8 fl.oz*			
Original	120	0	29
Natural	110	0	27
100% Juice Singles: *Per 14 fl.oz*			
Apple	200	0	48
Fruit/Grape Medley	230	0	55
Sunkist Orange Sensation	210	0	50
Veggie Blend	90	1	15
100% Juice Boxes: Avg. all flavors			
6.75 fl.oz box	100	0	25
4.23 fl.oz box	60	0	15
Mott's Plus Light,			
All flav., 8 fl.oz	130	0	15
Mott's Plus for Kids, 8 fl.oz	130	0	32
Mott's For Tots (47-54% Juice),			
All flavors, 6.75 fl.oz box	50	0	13
Naked Juice: *Per 8 fl.oz Unless Indicated*			
Just Fruit (100%): Carrot	80	0.5	17
O-J	110	0	27
Tangerine Scream	130	0	30
Apple, 10 fl.oz bottle	160	0	38
Protein Zone: Banana Choc.	240	1.5	39
P'apple, Coconut & Banana	220	2	34
Antioxidants: Berry Blast	130	0	29
Mighty Mango	150	0	35
Pomegranate Blends, avg.	160	1	36
Bare Breeze, avg. all flavors	130	0	31
Energy: Black & Blueberry	130	0	31
Plentiful Pomegranate Rush	150	0	35
Probiotics, avg., 10 fl.oz	180	0	43
Well Being: Tropical C	130	0	31
Power C; Strawb. Banana	120	0	29

Juice Brands (Cont)	C	F	Cb
Naked Juice (Cont)			
Superfood Smoothies:			
Blue Machine, avg.	170	0	40
Gold/Green Machine, avg.	140	0	32
Purple Machine	160	3	31
Red Machine	170	4.5	31
Nantucket Nectars			
Juice Cocktails: *Per 17.5 fl.oz*			
Carrot Orange Mango	260	0	65
Cranberry	280	0	70
Grapeade; Guava; Orange Mango	280	0	70
Other varieties, avg.	260	0	65
100% Juice: *Per 17.5 fl.oz*			
Apple	260	0	65
Peach Orange	280	0	70
Pineapple Orange Cherry	280	0	70
Pomegranate Cherry	260	0	65
Premium Orange Juice	240	0	60
Nectar Lemonades, avg., 17.5 fl.oz	240	0	60
Newman's Own			
Lemonade (Reg./Pink), 8 fl.oz	110	0	27
Fruit Juice Cocktail: Gorilla Grape	140	0	34
Orange Mango Tango	150	0	37
Razzma Tazz Raspberry	120	0	28
Northland			
100% Juice: *Per 8 fl.oz*			
Cranb./Peach/Blackberry; Raspb.	140	0	34
Cranberry Grape	140	0	36
Ocean Spray *Per 8 fl.oz*			
Juice Cocktails:			
Cranberry Juice Cocktail	130	0	33
with Calcium	150	0	37
Grapefruit Tangerine	120	0	31
Ruby Red Grapefruit	120	0	30
100% Juice Blends:			
Cranberry & Concord Grape	150	0	37
Cranberry & Mixed Berry	150	0	38
White Cranberry Blend	150	0	38
Cranberry Blends			
CranApple; CranTangerine, avg.	135	0	35
CranCherry	130	0	32
CranGrape	140	0	35
CranRaspberry/Strawberry	120	0	30
Light Juice Drinks, all flavors	40	0	10
Diet Juice Drinks:			
Cranberry Spray	7	0	2
Cranberry Grape Spray	5	0	2

Odwalla *Per 16 fl.oz Bottle*	C	F	Cb
AntioxiDance; Grapefruit, avg	180	0	45
B Berrier; Quencher	260	0	60
Carrot Juice	140	0	30
Carrot, Orange, Apple	200	0	46
Glorious Morning; B Monster	280	0	66
Mo'Beta	300	0	74
Poma Grand, average	320	0	80
Strawberry Lemonade	220	0	56
Super Protein, average	350	8	48
Wellness Echinacea	300	2	66
Smoothies:			
Blueberry B Monster	280	0	66
Blackberry Fruitshake	300	0	72
Mango Tango	300	2	68
Strawberry Banana	260	0	62
Strawberry C Monster	320	0	76
Orange Julius			
Originals, Orange:			
Small, 16 fl.oz	220	0	54
Medium, 20 fl.oz	270	0.5	68
Large, 32 fl.oz	440	1	108
Smoothies: *See Fast-Foods Section*			
Pom Wonderful			
100% Juice: *Per 8 fl.oz*			
Blueberry; Pomegranate	160	0	40
Cherry	150	0	38
Mango; Tangerine	140	0	34
Purely Juice: *Per 8 fl.oz*			
Berry Extreme with Acai	110	0	27
Pomegranate (100%)	150	0	36
Totally Tropical	120	0	30
R.W. Knudsen: *Per 8 fl.oz*			
Fruit Juices: Apple	120	0	30
Black Cherry	190	0	47
Blueberry	100	0	24
Cranberry Raspberry	130	0	32
Creamed Papaya	40	0	10
Grapefruit	100	0	23
Guava Strawberry	120	0	28
Hibiscus Cooler	90	0	24
Just Concord	160	0	40
Tomato	60	0	14
Other varieties, average	120	0	30
Sparkling Juice, avg., 8 fl.oz	120	0	30
Nectars: Coconut	140	5	27
Papaya; Peach	130	0	31
Boysenberry, average	130	0	31
Very Veggie, 8 fl.oz	50	0	11
Simply Nutritious: Mega C	140	0	34
Average other varieties	125	0	30

Juice Brands (Cont)

	C	F	Cb
Ralphs			
Lemonade (Premium Juice), 8 fl.oz	110	0	29
Orange Juice, 8 fl.oz	120	0	30
Pineapple Juice, 8 fl.oz	130	0	33
ReaLemon - ReaLime (Borden)			
Lemon/Lime Juice (from concentrate)			
1 teaspoon	0	0	0
2 Tbsp, 1 fl.oz	8	0	2.5
Santa Cruz (Organic)			
Apple Juice; Cider & Spice	120	0	30
Concord Grape; White Grape	160	0	40
Orange Mango	130	0	32
Tropical Blend	140	0	33
Average other varieties	100	0	24
Nectars: Cranberry	110	0	27
Average other varieties	115	0	30
Sodas: Per 12 fl.oz			
Cherry	140	0	34
Concord Grape	150	0	36
Lemonade; Champagne Style	100	0	26
Raspberry Lemonade; Apricot	120	0	29
Other varieties	130	0	33
Juice Boxes: Per 8 fl.oz			
Lemon	120	0	29
Orange; Grape, average	100	0	24
Tropical Punch	110	0	27
Seismic Super Juices (Quixtar): Per 12 fl.oz Bottle			
Citrus/Berry	200	0	49
Low Sugar Cherry	60	0	15
Simply Orange			
Lemonade; Limeade	120	0	31
Orange Juice, all varieties	110	0	26
Snapple			
Fruit Drink Blends, 8 fl.oz	120	0	29
Grapeade; Orangeade, 8 fl.oz	120	0	29
Lemonade, all types, 8 fl.oz	110	0	28
Diet: Snapple Apple	15	0	4
Kiwi Strawberry	20	0	5
Avg. other flavors	10	0	2
100% Juiced,			
(added vitamins), 11.5 fl.oz	160	0	40
Snap.E Tom			
Tom. & Chile Cocktail, 11 oz can	80	0	16
Ssips			
Juice Drinks, avg., 6.75 fl.oz box	100	0	25
Stonyfield Farm: Per Bottle (10 fl.oz)			
Peach Smoothie	250	3	49
Wildberry; Strawberry Smoothie	250	3	46
Light Smoothies, 10 fl.oz	130	0	41

	C	F	Cb
SunnyD			
Baja Juice: Per 12 fl.oz Bottle			
Orange	190	0	46
Orange Berry	190	0	46
Orange Pineapple	190	0	46
Red Punch	170	0	43
SunnyD Blends: Per 8 fl.oz			
Fruit Punch	120	0	29
Lemonade; Mango	130	0	32
Smooth Style	130	0	32
Tangy Original Style	130	0	32
Reduced Sugar (35% less)	50	0	15
With Calcium	140	0	35
Orange Fused Drinks, (5% Juice):			
Mango; Peach	80	0	20
Pineapple; Strawberry	80	0	20
Sunsweet			
Prune Juice/w. Pulp, 8 fl.oz	180	0	43
Tampico: Citrus Punch, 1 cup	110	0	25
Mango/Trop. Frt. Punch, 1 cup	110	0	28
Tang			
Pouches, average all flavors (1)	90	0	24
Mix: Prepared as Directed			
Regular (2 Tbsp dry), 6 fl.oz	110	0	27
Sugar Free, 8 fl.oz	5	0	0
Trader Joe's			
Refrigerated			
Small Bottles (16 fl.oz):			
Carrot Juice	150	0	33
Ginger Limeaid	120	0	31
Mango Antioxidants	240	0	60
Protein w. Pzazz	450	7	60
Strawberry Smoothie	240	0	58
Large Bottles (32 or 64 fl.oz):			
Original Lemonade, 8 fl.oz	110	0	27
Strawberry Lemonade, 8 fl.oz	120	0	29
100% Juice (64 fl.oz Bottle):			
All varieties, 8 fl.oz	110	0	25
All Natural Pasteurized: Per 8 fl.oz			
(32 fl.oz or 64 fl.oz Bottle):			
Concord Grape,	160	0	39
Cranberry Blend	150	0	38
Cranberry Harvest	130	0	36
Garden Patch; Vege -10	50	0	12
Hawaiian Pineapple	110	0	29
Just Pomegranate	150	0	37
Lemon Ginger w. Echinacea	140	0	36
Mango Lemonade	140	0	35
Mango Passion Fruit Blend	130	0	33
Rio Red Grapefruit	140	0	35
White Grape	160	0	40

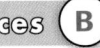

Juice Brands (Cont) C F Cb

Per 8 fl.oz Unless Indicated

Tree Top

	C	F	Cb
Apple Reserve/Fruit Punch	120	0	31
Apple Berry/Grape	130	0	32
Apple/Spiced Cider	120	0	31
Fiber Rich: Apple	140	0	35
Apple Apricot/Orange Banana	160	0	37
Grapefruit	130	0	30
Grower's Best, Apple NSA	120	0	29
Orange	120	0	28
Orchard Blends	130	0	31
Boxes: Average, 6.8 fl.oz	100	0	26
Chilled Juices: Grape	155	0	38
Cranberry; Cranberry Cocktail	140	0	34
Orchard Berry/Apple, avg.	115	0	29
Essentials: Fiber, 8 fl.oz	120	0	29
Healthy Heart	120	0	26
Healthy Kids	110	0	26
Immunity Defense; Low Acid	110	0	26
Light 'n Healthy varieties	50	0	13
Non-Refrigerated Juice Drinks:			
100% Fruit Punch	135	0	32
100% Grape	150	0	38
100% Orange; Apple; Ruby Red	110	0	27
100% Pineapple Orange	130	0	32
Light 'n Healthy, average	50	0	14
Refrigerated Juice Drinks:			
Average all flavors, 8 fl.oz	130	0	32
Light varieties, average	10	0	3
Twisters: Average, 8 fl.oz	120	0	29
20 fl.oz bottle	300	0	74
Fruit Smoothies, avg., 11 fl.oz	220	0	54
Tropicana Twister, avg., 12 fl.oz	180	0	32

V8® Juices & Drinks

V8 100% Vegetable Juice:

	C	F	Cb
5.5 fl.oz can	30	0	7
8 fl.oz cup	50	0	10
11.5 fl.oz can	70	0	14
12 fl.oz bottle	75	0	15
V-8 Splash, average, 8 fl.oz	75	0	19
V-8 Splash Smoothies: Strawb. 8 fl.oz	90	0	20
Tropical Colada, 8 fl.oz	100	0	21
Diet V-8 Splash, all flavors, 8 fl.oz	10	0	3
Fusion, all flavors, 8 fl.oz	120	0	28
12 fl.oz bottle	180	0	42

Per 8 fl.oz Unless Indicated C F Cb

Veryfine

	C	F	Cb
Apple Juice (100%)	110	0	27
Orange Juice (100%)	120	0	30

Walnut Acres: *Per 8 fl.oz*

	C	F	Cb
Organic: Apple	110	0	27
Apricot; Raspberry	130	0	32
Cherry	140	0	34
Cranberry	110	0	26
Incredible Vegetable	50	0	12
Other varieties, avg.,	120	0	30

Welch's: *Bottled Juices*

	C	F	Cb
100% Red Grape	170	0	42
100% White Grape/Peach			
8 fl.oz	160	0	39
14 fl.oz	280	0	68
Tomato Juice, 8 fl.oz	50	0	10

Concentrates: *Per 8 fl.oz*

	C	F	Cb
100% Grape	170	0	42
American White Grape	160	0	39

Cocktails: *Per 8 fl.oz Made Up*

	C	F	Cb
Concord Grape Concord Red	150	0	36
Mountain Berry	140	0	34
Strawberry Breeze	130	0	33
Light: Grape/Peach	70	0	18

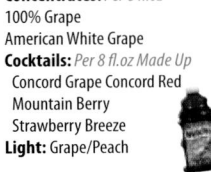

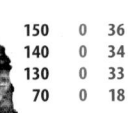

CALORIEKING PORTION WATCH

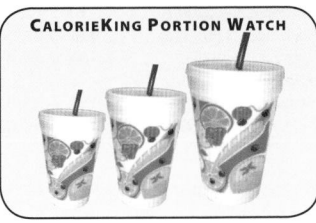

ORANGE JUICE	C	Cb
8 fl.oz	110	26
16 fl.oz	220	52
24 fl.oz	330	78
32 fl.oz	440	104

Quick Guide   C   F   Cb

Cow's Milk ~ *Average All Brands*

Whole (3.25% fat):

	C	F	Cb
2 Tbsp, 1 fl.oz	20	1	1.5
1 Cup, 8 fl.oz	150	8	12
1 Large Glass, 12 fl.oz	220	12	17
1 Pint, 16 fl.oz	295	16	22
1 Quart, 946 ml	590	32	44

Reduced-Fat (2% fat):

2 Tbsp, 1 fl.oz	15	0.5	1.5
1 Cup, 8 fl.oz	120	5	12
1 Large Glass, 12 fl.oz	180	7.5	18
1 Pint, 16 fl.oz	245	10	23
1 Quart, 946 ml	490	20	46

Light/Low-Fat (1% fat):

2 Tbsp, 1 fl.oz	13	0.3	1.5
1 Cup, 8 fl.oz	100	2.5	12
1 Large Glass, 12 fl.oz	150	4	18
1 Pint, 16 fl.oz	205	5	25
1 Quart, 946 ml	410	10	49

Fat Free/Skim:

2 Tbsp, 1 fl.oz	10	0	1.5
1 Cup, 8 fl.oz	90	0.5	13
1 Pint, 16 fl.oz	180	1	26
w. Oatrim Fiber (for replacement), 1 cup	85	0	22

Buttermilk: *Average All Brands*

Reduced-Fat (2%), 1 cup	120	5	10
Low-Fat (1%): 1 cup	100	2.5	12

Lactose-Free: *Per 8 fl.oz*

Lactaid 100: Whole

Lactaid 100: Whole	150	8	12
2% Reduced-Fat	130	5	12
1% Low-Fat	110	2.5	13
Fat-Free	80	0	13
Calcium-Fortified	80	0	13
Dairy Ease: Whole	160	9	11
2% Reduced-Fat	130	5	12
Fat-Free	90	0	12

Lower Carb Dairy Drinks: *Per 8 fl.oz*

Carb Countdown (Hood):

Whole	130	8	3
2% Reduced-Fat, 1 cup	90	5	3
Fat-Free, 1 cup	45	0	3

Goat/Sheep Milk, Kefir

Goat's Milk (Meyenberg):   C   F   Cb

	C	F	Cb
Whole, 1 cup, 8 fl.oz	140	7	11
Light/Low-Fat (1%), 8 fl.oz	100	2.5	11
Evaporated, reconst., 8 fl.oz	150	8	11

Kefir (Cultured Milk):

Nancy's: Plain, 8 fl.oz	110	3	14
Fruit flavors, avg, 8 fl.oz	180	2.5	34
Trader Joe's: Plain, 8 fl.oz	110	2.5	8
Strawberry, 8 fl.oz	160	2	21
Sheep's Milk: Whole, 1 cup	265	17	13

Canned & Dried Milk

Condensed: Reg. 2 Tbsp, 1 fl.oz	130	3	23
Low-Fat (Eagle), 2 Tbsp	120	1.5	23
Fat-Free (Eagle), 2 Tbsp	110	0	24
Evaporated: Whole, 2 Tbsp	40	3	3
Whole, ½ cup	170	10	13
Low-Fat (Carnation), 2 Tbsp, 1 oz	25	0.5	3
½ cup, 4 fl.oz	115	2.5	14
Fat-Free, 2 Tbsp, 1 oz	25	0	4
Dried: Whole, ¼ cup, 1 oz	160	9	12
Skim/Non-Fat, ⅓ cup	80	0	12
Made-up, 1 cup, 8 fl.oz	80	0	12
Buttermilk (sweet cream), 1 oz	110	2	14
Non-Fat, 1 Tbsp	25	0	3
Malted (Carnation), dry, 1 Tbsp	30	0.5	6

Soy/Non-Dairy Drinks ~ *See Page 48*

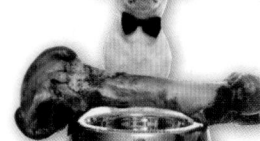

' What ever happened to sensible portion size?! '

Quick Guide

Chocolate Milk C F Cb

Average All Brands: Per Cup (8 fl.oz)

		C	F	Cb
Whole Milk (3.3%): 1 cup		210	8	26
1 Pint		415	17	52
Reduced-Fat (2%), 1 cup		190	5	30
Low-Fat (1%), 1 cup		160	2.5	26

Brands ~ Flavored Milk

Ready-To-Drink: Per 8 fl.oz Cup Unless Indicated

	C	F	Cb
Albertson's, low-fat	200	3	32
Alta Dena: Chocolate	260	9	37
Low-Fat Chocolate	200	3	32
Bravo!:			
Blenders Dble Choc., 11 fl.oz	180	4	20
Slammers: Starburst, 8 fl.oz	170	8	21
3 Musketeers, 8 fl.oz	140	3	17
Milky Way, 8 fl.oz	170	5	22
Cool Moos: Chocolate, 8 fl.oz	180	2.5	32
Strawberry, 8 fl.oz	160	2.5	2
Dominick's Low-Fat, 1 cup	170	2.5	28
Golden Guernsey, 1 cup	130	2.5	15
Hershey's: *Per 14 fl.oz Bottle*			
Choc Milk: 1% No Sugar Added	210	4.5	26
Reduced Fat Chocolate	350	9	54
Shakes, Creamy Chocolate	470	14	75
Boxes (8 fl.oz): Choc Milk	200	5	30
Chocolate Shake	230	4.5	42
Chocolate drink	130	1	29
Hood: Chocolate	230	9	31
Low-Fat (1%), Chocolate	170	3	28
Horizon Organic:			
Chocolate, Low-Fat, 1 cup	170	3	27
Reduced-Fat flavors, avg., 1 cup	180	5	27
Kroger/Ralphs, Low-Fat, 8 fl.oz	200	2.5	34
Muscle Milk, (Hi Prot.), avg., 17 fl.oz	350	17	17
Nesquik: Chocolate, 16 fl.oz	400	10	64
Banana, 16 fl.oz	400	10	60
Choc. Fat Free, 16 fl.oz	320	0	64
Double Choc., 16 fl.oz	400	10	60
Very Vanilla, 16 fl.oz	400	10	60
Quaker Milk Chillers, 14 fl.oz bottle	250	9	32
Skinny Cow, Fat-Free Chocolate, 1 c.	150	0	26
Starbucks, Strawb. & Creme, 12 fl.oz	320	2	66
Yoo-Hoo:			
Choc Drink, 6½ fl.oz box	110	1	24
Choc., 16 fl.oz pkg	250	2	56
Lite Choc., 9 fl.oz bottle	70	1	15

Shakes

C F Cb

Burger King:
Chocolate/Strawberry, avg.

	C	F	Cb
Small, 16 fl.oz	475	15	76
Medium, 22 fl.oz	655	20	104
Large, 32 fl.oz	950	29	151

McDonalds:
Average all flavors:

	C	F	Cb
12 fl.oz cup	430	10	75
16 fl.oz cup	570	13	101
21 fl.oz cup	760	18	132
32 fl.oz cup	1140	26	200

Nutrition/Meal Shakes ~ *See Page 50*

Smoothies

Smoothies C F Cb
Made Up Ready-To-Drink
(8 fl. oz Milk/Soy + Fruit): *Per 12 fl.oz*
Average all types:

	C	F	Cb
w. Whole Milk	300	8	50
+ Ice Cream, 1 scoop	400	13	62
with Non-Fat Milk	240	0	50

Fruit Smoothies ~ *See Page 40*
Freshens; Jamba Juice; TCBY: *See Fast-Foods*

Bottle Coffee Drinks ~ *See Page 39*

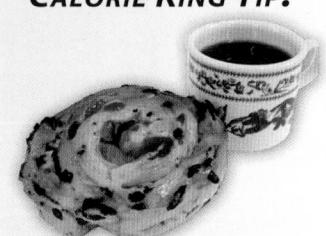

CALORIE KING TIP!

'Low-Fat' does not mean 'Low-Calorie'.
This low-fat Apricot Sticky Bun
has only 2g fat but has
over 400 calories!

Rice & Cereal Drinks

Per 8 fl.oz Cup	C	F	Cb
Almond Breeze (Blue Diamond)			
Original	60	2.5	8
Chocolate	120	3	22
Vanilla	90	2.5	16
Almond Dream			
Original Enriched	50	2.5	6
Unsweetened	30	2.5	1
Amazake, Original	150	0	34
Better Than Milk			
Rice Vegan Mix:			
Original, 2 Tbsp powder, 19g	70	1	16
Vanilla, 2 Tbsp powder, 19g	75	2	15
Don Jose: Horchata	140	4	25
Cereal Match	100	3	17
Eden Blend, Rice & Soy	120	3	18
Lundberg: Rice Drink	120	2.5	22
Vanilla Rice Drink	120	2.5	23
Pacific			
Rice Drinks: Multigrain	160	2	30
Low-Fat Plain/Vanilla	130	2	27
Organic Oat: Original	130	2.5	24
Vanilla	130	2.5	25
Nut Drinks: Hazelnut Original	110	3.5	18
Almond: Original Low-Fat	60	3	9
Vanilla Low-Fat	90	2.5	16
Unsweetened: Original	35	2.5	2
Vanilla	40	2.5	3
Rice Dream			
Carob	150	2.5	30
Heartwise: Original	130	2	27
Vanilla	140	2	30
Horchata	160	2.5	32
Vanilla/Vanilla Enriched	130	2.5	27
Original/Original Enriched	120	2.5	24
Supreme Vanilla Hazelnut	140	2.5	29
WestSoy:			
Plain Rice	110	2.5	20
Vanilla Rice	110	2.5	20

Note: Rice/oat/nut drinks are very low in protein. Unless enriched with protein (and calcium), they are not suitable for infants as a substitute for milk or calcium-enriched soy drinks

Soy Milk ~ Ready-To-Drink

Per 8 fl.oz Cup	C	F	Cb
365 Organic (Whole Foods):			
Original	90	3.5	10
Plain, unsweetened	70	3.5	5
Chocolate	150	3.5	24
Vanilla	100	3.5	11
Edensoy:			
Original	140	5	14
Vanilla	160	3	25
Light: Original	100	2	15
Vanilla	110	1	22
Extra Original	130	4	13
Extra Vanilla	150	3	23
Carob; Chocolate, average	175	4	28
8th Continent:			
Antioxidant Smoothie, Pomegranate Blueberry	110	0	23
Soymilk: Original	80	3	7
Chocolate	140	3	22
Vanilla	100	3	11
Light, Original	50	2	2
Fat-Free: Original	60	0	8
Vanilla	70	0	11
Kidz Dream Smoothie			
Berry Blast	100	2	17
Orange Cream	120	2	21
Lifeway			
Slim 6 Kefir	110	2	8
SoyTreat	160	4	23
Naturally Preferred (Ralph's/Kroger)			
Regular, Plain	80	3	8
Low-Fat: Plain; Vanilla	100	2.5	11
Odwalla:			
Single Serve Bottles, 450ml (15.2 fl.oz)			
Soy Smart, Chai	285	8	42
Chocolate Mint	305	8.5	40
Super Protein, Vanilla Al'Mondo	360	12	48
O Organics (Safeway):			
Plain	90	3.5	10
Chocolate	150	4	23
Vanilla Soy	100	3	9
Pacific: Select Plain, Low-Fat	70	2.5	9
Select Vanilla, Low-Fat	80	2.5	9
Organic, Original Unsweetened	90	4.5	4
Ultra (Extra Protein/Calcium): Plain	120	4	12

Soy Milk ~ Ready-To-Drink

Per 8 fl.oz Cup	C	F	Cb
Power Dream *(Imagine Foods)*:			
Java Jolt; Soy High Chai, avg., 11 fl.oz	245	4.5	42
X-Treme Choc, 11 fl.oz	260	5	48
Vanilla Blast, 11 fl.oz	240	5	39
Silk			
Plain	100	4	8
Chocolate	140	3.5	23
Enhanced	110	5	8
Light: Chocolate	120	1.5	22
Plain	70	2	8
Vanilla	80	2	10
Plus for Bone Health	100	3.5	11
Unsweetened	80	4	4
Vanilla	100	3.5	10
Vanilla Plus DHA Omega-3	110	5	8
Vanilla Plus Fiber	100	3.5	14
Very Vanilla	130	4	19
Slim-Fast (Soy-Based) ~ See Page 52			
Soy Dream			
Original; Enriched	100	4	8
Classic: Original	130	4	16
Vanilla	140	4	18
Chocolate Enriched	150	4	21
Vanilla Enriched	120	4	20
So Nice:			
Natural	70	3.5	3
Original	70	3	7
Chocolate	135	3	22
Omega Plus: Original	100	3.5	9
Vanilla	120	3.5	14
Vitasoy			
Classic Original	120	4.5	11
Chocolate Banana	130	4	21
Creamy Original	110	4	11
Green Tea	120	4	13
Peppermint Chocolate	140	4	19
Rich Chocolate	160	4	24
Smooth Vanilla; Vanilla Delight	120	4	13
Strawberry Banana	140	4	19
Light: Chocolate	100	2	17
Original	60	2	7
Vanilla	70	2	10
Unsweetened: Original	90	4.5	5
Single Serve Bottle:			
Plain, 11.5 fl. oz	140	6	12
Chocolate, 11.5 fl. oz	230	6	33
Vanilla, 11.5 fl. oz	160	5	18

Soy Milk ~ Ready-To-Drink (Cont)

Per 8 fl.oz Cup	C	F	Cb
WestSoy			
Lite: Plain	80	2	10
Vanilla	95	2	14
Low-Fat: Plain	110	2.5	20
Vanilla	120	1.5	21
Non-Fat: Plain	65	0	10
Vanilla	75	0	12
Plus: Plain	100	4	10
Vanilla	130	4	16
Soy Shakes, Chocolate/Vanilla	170	3.5	30
Soy Slender: Plain	60	3	3
Other varieties, average	70	3	4
Zen Soy			
Plain	90	3.5	9
Chocolate	170	4	27
Cappuccino	150	3.5	22
Vanilla	110	3.5	14

Soy Powder Mix

1 oz (¼ cup) mix makes 8 fl.oz Cup	C	F	Cb
Soy Protein Isolate, 1 oz dry	95	1	0
Better Than Milk:			
Original, 2 Tbsp	100	2.5	16
Vanilla, 2¾ Tbsp	80	2	8
Light, 2 Tbsp	75	2.5	7
Genisoy (Powder Shakes):			
Per 3 Rounded Tbsp			
Plain; Natural: 1 oz	110	1.5	0
Ultra-X, 1.3 oz	130	1.5	5
Chocolate: 1.2 oz	130	0.5	16
Ultra-X, 1.4 oz	150	1	20
Vanilla: 1.2 oz	130	1	17
Ultra-X, 1.4 ox	150	1	20
Joy Soy, Soy Melk, avg., 1 oz	90	2.5	10
Now Soy, ¼ cup, 22g	95	4.5	6.5
Revival Soy Shakes: *Per Packet*			
Plain; Unsweetened	130	2.5	3
Flavors, average: with Fructose	240	2.5	36
Unsweetened or Splenda	120	2.5	7
Whole Foods			
Choc.w. Spirulina, 1 oz	110	0	11
Vanilla w. Spirulina, 1 oz	110	0	11

Energy/Protein Drinks

	C	F	Cb
180 Energy/180 Blue, 8.2 fl.oz	120	0	30
Blue Low-Calorie, 8.2 fl.oz	15	0	4
24-7 Energy, Avg, 16 fl.oz can	260	0	60
ABB Energy: Turbo Tea, 18 fl.oz	150	0	38
Adrenalyn Stack, 18 fl.oz	25	0	6
Ripped Force, 18 fl.oz	90	0	23
Hi-Pro: Extreme Body, 15 fl.oz	250	2	9
Pure Pro, 22 fl.oz	150	0.5	3
Pure Pro Shake, 11 fl.oz	160	0.5	5
Power: Blue Thunder, 22 fl.oz	290	0.5	40
Extreme XXL, 22 fl.oz	980	1	197
Accelerade, all flavors, 20 fl.oz	200	0	35
AdvantEdge (EAS): Per Container (11 fl.oz)			
Carb Control	110	3	2
Complete Nutrition	200	3	28
AllSport, all flav., 8 fl.oz	60	0	16
AMP Energy Drink, 8.4 fl.oz	110	0	29
Relaunch/Elevate, 16 fl.oz	220	0	58
Tall Boy Overdrive, 16 fl.oz can	220	0	58
Arizona: Caution Energy, 8.3 oz	130	0	34
Green Tea Energy, 8 oz	100	0	26
Lite Tea Energy, 8 oz	70	0	17
Atkins: Advantage Shake, 11 oz can	160	9	4
Bally Total Fitness, Whey Pro, 1 scoop	100	1.5	2
Blast, 8.3 oz	120	0	29
Bariatrix Shakes, 1 serving	100	2	6
Anytime Drinks, 8 oz, average	90	4	3
Proti 15 Drink, avg., 1 pkg	75	1	4
Bawls Guarana, 10 fl.oz	120	0	32
Blue Energy, 8.3 fl.oz	120	10	30
Blue Sport, 8.3 fl.oz	90	0	23
Body Fuel (w. NutraSweet), 1 scoop	80	0	20
Bolthouse: Per 15.2 fl.oz			
Perfectly Protein:			
Mocha Cappuccino	340	5	55
Vanilla Chai Tea	305	6	48
Boo•Koo Energy, avg., 16 fl.oz	240	0	60
Boost: High Protein, 8 fl.oz	240	6	33
Nutritional Energy, 8 fl.oz	240	4	41
Boost Plus, 8 fl.oz	360	14	45
Boost w. Benefiber, 8 fl.oz	240	4	42
Boost Smoothie, 8 fl.oz pkg	240	3	44
Glucose Control, 8 fl.oz	190	7	16
Carnation Instant Breakfast			
Powder: 1 envelope, 1.3 oz	200	1	39
Carb Conscious, 1 envelope, 21g	150	1	24
Ready-To-Drink, avg., 11 fl.oz	250	5	40
Celebrity Juice Diet, 4 fl.oz	60	0	14
CeraSport: Liquid, 11 fl.oz	70	0	17
Champion Lyte, Sports Drink	0	0	0

Champion Nutrition	C	F	Cb
Heavywt Gainer 900, 4 sc., 5.4 oz	630	10	101
Ultramet: Original, 1 pkt, 2.7 oz	280	2	24
Ultramet Lyte, 1 pkt, 2 oz	190	1	17
Ultramet Low Carb, 1 pkt, 2 oz	230	6.5	6
Citrucel Fiber Shake, 1 pkg	50	2	6
Clif Shot Energy Gel, 1.1 oz pkt	100	0	24
Cocaine Energy, 8 fl.oz can	70	0	18
Curves Protein Drink:			
Chocolate; Vanilla, 2 scoops	100	1.5	8
made with skim milk, 8 fl.oz	190	2	23
CytoSport Muscle Milk, 2 scoops	350	18	12
Designer Whey Protein Van., 1 scp	90	1.5	2
EAS ~ See AdvantEdge/Myoplex			
Endura (Unipro), 2 scoops, 1.3 oz	120	0	29
Ensure: High Protein, 8 oz bottle	230	6	31
Ensure Fiber/Regular, 8 fl.oz can	250	6	42
Ensure Plus, 8 fl.oz bottle	350	11	50
Glucerna, 8 fl.oz can, average	200	7	27
Weight Loss Shake, 11 fl.oz	290	11	39
High Calcium, 8 fl.oz	220	6	31
Enterex Glucose Control, 8 fl.oz			
(Carbohydrates as Maltodextrin)	237	9	27
Equaline (Albertson's): Plus, 8 fl.oz	350	11	50
Advanced, 8 fl.oz	250	6	40
FRS Energy, 11.5 fl.oz can: Regular	140	0	35
Fruit20 (Veryfine), 8/16/20 fl.oz	0	0	0
Full Throttle			
Energy: Original, 16 fl.oz	220	0	57
Blue Demon/Fury, 16 fl.oz	220	0	57
Coffee & Energy:			
Caramel/Vanilla, 15 fl.oz	260	0	45
Mocha, 15 fl.oz	280	0	50
Hydration + Energy, 16 fl.oz	140	0	36
Fuze: Slenderize, 8 fl.oz	5	0	2
Refresh, 8 fl.oz	90	0	25
Vitalize, 8 fl.oz	100	0	25
Gatorade			
Thirst Quencher:			
(Lemon/Lime, AM, Fierce, Rain)			
1 Cup, 8 fl.oz	50	0	14
12 fl.oz Bottle	75	0	20
20 fl.oz Bottle	125	0	32
32 fl.oz Bottle	200	0	50
Endurance: Same as Thirst Quencher			
G2 (Low Calorie), 1 cup, 8 fl.oz	30	0	7
20 fl.oz Bottle	70	0	17
Nutrition Shake, all flavors, 11 oz	370	8	54
GazZü, all flavors, 16 fl.oz	220	0	54
Genisoy: Ultra XT, 3 Tbsp	150	1	20
Protein Powder, 3 Tbsp	130	1	17
Glaceau: Smartwater	0	0	0
Fruitwater, 20 oz bottle	20	0	5
Vitaminenergy, 16 oz can	100	0	25
Vitaminwater, 20 fl.oz	125	0	31

Energy/Protein Drinks (Cont)

	C	F	Cb
Glucerna Wt Loss Shakes, 11 oz	200	7	27
GNC Lean Shake, 2 scoops	180	2	30
GNC Pro Performance:			
Mega MRP: 3 scoops, 3.3 oz	290	3	11
24 Hour Pro Complex, 39g	150	5	7
100% whey Protein, 29g	130	2.5	5
50 Gram Slam, 15 oz	240	1	6
Crea Drive, 45g	140	0	34
Mass XXX, 7 oz	750	5	126
Weight Gainer 2200 Gold, 17 oz	1840	30	402
Wheybolic Extreme 60, 82g	270	1	6
GU Energy Gel, 1 packet	100	0	25
Guru Energy: Regular, 8.3 oz can	100	0	25
Lite, 8.3 oz can	10	0	2
Hammer Gel, avg. all flav., 2 T., 1¼ oz	90	0	23
Hansen's: Energade Citrus/Orange	60	0	16
Energy Pro	120	0	32
Rumba, 8 fl.oz	120	0	28
Herbalife: Shapeworks Mix, 2 sc, 25g	90	1	13
with 8 fl.oz non-fat milk	180	1	20
HMR: 70 Plus, 1 package	110	0.5	13
500	100	0	17
Hollywood Celebrity Diet, ½ cup	100	0	25
Impulse Energy Drink, 8.3 oz	110	0	28
Jarrow: Whey Protein, 1 scoop	100	1	5
Berry High, 1 scoop, 6g	20	2	5
Muscle Optimal, 2 scoops, 47g	230	2	17
Java Monster Energy: *Per 15 fl.oz Can*			
Lo-Ball/Mean Bean	95	3	10
Loca Moca	190	0	48
Orig./Irish/Nut-Up/Russian	190	3	32
Jolt: Cola, 16 fl.oz can	200	0	52
Blue Raspberry, 16 fl.oz	240	0	60
Power Cola, 23.5 fl.oz	300	0	75
Jones: Energy,16 fl.oz	260	0	64
Kashi GoLEAN Shakes, 2 scoops	220	1	30
Knudsen: ReCharge, 8 fl.oz	70	0	18
Simply Nutritious, 8 fl.oz	130	0	30
Kombucha, Wonder Drink, 8.5 fl.oz	60	0	16
La Brada			
Drink: Lean Body, (40g Pro.), 17 fl.oz	260	9	9
Powders: Lean Body, 79g	330	8	24
Lean Body Mass 60, 6 oz	610	7	77
Breakfast, 92g	360	7	35
Carb Watchers, 65g	240	4	12
Lightfull: *Per 8.25 fl.oz*			
Cafe Latte	90	0.5	37
Chocolate Satisfaction	90	0.5	38
Fruit Flavors, avg.	90	0	37
(Note: Carb figures include Erythritol natural sweetener)			
Lipovitan EB3, 8.6 fl.oz	115	0	26
Liquid Lightening, Reg., 8.4 fl.oz	90	0	22

	C	F	Cb
Max Velocity (Albertson's), 8.45 fl.oz	130	0	33
Lite, 8.45 fl.oz	15	0	0
MDX (Mountain Dew), 8 fl.oz	120	0	32
Met-Rx: Original, 1 pkt, average	260	3	21
Protein Plus, 2 scoops	110	1	4
Nutri Shake, 1 can	240	2	39
RTD 40, 15 fl.oz can	240	3	13
Metabolol: Endurance, 2 scp, 52g	200	5	24
Met, 2 scoops, 66g	200	3	40
Met Max, mix, 2 scoops, 62g	230	2.5	11
Creatinine Extreme, 2 sc. 92g	280	0	68
Monster Energy: 16 fl.oz can	200	0	50
XXL, 24 fl.oz can	300	0	75
Lo-Carb, 16 fl.oz can,	20	0	5
MRM: Low Carb Protein, 1 sc. 30g	120	2.5	3
Iso-bolic, 1 scoop, 1 oz	115	1.5	1
Whey Pumped, 1 scoop	90	1	5
Muscle Milk (Hi Protein): avg., 17 fl.oz	350	17	17
14 fl.oz bottle	230	9	12
Light, 8.5 fl.oz pkg	160	5	9
Muscle Tech Nitro: Complete	280	3	32
Cell Tech RTD, 14½ oz	300	0	75
Mass Tech Weight Gain, 5 scoops	830	5	150
Nitro Tech, 15 fl.oz	210	1	9
Myoplex: Original Shake, 17 fl.oz	280	2	24
Carb Control, 11 fl.oz	150	3.5	5
Deluxe Powder, 1 pkt, 3.4 oz	340	4.5	28
Lite (Ready to Drink), 11 fl.oz pkg	170	2	20
Lite Powder, 1 pkt, 2 oz	190	1.5	20
Naturade: Power Shake, 1 scoop	100	1	10
Protein Booster, avg., ⅓ c. dry	110	1	3
Total Soy, Orig., 1 scoop, 1.3 oz	150	2	20
Nature's Best: Isopure	300	0	25
Isopure Endurance, 3 scoops	330	0	60
Carbo Power, 16 fl.oz	400	0	100
Zero Carb, 2 scoops, 2.1 oz	220	0	3
Pro Smoothie, 15 oz	240	1.5	7
No Fear: 16 fl.oz	270	0	67
Sugar Free, 16 fl.oz	20	0	2
Noní: Tahitian/Pacific, 2 Tbsp	10	0	3
Noni Juice, 1 fl.oz	10	0	3
Liquid Hawaiian/Tahiti, 1 Tbsp	30	0	8
Nutrament (Mead Johnson), 12 fl.oz	360	10	52
Nutrilite (Quixtar):			
Protein Shakes, 11.5 fl.oz	170	6	6
Sports Drinks, Regular, 16 fl.oz	120	0	28
Whey Protein Powder:			
Chocolate, 1.27 oz pouch	130	2	5
Vanilla, 1.16 oz pouch	120	1.5	3
Odwalla **Serious Energy,** 15.2 fl.oz	305	0	74
Optimum Nutr.: 100% Whey, 1.1 oz	120	1	3
100% Soy Protein, 1.1 oz Scoop	120	1.5	2
Pedialyte (Abbott)	25	0	5
Piranha Energy (EAS), 8.4 oz	130	0	33

Energy/Protein Drinks (Cont)

	C	F	Cb
PowerAde			
Regular: 12 fl.oz bottle	90	0	25
20 fl.oz bottle	160	0	41
PowerAde Zero	0	0	0
PowerBar			
Recovery: Choc shake, 1 scoop	250	5	40
Vanilla shake, 10.6 oz	240	5	34
Endurance, 1 scoop, 0.7 oz	170	0	42
Power Gel, avg., 1.5 oz pkg	110	0	27
ProBalance, 8.45 fl.oz	300	10	39
Pro-Cal 100 (R-Kane), 1 pkt	100	1.5	7
Propel Fitness Water,			
all flavors, 23.7 oz bottle	40	0	10
Red Bull Energy, 8.3 fl.oz	110	0	28
12 fl.oz	160	0	40
Sugar-Free, 8.3 fl.oz	10	0	3
Red Devil Energy Drink, 16 fl.oz	230	0	58
Redline Energy	0	0	0
Resource (Novartis): Shake, 6 fl.oz	270	6	45
Shake Plus, 8 fl.oz	480	16	69
Health Shake: 4 fl.oz	200	4	35
No Added Sugar, 4 oz	200	9	22
Diabetishield, 8 fl.oz	150	0	30
Breeze, 8 fl.oz	250	0	54
Benefiber Juice, 4 oz	70	0	18
Revenge Pro (Champ. Nutr.), 1 oz	100	0.5	30
Pro-Score 100, 2 scoops	160	2	1.5
Revival Soy Mix: Plain Soy, 1 pkg	120	3.5	3
Chocolate Day Dream, 1 pkg	240	2.5	36
Other varieties, avg., 1 pkg	225	2	33
Rhino's Energy Drink, 100ml	50	0	13
Rip It Energy, 16 fl.oz	260	0	66
Chic (Sugar Free), 12 fl.oz	5	0	1
Rite Aid: Nutritional, 8 fl.oz	250	6	40
Plus, 8 fl.oz	350	11	50
Rockstar:			
Energy Drink, 16 fl.oz	280	0	62
Diet Energy Drink, 16 fl.oz	20	0	4
50% Juice, 16 fl.oz can	200	0	48
Rush Energy Lite, 8 fl.oz	0	0	0
Regular, 8 fl.oz	120	0	30
Sav-on Nut'l: Plus, 8 oz	350	11	50
Equaline Advance, 8 oz	250	6	40
High Protein, 8 oz	230	5	31
Slim-Fast Shake (Ready To Drink):			
Original, 10.8 oz	220	3	40
High Protein, 11 oz	190	5	24
Easy To Digest, 11 oz	180	5	24
Optima Shake, 10.8 oz can	180	6	24
Low Carb Diet, 11 oz	190	9	6
Powder Shake Mix: 1 scoop, 26g	110	3	18
w. 8 fl.oz fat-free milk	200	5	30
Snapple: Antioxidant Water			
Average all flavors, 20 fl.oz bottle	125	0	31

SoBe: Per Can/Bottle

	C	F	Cb
Adrenaline Rush: 8.3 fl.oz can	140	0	37
16 fl.oz can	260	0	68
Sugar Free, 16 fl.oz	20	0	2
Coolata Energy, 16 fl.oz	250	0	62
Courage, 20 fl.oz	280	0	70
Elixir 3C: Per 20 fl.oz			
Cranberry Grapefruit	260	0	65
Orange-Carrot	230	0	58
Pomegranate-Cranberry	250	0	63
White Concord Grape	300	0	75
Energy, 20 fl.oz	270	0	67
Fuerte, 20 fl.oz	320	0	80
Lean, all flavors, 20 fl.oz	10	0	2
Life Water, all flav., 20 fl.oz	100	0	25
Lizard: Tsunami, 20 fl.oz	250	0	61
Other flavors, avg., 20 fl.oz	310	0	77
Power, 20 fl.oz	260	0	65
Synergy, all flavors, 11.5 fl.oz can	120	0	30
Solaray Soytein (Protein Energy Meal):			
Natural (No Sugar Added), 24g	70	1	2
Flav., avg., 1 heaped scoop, 25g	80	1	6
Sparks (Alcoholic) ~ Page 29			
Spiru-Tein			
Powder, 1 scp, avg., 34g	100	0	10
Steaz Energy, 12 fl.oz	130	0	34
Diet Berry Energy, 12 fl.oz	60	0	14
The Sports Club/LA, PTS Protein Powder,			
Choc/Mocha/Van., 2 scoops, 1 oz	110	3	5
Trader Joe's, Energy, 8 fl.oz	130	0	33
Trim Advantage (Quixtar) Meal Shake:			
Chocolate, 11.2 fl.oz pkg	150	3	16
French Vanilla, 11.2 fl.oz pkg	140	3	14
Twin Lab: Ultra Fuel, 16 fl.oz	400	0	100
Energy Fuel, 250ml can	0	0	0
Vault: Regular/Red Blitz, 12 fl.oz	180	0	47
Vault Zero	0	0	0
Verve Energy, 8.3 fl.oz can	70	0	18
Sugar Free	5	0	1
Vitamin Water ~ See Glaceau			
Walgreens: Nutri' Drink; Theragran-M	250	6	40
Plus; Theragran-M Plus, 8 oz	350	11	50
Weider (Powders)			
Creatine ATP, ½ cup, 1.7 oz	210	0	37
Mass 1000, 1⅓ cups	740	4	146
Ultra Whey Pro, ⅓ cup, 1 oz	110	1.5	6
Dynamic: Muscle Builder, 1½ oz	170	1	22
Weight Gainer, 4 scps, 3.4 oz	380	2	67
Worldwide: Carbo Rush, 20 fl.oz	270	0	67
Pure Protein Shakes, 11 fl.oz, avg.	160	1	2
Rapid Recovery, 20 fl.oz, avg.	275	0	32
Xtreme Trim, 20 fl.oz	25	0	7
Supercharged tea, 20 fl.oz	15	0	4
XS (Quixtar): Energy Drink, 8.4 oz	10	0	1
Power Protein Shake, 11 fl.oz	220	6	4
Zola Acai, 11 fl.oz pkg	170	2	38

Quick Guide

Cola Drinks
Average All Brands

		C	**F**	**Cb**
Includes *Coca-Cola* **and** *Pepsi*				
8 fl.oz Cup/Can		100	0	26
12 fl.oz Can		150	0	39
16 fl.oz Bottle		200	0	52
20 fl.oz Bottle		250	0	65
24 fl.oz (Pepsi)		300	0	84
1-Liter Bottle (34 fl.oz)		400	0	100
2-Liter Bottle (68 fl.oz)		800	0	200

Other Soda Drinks *(Average All Brands)*

	C	**F**	**Cb**
Club Soda, 12 fl.oz	0	0	0
Cream Soda, 12 fl.oz	190	0	48
Diet/Low Cal Drinks, 12 fl.oz	5	0	1
Ginger Ale, 12 fl.oz	125	0	31
Lemon Lime, 12 fl.oz	150	0	37
Orange, 12 fl.oz	180	0	45
Pink Lemonade, 12 fl.oz	180	0	45
Root Beer, 12 fl.oz	150	0	39
Tonic Water, 12 fl.oz	125	0	2
Mineral Water: Plain, 12 fl.oz	0	0	0
Sweetened/flavored, 12 fl.oz	150	0	37
w. Fruit Juice, 12 fl.oz	120	0	30
Soda Water/Seltzer: Plain/Diet	0	0	0
Sweetened/flavored, 12 fl.oz	155	0	39
w. Fruit Juice, 12 fl.oz	160	0	40
Soft Frozen Lemonade, 12 fl.oz	300	0	75

Fountain, Movie Theater & Take-Out

Average All Flavors

	C	**F**	**Cb**
Small Cup, 12 fl.oz: No Ice	160	0	40
With ⅓ Ice	120	0	30
Regular, 16 fl.oz: No Ice	215	0	53
With ⅓ Ice	160	0	40
Medium, 22 fl.oz: No Ice	295	0	73
With ⅓ Ice	220	0	55
Large, 32 fl.oz: No Ice	430	0	105
With ⅓ Ice	320	0	80

(Note: ⅓ Cup of Ice = ¼ Cup Liquid)

Soft Drinks Brands

Per 12 fl.oz Unless Indicated

	C	**F**	**Cb**
A&W: Cream Soda	180	0	46
Float, 11.5 fl.oz bottle	260	1.5	64
Root Beer	170	0	46
Diet Cream Soda/Root Beer	1	0	0
Albertson's: Max Cola	165	0	44
Lemon Lime	150	0	41
Other flavors, average	180	0	48

Soft Drink Brands (Cont)

Per 12 fl.oz Unless Indicated

	C	**F**	**Cb**
Barq's: Root Beer	165	0	45
Floatz, 12 fl.oz	190	0	51
Big Red, 12 fl.oz	150	0	38
Blue Sky: Cola; Orange Cream	160	0	43
Cherry; Raspberry; Root Beer	155	0	42
Grape; Lemon Lime; Dr Becker	130	0	36
Organic, all flavors, avg.	165	0	40
Other varieties, average	145	0	43
Bubble Up, 12 fl.oz	165	0	42
Cactus Cooler, 12 fl.oz	150	0	40
Canada Dry: Club Soda	0	0	0
Ginger Ale, all flavors	120	0	33
Tonic Water	90	0	24
Diet, 12 fl.oz	0	0	0
Capri Sun:			
Roaring Waters, 6.75 fl.oz	35	0	9
Sport, all flavors, 6.75 fl.oz	60	0	15
Coca-Cola: *Per 12 fl.oz*			
Classic/Caffeine Free	145	0	41
Diet Coke, all flavors	0	0	0
Cherry Coke/Vanilla Coke	155	0	42
Coca-Cola Zero	0	0	0
Country Time, Lemonade, 333 ml	180	0	35
Crush, all flavors	185	0	51
Dad's: Orange Cream Soda, 12 fl.oz	180	0	45
Root Beer, 12 fl.oz	165	0	41
Diet Rite, Pure Zero	0	0	0
Dr Pepper: Regular	140	0	40
Cherry Vanilla	150	0	39
Diet, all flavors	0	0	0
Fanta, all flavors	110	0	27
Fresca: Orig. Citrus	0	0	0
Blackcherry Citrus	0	0	0
Peach Citrus	0	0	0
GuS, average all flavors	95	0	23
Hansen's: Diet Soda	0	0	0
Natural Orange Mango	160	0	44
Other flavors, average	150	0	44
Hawaiian Punch, Fruit Juicy Red	120	0	30
Henry Weinhard's: Root Beer	170	0	43
Cream flavor, average	175	0	42
Hires, Root Beer	170	0	45
IBC: Root Beer	160	0	43
Cherry Limeade	170	0	44
Cream Soda; Black Cherry	180	0	48
Diet Root Beer	0	0	0

Per 12 fl.oz Unless Indicated	C	F	Cb
Icee: Coca-Cola	100	0	27
Barq's; Minute Maid	200	0	52
Smoothee Lemonade	255	0	64
Jolt Cola, 16 fl.oz	200	0	52
Blue Raspberry , 16 fl.oz	240	0	60
Cherry Cola, 16 fl.oz	180	0	46
Grape, 16 fl.oz	210	0	54
Orange, 16 fl.oz	210	0	52
Passionfruit, 16 fl.oz	240	0	58
Ultra Citrus, 16 fl.oz	10	0	0
Jones Soda: Cola, 16 fl.oz	260	0	64
Whoopass, 16 fl.oz	200	0	50
Other flavors, average	185	0	46
MDX Energy Soda (Sugar Free)	0	0	0
Mello Yello, Regular	180	0	48
Minute Maid: Fruit Punch	170	0	42
Lemonade Reg./Pink			
12 fl.oz can/bottle	150	0	38
20 fl.oz Bottle	250	0	63
Orangeade	160	0	40
Mountain Dew:			
Live Wire; Code Red	165	0	47
Diet flavors	0	0	0
Mug Root Beer	150	0	44
Natural Brew: Vanilla, Cream	170	0	42
Ginseng Cola, Ginger Ale	170	0	42
Root Beer	180	0	44
Nehi, Royal Crown Peach	190	0	51
Orangina: 10 fl.oz bottle	110	0	28
Pepsi: Regular/Blue/Caffeine Free	150	0	42
Diet Pepsi; Jazz	0	0	0
One, 12 fl.oz	2	0	0
Wild Cherry; Vanilla	150	0	42
Perrier, Carbonated Water	0	0	0
Pibb Xtra	145	0	39
RW Knudsen, Spritzers, average	180	0	43
RC Cola: Regular; Cherry	165	0	45
Diet Cola	0	0	0
Reed's, Ginger Brew, avg. all var.	145	0	38
7•UP: Regular	150	0	39
Cherry, Gold	150	0	39
Diet varieties, 12 fl.oz	0	0	0
7•UP Plus, 12 fl.oz	15	0	3
Safeway/Vons: Go 2 Cola	160	0	44
Cherry Cola	160	0	43
Ditto Lemon Lime	165	0	41
Parker's Cream Soda	170	0	42
Parker's Root Beer	170	0	47
Diet flavors	0	0	0
Santa Cruz, Sparkling, average	135	0	32
Schweppes: Seltzer	0	0	0
Tonic Water; Ginger Ale, average	130	0	35

Per 12 fl.oz Unless Indicated	C	F	Cb
Shasta: Cream Soda	190	0	47
Cherry Cola; Doc Shasta	160	0	39
Club Soda; Diet, all flav.	0	0	0
Fr. Punch, Pineapple; Or.	200	0	50
Ginger Ale	130	0	32
Other flavors, average	175	0	45
Sierra Mist, Lemon Lime	150	0	39
Sprite: Regular	145	0	40
Tropical Remix	0	0	0
Zero	4	0	0
Squirt, Citrus Burst	150	0	40
Star Ruby (GUS): Valencia Orange	95	0	24
Other flavors	90	0	22
Stewarts: Root Beer	160	0	41
Grape	190	0	48
Key Lime	180	0	46
Sun Drop: Regular, 20fl.oz bottle	325	0	81
Cherry Lemon, 20 fl.oz bottle	300	0	75
Diet Sun Drop, 20 fl.oz bottle	10	0	2
Sunkist: Orange	195	0	53
Diet Sunkist	0	0	0
Cherry Limeade	180	0	45
Sunkist Float, 11.5 fl.oz	260	1.5	64
Sunny D, 12 fl.oz	180	0	44
TAB, 12 fl.oz	0	0	0
Thomas Kemper: Root Beer	140	0	34
Other flavors, average	160	0	40
Vernor's, Ginger Ale	150	0	39
Walgreens: Grape Soda, 20 fl.oz	300	0	75
Cola; Lemon Lime, 20 fl.oz	225	0	60
Red Soda; Root Beer, 20 fl.oz	225	0	60
Diet Cola	0	0	0
Welch's: Soda, 12 fl.oz	190	0	51
Sparkling	240	0	60
365 Organic (Whole Foods):			
Spritzers, all flavors	110	0	27

Powdered Soft Drink Mix

Per 8 fl.oz Prepared	C	F	Cb
All-Bran Fiber Drink Mix,			
Pink Lemonade, 1 pkt	20	0	12
(Note: Carbs include Polydextrose)			
Capri Sun, Sport ½ pk	25	0	5
Cool Splashers, 8 fl.oz	60	0	16
Country Time: Lemonade	60	0	16
Other flavors, average	80	0	19
Lite	35	0	9
Crystal Light, 8 fl.oz	5	0	1
Flavoraid, ⅛ pkg	0	0	0
Kool-Aid: All flavors	60	0	16
Unsweetened, 6 fl.oz	5	0	0
Propel, ½ pkg	10	0	3
Tang, 8 fl.oz, average	40	0	10

Quick Guide

Teas

	C	F	Cb
Regular: Bag, Loose or Instant			
Brewed, 1 cup, 8 fl.oz	2	0	0.5
(Add extra for sugar/milk)			
Herbal: Average all varieties, 1 cup	2	0	0
Bigelow, all flavors	0	0	0
Celestial Seasonings:			
All flavors	0	0	0
Bubble Tea, average, 12 fl.oz	175	0	41
Chai Tea: *Café D' Vita,* 2 Tbsp	120	3.5	21
Starbucks: See Fast-Foods Section			

Iced Tea

	C	F	Cb
Average All Brands			
Sweetened: 8 fl.oz	100	0	25
12 fl.oz	150	0	38
16 fl.oz	200	0	50
Unsweetened: 8 fl.oz	2	0	0

Iced Tea Mixes

Per 1 Cup Made-Up

	C	F	Cb
4C Instant	70	0	18
All-Bran Fiber Drink Mix, 1 pkt	20	0	12
(Note: Carbs include Polydextrose)			
Carb Options, 1 cup	0	0	0
Crystal Light Sugar Free	5	0	0
Lipton: Instant, unsweetened	0	0	0
Instant Raspberry	80	0	19
Lemon	70	0	18
Peach/Raspb, Sugar Free	5	0	1
Iced Tea To Go	0	0	0
Nestea			
Lemonade Tea, 1⅓ Tbsp	60	0	15
Lemon flavored Iced Tea, 1⅓ Tbsp	60	0	15
Sugar Free Lemon Iced Tea, 2 tsp	5	0	2
Unsweetened Tea, 2 tsp	0	0	0
Concentrate: Green Tea, 2 Tbsp	80	0	18
Lemon Tea, 2 Tbsp	80	0	19
Raspberry, 2 Tbsp	90	0	19

Bottled & Canned Teas

	C	F	Cb
Arizona: *Per 8 fl.oz Cup*			
Black with Ginseng	70	0	18
Green Tea(s)/Asian Plum	70	0	18
Diet Green Tea (w. Sorbitol)	5	0	2
Peach/Raspberry	70	0	18
Sweet Tea	90	0	23

Bottled & Canned Teas (Cont)

	C	F	Cb
Fuze, all flavors, 16 fl.oz	120	0	30
Gold Peak, 16.9 fl.oz bottle	170	0	46
Hansen's: Green Tea, 16 fl.oz	120	0	30
Peach/Pomegr. Green, 16 fl.oz	180	0	44
Honest Tea, avg., all flav., 16.9 fl.oz	85	0	21
Lipton Brisk			
Avg. all flavors, 12 fl.oz can	130	0	33
20 fl.oz bottle	215	0	55
Lipton Iced Tea			
Lem./White w. Raspb., 16.9 fl.oz	125	0	31
Green Tea w. Citrus:			
16.9 fl.oz bottle	170	0	42
20 fl.oz bottle	200	0	50
Diet, all flavors	0	0	0
Nantucket			
Lemon Tea 17.5 fl.oz	175	0	44
Nestea Iced Tea			
Lemon/Peach/Raspb.	90	0	23
Green Tea, 20 fl.oz	210	0	56
Diet Green/Lemon Tea	0	0	0
Pom Pomegranate:			
Pomegranate Tea, 16 fl.oz	140	0	35
Lychee Green, 16 fl.oz	140	0	35
Light flavors, 16 fl.oz	70	0	34
Note: Carbs figure for Light flavors includes Erythritol natural sweetener which has negligible calories .			
Sbarro, 16 fl.oz Bottle	180	0	48
Shasta, Lemon, 16 fl.oz	140	0	35
Snapple: Iced Tea, all flavors, 16 fl.oz	200	0	50
Black Teas, avg., 17.5 fl.oz	75	0	19
Diet/Unsweetened Teas	0	0	0
Green/White, 17.5 fl.oz	130	0	32
Red Tea, 17.5 fl.oz	100	0	25
SoBe: Green; Oolong, 20 fl.oz	240	0	60
Dragon; Zen Tea, 20 fl.oz	270	0	70
Special K20 Protein			
Iced Tea, 16 fl.oz	50	0	12
Ssips, Lemon Iced, 8 fl.oz	100	0	24
Steaz, Organic Green, 12 fl.oz	135	0	34
Tazo: *Per 13.8 fl.oz Bottle*			
Berryblossom White Tea	60	0	15
Lemon Ginger; Peach	120	0	30
Mojito Green (Diet)	0	0	0
White Cranberry	140	0	35
TeaZazz: Peach Tea, 20 fl.oz	50	0	12
Turkey Hill: Iced Tea, 16 fl.oz	180	0	44
Fruit flavors, avg., 16 fl.oz	220	0	55
365 Organic *(Whole Foods):*			
Berry Black Tea, 16 fl.oz	60	0	14
Lemon Green Tea, 16 fl.oz	40	0	10
White Jasmine Tea, 16 fl.oz	30	0	8

Note: Most breads have similar calories on a weight basis. However, volume may vary.

For example, 1 oz of bread may equal 1 slice regular bread or 2 slices of a lighter bread. It is best to weigh bread used and calculate using: 1 oz bread = 70 calories, 14g carb.

Quick Guide

Bread

	C	F	Cb
White or Wheat ~ Average Per Slice			
Thin or Light, ¾ oz	50	0.5	10
Sandwich slice, 1 oz	70	1	14
Thick or Large slice, 1½ oz	105	1.5	21
Thick/Home-made, 2 oz	140	2	28
Extra Thick/Home-made, 3 oz	210	3	42
Whole Loaf, 16 oz	1120	16	224
Whole Loaf, 24 oz	1680	24	336
With Seeds or Nuts:			
Sandwich slice, 1½ oz	130	5	18
Thick slice/Home-made, 2½ oz	215	8	30
Toast ~ Has same calories as bread used			
1 Slice (1 oz fresh)			
w. 2 tsp regular spread	140	9	12
w. 2 tsp "light" spread	105	5	12
w. 1 Tbsp regular spread	170	12	12
w. 1 Tbsp "light" spread	120	7	12

Breads

	C	F	Cb
12-Grain, 1½ oz slice	110	1.5	22
Batard (8 oz), thick slice, 2 oz	150	0.5	28
Bran style/Dark, 1 oz slice	70	1	14
Bread w. Soy Isoflavones, 1.2 oz	80	2.5	13
Buttermilk, average, 1½ oz slice	110	1	22
Caraway Rye, 2 oz slice	150	2	28
Challah, ¾ oz slice	85	1.5	17
Chapati, 1 oz	110	3	18
Ciabatta, 1 slice, 2 oz	130	1	26
Cornbread, average, 1 pce, 3 oz	220	6	37
Cracked Wheat Sourdough, 1½ oz	130	0.5	27
Croissants: See Page 113, 173			
Crustless Bread, regular slice ¾ oz	40	0.5	8.5
Crusts Only, regular slice, ¼ oz	30	0	7
English Toasting, slice, 2 oz	140	1.5	27
'Enriched' Breads, average, 1 oz sl.	60	1	12
Flax & Sunflower Round, 1.2 oz	90	2	18

Breads (Cont)

	C	F	Cb
Foccacia: Plain, 2 oz portion	150	2.5	28
Cheese & Garlic; Pesto, 2 oz	160	6	21
Tomato & Olive, 2 oz	150	5	21
French Stick/Baguette, 1 oz slice	70	1	15
French Toast, 1 slice, 1.6 oz	140	2	26
Sticks *(Aunt Jemima)*, 1 pce, 1 oz	90	2	17
Garlic Bread/Toast:			
Small slice + 1 tsp spread, ¾ oz	80	5	7
Med. slice + 2 tsp spread, 1½ oz	160	10	14
Thick slice + 3 tsp spread, 1.8 oz	220	14	20
Pepperidge Farm, 1 slice, 1.4 oz	160	10	15
Hemp Bread, 1.2 oz	95	2	12
Italian Bread, 2 oz slice	140	1	28
Light Bread, avg., 0.8 oz slice	40	0.5	8
Lower Carb (higher Protein/fiber),			
average all brands, 1 oz	60	1.5	9
MultiGrain, 1 slice, 1.3 oz	60	1.5	17
Nut/Health Nut, 1.35 oz slice	90	1.5	18
Oatmeal/Oatbran Bread, 1½ oz	90	1.5	19
Pita: Average all types,			
Small (4" diam) 1.1 oz	90	0	18
Large (6½" diam) 2 oz	140	1.5	27
Extra Large (9" diam) 4 oz	300	1.5	60
Popovers (1), no butter	130	2	18
Poppyseed (Vienna), 0.8 oz sl.	55	1	10
Pumpernickel: Large slice, 1.35 oz	80	0	15
Cocktail/Party size	30	0.5	6
Raisin Bread, 1 oz slice	80	1.5	14
Raisin Walnut, 1 oz slice	70	1.5	15
Roman Meal, 1.1 oz slice	80	1	15
Rye: Average, 1 thin slice, 1 oz	80	1	14
1 thick slice, 2 oz	150	2	25
Cocktail size, 0.4 oz	25	0.5	4
Sandwich Bread, 1 oz slice	70	1	12
Sandwich Pockets, 2 oz	140	1.5	27
Sourdough, 1½ oz slice	120	1	25
Sourdough French, 1 oz	75	0	14
Spelt, 1.6 oz	130	1	26
Sprouted 7-Grain, 1.5 oz slice	110	0.5	18
Squaw, 1.1 oz slice	85	0.5	13
Sweet Hawaiian Bread, 1.3 oz	110	2	18
Tacos/Tortillas: See Page 104			
Turkish/Middle Eastern, 1 oz sl.	80	1.5	16
Wheat-Free Breads: Spelt, 1.6 oz	130	1	26
Healthseed Rye, 1.6 oz	90	1	20
Kamut, 1.2 oz	80	2	16
Millet, 1.5 oz	100	1	20

Bread Brands

	C	F	Cb
Controlled Carb Gourmet			
High Fiber, 1 slice, 1 oz	80	2.5	11
Zero Net Carb Bagel, 1 oz	120	2	14
Ener-G: Gluten-Free Breads			
Brown Rice Bread, 1 slice, 1.3 oz	130	6	18
Light Brown Rice, 1 slice, ¾ oz	50	2	7
Corn Loaf, 1 slice, ¾ oz	40	1.5	8
Light Tapioca, 1 slice, ¾ oz	45	1.5	7
Ezekiel			
Low Carb: Wheat, 0.8 oz	70	4	4
Savory Herb, 0.8 oz	60	2.5	4
Genesis 1: 29, 0.8 oz	80	2	14
Francisco International			
Bavarian Sweet Wheat, 1 slice, 1.7 oz	130	2	24
Sheepherder's, 1slice, 1½ oz	120	1	22
Sourdough,1 slice, 1½ oz	110	0	23
Nature's Path: Per Slice (2 oz)			
Manna: Carrot Raisin; Millet Rice	130	0	27
Cinnamon Date	150	0	29
Fruit & Nut	140	1	27
Sun Seed	160	2	29
Whole Rye	150	0	32
Oroweat: Per Slice			
100% Whole Wheat, 1.3 oz	100	2	19
Sugar Free Whole Grain, 1 sl., 0.8 oz	50	1	9
Pepperidge Farm: Per Slice			
100% Whole Wheat, Thin	70	1	12
Carb Style 7-Grain	60	1.5	8
Cinnamon Swirl	80	1.5	15
Farmhouse Soft	110	2	19
Light Style, average	45	0	9
Raisin Cinnamon Swirl	80	1.5	15
Ralph's, Breakfast Bread: Per Slice (2 oz)			
Cranberry Orange, 1 sl., 2 oz	180	4	32
Wild Berry, 1 sl., 2 oz	180	3	33
Sara Lee: Per Slice			
Delightful White, 0.8 oz	45	0.5	9
Honey Wheat, 1 oz	80	1	16
Heart Healthy, Multi Grain, 1.4 oz	80	1	14
Schwan's: Per Serving			
Chse Stuffed Bread w. Sauce, 2 oz	160	5	20
Five Chse Garlic French Bread (1), 3.3 oz	330	20	26
Fr. Baguette Bread, ¼ loaf, 1.7 oz	130	0	25
Southern Style Biscuits (1), 2.2 oz	200	10	23
Trader Joe's			
Fat-Free Multi-Grain, 1.1 oz	70	0	15
Mom's White, 1.1 oz	90	1	15
Seeded Harvest, 1 oz	65	1	12
Pumpernickel, 1.3 oz	100	0	21
Wonder: Sandwich, 1 slice, 1 oz	60	0.5	13
Light Wheat, 1 slice, ¾ oz	40	0.5	9

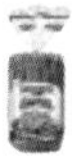

Bread Rolls & Buns

	C	F	Cb
6" Roll, Plain, average 2½ oz	200	1	38
Brown 'n Serve, average, 1 oz	70	1	13
Ciabatta Roll, 3½ oz	230	4	41
Dinner Rolls:			
1 small, 1 oz	90	1.5	17
1 medium (3" diam),1½ oz	110	1	23
Frankfurter/Hot Dog: 1¼ oz	110	1.5	21
1½ oz size	130	2	25
French: 1 med, 1.3 oz	110	1.5	22
1 large, 3 oz	230	2.5	42
Hamburger: Regular, 1½ oz	110	1.5	22
Large, 3 oz	210	3	40
Hoagie/Submarine, Plain, 2⅓ oz	200	1	38
Kaiser Roll:			
Small, 2 oz	200	2.5	35
Large, 3½ oz	350	4	61
Onion Roll, 2.4 oz size	180	2.5	34
Party Roll, 0.6 oz	45	0.5	9
Sandwich Roll:			
Small, 2½ oz	190	1.5	37
6" size, 4 oz	300	2.5	57
Sourdough Roll, 1¼ oz	110	1	21
Wheat Roll:			
Small, 1.2 oz	100	1	17
Medium, 1¾ oz	130	1.5	23
Large, 3½ oz	260	3	46

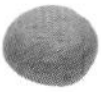

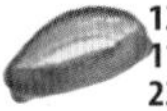

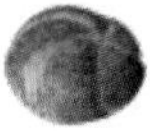

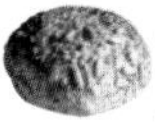

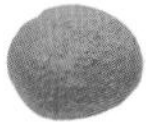

Breadsticks, Croutons

	C	F	Cb
Breadsticks: Salt Sticks, plain, 1 oz	110	1	20
Fresh baked (1), 2 oz	180	2.5	34
Stella D'oro: Sesame (1)	50	2	7
Original, 1 piece	45	1	7
Croutons: Seasoned, 2 Tbsp, ¼ oz	35	1.5	4
9 small or 6 large, ¼ oz	35	1.5	4
Fat-Free (Pepp. Farm), 2 Tbsp	30	0	5

Bread Products

	C	F	Cb
Bread Crumbs, dry:			
Plain or seasoned, 1 oz	110	1.5	20
1 cup, 3½ oz	385	5	70
Corn Flake Crumbs, 1.1 oz	120	0	29
Graham Cracker Crumbs, 1 oz	110	2.5	20
Keebler, 3 Tbsp, ½ oz	70	1.5	13
Bread Dough: Frozen, 1 slice, 2 oz	140	2	26
Refrigerated, French, 1" slice	60	1	13
Wheat/White, 1" slice	80	2	14
Coating Mixes: Avg., 2 Tbsp., 1 oz	100	0.5	20
Stuffing: Average, dry mix, 1 oz	110	1	10
Made-up, ½ cup, 4 oz	180	9	11

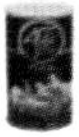

Quick Guide

Bagels
Average All Brands

Plain/Onion: **C**   **F**   **Cb**

	C	F	Cb
1 mini/bagelette, 1 oz	75	0.5	15
1 small bagel, 2 oz	145	1	29
1 medium bagel, 3 oz	230	1.5	45
1 large bagel, 4 oz	285	2	56
Bagel Chips (New York Style), 4 slices, ¾ oz	100	4.5	12
Pizza Bagel Bites, 4 pces, 3.1 oz	200	6	29
Bagel Bites (Ore-Ida), 4 pces	190	7	25
Bagel Crisps (New York Style), 7 pces	140	6	17

Bagel Brands

	C	F	Cb
Controlled Carb Gourmet			
High Fiber Bagel (1), 2 oz	160	5	22
Individual Wrapped (1), 2 oz	80	6	20
Zero Net Carbs (1), 2 oz	60	1	1
Costco Bakery: Plain, 4 oz	300	1	61
Everything, 4 oz	330	3.5	62
Enjoy Life, all types, 3.2 oz	270	6	50
Lenders: Original, frozen, 2 oz	140	0.5	29
New York, frozen, 3.3 oz	230	1	47
Plain, refrigerated, 2.9 oz	210	1.5	42
Oroweat: Oatmeal, 3.4 oz	270	4	49
Whole Wheat, 3.4 oz	250	1.5	52
Sara Lee: Mini, average, 1.3 oz	100	0.5	22
Toaster Size, all types, 2.2 oz	170	0.5	35
Apple Cinnamon	310	1.5	64
Banana Walnut	350	7	61
Cranberry Orange	310	1.5	64
Western: All flavors, avg., 2 oz	110	0	25

Fast-Food Stores: See Page 182

Bagel Spreads

Cream Cheese:

	C	F	Cb
Plain: 2 Tbsp, 1 oz	80	8	2
2 oz mini-tub	160	16	4
Reduced Fat: 2 Tbsp, 1 oz	60	5	2
2 oz mini-tub	120	10	4
Flavors: Lox, 1 oz	75	6	1
Raisin Walnut, 1 oz	90	6	8
Strawberry, 1 oz	60	3	7
Sundried Tomato, 1 oz	80	7	2
Vegetable, 1 oz	60	6	1

English Muffins   **C** **F** **Cb**
Average All Brands

Plain/Whole Wheat:	C	F	Cb
Regular, 2 oz	133	1.5	26
Heavier, 2.5 oz	155	2	31
Super Size, 3.2 oz	190	2	38
Raisin-Cinnamon, 2.2 oz	140	1	29

Note: Actual weight of packaged muffins can be 10-15% heavier than stated net weight.

Rice Cakes

	C	F	Cb
Reg. size, avg. 1 cake, 9g	35	0	7.5
Hain, Mini, average, 9 pieces	70	2	12
Lundberg, all types, 15g each	60	0.5	14
Quaker, Large, all flavors, 13g each	50	0	11
Westbrae, 1 cake, 7g	25	0	5

Taco Shells & Tortillas

	C	F	Cb
Tacos: Mini Size (1)	25	1.5	2
Regular size, all types (1)	50	2	7
Large (1)	90	4	13
Salad Shell, flour (Del Oro), 1.4 oz	230	17	10
Tortilla (Soft Taco), each	85	2	15
Corn Tortilla: 6", 1 oz each	55	0.5	11
Flour Tortilla: 8", 1.75 oz	145	3	26
Low-Fat	110	1.5	22
Burritos, 1 tortilla, 2.3 oz	190	5	32
Low-Fat	110	1.5	22
Tostada Bowl (Rio Rancho), 6" 1.25 oz	180	9	22
Tostada Shells, each	55	3	6
La Tortilla Factory			
Fat Free Flour Tortillas:			
Burrito size, 2.5 oz	120	0.5	34
Soft Taco, 1.8 oz	90	0	24
Low Carb Low-Fat Tortillas:			
Large, 1.26 oz	80	3	19
Original, Flavors, 1.26 oz	50	2	11
Mission Foods			
Tortillas: Per 6" Tortilla			
Flour, 1 oz	80	1.5	13
Low Carb Flour, 1 oz	80	2	12
Low Carb Whole Wheat, 1 oz	80	2	12
White Corn, 0.8 oz	45	0.5	8.5
98% Fat-Free Burrito, 10", 2.4 oz	180	1.5	37

Crispbreads & Matzos ~ Page 90

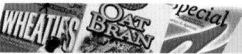
Quick Guide

Cooked Cereals
	C	F	Cb
Buckwheat Groats, roasted:			
Dry, ½ cup, 3 oz	285	2	61
Cooked, 1 cup, 6 oz	155	1	34
Bulgur: Dry, ½ cup, 2½ oz	240	1	53
Cooked, 1 cup, 6½ oz	150	0.5	34
Corn/Hominy Grits:			
Dry: ¼ cup, 1.4 oz	145	0.5	31
3 Tbsp, 1 oz	110	0.5	23
Cooked, ¾ cup, 6½ oz	110	0.5	23
Instant, 1 pkt, dry, 0.8 oz	75	0	18
w. Imitation Bacon Bits, 1 oz	100	0.5	22
Cream of Rice, ckd, ¾ cup, 6½ oz	95	0	21
Cream of Wheat:			
Regular, ckd, ¾ cup, 6½ oz	100	0.5	21
Quick, ckd, ¾ cup, 6½ oz	95	0.5	20
Instant, ckd, ¾ cup, 6½ oz	110	0.5	24
Farina: Cooked, ¾ cup, 6 oz	85	0	18
Millet, dry, ¼ cup, 1¾ oz	190	2	36
Oat Bran: Dry, ⅓ cup, 1 oz	70	2	13
Cooked, ½ cup, 3¾ oz	45	1	9
Oatmeal: Dry, ⅓ cup, 1 oz	105	1.5	18
Regular, ckd, ¾ cup, 6 oz	110	2	19
1 cup, 8 oz	145	2.5	25
Instant: Regular, dry, avg., 1 oz	105	1.5	18
Flavored, dry, average, 1½ oz	150	2	32
Wheat Hearts, 1 oz dry, ¾ c. ckd	110	0.5	24

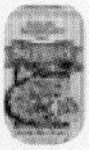

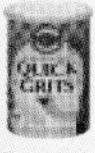

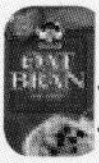

Brans, Wheat Germ, Add-Ons
	C	F	Cb
Bran: Wheat, unprocessed,			
1 Tbsp, 3g	5	0	2
Rice Bran: Raw, 1 Tbsp, 5g	15	1	2.5
¼ cup, 1 oz	95	6	15
Oat Bran: Raw, 1 Tbsp, 5g	10	0.5	4
⅓ cup, 1 oz	70	2	19
Wheat Germ: Raw, 1 Tbsp, ¼ oz	25	0.5	4
¼ cup, 1 oz	105	3	15
Fruit: Dried, average, 1 oz	70	0	18
Banana, ½ medium	55	0	14
Prunes in Syrup (5), 3 oz	90	0	23
Honey, 1 Tbsp, ¾ oz	65	0	17
Lecithin Granules, 1 Tbsp, 10g	55	4	0.5
Nuts, Almonds (6), ¼ oz	40	1	1.5
Bee Pollen Granules, 1 T., 8g	25	1	2
Psyllium Husks, 1 Tbsp, 5g	15	0	4

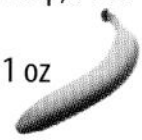

Hot/Cooked Cereals ~ Brands
Per Serving
	C	F	Cb
Albers Grits, ¼ cup, 1.4 oz	140	0.5	31
Bobs Red Mill-10 Grain, ¼ c., 40g	140	1	28
Country Choice Oats, 1 pouch, avg.	110	2	19
Dr McDougall's			
Oatmeal: *Per Package*			
& Barley, Peach Raspb., 3 oz	300	4	62
& Wheat, Apple Cinn., 2.32 oz	250	3	50
Organic, Maple 4 Grain, 2.57 oz	260	3	52
Organic Instant Oatmeal: *Per Packet*			
Original, 1 oz	120	2	21
Light Apple Cinnamon, 1.95 oz	120	1.5	24
Light Maple Brown Sugar, 1.34 oz	150	2	28
4 Grains w. Maple Sugar, 2.2 oz	220	4	44
Erewhon: Barley Plus, ¼ c., 1.7 oz	170	1	37
Brown Rice Crm, ¼ cup, 1.6 oz	170	1	36
Instant Oatmeal, 1.2 oz avg.	130	2.5	25
McCann's Instant Irish Oatmeal			
Apple & Cinnamon, 1.23 oz	130	1.5	27
Maple & Brown Sugar, 1.5 oz	160	2	32
Original, 1 oz pkg	100	1.5	18
Steel Cut Oats, ¼ cup, 1.4 oz	150	2	26
Mother's Oat Bran, ½ cup, 1.4 oz	150	3	25
Nabisco: Cream of Wheat, 1 oz	120	0	23
Malt-O-Meal: Orig., 3T., 1.2 oz	120	0.5	26
Maple Brown Sugar, ¼ cup	170	0	37
Natures Path: Apple Cinn.1.7 oz	210	2.5	40
Average other varieties	200	4	40
Quaker: Oatbran, ½ cup, 1.4 oz	150	3	25
Honey Nut, 1 cup, 1.5 oz	170	3.5	31
Maple Brown Sugar, 1.9 oz ctn	160	2	33
Multigrain, ½ cup, 1.4 oz	135	1.5	29
Old Fashioned Oats, ½ cup, 1.4 oz	150	3	27
Sun Country Quick Oats, ½ c.,1.4 oz	150	3	27
Grits: Reg. all types, 1 pkg, avg.	130	1.5	29
Instant, all types, 1 pkg, 1 oz	100	0	22
Instant Oatmeal: *Per Package*			
Oatmeal Regular, 1 oz	100	2	19
Bakery Favorites, avg., 1½ oz	160	2	31
Fruit and Cream, avg. all flavors	130	2.5	26
Oatmeal Express, avg. all flavors	200	2.5	42
Supreme, avg. all flavors	160	3	31
Silver Palate Oatmeal, ⅓ c., 40g	160	3	26
Uncle Sam Oatmeal, 1.2 oz	130	3	24

B Breakfast Cereals

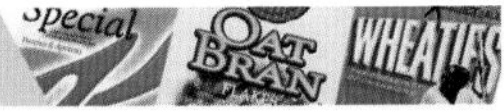

Quick Guide

Cold Cereals	C	F	Cb
Average All Brands			
Bran Flakes, ¾ c., 1 oz	95	0.5	24
Corn Flakes, 1 c., 1 oz	100	0	24
Granola, ¼ c., 1 oz	150	7.5	16
Oat Bran Cereal, ½ cup, 1½ oz	145	3	25
Puffed Rice, 1 cup, ½ oz	55	0	13
Puffed Wheat, 1 cup, ½ oz	45	0	10
Raisin Bran, ½ cup, 1 oz	90	0.5	22
Rice Crisps, 1 cup, 1 oz	105	0.5	24
Shredded Wheat, 1 bisc., 1 oz	85	0.5	20
Sugar-frosted Flakes, ¾ c, 1 oz	115	0	28
Wheat Flakes, ¾ cup, 1 oz	105	1	24

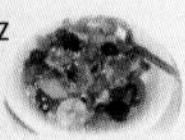

Breakfast/Cereal Bars/Pop Tarts: *See Page 33*

Ready-To-Eat Cereal

	C	F	Cb
Arrowhead Mills			
Amaranth Flakes, 1 cup, 1.2 oz	140	2	26
Bran Flakes, 1 cup, 1 oz	140	2.5	24
Corn Flakes, 1 cup, 1.2 oz	120	0	27
Kamut Flakes, 1 cup, 1.1 oz	120	1	25
Multi Grain Flakes, 1 cup, 1½ oz	170	2	33
Nature O's, 1 cup, 1.1 oz	130	2	25
Oat Bran Flakes, 1 cup, 1.2 oz	140	2.5	24
Puffed Kamut, 1 cup, ½ oz	50	0	11
Rice Flakes, 1 cup, 1.7 oz	180	1	40
Shredded Wheat, 1 cup, 1.7 oz	200	1	42
Spelt Flakes, 1 cup, 1.1 oz	120	1	24
Atkins			
Morning Start: Blueberry, ½ cup	90	2	12
Crunchy Almond Crisp, ½ cup	90	2	10
Triple Berry, ½ cup	90	2	10
Back to Nature			
Energy Start:			
Hi-Protein Crunch, ½ cup 1.7oz	170	1.5	28
Organic Oat & Soy Crisp, ¾ c. 1.9oz	200	3	37
Granola: Apple Blueb., ½ cup 2oz	200	2.5	39
Apple Cinn.; Classic, ½ c. 1.8oz	180	2.5	36
Apple Strawb., ½ cup 1.9oz	190	2.5	37
Cranb. Pecan, ½ cup 1.6oz	180	5	35
French Van., ½ cup 1.9oz	220	6	35
Hi-Protein, ½ cup 2.2oz	260	6	41
Raisin, ½ cup 1.9oz	190	2	35
Muesli, ¾ cup 2.3 oz	230	4	48

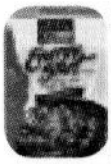

Back to Nature (Cont)	C	F	Cb
Heart Basics:			
Banana Nut Multibran, ¾ cup 1.9oz	170	1.5	46
Flax & Fiber Crunch, ¾ cup 1.8 oz	180	2.5	37
Hi-Fiber Multibran, ¾ cup 1.7oz	140	1	40
Organic Apple Cinn. Harvest, ¾ c.	180	1.5	45
Barbara's Bakery			
Brown Rice Crisps, 1 cup, 1.1 oz	120	1	25
Corn Flakes, 1 cup, 1.1 oz	110	1	25
Crispy Wheats, ¾ c., 1.1 oz	110	0.5	25
Honey Crunch'n Oats. 1 c. 2 oz	210	3	48
Organic O's, avg., ¾ cup, 1 oz	120	2	24
Wild Puffs, avg. all flavors, 1 c., 1½ oz	170	1.5	35
Puffins: Original, 1 cup, 1½ oz	135	1.5	36
Cinnamon, 1 c., 1¾ oz	175	1.5	45
Honey Rice, 1 c., 1½ oz	180	2	37
Peanut Butter, 1 c., 1½ oz	165	3	34
Shredded Oats:			
Cinnamon Crunch, 1 cup, 2 oz	230	3	43
Bite Size: 1¼ cup, 2.1 oz	220	2.5	46
Vanilla Almond, 1 cup, 2 oz	220	3	42
Ultima Organic:			
Flax & Granola, 1 cup, 2 oz	210	3	43
High Fiber, 1 cup, 2 oz	180	2	48
Pomegranate,1 cup, 2 oz	200	2	48
Bob's Red Mill			
Heartland's Ceros, Gluten-Free:			
Original Flavored, 1 cup, dry	120	0	24
Cinnamon Flavored, 1 cup, dry	110	0	23
Breadshop Granola:			
Triple Berry Crunch, ⅔ cup	210	8	34
Cinnamon Raisin ½ cup, 1.9oz	220	6	37
Crunchy Oat Bran w. Alm., ½ cup	210	8.5	31
Honey Gone Nuts, ½ cup, 1.8oz	240	10	33
Mocha Almond Crunch, ½ c., 1.7oz	210	7	34
Pralines 'n Cream, ½ cup, 1.7oz	210	7	34
Raspberry 'n Crm, ½ cup, 1.8oz	220	7.5	34
Super Natural w. Alm.,½ cup	220	9	31
Triple Berry Crunch, ½ cup 1.8oz	220	7	36
Vermont Maple, ½ cup 1.8oz	210	7	33
Cascadian Farms			
Honey Nut O's, 1 cup, 1 oz	120	2	24
Multi-Grain Squares, ¾ c., 1 oz	110	1	25
Oats & Honey Granola, ⅔ c., 2 oz	230	6	42
Purely O's, 1 cup, 1.1oz	110	2	22
Hearty Morning, ¾ cup, 1.9 oz	200	3	43
Raisin Bran, 1 cup, 1.9 oz	180	1	43
Dr McDougall's, Muesli, 1½ oz	160	2	31
Ener-G: Crumbles, ¼ cup, 1.1 oz	100	3	16
Rice Bran, ½ cup, 2.4 oz	220	14	34

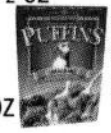

Ready-To-Eat (Cont)

	C	F	Cb
Erewhon			
Aztec, 1 cup, 1 oz	110	0	26
Corn Flakes, 1¼ cups, 2 oz	210	2.5	45
Crispy Brown Rice: 1 cup, 1 oz	110	0	25
w. Mixed Berries, 1 cup,1 oz	120	0.5	27
Gluten Free, 1 cup, 1 oz	110	0.5	25
No Salt Added, 1 cup, 1 oz	110	0	25
Kamut Flakes, ⅔ cup, 1.2 oz	110	0	25
Raisin Bran, 1 cup, 1.8 oz	170	1	40
Rice Twice, ¾ cup, 1 oz	120	0	26
General Mills			
Basic 4, 1 cup, 1.9 oz	210	3	44
Boo Berry, 1 cup, 1.1 oz	130	1	29
Cheerios: *Per ¾ Cup*			
Apple Cinnamon, 1 oz	120	1.5	25
Berry Burst, all flavors, 1 oz	100	1	22
Frosted, 1 oz	110	1	23
Fruity, 1 oz	100	1	23
Honey Nut, 1 oz	110	1.5	22
Multi Grain, 1 cup, 1 oz	110	1	23
Oat Cluster Crunch, 1.1 oz	110	1	22
Original, 1 cup, 1 oz	100	2	20
Yogurt Burst, all flavors, 1 oz	120	1.5	24
Chex: Corn, 1 cup, 1 oz	120	0.5	26
Chocolate, ¾ cup, 1.1 oz	130	2.5	25
Honey Nut, ¾ cup, 1.1 oz	120	0.5	28
Multi-Bran, ¾ cup, 1.1 oz	160	1.5	39
Rice, 1 cup, 1 oz	100	0.5	23
Strawberry, ¾ cup, 1.1 oz	130	2	26
Wheat, ¾ cup, 1.7 oz	160	1	38
Cinnamon Tst Crunch, ¾ c., 1 oz	130	3	25
Cocoa Puffs, ¾ cup, 1 oz	110	1.5	23
Count Chocula, ¾ cup, 1 oz	100	1	22
Country Corn Flakes, 1 cup, 1.1 oz	120	0.5	28
Fiber One, ½ cup, 1 oz	60	1	15
Fiber One Honey Clusters, 1¼ cup	160	1.5	42
French Toast Crunch, ¾ c., 1 oz	130	3	24
Golden Grahams, ¾ cup, 1 oz	120	1	26
Honey Nut Clusters, 1 cup, 2 oz	210	1	49
Kix: 1¼ cup, 1.1 oz	110	1	25
Berry Berry, ¾ cup, 1 oz	100	1.5	22
Lucky Charms, avg., ¾ cup, 1 oz	110	1	22
Oatmeal Crisp, Almond, 1 c., 2 oz	240	4.5	47
Raisin Nut Bran, 1¼ cups, 2 oz	180	3	38
Reese's Puffs, ¾ cup, 1 oz	120	3	22
Total: Honey Clusters, ¾ cup, 1.7 oz	170	1.5	37
Raisin Bran, 1 cup,	160	1	40
Trix, avg., 0.63 oz pkt	110	1.5	21
Wheaties, ¾ cup, 1 oz	100	0.5	22

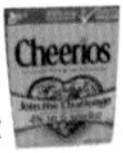

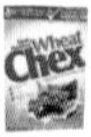

	C	F	Cb
Health Valley			
Organic Flakes:			
Amaranth Flakes, ¾ cup, 1 oz	100	0	23
Corn Flakes, ¾ cup, 1.1 oz	110	1	24
Cranberry Crunch, ¾ cup, 1.8 oz	190	4	38
Fiber 7, Multigrain Flakes, 1 c., 1.7 oz	160	1	37
Golden Flax, ¾ cup, 1.8 oz	190	3	38
Oat Bran Flakes: ¾ cup, 1 oz	110	1	19
w. Raisins, ¾ cup, 1 oz	110	0.5	23
Crunch-Ems!, avg., 1 cup, 1 oz	110	0	27
Granola, ⅔ cup, 2 oz	190	2	42
Heart Wise, 1 cup, 2 oz	200	3	37
Heartland			
Granola: Original, ½ cup, 2 oz	240	6	40
Low-Fat Raisin, ½ cup, 1¾ oz	200	3	40
Jewel			
Cornflakes, 1 cup, 1 oz	100	0	24
Crunchy Wheat & Barley, ½ c., 1.7 oz	170	1	38
Nutty Nuggets, ½ cup, 1.7 oz	170	1	38
Oats & Flakes w. Honey, ¾ c., 1.1 oz	130	1	27
Kashi			
7 Whole Grain: Flakes, 1 cup, 1.8 oz	180	1	41
Honey Puff, 1 cup, 1.1 oz	120	1	25
Nuggets, ½ cup, 2 oz	210	1.5	47
Pilaf, ½ cup, cooked	170	3	30
Puffs, 1 cup, ½ oz	70	0.5	15
Kashi U, 1 cup, 2 oz	200	3.5	42
GoLEAN: 1 cup, 1.8 oz	140	1	30
Creamy Truly Vanilla, 1 pkt, 40g	150	2	25
GoLean Crunch! Orig., 1 c., 1.9 oz	190	3	36
Honey Almond Flax, 1 cup, 1.9 oz	200	5	34
Good Friends: 1 cup, 1.9 oz	170	2	43
Cinna-Raisin Crunch, 1 c., 1.8 oz	170	1.5	41
Granola: Cocoa Beach, ½ cup, 2 oz	230	9	33
Mountain Medley, ½ cup, 2 oz	220	7	37
Orchard Spice, ½ cup, 1.9 oz	220	7	37
Summer Berry, ½ cup, 2 oz	210	6	37
Heart to Heart:			
Honey Toasted Oat, ¾ cup, 1.2 oz	110	1.5	25
Oat Flakes & Blueb. Clusters, ¼ c	200	2.5	42
Oatmeal, avg. all flav., 1.5 oz pkg	160	2	33
Mighty Bites, Honey Cr., 1 c., 1.2 oz	110	1.5	23
Organic Promise:			
Autumn Wheat, 1 cup, 1.9 oz	190	1	45
Cinnamon Harvest, 1 cup, 1.9 oz	190	1	44
Strawberry Fields, 1 cup, 1.1 oz	120	0	28
Vive Probiotic, 1¼ cup, 2 oz	170	2.5	43

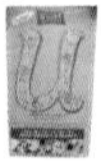

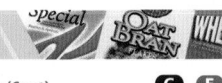

B — Breakfast Cereals

Ready-To-Eat (Cont)

	C	F	Cb
Kellogg's			
All-Bran: Bran Buds, ⅓ cup, 1.1 oz	70	1	24
Complete Wheat Flakes, ¾ c., 1.1 oz	90	0.5	23
Extra Fiber, ½ cup, 0.9 oz	50	1	20
Original, ½ cup, 1.1 oz	80	1	23
Strawberry Medley, 1 cup, 1.9 oz	170	1.5	44
Yogurt Bites, 1¼ cups, 2 oz	190	3	44
Apple Jacks, 1 cup, 1.2 oz	120	0.5	28
Berry Krispies, 1 cup	120	0	27
Cereal Straws, all flav. (3), 1.1 oz	140	3.5	24
Cocoa Krispies, ¾ cup, 1.1 oz	120	1	27
Complete, Oat Bran Flakes, ¾ cup	110	1	23
Corn Flakes, Original, 1 cup, 1 oz	100	0	24
Corn Pops, 1 cup, 1 oz	120	0	28
Cracklin' Oat Bran, ¾ cup, 1.8 oz	200	7	35
Crispix, Original, 1 c., 1 oz	110	0.5	25
Crunch: Caramel Nut, 1¼ cups	210	3.5	41
Raisin Bran, 1 cup, 1.9 oz	190	1	45
Toasted Honey, 1¼ cups, 2 oz	220	1.5	50
Froot Loops: Original, 1 cup, 1.1 oz	120	1	26
Reduced Sugar, 1¼ c.	120	1	28
Grab'N Go Pack, 1 pouch	90	0.5	20
Marshmallow, 1 cup, 1.1 oz	120	1	27
Frosted Flakes, 1 cup, 1 oz	110	0	27
Fruit Harvest, Banana Berry, ¾ cup	120	2	25
Granola, Low-Fat:			
with Raisins, ⅔ cup, 2.1 oz	230	3	49
without Raisins, ½ cup, 1.7 oz	190	2.5	40
Honey Smacks, ¾ cup, 1 oz	100	0.5	24
Mini Swirlz Cinnamon Bun, 1 cup	120	2	25
Mini-Wheats: Frosted Big Bite (5)	180	1	41
Frosted Bite Size (24), 2.1 oz	200	1	48
Frosted Vanilla Creme (24), 1.8 oz	180	1	43
Unfrosted (30), 2.1 oz	200	1.5	46
Mueslix, ⅔ cup, 2 oz	200	3	40
Nutri-Grain Bars: *See Page 33*			
Pops, Choc. P'nut Butter, 1 c., 1¼ oz	160	4	28
Product 19, 1 cup, 1 oz	100	0	25
Raisin Bran: Regular, 1 c., 2.1 oz	190	1.5	45
Rice Krispies: Orig, 1¼ cup, 1.1 oz	120	0	29
Berry, 1 cup, 1.1 oz	120	0	27
Frosted, ¾ cup, 1.1 oz	110	0	27
Cocoa, ¾ cup, 1.1 oz	120	1	27
with Strawb., 1 c., 1.1 oz	110	0	27
Treats, ¾ cup, 1.1 oz	120	1.5	26
Smart Start:			
Healthy Heart, avg., 1 c., 1¼ cup, 2.1 oz	190	2.5	38
	230	3	46
Antioxidants, 1 c., 1¾ oz	190	0.5	43
Smorz, 1 cup, 1.1 oz	120	2	25

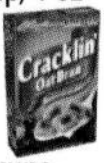

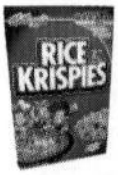

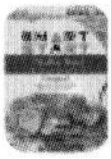

	C	F	Cb
Kellogg's (Cont)			
Special K: Original 1 cup, 1.1 oz	120	0.5	22
Fruit & Yogurt, ¾ cup, 1.1 oz	120	1	27
Low Carb Lifestyle, ¾ cup, 1 oz	100	3	14
Red Berries, 1 cup, 1.1 oz	110	0	25
Vanilla Almond, ¾ cup	110	1.5	25
Grab'N Go, avg., 1 pouch	100	1	22
Malt-O-Meal			
Apple Zings, 1 cup, 1.1 oz	130	1	30
Blueb. Muffin Tops, ⅔ cup, 1.1 oz	130	3.5	24
Coco Roos, ¾ cup, 1.1 oz	120	1.5	26
Colossal Crunch, ¾ cup, 1.1 oz	120	1.5	26
Dyno-Bites, ¾ cup, 1 oz	110	0.5	27
Frosted Flakes, ¾ cup, 1.1 oz	120	0	28
Frosted Mini Spooners, 1 c., 1.9 oz	190	1	45
Golden Puffs, ¾ cup, 1 oz	110	0	24
Raisin Bran, 1 cup, 1.7 oz	220	1.5	49
Mother's			
Bumpers: Cocoa, 1 cup, 1.2 oz	120	0.5	29
Grahams, ¾ cup, 1 oz	100	1	24
Honey Round-Ups, ¾ cup, 1 oz	110	0.5	25
Oat & Honey Granola, ¾ cup, 2½ oz	315	9	52
Peanut Butter, 1 cup 1.2 oz	130	2.5	24
Nature's Path			
Corn Flakes, all types, ¾ cup, 1 oz	110	1	24
Flax Plus Multibran, ¾ cup, 1 oz	110	1.5	23
Heritage, all types, ¾ cup, 1 oz	110	1	23
Multigr. Oatbran Flakes, ¾ c., 1 oz	110	1	24
Toaster Pastries (1), 1.83 oz, avg.	210	4.5	39
Granola: Ginger Zing; Hemp, 1 oz	140	5	21
Pumpkin Flax Plus, ½ cup, 1 oz	150	3.5	21
Average, other varieties	135	4	21
Kamut Crisp Flakes, ¾ c.	100	0.5	23
Power Breakfast, 1 cup	190	2.5	40
Koala Crisp, ⅔ cup	120	0.5	26
Gorilla Munch, ¾ cup, 1 oz	115	1	26
New England Natural Bakers			
Muesli, ½ cup, 2.1 oz	220	5	40
Granola: Almond Raisin Crisp, ½ c.	220	9	36
Apple Sunrise, ½ cup	210	7	34
Berry Good, ⅔ cup, 2.1 oz	250	6	44
Grateful Date, ½ cup, 1.7 oz	210	7	33
Honey Crunch; Pecan, ½ cup	285	13	37
Low-Fat Granola, ½ cup, 1.7 oz	200	2.5	41
Save The Forest: Chocolate Mix	160	10	18
Fruit & Nut Mix, ½ cup, 2.1 oz	270	12	35
Nut Granola, ½ cup, 2.1 oz	270	12	35
Granola: Absolutely Nuts, ⅔ cup	220	9	30
Raspberry Razzmatazz, ¾ cup	250	9	37

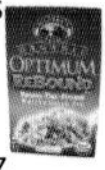

Ready-To-Eat (Cont)

	C	F	Cb
New Morning			
Cocoa Crispy Rice, ¾ cup, 1 oz	**120**	0.5	26
Cocomotion, ¾ cup, 1 oz	**100**	0.5	22
Fruit-e-O's, Organic, 1 cup, 1 oz	**120**	1.5	25
Oatios: Original, 1 cup, 1 oz	**110**	2	22
Apple Cinn/Honey Almond, 1 oz	**120**	1	17
NutriSystem: *Per Package*			
Granola, Low-Fat	**160**	2.5	31
NutriCinnamon Squares	**120**	1	22
NutriFlakes (40% Bran Flakes)	**110**	1	23
NutriFrosted Crunch	**110**	1	19
Oatmeal, Apple Cinnamon	**150**	1.5	28
Peace			
Banana Nut Rainforest, 1 cup, 2 oz	**220**	7	36
Essential 10, 1 cup, 2 oz	**170**	3	35
Granola, avg. all flavors, ⅔ cup	**240**	6	40
Hearty Raisin Bran, 1 cp, 2 oz	**180**	2	43
Maple Pecan; Vanilla Alm., 1 c. 2 oz	**210**	5	39
Post			
Alpha Bits, No Sugar, 1 cup	**110**	2	22
Bran Flakes, ¾ cup	**100**	0.5	24
CarbWell: Cinnamon Crunch	**110**	2	14
Golden Crunch, 1/10 package	**110**	1	14
Grape-Nuts, 2 oz	**200**	1	48
Grape-Nuts Flakes, ½ cup	**110**	1	24
Honey Bunches of Oats, 1.1 oz	**120**	1.5	25
Just Bunches: Caramel, ⅔ cup	**250**	7	43
Honey, Rstd, ⅔ cup	**250**	7	43
Live Active Crunch:			
Mixed Berry, 1 c. 2 oz	**190**	1.5	43
Nut Harvest, 2 oz	**210**	7	38
Oreo O's w. Marshmallow, ¾ cup	**110**	2	22
Pebbles: Cocoa, ¾ cup, 1.1 oz	**110**	1.5	26
Fruity, ¾ cup, 1.1 oz	**110**	1	26
Raisin Bran, 1 cup, 2.1 oz	**190**	1	46
Selects: Banana Nut Crunch 2.1 oz	**240**	6	44
Cranberry Almd Crunch, 1 cup	**200**	3.5	39
Great Grains, Crunchy Pecan, ⅔ c.	**220**	6	38
Shredded Wheat, Orig., 2 biscuits	**160**	1	37
Trail Mix Crunch, avg., 1.7 oz	**180**	3	37
Quaker			
100% Natural Granola: ½ cup, 1.8 oz	**220**	6.5	37
w. Raisins, ½ c., 1.8 oz	**215**	6	38
Low-Fat: ⅔ cup	**215**	3	45
Oat Bran, ½ cup, 1.4 oz	**150**	3	25
Oatmeal Squares, 1 cup	**210**	2.5	44
Captain Crunch: Regular, ¾ cup, 1 oz	**110**	1.5	23
Crunch Berries, ¾ cup, 1 oz	**100**	1.5	22
Peanut Butter, ¾ oz, 1 oz	**110**	2.5	21

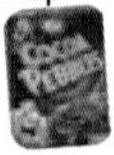

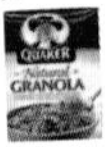

	C	F	Cb
Quaker (Cont)			
Crunchy Corn Bran, 1 c., 1 oz	**90**	2.5	23
Honey Graham Oh's, ¾ c.	**110**	2	23
King Vitaman, 1 c., 1.1 oz	**120**	1	26
Life, all types, ¾ c., 1.1 oz	**120**	1.5	26
Instant Oatmeal: *See Page 59*			
Bars: *See Page 33*			
Sweet Home Farm			
Honey Nut Granola, ½ cup, 1.9 oz	**200**	7	34
Low-Fat Granola, ½ cup, 1.9 oz	**180**	3	38
Trader Joe's			
Clusters: Raisin Bran, 1 cup, 3 oz	**300**	4	63
Super Nutty Toffee, 1 cup, 3 oz	**370**	13	57
Avg. all other flavors			
⅔ cup, 2 oz	**230**	6	38
1 cup, 3 oz	**340**	9	57
Cornflakes, 1 cup, 1.1 oz	**110**	0	26
Golden Flax Cereal, ¾ cup, 1.7 oz	**200**	3.5	37
Granola, avg., ⅔ cup, 2 oz	**240**	8	37
High Fiber Cereal, ⅔ cup, 1.1 oz	**80**	0.5	23
Honey Nut O's, ¾ cup, 1 oz	**120**	1.5	24
Joe's O's, 1 cup, 1 oz	**110**	1.5	22
Morning Lite, 1 cup, 1.4 oz	**130**	2	32
Shredded Wheats, 1 cup, 1.7 oz	**180**	1	38
Soy Flax Clusters, 1 cup	**190**	3	38
Triple Berry O's, ¾ cup, 1 oz	**110**	1	25
Toasted Oatmeal Flakes, ¾ c., 1.1 oz	**110**	1	23
Wheats, avg., 1 cup, 2 oz	**200**	1	42
Udi's, Granola, Au Naturel, ½ c., 2 oz	**240**	8	38
Uncle Sam			
Cereal w. Real Mixed Berries, 1 cup	**190**	4.5	39
Original, ¾ cup, 1.5 oz	**190**	5	38
Weetabix: 2 biscuits, 1.3 oz	**120**	1	28
Crispy Flakes: ¾ cup, 1.1 oz	**110**	0.5	24
& Fiber, 1¼ cup, 2 oz	**170**	1.5	44
Weight Watchers			
Banana Almond Medley, ¾ cup	**170**	3	31
Cinnamon Cluster Crunch, ¾ cup	**150**	1	32
Flakes'n Fiber, ½ cup, 1.1 oz	**90**	2	17
Honey Almond Crisp, ¾ cup, 1½ oz	**140**	2	32
Puffed Vanilla Wheat, 1 cup, 1.1 oz	**110**	0.5	25
Whole Foods (365)			
Corn Flakes, 1 cup, 1 oz	**100**	0	24
Honey Puffed Wheat, 1 oz	**110**	0	26
Frosted Flakes, ¾ c., 1 oz	**110**	0	26
Oat Bran Flakes, 1 c., 2 oz	**220**	3	45
Raisin Bran, 1 cup, 2 oz	**210**	1	44
Shredded Wheat, 1 cup, 1.7 oz	**180**	1	32
Frosted, 1 cup, 2 oz	**210**	1	45

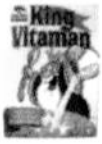

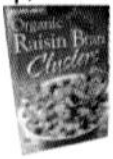

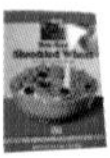

C Cakes, Pastries ~ Ready to Eat

Ready-to-Eat

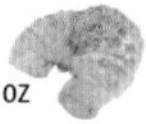
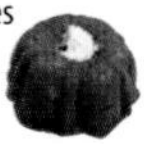
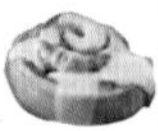
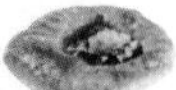

Ready-to-Eat	C	F	Cb
Angel Food: Plain, no oil, 2 oz	145	0	33
Plain with oil, 2 oz	145	1	27
w. Cream Frosting	255	7	45
Almond Croissant, 5 oz	620	35	67
Apple Danish, 5 oz	450	18	67
Apple Pie: *See Pies/Tarts Page 136*			
Baklava, 1½" square, 1.75 oz	200	10	27
Banana w. Butter Cream, 2 oz	230	9	37
Banana Walnut, 3 oz	270	11	40
Bear Claw, 4½ oz	540	24	71
Black Forest, 3 oz (1/12)	345	11	59
Brownie: Small, 2" Square, 1 oz	130	8	14
Large, 3 oz	390	24	42
Bundt, average all types			
1 slice 3 oz (1/10)	300	13	42
Mini-Bundt, 5 oz	500	22	70
Cannoli	375	17	44
Carrot Cake: Plain, 3 oz	300	16	37
w. Cream Cheese Frosting	400	22	48
Cheesecake: Small serving, 3 oz	235	13	26
Large serving, 5 oz	395	21	44
w. Low-Fat Cheese/Fruit, 3 oz	170	4	28
Cheesecake Factory: 1 slice	630	45	53
Denny's Cheesecake, 1 slice	580	38	51
Chocolate Cake:			
Plain, no frosting, 1/12 of 9", 3½ oz	340	14	51
with chocolate frosting, 4 oz	415	18	62
Chocolate Croissant, 4¼ oz	470	26	54
Chocolate Eclair w. Custard, 3½ oz	260	16	24
Chocolate Fudge Cake, 3 oz	270	12	40
Chocolate Meringue, 1/6 pie	320	13	48
Churros, 1 stick, 1½ oz	125	5	18
Cinnamon Crumb Cake, 2½ oz	260	9	40
Cinnamon Roll: Small, 2 oz	220	8	34
Regular, 4 oz	440	16	68
Large, 6 oz	660	24	102
Brands ~ *See Page 69*			
Coffee Cake, 2 oz	180	6	30
Concha: Small, 2 oz	240	9	33
Large (5" diameter), 5½ oz	615	23	85
Cream Puff (custard fill), 4.6 oz	335	20	30
Creme Horns, each, 3 oz	210	5	36
Crumble Coffee Cake, 4½ oz	500	25	65
Danish Pastry:			
Small, 2½ oz	250	14	25
Large, 5 oz	500	28	50
Donuts: *See Page 68*			
Eclair, Choc., Cust. fill, 3½ oz	260	16	24
Fig Bars, average, each	160	3	31

Ready-to-Eat (Cont)

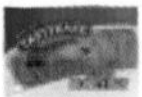
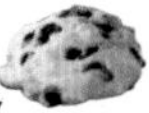
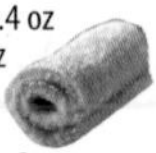

Ready-to-Eat (Cont)	C	F	Cb
Fruit Cake, Dark/Light, 2 oz	185	5	34
Fudge Nut Brownie, each, 3½ oz	380	18	54
Gingerbread: From mix, 3" sq.	210	4	41
Honey Bun, each, 2.7 oz	310	15	39
Jelly Roll, 1/12 roll, 1.8 oz	150	2	32
Key Lime Pie, 4.3 oz	400	25	41
Kolacky, Apricot/Rasp., ½ oz (1)	60	3.5	8
Lady Fingers, 3 oz	310	4.5	59
Lemon Cake, 4 oz	440	24	49
Lemon Poppy Seed Creme, 1.6 oz	180	9	23
Marble Cake, 1 slice, 4 oz	430	23	50
Mississippi Mud Pie, 4 oz	480	22	67
Mud Cake, 1 piece, 4½ oz	380	20	44
Muffins: *See Page 69*			
Palmier Cookie, large, 4½ oz	490	25	62
Pineapple Upside Down, 2½ oz	230	9	36
Peach Melba, 3½ oz	300	8	52
Pecan Sticky Roll, 6½ oz	690	22	91
Pecan Twirls, 1 piece, 1.3 oz	170	7	26
Pies & Tarts: *See Page 136*			
Pound Cake, 3 oz	330	17	40
Raspberry Rugulah,			
1 pce, 1.2 oz	110	9	7
Scone, fruit, 2 oz	200	9	30
Sponge: Plain, 2½ oz	220	10	33
w. Cream & Strawberry Jam	390	12	69
w. Chocolate Frosting	290	12	45
Strawberry Creme, 4.7 oz	400	27	33
Strudel Bites, ¾ oz	60	2.5	9
Strudel, fruit, avg., 4.4 oz	300	17	32
Sweet Roll, avg., 1½ oz	150	6	23
Swiss Rolls, (2)	270	12	38
Tiramisu, 4.4 oz	440	22	34
Turnovers, fruit, avg., 3 oz	290	15	35

Cupcakes

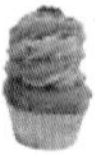
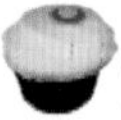
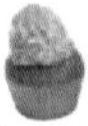

Cupcakes	C	F	Cb
Average all Varieties			
Regular:			
Cake only, 1½ oz	140	5.5	20
Cake + Icing, 2½ oz	260	13	34
Large *(Muffin Size):*			
Cake only, 2½ oz	235	9	34
Cake + Icing, 5 oz	520	27	67
Mini (2-Bite):			
Cake only, 0.4 oz	40	1.5	5.5
Cake + Icing, 1 oz	110	5.5	13
Icing Only: Per 1 oz	115	7	13
Thick/Tall amount, 2½ oz	290	17	32
Starbucks Cupcakes:			
Triple Chocolate, 3¼ oz	360	20	46
Vanilla, 3 oz	320	16	43

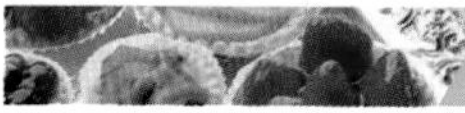

Cakes ~ Brands

	C	F	Cb
Albertson's Bakery			
Butter Ring Cake, ⅛, 3 oz	**310**	16	39
Sock it to me Ring Cake, ⅛, 3 oz	**290**	12	42
Cake Slices: *Per Slice (1½ oz)*			
Cinnamon Butter Streusel Creme	**140**	9	20
Butter Creme Cake	**110**	6	20
Lemon Creme Cake	**130**	9	19
Blueberry Creme Cake	**120**	8	18
Bimbo			
Concha, avg., 2.1 oz	**240**	9	33
Homestyle Pound Cake, 2.6 oz	**300**	15	37
Pecan Pound Cake, 2.9 oz	**330**	16	41
Raisin Pound Cake, 2.9 oz	**340**	16	43
Buon Appetite			
Sliced: Cheesecake, 4 oz	**440**	24	49
Lemon Cake; Pound Cake, 4 oz	**440**	24	49
Marble Cake, 4 oz	**430**	23	50
Walnut Brownie, 3.5 oz	**380**	18	54
Cheese Coffee Cake, 2.2 oz	**270**	15	31
Banana Bread	**450**	25	49
Claim Jumper: Carrot Cake, 4.6 oz	**450**	24	54
Choc. Motherload Cake, 5.3 oz	**520**	27	73
Cheesecake Factory: *See Fast-Foods Section*			
Entenmann's			
All Butter Loaf, ⅙ loaf, 2 oz	**220**	10	31
Cheese-Filled Crumb Coffee, 2 oz	**200**	9	25
Chocolate Fudge, ⅙ cake, 3 oz	**270**	12	40
Coffee Cake, Cheese Topped, ⅑, 2 oz	**200**	9	26
Gourmet Cinn. Rolls, ½ roll	**220**	8	34
Louisiana Crunch, ⅑, 3 oz	**330**	15	47
Pecan Danish Ring, ⅛ cake	**250**	15	26
Raspberry Danish Twist, ⅛ cake	**220**	11	28
Enten-Minis: Brownie Frosters, 1.8 oz	**230**	10	32
Caramel & Creme Squares, 1 oz	**135**	7	19
Carrot Cakes, 1½ oz	**160**	7	22
Chocolate ½ Rounds 1 oz	**140**	7	18
Chocolate Rounds, 2 oz	**290**	14	40
Napolean, 2 oz	**270**	14	34
Roundabouts, 1 oz	**115**	6	15
Muffins/Sweet Rolls: *See Page 69*			
Hostess: *Per Cake Unless Indicated*			
100 Calorie Packs,			
Coffee Cakes, Muffins, avg.	**100**	3	20
Cinnamon Streudel Cake (1)	**170**	5	29
Chocodiles	**230**	11	36
Cup Cake (1), 45g	**190**	9	26

Hostess (Cont)	C	F	Cb
Ding Dongs (1)	**180**	9	23
Ho Ho's, each	**125**	6	18
Pound Cake, 1½ oz	**150**	7	20
Shortcake (1)	**110**	2	21
Snoballs (1)	**170**	5	32
Suzy Q , 2 cakes, 4 oz	**440**	17	70
Twinkies, 1 cake, 1.5 oz	**150**	4.5	27
Fried Twinkie *(Page 175)*			
Zingers:			
Raspberry (1)	**160**	7	24
3-Pack, 4.5 oz	**480**	20	71
Chocolate (1)	**150**	5	25
Vanilla (1)	**160**	5	27
Little Debbie			
Boston Crème Rolls (1), 2.2 oz	**270**	12	40
Brownies (1)	**290**	13	40
Choc Chip Snack Cake (2), 2.4 oz	**300**	14	42
Chocolate Cup Cake	**190**	9	26
Coffee Cakes (1)	**200**	6	35
Devil Cremes (1) 1.65 oz	**200**	9	29
Devil Squares, 2 cakes, 2.2 oz	**270**	12	38
Fancy Cakes (2)	**310**	15	43
Frosted Fudge , 1.5 oz cake	**190**	9	26
Orange Cup Cake (1)	**210**	10	29
Smores (1)	**190**	7	30
Strawberry Shortcake Rolls, 2.1 oz	**240**	9	39
Swiss Cake Rolls, 2 cakes	**270**	12	38
Zebra Cakes, 2 cakes, 2.6 oz	**320**	14	48
Mrs Smith's			
Butter Pound Cake, ¼ cake	**290**	14	38
Carrot Cake, ⅙ cake	**300**	16	37
Cinnabon Cinn. Pecan Coffee Cake, ⅙	**270**	17	25
Mrs Smith's Heavenly 100:			
Chocolate Cake, 1 pce	**100**	4	15
Mousse, 1 cup	**100**	3	17
Nemo's			
Banana Cake, 3 oz	**300**	12	45
Chocolate Cake, 3 oz	**290**	12	44
Carrot Cake, 3.6 oz	**380**	20	46
Zucchini Cake, 3.6 oz	**400**	21	47
Nilla			
Caksters, 3-Pack, 2.65 oz	**330**	15	49

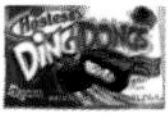

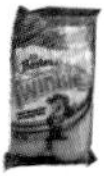
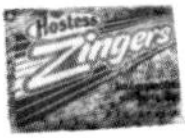

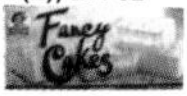

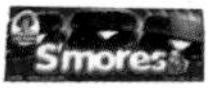

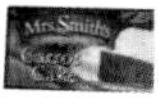

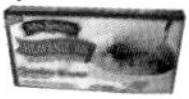
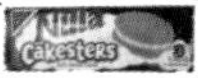

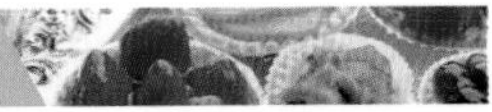

Cakes ~ Brands (Cont)

Oreo	C	F	Cb
Cakesters			
2 cake pkg, 2 oz	250	12	36
Pepperidge Farm			
Turnovers (Frozen): Apple, 3.2 oz	290	15	36
Raspberry, 3.2 oz	290	15	35
3-Layer Cakes:			
Coconut, ⅛, 2.5 oz	240	10	35
Chocolate Fudge, ⅛ cake, 2.5 oz	230	10	33
Golden, ⅛ cake, 2.5 oz	230	9	34
Apple Dumpling	250	11	33
Peach Dumpling	320	11	50
Rich's: Mini Eclairs (7)	335	21	32
Mini Creme Puffs (6)	290	24	15
Safeway Select			
Molten Chocolate Lava Cake, 4½ oz	440	26	50
Sara Lee (Frozen)			
Cheesecake: *Per Slice*			
French Classic, ⅕ cake	410	25	41
French Strawberry, ⅙	320	14	43
New York Style Classic, ⅙ cake	350	21	35
Original Cream Cherry, ¼ cake	350	12	55
Original Cream Classic, ¼ cake	340	18	38
Original Cream Strawberry, ¼ cake	330	12	49
Coffee Cakes: *Per Slice*			
Butter Streusel, ⅙ cake	190	9	24
Crumb Cake, ⅛ cake	190	8	30
Deluxe Cinnamon Rolls w. Icing (1)	320	15	41
Pecan Cake, ⅙ cake	140	13	23
Layer Cakes: *Per ⅛ Whole*			
Layer Coconut, ⅛ cake	260	14	33
Layer Double Chocolate, ⅛ cake	260	13	33
Layer Fudge Golden, ⅛ cake	260	13	34
Layer Vanilla, ⅛ cake	260	14	32
Pound Cakes: *Per ¼ Whole*			
All Butter, 2.6 oz, ⅙ cake	220	15	34
Free & Light	200	4	39
Strawberry Swirl	290	11	44
Bites: *Per Serving*			
Choc. Dipped Orig. Cheesecake	100	7	8
Choc. Dipped Praline Pecan (5)	90	6	8
Triple Choc. Fudge Brownie (1)	90	4	1

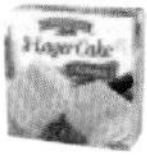

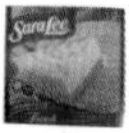

Smart Ones (Weight Watchers)	C	F	Cb
Brownie à la Mode	200	4	36
Carrot Cake (1) 1 oz	80	2.5	16
Chocolate Cake (1) 1 oz	80	3	15
Chocolate Mousse	180	4	28
Chocolate Eclair	140	4	24
Choc. Chip Cookie Dough Sundae	170	3	32
Double Fudge Cake	220	7	35
Key Lime Cheesecake, 2½ oz	150	5	20
Key Lime Pie, 3.3 oz	190	4.5	33
Lemon Cake (1) 1 oz	80	2.5	14
Mint Choc Chip Sundae, 2½ oz	150	3	28
Mocha Fudge Sundae, 2½ oz	160	4	27
New York Style Cheesecake	150	5	21
Strawberry Shortcake, 3½ oz	170	6	25
Tastykake: Chocolate Jnr, 3.3 oz	340	12	55
Creme Filled Koffee Kakes, 3 oz	390	19	51
Koffee Kake Junior, 2.53 oz	270	10	42
Trader Joe's			
Bakery: Apricot Tea Loaf 2 oz	160	2	34
Choc Bundt Cake, 1/12 cake	340	21	34
Mini Bundt Cake, ½ cake	190	4	35
Marble Tea Loaf, ⅛, 2 oz	160	2.5	31
Mini Carrot Cake, 5 oz	400	16	58
Cupcakes: Chocolate, 3.2 oz	430	23	54
Vanilla, 3 oz	400	20	52
Frozen Dessert:			
Cheesecake Brownie Bites (1)	110	7	9
Choc Celebration Cake, 2.8 oz	270	11	42
Choc Lava Cake, 1/10, cake, 3.8 oz	360	23	40
Karat Cake, ⅛ cake, 3 oz	320	19	37
Low-Fat Cranb. Orange Brd, 2 oz	160	2	33
Mango Passion Exotique, ⅛, 1.9 oz	150	8	18
N.Y Style Cheesecake, ⅐, 4½ oz	400	28	32
Old Fash'd Cheesecake, 1/12, 4.6 oz	470	29	40
Peppermint Cheesecake, ⅙ cake	310	19	30
Tiramisu, ⅛ cake, 2.2 oz	220	11	17
Tiramisu Torte, ⅐ cake, 3.2 oz	230	12	24
Van de Kamp's			
Angle Food Ring, ⅛ cake	130	0	29
Banana Square Cake, ¼ cake	410	18	60
Bear Claw, 1 pce, 2 oz	250	14	26
Carrot Square Cake, ¼ cake	520	33	54
Cinn. Raisin Danish, 1 pce, 2 oz	230	11	32
Crumb Cake, ⅛ cake, 2.5 oz	330	18	39
Fruit Danish, 1 pce, 2 oz	220	11	28
German Chocolate Cake, ¼ cake	290	16	36

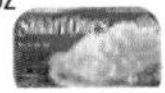

Cakes ~ Mixes

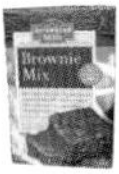
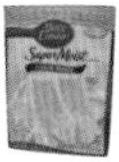
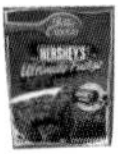
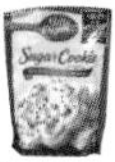

Made As Directed	C	F	Cb
Arrowhead Mills			
Choc Chip	**90**	3	16
Cookie (1), avg. all types	**100**	4	16
Oatmeal Raisin	**90**	2	16
Wheat Free Brownie, 1/20 pkg	**160**	7.5	21
Banquet			
Dessert Bakes: *Per Serving*			
Apple Crisp, ⅙ pkg	**220**	4	44
Chocolate Lava Cake, ⅐ pkg	**370**	7	73
Cherry Cobbler, ⅙ pkg	**250**	4	53
Peach Cobbler, ⅙ pkg	**240**	3.5	51
Betty Crocker			
Cakes (Super Moist): *Per 1/12 Cake*			
Butter Recipe Yellow	**240**	12	35
Chocolate varieties	**240**	12	33
Cinnamon Swirl	**280**	11	42
Devil's Food	**270**	14	33
White	**230**	10	33
Other flavors, average	**270**	13	35
Per 1/10 Cake (Prepared): Carrot	**320**	16	41
Sour Cream Cake	**280**	12	43
If using No Cholesterol Recipe, deduct 40 cals and 4g fat.			
Other Cakes: Pound Cake, ⅛	**260**	8	45
Angel Food Cake, 1/12 mix	**140**	0	32
Gingerbread Cake, ⅛	**220**	6	39
Pineapple Upside Down, ⅙	**390**	13	65
Sunkist Lemon Bar (1)	**140**	4	24
Wild Blueberry:			
Brownie Mixes: *Per 1/20 Pkg*			
Chocolate Chunk	**180**	9	25
Dark Chocolate	**170**	7	25
Fudge	**170**	9	22
Low-Fat Fudge Brownie, 1/18 cake	**130**	2.5	27
Original Supreme	**160**	5	27
Peanut Butter; Walnut, avg.	**180**	9	23
Turtle (Caramel & Pecan)	**170**	9	23
Cookie Mix: *Per 2 Cookies*			
Chocolate Chip	**170**	8	21
Double Chocolate Chunk	**150**	6	21
Oatmeal	**160**	7	22
Oatmeal Chocolate Chip	**160**	8	21
Peanut Butter	**150**	8	20
Rainbow Chocolate Candy	**160**	7	22
Sugar Cookie	**170**	8	22
Walnut Chocolate Chip	**170**	9	21

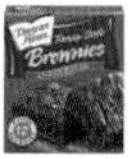
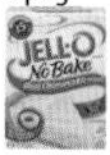
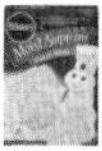

Duncan Hines	C	F	Cb
Brownie Mix: *Per 1 oz Brownie, Prepared*			
Candy Shop Peanut Butter Cup, 1 oz	**170**	8	23
Chewy Fudge/Marble Swirl	**180**	9	24
Dark/Milk Choc. Fudge	**170**	7	25
Turtle	**160**	7	23
Cake Mix: *Per 1/12 Cake*			
Angel Food Fat-Free,1.3 oz	**140**	0	30
Moist Deluxe Cake:			
Ban. Supreme/Yellow Cake, 1½ oz	**270**	12	36
Classic White, 1½ oz	**210**	6	36
Dark Choc./Devil's Food, 1½ oz	**290**	15	35
French Vanilla, 1½ oz	**250**	12	34
Jell-O No Bake Cheesecakes: *Prep'd As Directed*			
Chocolate Silk Dessert, ⅙ pkg	**290**	14	36
Homestyle Cheesecake, ⅙ pkg	**370**	17	51
Oreo, ⅙ pkg	**370**	17	51
Peanut Butter Cup, ⅛ pkg	**360**	20	42
Pumpkin Pie, ⅛ pkg	**250**	10	36
Real Cheesecake, ⅙ pkg	**350**	16	48
Krusteaz: Cinn. Crumb Cake, 1"	**230**	7	38
Lemon/Key Lime Bar, 2" bar	**160**	3.5	29
Bakery Style Cookie Mix: *Per Cookie*			
Chocolate Chip, 2½"	**140**	5.5	19
Gingerbread, ⅛ cake	**210**	3.5	41
Snickerdoodle	**130**	5	20
Pillsbury			
Moist Supreme: *Per 1/12 Cake*			
Devils Food	**260**	13	35
Pineapple, Classic Yellow	**250**	11	35
Brownie Mix: Choc. Extreme, 1/16	**160**	8	22
Funfetti, 1/12	**250**	11	36
Traditional Fudge, 1/20	**170**	8	23

Cake Frostings

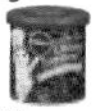

Betty Crocker			
Drizzlers, 2½ Tbsp	**220**	13	26
Rich & Creamy, average, 2 Tbsp	**140**	5	23
Whipped, all flavors, 2 Tbsp	**110**	5	15
Easy Flow Icing, 1 Tbsp	**75**	3	12
Duncan Hines: *Per 2 Tbsp (1.2 oz)*			
Creamy Homestyle, avg all flavors	**140**	6	23
Homestyle Fat-Free, 6 tbsp	**100**	0	24
Whipped, avg., 3 Tbsp	**160**	9	20
Pillsbury: *Per 2 Tbsp (approx. 1/12 Tub)*			
Creamy Supreme: Choc Fudge	**140**	6	21
Classic White	**140**	5	22
Milk Choc	**140**	6	21
Vanilla; Vanilla Funfetti	**150**	6	25
Reduced Sugar: Choc., 2 Tbsp	**120**	8	16
Vanilla, 2 Tbsp	**120**	7	18
Whipped Supreme, avg all flavors	**100**	5	14

Quick Guide

Donuts
Average All Brands

	C	F	Cb
Plain, 1¾ oz	210	12	25
Sugared, 1¾ oz	220	11	27
Glazed, 2 oz	250	12	34
Chocolate Iced, 2 oz	260	14	29

Donuts ~ Brands

	C	F	Cb
Albertson's			
Donut Holes: Assorted	150	8	18
Powdered Sugar (4) 1.7 oz	180	7	26
Gem Donuts: Plain Cake (3) 1.6 oz	190	12	20
Chocolate (3)	260	16	25
Sticky Donuts, 2.2 oz	230	10	32
Bon Appetite			
Cherry Donuts (1) 2 oz	260	15	30
Mini Donuts: Chocolate (4)	270	16	30
Powdered; Crumb, avg. (4)	240	12	32
Cloverfield			
Donut Holes (4)	260	15	30
Dolly Madison			
Regular, 1¾ oz	270	12	40
Gem varieties, ½ oz each	65	3	8
Powdered Mini, ½ oz each	60	3	8
Dunkin' Donuts			
Apple N' Spice Donut	200	8	29
Blueberry Cake Donut	290	16	33
Boston Kreme Donut	240	9	36
Chocolate Frosted Cake Donut	360	20	40
Chocolate Glazed Cake Donut	290	16	33
Cinnamon Cake Donut	330	20	34
Glazed Cake Donut	350	19	41
Jelly Filled Donut	210	8	32
Kreme Filled (Choc./Vanilla)Donut	270	13	25
Old Fashioned Cake Donut	300	19	28
Powdered Cake Donut	330	19	36
Sugar Raised Donut	170	8	22
Entenmann's			
Dark Choc. Frosted	280	19	28
Frosted Devil's Food	320	19	35
Glazed Buttermilk, 2¼ oz	270	14	34
Milk Chocolate Frosted, 2.4 oz	310	19	35
Powdered, 1¾ oz	230	14	25
PopEms (bite size): *Per 4 pieces*			
Glazed (4) 2 oz	240	12	31
Glazed Devil's Food (4) 2 oz	240	11	33
Popettes (bite size), 3 pces, 1.8 oz	240	15	24

Donuts ~ Brands (Cont)

	C	F	Cb
Hostess			
Dunkin Stix (3)	490	25	63
Donut Bites, 1 pouch, 2.3 oz	300	15	38
Regular: Plain, 1.4 oz	160	9	18
Chocolate Frosted, 2 oz	230	13	26
Powdered, 1.7 oz	190	9	25
Old Fashioned Glazed, 2.1 oz	240	11	33
Donettes: Frosted (3) 1.76 oz	220	13	23
Crumb (4) 2 oz	220	9	32
Powdered (4) 2.1 oz	240	12	31
Jewel: Cinnamon Spiced, 2 oz	230	15	24
Krispy Kreme			
Chocolate Glazed Cruller	290	15	37
Chocolate Iced Glazed	250	12	33
Chocolate Iced Kreme Filled	350	20	38
Chocolate Iced w. Sprinkles	260	12	38
Cinnamon Twist	230	9	33
Glazed Cruller	240	14	26
Glazed Kreme Filled	340	20	38
Maple Iced Glazed	240	12	32
New York Cheesecake	320	19	35
Original Glazed	200	12	22
Powdered Cake	280	14	37
Traditional Cake Doughnut	230	13	25
Doughnut Holes, Glazed (5)	200	11	24
Little Debbie			
Donut Sticks, 1.65 oz pkg	230	14	25
Mini Donuts, Frosted (4)	230	13	27
Tastykake			
Cinnamon, 1.8 oz	220	13	25
Mini: Frosted Rich (6)	380	22	42
Cinnamon (4) 1.8 oz	210	10	28
Powdered Sugar (6) 2½ oz	280	13	37
Van De Kamp's			
Plain (1) 1.25 oz	150	9	17
Chocolate (1) 1.4 oz	170	9	22
Powdered (1) 1.5 oz	160	8	22
Crumb (1) 1.6 oz	180	7	26
Old Fashioned Glazed: 2.3 oz	270	12	39
Chocolate, 2.3 oz	300	15	36
Glazed Choc. Donut Holes (4)	250	11	37
Mini Donuts: Powdered (3)	210	11	26
Chocolate (3)	250	15	27
Crumb (3)	200	8	28
Zingers			
Devil's/Vanilla Food, avg. (1)	155	5	26

Quick Guide   C F Cb

Muffins: Ready-To-Eat
Average All Types:

	C	F	Cb
Small, 1 oz	80	3	12
Medium, 2 oz	160	6	24
Large, 3 oz	240	9	36
Extra Large, 4 oz	320	12	48
Giant, 6 oz	480	18	72
Super Size, 8 oz	640	24	96

Brands ~ Ready-To-Eat

	C	F	Cb
Awreys: Blueberry, 2.25 oz	240	12	31
Raisin Bran, 1.5 oz muffin	160	8	21
Controlled Carb Gourmet			
Almond Muffins, 3 oz	210	15	28
Entenmann's: Golden, 2.4 oz	240	12	29
Little Bites, Blueberry, 1 pouch	190	9	27
Hostess: Mini, 1 pouch, avg.	260	15	30
Fruit Pie/Tart, avg., 4.5 oz	475	20	68
Hearty Muffin: Blueberry, 6 oz	690	42	72
Banana Nut, 6 oz	750	48	72
Muffin Loaf: Blueberry, 3.8 oz	420	19	58
Banana Nut, 3.8 oz	460	24	56
100 Calorie Packs:			
Banana Streusel (3) 1 oz	100	3.5	19
Blueberry Streusel (3) 1 oz	100	3	20
My Favorite Muffin: Plain, 6 oz	660	30	75
Chocolate Chip, 6 oz	635	33	81
Fat Free, avg., 6 oz	325	0	78
Otis Spunkmeyer: *Per Whole Muffin (4 oz)*			
Banana Nut, 4 oz	460	22	58
Cheese Streusel	420	18	62
Wild Blueberry	420	22	52
Our Daily Muffin: Each, 3 oz	140	0.5	31
Starbucks: *See Fast-Foods Section*			
Trader Joe's: Banana, 4 oz	280	12	39
Chocolate Chip, 4 oz	430	17	65
Mini: Blueberry, 0.8 oz	110	6	12
Bran w. Raisin, 0.8 oz	80	3	13
Weight Watchers: Blueb., 2.5 oz	180	3	35
Double Chocolate, 2.5 oz	190	4	35
Fast-Food Restaurants: *See Page 183*			

Muffin Mixes   C F Cb
Prepared: Per Muffin

	C	F	Cb
Betty Crocker: Apple Streusel (1)	200	6	34
Blueberry (1)	190	7	27
Choc Chip; Cinnamon Streusel (1)	220	8	30
Water Muffins: Choc Chip (1)	160	5	26
Blueb.; Lemon Poppyseed, avg.	130	3.5	24
Cornbread (1)	180	6	24
Wild Blueberry (1)	130	1.5	26
Pillsbury: Hot Roll Mix, 1 roll	130	3	21
Just Add Milk Blueb. Muffin (1)	170	5	30
Ultimate: Blueberry Streusel (1)	190	12	35
Choc Fudge Choc Chip (1)	270	13	34
Sunmaid: Honey Raisin Bran (1)	280	9	47
Trader Joe's: Pumpkin Muffin (1)	250	11	35

Sweet Rolls & Buns   C F Cb

Note: It is best to weigh for accuracy as actual weight can be 10-50% higher than label weight·

	C	F	Cb
Bon Appetite: Cinn. Roll, 5 oz	580	34	64
Mammoth Cinnamon Roll, 5 oz	560	28	70
Cinnabon: Classic	815	32	117
Caramel Pecanbon, 1 roll	1100	56	141
Minibon, 1 roll	340	13	49
CinnaPretzel	755	6	156
Cinnabon Stix (5) no frosting	380	21	41
Cloverhill Bakery			
Jumbo Honey Bun, 4.75 oz	540	26	70
Entenmann's: Cinn. Roll (½) 2 oz	220	8	34
Hostess:			
Honey Bun, Glazed, 2.7 oz	310	15	39
Actual weight up to 3.6 oz	415	20	52
Iced/Frosted, 3.5 oz	395	5.5	50
Cinnamon Sweet Roll (1)	205	5.5	35
Little Debbie:			
Pecan Spinwheels, 1 oz	110	4	16
Honey Buns, 1.76 oz	220	12	26
McDonald's: Cinnamon Melts, 4 oz	460	19	66
Pillsbury: Cinnamon Roll, 1.5 oz	150	5	23
Sugar Free (1) 1.5 oz	110	3.5	22
Ralph's: Cinnamon Roll, 2.5 oz	290	11	44
Trader Joe's: Cinn. Roll, 2.35 oz	250	7	41
Low-Fat Cinn. Roll, 2.35 oz	180	2	36
Frosted Cinnamon Bun, 4 oz	400	9	66
Van de Kamp's: Cinn. Roll, 1.1 oz	130	7	16
Zen Bakery: Cinn. Raisin Roll, ½	100	1	21

Quick Guide

Chocolate
Average All Brands

	C	F	Cb
Milk Chocolate, regular:			
Plain/Nuts/Fruit, average, 1 oz	150	10	13
1½ oz Bar	225	15	23
2 oz Bar	300	20	30
4 oz Block	600	40	60
8 oz Block	1200	80	120
1 Pound, 16 oz	2400	160	240
Dark/White Chocolate, 1 oz	150	10	16
Sugar Free (Hershey's) 1 pce, 0.3 oz	40	3	5
Chocolate-coated:			
Almonds, 5-6, 1 oz	160	11	14
Clusters, Nut, 3 pces, 1.2 oz	200	18	16
Coffee Beans, 1.4 oz	180	9	22
Creme/Cordial Centers, 1 oz	120	5	20
Fudge, 1 oz	125	4	20
Macadamias, 9 pces, 1.3 oz	220	15	18
Mints, 1 med., ½ oz	55	1	11
Nougat & Caramel, 1 oz	125	5	18
Peanuts, 12 med., 1 oz	145	9	14
Raisins, 28 med., 1 oz	110	4	19
Cooking Chocolate:			
Sweet/Semi-sweet, 1 oz	140	8	18
4 oz Bar (Baker's)	520	35	68
Chips, 1 Tbsp, ½ oz	70	4	9
½ cup, 3 oz	420	24	54
Unsweetened, 1 oz	140	14	8
Carob: Plain, 1 oz	150	9	16

Brands & Generic

Per Piece/Serving

	C	F	Cb
100 Grand: 1.5 oz bar	180	8	29
King Size, 2.8 oz	350	14	57
Snack Size (2), 1½ oz	180	8	29
Abba Zaba, 2 oz bar	250	5	48
Absolutely Almond, 2.5 oz bar	380	23	40
Aero Bar (Nestlé), 1.45 oz bar	210	13	26
After Dinner Mints, 1 small	25	1.5	3
After Eight Mint (Nestlé), each	35	1	6
Air Head, 1 bar, 15.6g	60	0	15
Allen Wertz: Simply Sugar Free			
Coffee Time (decaf), 4	45	1.5	8
Coffee Toffee, 6	120	3	23
Other types, 4	120	2.5	23
Almond Joy: 1.6 oz bar	220	13	26
King Size, 4 pces, 3.1 oz	450	24	54
Snack, 17g bar	80	4.5	10
Cookies (2), 1 oz	140	8	17
Almond Roca: 3 pces	220	15	17
Sugar Free, 3 pces	150	15	16
Almonds, sugar-coated (15), 40g	175	4	29

Brands & Generic (Cont)

Per Piece/Serving

	C	F	Cb
Almond Clusters (Trader Joe's), 2 pce, 1.2 oz	210	14	5
Altoids (C & B), 10 pces	10	0	2
Amazin' Fruit, 1 bag, 1.9 oz	180	0	41
Andes, Thins, avg. all flav. (8), 1.4 oz	200	13	22
Anthon Berg: Cognac, each	180	8	25
Marzipan w. Madeira, 1.4 oz	175	7.5	26
Marzipan Brod	120	7	13
Asteroid (Nestlé), 1.9 oz	260	10	40
Atomic Fireball, 1 piece	4	0	1
Baby Ruth: King Size, 3.7 oz bar	500	24	66
2.1 oz bar	280	14	39
Fun size, 2 bars	170	8	24
Minis, 4 bars	200	9	30
Carb Select, 2 bars	180	8	26
Baci (Perugina): 1 pce, ½ oz	75	6	7
Bar, 1.58 oz	230	15	27
Barley Sugar, 1 pce, 0.2 oz	25	0	6
Baskin-Robbins: 3 pce, 0.5 oz	60	1	13
Sugar Free, 4 pces	40	1	14
Big Hunk, 2 oz	230	3	47
Bit-O-Honey, 1.7 oz	180	3.5	38
Chews, 6 pces, 1.4 oz	150	3	32
Bliss (Hershey's), avg., 1 piece	35	2.5	4
Blow Pops, each, 0.6 oz	60	0	15
Bon Bons, 2 pieces	45	0	12
Boston Baked Beans, 11 pces, 15g	70	2.5	10
Brach's: Almond Supremes (11)	220	13	22
Butterscotch Hard (3), 0.6 oz	70	0	17
Caramel Clusters (2), 36g	180	10	20
Circus Peanuts (5), 1.4 oz	160	0	39
Double Dippers (15), 1.4 oz	210	12	23
Golden Butter Toffee (3), 0.6 oz	80	2	15
Malted Milk Balls (15), 1.3 oz	190	7	30
Milk Maid Caramel (4), 1.37 oz	160	4.5	27
Orange Slices (3), 45g	150	0	38
Breath Savers, all types, each	5	0	2
Brite Crackers, 1 bag, 1.5 oz	140	0	32
Bubble Gum: See 'Gum' Page 131			
Buncha Crunch, ⅓ cup, 1.4 oz	180	8	26
Movie Box, 3.2 oz	440	20	64
Burnt Peanuts, 15 pces, 40g	70	3	10
Butterfinger: 2.1 oz bar	270	11	43
King Size, 3.7 oz bar	480	18	75
Fun size, 0.75 oz	100	4	15
Giant (5 oz pkg), pieces in choc., ½ pkg, 2½ oz	340	16	48
Beast, 140g	640	24	100
Miniatures: 1 pce, 10g	45	1.5	7
4 pieces, 40g	180	7	29
Stix, 1 stick, 17g	90	4.5	11

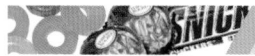

Brands & Generic (Cont)

Per Piece/Serving **C** **F** **Cb**

Butterfinger (Cont):
Crisp Bar: 1.76 oz bar	250	13	33
King Size, 90g	500	28	62
Minis, 4 pieces	220	11	29
Butterfinger B.B.'s, 1.7 oz bag	220	9	34
Buttermints, 7 pces, 13g	50	0	13
Butterscotch: 3 pces	70	0	19
Buttons *(Walgreens),* 3, 18g	70	0	17
Chips *(Hershey's),* 1 Tbsp	80	4	10
Discs *(Sathers),* 3 pces	70	0	17
Cadbury: Creme Egg	170	6	28
Dairy Milk, 7 pces, 1.4 oz	200	11	23
Mini Eggs, 12 pces,1.4 oz	190	8	28
Candy Apple, medium, 6.5 oz	280	0	60
Candy Cane, medium, 5", ½ oz	50	0	13
Candy Corn, 1 oz	100	0	26
Candy Jar Mix *(Jewel),* 3, 0.6 oz	70	0	17
Candy Necklaces, 20g each	80	0	20
Caramels: each	40	1	8
Chocolate, each	25	0.2	6
Creams: 3 pces, 1¼ oz	130	3	23
2.75 oz pkt, 5 pces, 1½ oz	160	3.5	30
Caramel Nips: 2 pces	60	1.5	11
Chocolate Parfait, 2 pces	60	2	11
Peanut Butter, 2 pces	60	2	11
Sugar Free Caramel, 2 pces	60	1.5	12
Caramel Popcorn, ⅔ cup	150	6	23
Caramello *(Hershey's),* 1.6 oz bar	210	10	29
Snack, 0.66 oz	80	4	11
Cadbury: 6 pces	200	9	27
Kingsize, 2.7 oz bar	360	16	49
Certs, Breath Mints, 1 pce	5	0	2
Charleston Chew,1 bar, 60g	260	7	49
Charms: Blow Pop	60	0	15
Flat Pop	50	0	13

Chew-ets Peanut Chews:
Original, 6 pces, 56g	260	13	25
Chocolate, 6 pces	270	14	34
Chews, 1 roll	120	1	28
Chick O Stick, 2 oz	260	6	44
Chocolate Mints *(Hershey's),* each	10	0.1	2
Chocolate Parfait Nips, 2 pces	60	2	11
Chuckles Jelly: each	35	0	9
Jujubes *(Hershey's),* 55 pces, 40g	110	0	28
Chunky Bar *(Nestlé):* 1.4 oz	190	11	24
King Size, 2½ oz	340	19	43
Giant, 5 oz	680	40	84
Chupa Chups, 1 Pop,	50	0	12
Cinnamon Bears *(Walgreens),* 5	130	0	34
Cinn. Buttons *(Walgreens),* 3 pce	70	0	17

Per Piece/Serving **C** **F** **Cb**
Cinnamon Disks *(Walmart),* 3 pces	70	0	19
Cinnamon Drops *(Sathers),* 19 pce	150	0	36
Circus Peanuts, Marshmallow *(Spangler),*			
6 pieces, 1.5 oz	160	0	40
CocoaVia Crunch Bars, 0.7 oz	90	5	11
Coconut Stacks, 8 pieces	260	13	37
Coffee Go Coffee/Cappuccino, ea.	18	0.5	4
Coffee Rio-Gold, each	15	0.5	3
Collard & Bowser, Eng. Toffee (2)	80	4	12
Conversation Hearts *(Necco),* 1 lge	10	0	4
Cote d'Or: Bouchee, each	130	8	12
Chokotoff, each	210	9	30
Nougatti	150	8	19
Bar & Nuts, 1.3 oz	220	18	12
Cotton Candy, 1 oz	110	0	28
Cough Drops: *See Page 77*			
Cracker Jack, ½ cup, 1 oz	120	2	23
Creme Savers: *See Lifesavers*			
Crisped Rice: Almond, 1 bar	130	6	18
Choc Chip, 1 bar	115	4	18
Crows, 12 pieces, 1.5 oz	140	0	35
Crunch: Original, 1.55 oz bar	220	12	29
Fun Size, 1.5 oz	210	10	29
Miniatures: 1 pce	30	1.5	4
Dark, 1 pce	50	3	6
Buncha Crunch, 3.2 oz box	440	20	64
Crunch Crisp, 1.74 oz bar	240	13	32
Crunch White: 1.4 oz Bar	220	13	23
Giant, 4.5 oz bar	710	42	74
Stix, 1 stick	90	6	12
Dots, 12 dots, 1.5 oz	140	0	35
Double Dip Stick, 1 stick	16	0.5	3
Dove			
Milk Choc: Singles Bar	200	12	22
Large Tablet Bar, 3.53 oz	540	33	60
Dark Choc: Singles Bar, 1.3 oz	190	12	22
Large Tablet Bar, 3.53 oz	510	33	60
Miniatures: Milk Choc, 1 piece	45	2.5	5
with Caramel, 1 piece	40	2	5
Dark Choc, 1 piece	40	2.5	5
Choc Covered Almonds:			
Dark, 10 pieces	160	12	15
Milk, 10 pieces	170	12	15
Sugar Free: Dark (3.4 oz bag),			
All flavors, 1 piece	40	3	4
Double Buble Ball Gum	20	0	5
Dum Dum Pops *(Spangler),* 1 pop	25	0	6
Endulge *(Atkins):* Per Serving			
Caramel Nut Chew Bar, 34g	130	8	17
Peanut Caramel Cluster, 34g	140	9	12

Brands & Generic (Cont)

Per Piece/Serving	C	F	Cb
English Toffee, 1 pce	48	3	5
Eda's Sugar Free, all flav., 5, ½ oz	40	0	15
5th Avenue: 2 oz bar	260	12	37
King Size bar	480	24	60
Snack Size, 0.58 oz	80	4	10
Fanny May: Single Wrapped Pieces			
Mint Meltaway Patty, 3 pces, 40g	230	15	30
Pixie, 2 pces, 45g	240	14	26
Trinidad, 1 pce, 42.5g	310	12	25
Fast Break (Reese's): 2 oz bar	260	13	35
Ferrero Rocher: each	75	5	6
3 pces, 1.3 oz	220	15	17
Fifty 50 Snack Bars:			
Peanut Butter, 1.2 oz	190	14	17
Almond Choc., 7 pce, 1½ oz	200	17	18
Crunch Bar, 7 pce, 40g	140	11	16
Dark Choc, 7 pce, 40g	170	14	21
Milk Choc., 7 pce, 40g	190	16	19
Fluffy Stuff (Charms), 0.6 oz bag	70	0	17
Fondant: Choc-coated, 1.2 oz	120	3	27
Mint, 1 oz	105	4	27
Fran's: Gold Bar, 45g	250	14	17
Gold Bites (Almonds), 23g	120	7	13
Footsies, 12 pces	140	3	29
Fruit Crystals (Walgreens), 3 pces	70	0	17
Fruit Drops, each	6	0	1
Fruit Gems (Sunkist), 3, 1.2 oz	105	0	26
Fruit Leathers, average, 0.5 oz	45	0	12
Fruit Pastilles, 1 roll, 1.4 oz	100	0	26
Fruit Rolls, 1 roll	70	0	18
Fruit Roll-Ups, ½ oz	50	1	12
Fruit Runts (Walgreens), 12 pces	60	0	14
Fudge: Chocolate/Vanilla (1), 21g	90	5	13
with Nuts (1), 21g	100	6	12
Choco. Marshmallow, 1 oz	120	5	18
w. Nuts, 1 oz	115	3	19
Peanut Butter, 1 oz	115	3	19
Ghirardelli:			
Squares: Dark Choc. (4), 43g	220	17	23
Other varieties (3), 45g	215	12	28
3 oz Bars: Dark Choc., 12 pieces	440	34	46
Other varieties avg., 12 pces	440	28	52
Intense Dark: Twilight, 3 pces	200	17	17
Other varieties, avg., 3 pces	200	15	21

Per Piece/Serving	C	F	Cb
Godiva: Hearts, 7 pieces, 1.4 oz	210	13	23
Bars: Milk/Dark, avg., 1½ oz	230	14	26
Extra Dark 72%, 1½ oz	230	17	18
Assorted Chocs: 2 pieces, 31g	160	10	17
Sugar Free, 3 pieces	200	15	23
Bouchee au Chocolate, 2 pces	220	13	23
Chocolate Pretzels, 6 pces, 1.4 oz	200	10	26
Go Lightly: Box Candies, 2-3 pces	220	16	28
Bags: Assorted Taffy, 5 pieces	130	3	36
Vanilla Caramels, 5	150	6	31
Super Free Creme Crunch (4)	150	5	33
Goobers Peanuts, 1 pkg, 1.4 oz	200	13	21
Good & Plenty (Hershey's): 50g	170	0	43
Snack Size, 1 box, 17g	60	0	14
GooGoo Cluster, 1 bar, 1.75 oz	240	11	32
Gum Drops: 1 small, 9g	10	0	7.5
5 pces, 44g	150	0	37
Gummi Bears, 9 bears, 42g	120	0	29
Gummi Novelties (Walgreens), 6	150	0	22
Gummi Savers, 10 pieces	120	0	30
Gummi Sweet Tarts, 1 bug, 1.5 oz	150	0	34
Gummi Watch, 1, 2 oz	105	0	24
Gummi Worms (1), 8g	25	0	6
Guylian: Milk Choc., 8 squares, 1 oz	120	9	16
Dark Choc., 8 squares, 1 oz	130	9	16
Guylian Twists, 4 pces, 35g	200	3	23
Halvah (Joyvah): Plain, 1 bar, 2 oz	390	25	18
Choc.coated Sesame, ½ bar, 2 oz	380	23	20
Hard Candy: All flavors, 16g	60	0	15
1 regular piece	20	0	5
Heath: Original, 39g	210	13	24
Bites, 15 pces, 39g	210	12	25
King Size, 2.8 oz	430	25	49
Minis, 6 pces	240	14	27
Hershey's:			
Milk Chocolate: 1½ oz bar	210	13	26
Cookies 'n' Creme, (2) 34g	170	9	21
Kingsize, 2.6 oz bar	400	23	42
7 oz bar, ⅓ bar	200	12	21
w. Almonds, 1.45 oz bar	210	14	21
Cacao Reserve:			
Milk Choc. (35% cacao), 4 blocks, 1.4 oz	220	15	21
Dark Choc. (65% cacao), 1.4 oz	230	15	21
Extra Dark (60% cacoa):			
Avg. all flavors: 3 pces, 1.6 oz	210	13	20
3.5 oz Bar	560	35	54
Candy-Coated Eggs:			
Milk Choc (4), 0.6 oz	90	4	12
w. Almonds (4) 0.6 oz	100	6	9

Brands & Generic (Cont)

Per Piece/Serving   **C** **F** **Cb**

Hershey's (Cont):
Pot of Gold Chocolate:

	C	F	Cb
Nut Assortment, 4 pces 1.4 oz	200	13	23
Caramel Assort., 4 pces 1.4 oz	190	10	26
Creme Assortment, 1.5 oz	170	4	32
Truffle Assortment, 1.5 oz	200	9	27
Special Dark Choc.: 1.45 oz bar	180	12	25
King Size, 2.5 oz	400	22	44
Large, 5 oz bar	780	43	86
Snack Size, ½ oz	70	4.5	9
Snacksters, 1 pkg, 20g	100	3.5	15
Sticks, avg. all varieties, 11g	60	3	7
Sugar Free: Milk Choc. Candy (5)	170	13	25
Dark Choc. Candy (5), 1.4 oz	150	13	24
Peanut Butter Cups Minis (5)	180	13	27
York Peppermint Patties, 3 pces	80	3.5	28
Honeycomb: Plain, 1 oz	115	0	27
Choc-coated, 2 pces	180	7	31
Hot Tamales, 1 box, 60g, 2.1 oz	220	0	55
Hugs ~ *See Kisses*			
Ice Blue Mints *(Walgreens)*, 3, 17g	70	0	17
Jawbreakers *(Sathers)*, 15, 17g	70	0	17
Jellies, 3 medium, 1 oz	130	0	33
Jells Raspberry *(Joyva)*, 3 pces, 44g	160	0	38
Jelly Beans: Small, 22 beans, 1 oz	100	0	24
Regular, 13 beans, 40g	150	0	37
1 bean	10	0	3
Sugar Free, 35 beans	110	0	36
Jumbo, 1 bean	20	0	5
Jewel, 13 beans, 1.4 oz	140	0	36
Sathers/Walgreens, 13 pces	150	0	37
Wonderbeans, 33 beans	100	0	24
Jelly Bellys: each	4	0	1
35 pces, 1.4 oz	140	0	37
Sugar Free Beans/Sours (37), 1.4 oz	120	0	30
Sugar Free Fruit Slices, 8 pces, 1.4 oz	60	0	30
Jelly Rings *(Jewel)*, 5 pces, 42g	120	0	30
Jolly Rancher:			
Fruit Chews, 3 pces	75	1	16
Gummies, 9 pces, 39g	120	0	29
Hard Candy (3), 18g	70	0	17
Blow Pop, 0.6 oz	60	0	15
Junior Caramels: 13 pces, 42g	190	6	33
Mini, 2 boxes, 24g	110	3	19

Per Piece/Serving   **C** **F** **Cb**

	C	F	Cb
Junior Mints: 52g box	220	4	45
16 pces, 1.4 oz	170	3	35
Juicefuls: Red Raspb., (3), 0.6 oz	60	0	15
Assorted Fruits, 1 pce	20	0	5
Jujubees, all types (55), 40g	110	0	28
Juju Bears, 5 pces	130	0	34
Juju Mix *(Sathers)*, 11 pce, 1½ oz	150	0	35
Jujyfruits, 16 pces, 40g	120	0	32
Kissables, 28 pces, 1 oz	125	6	19
Kisses, avg. all flavors:			
1 piece	25	1.5	2.5
6 pieces, 1 oz	155	9	17
Kit Kat: 4-piece bar, 1.5 oz	210	11	28
Big Cat, 1.94 oz	290	14	35
King Size, 3 oz bar	440	22	54
Snack Size, 2-piece bar, 0.9 oz	135	7	16
Caramel Bar (1), 41g	200	11	27
Extra Krispy Bar (1)	220	12	29
White Choc, 4 piece, 1½ oz	220	12	27
Krackel: 1.5 oz bar	210	11	26
Snack size, 0.6 oz	85	4.5	11
Kraft: Caramels, (5), 40g	160	3.5	30
Kudos: *See Page 139*			
Lance: Peanut Bar, 1.8 oz pkg	240	14	22
Lemon Drops (3) ½ oz	50	0	14
Sugar Free *(Walgreens)*, 4, 13g	25	0	13
Lemonhead, 10, ½ oz	50	0	14
Licorice: Average all types, 1oz	100	0	25
Bites *(Switzer)*, each	10	0	3
Chews *(Panda)*, each	10	0	3
Tid Bits, each	5	0	1
Twists: Black/Red, avg. 1 pce	35	0	8.5
Sugar Free, 1 pce	13	0	2.5
American Licorice Co.: Laces (1)	35	0	8
Jumbo Rope, 2 pces	140	0	34
Red Bites, 1.4 oz	140	0	33
Snaps, 31 pces, 40g	140	0.5	33
Stick, (1) 0.5 oz	35	0	8.5
Super Red Ropes (1), 66g	240	0	54
Superstring, 1⅓ pces	140	0	34
Vines, 2 pces	70	0	17
Sugar Free Red Twists (7)	90	0	25
Lifesavers: Large size, 1 candy	15	0	3.5
Regular, all flavors, 1 candy	10	0	2.5
1 Roll (14 candies), 1.14 oz	140	0	35
Creme Savers: 3 pces	60	0	11
Sugar Free, 4 pces	35	0	14
Gummi Savers (10), 39g	130	0	30
Peppermint (4)	60	0	15
Fruit Splosion, 10 pces	130	0	30
Sugar-Free Delites: *Per Candy*			
Orchard Fruits; Summer Blend	7	0	2.5
Butter Toffee; European Collect.	10	1	2.5

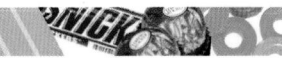

Brands & Generic (Cont)

Per Piece/Serving	C	F	Cb
Lik-m-aid (Nestlé), Wonka Fun Dip, 1 pkg	50	0	13
Lindt: Lindor, Balls, avg. (1)	75	6	5
70% Cocoa, 4 pces	220	17	13
Truffles (3)	220	17	16
Lollipops: Mini, 1/4 oz	25	0	6
Small, ½ oz	50	0	12
Medium, 1 oz	100	0	25
Giant (4" diam), 3½ oz	350	0	88
Look! Bar, 1.5 oz	190	6	49
M & M's:			
Milk Chocolate, 1 pce	5	0.1	0.5
20 pces, 0.6 oz	70	3	10
1.7 oz pkg	240	10	34
¼ cup, 1.8 oz	255	11	37
Dark Choc.: 3.14 oz pkg	440	20	60
Fun Size, 18g pkg	90	4	13
Almond Choc., 1.3 oz pkg	200	11	21
Minis, Mega Tube, 1.1 oz tube	150	7	21
Peanut: 1.74 oz pkg	250	13	30
Fun Size, 18g pkg	90	4.5	11
Peanut Butter, 1.6 oz pkg	240	14	26
Premiums: Choc./Raspb. Almond			
¼ cup, 1½oz	240	16	20
Mint/Mocha/Triple, avg., 1½ oz	230	14	25
Mamba, 9 pces, 1½ oz	170	2.5	36
Marathon (Snickers) Bar, 1.9 oz	220	7	26
M.Azing: 1 bar, 1.5 oz	230	12	27
Peanut Butter (1), 1.5 oz	230	13	25
Marshmallow Egg, 1 egg, 1 oz	120	3	22
Marshmallows: Firm/Soft, 1 oz	90	0	23
Regular size, 4 pces, 33g	100	0	24
Mini-Marshmallow, ⅔ c., 30g	100	0	24
Choc-coat. Twists (Joyva), each	95	2	10
Fluff, 2 Tbsp, 18 g	60	0	15
Kraft: Mini, ½ cup, 30g	100	0	24
Creme, 2 Tbsp	45	0	11
Jet-Puffed, 5 pces, 30g	100	0	24
Funmallows, ⅔ cup, 30g	100	0	24
Marzipan, 2 Tbsp, 39g	160	4	29
Mauna Loa, 1.76 oz	280	19	24
Mexican Hats (7), 38g	120	0	30
Mentos: Regular (1)	10	0	3
Sugar Free (1)	5	0	2.5
Mike & Ike: 1 pkg, 1.1 oz	120	0	30
23 pces, 40g	140	0	36
Milkfulls (Storck), 6 pces, 1.4 oz	170	3	35
Milk Chocolate: See Hershey's			
Milk Duds, 13 pces, 1.4 oz	170	6	28

Per Piece/Serving	C	F	Cb
Milky Way: Midnight Bar, 1.75 oz	220	8	36
Regular Bar, 2 oz	260	10	41
Fun size, 2 bars, 34g	150	6	24
Milky Way To Go, 51g	230	9	36
Miniatures: (5) 43g	190	7	30
Midnight Minis (5), 41g	190	7	29
Mints: Uncoated, 7 pces	60	0	17
1 mint (¾" diam.)	4	0	1
1 large mint (1½" diam.)	10	0	2
Mon Cheri (Ferrero), 4 pces, 45g	260	18	20
Mounds: 1.7 oz	230	13	29
Snack, 0.68 oz	90	5	11
King Size, 3½ oz	490	26	58
Minis, 3 pces, 41g	200	11	24
Mr Goodbar: 1.7 oz bar	260	17	26
King Size, 2.6 oz bar	400	24	40
Snack, 17g	80	4.5	10
Mrs Fields Choc, 2 pces, 33g	160	8	22
Necco Candy Wafers (40) 57g	220	0	56
Neuhaus, average all types	80	5	7
Newman's Own:			
Caramel Cups, 3 pces, 1.2 oz	160	9	21
P'Nut B. Cups (Milk/Dark), 3, 1 pkg	180	12	19
Sweet Dark Choc Bar, 79g	400	26	48
Nibs, all types, 1 pouch, 63g	215	2	49
Nips, all flavors, 2, 14g	60	2	11
Nite Bite (Glucose Bar)	100	3.5	10
Nougat: 3 pces, 1 oz	150	2.5	32
Choc. Covered, 1 oz	125	4	22
Now & Later (Nabisco), 9, 41g	120	1	29
Nutrageous Bar (Reese's), 1.8 oz	280	16	27
Oh Henry! 2 oz bar	265	13	37
Orange (Lindt), 5 slices	230	14	23
Orange Slices: Jewel, 3, 1½ oz	140	0	35
Walgreens, 3, 1½ oz	150	0	36
Pastel Mints (Walgreens), 20 pces	60	0	14
Patteez (Sweet n' Low), 4 pces	100	2	29
PayDay Bar: 1.8 oz bar	240	11	30
King Size, 3.4 oz bar	480	24	52
Snack Size, 0.7 oz	90	5	10
Avalanche, 1.8 oz bar	250	13	29
Peanut Bar, 1.6 oz bar	210	14	20
Peanut Butter Cups: See Reese's; Newman's Own			
Peanut Brittle, 1 piece, 1½ oz	220	15	20
Sugar Free (Judy's), ¾ cup, 1 oz	100	6	2

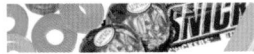

Brands & Generic (Cont)

Per Piece/Serving	C	F	Cb
Peanuts, choc-covered, 15 pces	210	12	23
Pearson's Mint Patties, (5), 38g	150	2.5	31
Pecan Roll, ⅓ bar, 40g	190	10	24
Peppermints, 7 small, 0.5 oz	60	0	15
Brach's, 3 pces	60	0	15
Peppermint Twists (2), 14g	60	0	14
Pez, 1 roll	35	0	9
Planters: Choc. Peanuts (25) 7 oz	220	13	20
Orig. Peanut Bar, 1.6 oz	230	14	22
Hersheys, 2½ oz	390	24	34
Pops ~ See Lollipops			
Poprocks, 9.5g pkg	35	0	9
Pralines: Small, 0.3 oz	38	2	5
1 large piece, 1.4 oz	180	10	24
Pretzels: Choc-covered, Mini (6), 38g	190	9	24
White Choc Bites (23), 40g	200	9	25
Pretzel Flipz (Nestlé), 8 pces, 1 oz	130	5	20
Raisinets: 1 pkg, 1.7 oz	205	8	34
King Size, 2.8 oz	330	13	56
Dark Raisinets, ¼ cup, 45g	130	8	32
Reese's			
Peanut Butter Cups: 2 cups, 1.8 oz	260	15	29
King Size (4), 2.8 oz	420	24	44
Mini, 5 pces, 39g	210	12	22
8-Pack, 1/2 oz	80	4.5	8
Snack Size, 1 pce, 21g	110	6	12
Sugar Free, 2 pces, avg., 39g	170	12	24
Caramel filled (2),1.4 oz	190	10	25
Big Cup: Regular, 1.4 oz	190	12	21
w. Nuts: 1.4 oz	220	13	21
King Size (2), 2.8 oz	430	26	41
White Chocolate (2), 1.5 oz	220	13	22
Reeses Pieces: 1.4 oz	190	9	24
King Size, 3 oz	400	20	46
Reeses Sticks: 1.5 oz	230	13	23
King Size (1), 3 oz	460	26	46
Snack Size (1), 17g	90	5	9
Reeses Whipps (40% less fat),1.5 oz	230	9	36
Clusters, 3 pces, 1½ oz	230	13	24
Crispy Crunchy Bar: 1.7 oz	240	14	27
2 pces, 1.2 oz	190	11	18
King Size, 3.1 oz bar	480	28	48
Fast Break, 2 oz bar	210	13	34
Nutrageous Bar, 1.8 oz	280	16	27
Snacksters, 1 pkg, ¾ oz	100	4	14
Peanut Butter Chips, 1 Tbsp, 15g	80	4	7
Chocolate Dipped Cookies (4), 2 oz	300	15	34
Rice Krispies Treats (Kellogg's):			
1 bar, average all varieties	110	3.5	19
Rice Crunchy Bars, 19g bar	70	0.5	15
Riesen Choc. Chew, 1.57 oz bag	180	7	29
Rocky Road, 2 oz bar	240	11	34

Per Piece/Serving	C	F	Cb
Robin Eggs, Large (2); Mini (10)	100	3.5	16
Rolo: All types (3), 0.64 oz	85	4	12
Mini Bites, 19 pieces, 1.4 oz	190	9	26
Root Beer Barrels (3) 0.5 oz	70	0	17
Ross Chocolate Bars, Avg, 1.2 oz	180	13	19
Russell Stover Candy: Creams (1)	65	3	11
Almond Delight, 15 pces	220	18	15
Chocolate Asst., 2 pces	140	6	21
Choc-covered Nuts, 3 pces	230	16	17
Cherry Blimps, 3 pces	170	12	24
Sugar Free: Mint Cremes (3)	190	14	22
Mint Patties, 3 pces	180	11	27
Pecan Delight (2), 1 oz	130	9	5
Cups (3), 1.2 oz	170	13	16
Mint Patties, 3 pces	180	11	27
Nett Carb: Choc. Candy Almond (15)	210	18	15
Mint Patties, 3 pces, 43g	180	11	27
Peanut Butter Cups (4)	180	14	18
Pecan Delight, 4 pces	180	13	22
Toffee Squares, 3 pces, 45g	170	11	22
Salt Water Taffy (Brach's), 5	170	2.5	36
Seashells (Guylian), 1 shell	70	4.5	6
See's Candies:			
Almond Royal, 5 pieces, 1.3 oz	190	13	18
Assorted Peppermints, 2 pieces	160	4.5	32
Krispy's: Caffe Latte, 5 pces 1.3 oz	180	8	27
Mint, 5 pieces, 1.3 oz	170	8	27
Little Pops: assorted, 4 pcs, 0.5 oz	60	2.5	11
Butterscotch, 4 pieces, 0.5 oz	50	1.5	10
Cafe Latte, 4 pieces, 0.5 oz	50	1.5	9
Vanilla, 4 pieces, 0.5 oz	50	2	11
Molasses Chips, 6 pieces, 1.4 oz	180	8	28
Peanut Brittle Bar, 1 bar, 1 oz	150	10	15
Sugar Sticks, 2 pieces	50	0	13
Toffee-ettes, 3 pieces, 1.6 oz	270	21	18
Sesame Crunch, 3 pces	80	4	7
Signature Treasures (Nestlé):			
Choc. Creme, 3 pieces, 1.2 oz	170	9	21
Creamy Caramel, 3 pieces, 1.3 oz	170	9	23
Dark Choc Caramel, 3 pieces	160	10	22
Milk Choc Caramel, 3 pieces	170	9	23
Peanut Butter, 3 pieces	180	12	20
Sixlets (Hershey's), 24 pces	90	3.5	14
Skittles: Sour, 1.2 oz bag	200	2	44
Orig./Trop./Wild Berry, 2.17 oz	250	2.5	56
Bubblegum, 2 pcs	10	0	2
Fun Size, 1 bag, 15g	60	1	14
King Size, 4 oz bag	440	4.5	102
Skor Toffee Bar, 1.4 oz	210	12	24
Smarties: Candy Rolls, 1 roll	25	0	6
Giant, 2 pcs, 7g	25	0	5

Brands & Generic (Cont)

Per Piece/Serving	C	F	Cb
Snack Barz (Hershey's), 25g	120	7	17
Snickers: 2.07 oz bar	280	14	35
King Size, 3.7 oz	510	24	63
Creme Egg (1), 1.2 oz	170	10	20
Fun Size, 2 bars, 34g	160	8	21
Miniatures, 4 pieces	170	9	22
Munch Bar, 1.4 oz bar	220	15	18
Adventure Bar, 1.87 oz	250	12	32
Cruncher, 1.56 oz	220	11	28
Cruncher To Go, 2.54 oz	350	18	45
Marathon Bar: avg., 1.9 oz bar	210	8	26
King size	440	22	60
Almond, 1.76 oz	240	11	32
Sno Caps, ¼ cup, 40g	180	8	30
Soft 'N Chewy Butter Toffee, ea.	30	0.5	5
Sorbee: Choc., ½ bar, 40g	200	14	20
Gummie Bears, 16 pces	120	0	30
Peanut Butter, 4 pces	210	15	19
Sour Punch: All types, 2 oz	200	1.5	46
1 straw	20	0	5
Spearmint Leaves: Jewel, 5, 40g	140	0	35
Walgreens, 4 pieces, 46g	160	0	39
Spree Candies: Original, 15 pces	50	0	13
Chewy Spree, 8 pces	60	0	13
Starburst: Candy Canes, 0.5 oz	70	0	18
Fruit Chews, each	20	0.4	4
2 oz pkg	240	5	48
Jellybeans, 1.5 oz	160	0	39
Jellybean Egg, 2 oz	200	0	51
Tropical Fruit, 2.07 oz pack	240	5	49
Starlight Mints, 3 pces, 16g	60	0	15
Suckers (Walgreens), 1 sucker, 11g	45	0	11
Sugar Babies, 30 pces, 40g	180	1.5	41
Sugar Coated Peanuts, 1 oz	120	8	10
Sunbursts Sunflowers (Kimmie):			
Candy Bar Bag, 1.3 oz	145	6.5	21
Coffee Break Tube, 3 oz	330	15	48
Sweet 'N Low: Chews, each	20	0.5	5
Coffee Cremes (1)	40	3	6
Wafer Bars, avg., 3 pces	140	7	23
Mint Cremes, 3½ pces	120	9	22
Mint Patteez, 4 pces	100	2	29
Sweet Escapes: See Hershey's			
Sweet Tarts (Nestlé), 5 pces, ½ oz	50	0	13
Symphony: 1.5 oz bar	230	14	24
Large, 5 oz bar	785	47	82
Snack: Chocolate (1), 0.6 oz	90	5	10
w. Almds & Toffee (1), 5 oz	230	14	23

Per Piece/Serving	C	F	Cb
Taffy, 1 pce, 23g	80	1	19
Take 5 (Hershey's): 1.5 oz bar	210	11	25
King Size, 2.25 oz bar	320	16	38
Marshmallow, 1.3 oz bar	180	9	22
Peanut Butter, 1.5 oz bar	220	11	23
3 Musketeers 2.13 oz bar	260	8	46
Fun size, 3 pieces	190	6	34
Mint Minis, 7 pieces	170	5	32
Pop'ables (15)	180	6	31
Tang-a-Roos, 1 roll	25	0	6
Terry's Choc Orange, (5), 1.5 oz	230	12	27
Tic Tac, all varieties, each	2	0	0
Toblerone: 50g (1.76 oz) bar	255	15	30
1 bar, 100g (3.5 oz)	510	30	60
⅓ bar, 33g	170	10	20
Mini, 3 pces	200	11	24
Toffees, Regular, 1 oz	160	9	18
Toll House Milk Choc. Morsels, 1Tbsp	70	4	9
Tootsie Pops, Mini	30	0	7
Tootsie Roll, 2.25 oz roll	245	2	55
Trolli: Gummies, 18 pieces, 40g	110	0	26
Cherry Bombers, 10 pieces	130	0	31
Truffles: Regular, 1 pce, 12g	60	4	6
Large (Godiva), 0.75 oz	110	6.5	12
Extra Large (J.Schmidt), 1½ oz	220	13	24
Turtles (Nestlé): Avg., each	80	4.5	9
Sugar Free, 3 pieces, 38g	150	11	20
Twists (Sugar Free): Licorice; Strawberry,			
7 twists, 40g	90	0	25
Twix: 2 oz pkg	280	14	37
King Size, 3 oz pkg	405	20	52
Fun Size, 0.5 oz	80	4	10
Twix To Go	480	24	64
Minis, 3 pces, 29g	150	7	20
Caramel, 24g	130	6	16
Peanut Butter To Go	480	28	48
Peanut Butter, 1.8 oz	280	17	26
Twizzlers: Bites (17), 40g	140	0.5	32
Cherry Nibs, 2.3 oz pkg	220	2	50
Pull 'n' Peel Cherry, 1.7 oz	160	1	36
Sourz Assorted, 1.8 oz	180	1.5	40
Twists Chocolate, 1.6 oz	160	1	36
Uno Bar 1.5 oz	250	17	22
Velamints Sugar Free, 2 pce	5	0	1
Weight Watchers (Whitman's):			
Butter Cream Caramel, 3 pces	150	8	23
Caramel Medallions, 3 pces	150	9	26
English Toffee Squares, 3 pces	160	10	23
Mint Patties, 3 pces	150	9	26
Peanut Butter Crunch, 4 pces	180	8	31
Pecan Crowns, 3 pces	150	9	22

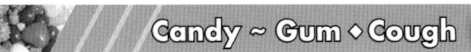

Brands & Generic (Cont)

Per Piece/Serving	C	F	Cb
Werther's: Original, 3 pce, 15g	60	1	13
Chewy Caramel (6), 37g	170	5	30
Caramelts (8), 40g	250	18	18
Sugar-Free, 5 pieces	40	1	14
Whatchamacallit Bar, 1.6 oz	230	12	28
King Size, 2.6 oz	370	18	46
Whitman's: Pecan Roll, 2 oz roll	300	20	26
Sampler, 3 pces, 1.4 oz	200	9	28
Assorted; Dark Chocolate, 3 pces	220	12	26
Snoopy Treats, 2 pces	190	10	24
Sugar Free: Choc. Almonds (4)	95	7.5	10
Sampler (7 oz Box), 3 pces	170	11	23
Whoppers, 9 pces, 21g	100	3.5	16
Wonka: Wonka Bar (1), 1.3 oz	180	10	25
Laffy Taffy: Orig., 5 bars, 1.5 oz	160	2	36
Stretchy & Tangy, 1½ oz	165	4	33
Nerds, 1 box	240	0	42
Gobstopper, Box, 1.77 oz	650	0	182
Runts Fruit Box, 1.8 oz	210	0	49
Tart 'N Tinys, 1.75 oz pkt	180	0	44
Yogurt Candy, Coated Raisins, 27 pces, 40g	180	8	28
York Peppermint Pattie: Regular, 1.37 oz	140	2.5	31
Fun Size, 0.6 oz	60	1	13
King Size, 2.86 oz	320	6	66
York Mints, 3	10	0	2
Zachary Old Fashioned Drops, 1 oz	100	0	26
Zagnut, 1.75 oz bar	230	10	31
Zero Bar: 1.8 oz bar	230	8	37
King Size, 3.4 oz	420	16	66
Zingos, 3 pce, 2g	5	0	2

Gum ~ Per Piece

	C	F	Cb
Bazooka, each	15	0	4
Beechies	6	0	2
Big League Chew	10	0	2
Bubble Yum	25	0	6
Sugarless	10	0	3
Candilicious	30	0	2
Carefree (Sugarless/Regular)	5	0	2
Chiclets, 1 piece	5	0	1
Clorets, 1 stick	10	0	2
Dentyne	5	0	0.5
Estee, bubble/regular	5	0	2
Extra (Wrigley's), Sugar-Free	5	0	2
Freshen-Up	10	0	3
Hubba Bubba: Regular	23	0	6
Sugar-free, average	14	0	0.5
Ice Breakers	0	0	0
Sonic Boom Bubble Gum	15	0	3
Sticklets	7	0	2
Super Bubble	15	0	4
Trident, Original/White	5	0	2
Wrigley's, all flavors	10	0	2

Carob Candy

Per Piece/Serving	C	F	Cb
Carob: Plain/Natural, 1 oz	160	11	9
Carob Coated: Raisins, 1 oz	130	8	15
Almonds/Peanuts, 1 oz	150	10	14
Malt Balls, 1 oz	135	8	14
Caramels, 1 oz	110	4	18
Dates, 1 oz	125	5	20
Soybeans	145	9	16
Trail/Party Mix, 1 oz	140	9	15
Carob Chips, unsweetened, 1 oz	140	7	19
Carob Bars: Plain/Nut, 1 oz	160	11	13
Fruit & Nut, 1 oz	155	10	13
Mint/Orange, 1 oz	160	11	14
Carafection: Cashew Coconut Crunch, ½ Bar, (42g) 1.5 oz	250	14	5
Caroby Natural Touch, 3 oz	450	27	36

Cough Drops

	C	F	Cb
Beech Nut, 1 drop	10	0	2
Diabetic Tussin, 1 drop	0	0	0
Halls Defense Vit. C, 1 drop	15	0	4
Halls Fruit Breezers, 1 drop	15	0	4
Halls Menthol Drops, 1 drop	15	0	4
Sugar Free, 1 drop	5	0	4
Halls Plus, 1 drop	20	0	5
Listerine Lozenge (Amer. Chicle)	10	0	2
Luden's Throat Drops, all flavors, 1	10	0	2
Sugar Free, 1 drop	0	0	0
Pine Bros, 1 cough drop	10	0	3
Ricola: Cough Drops (1)	10	0	3
Sugar-Free Lemon Mint (2)	0	0	1
Rite Aid, Menthol Cough (1)	10	0	3
Robitussin: Regular, 1 drop	15	0	3
Honey Cough, 1 drop	40	0	10
Sugar Free Throat, 1 drop	10	0	3
Sunny Orange Vit. C, 1 drop	10	0	3
Rolaids Sodium Free, 1	5	0	1
Sathers Peppermint Lozenges, 1	15	0	3
Squibb Cough/Throat Loz.'s, 1	15	0	4
Sucrets (Beecham) Lozenges, 1	10	0	2
Wintergreen Loz. (Walgreens), 1	15	0	3

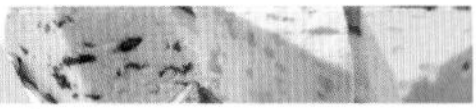

Quick Guide   C F Cb

Firm/Hard Cheeses
(American, Cheddar, Colby, Swiss)

Regular Cheese:	C	F	Cb
Thin Deli slice, ¾ oz	90	7	0
1 oz slice/piece	115	9	0.5
8 oz package	915	75	3
16 oz (1lb) package	1830	150	6
Cubes: 1" cube, ¾ oz	85	7	0.5
1¼" cube, 1 oz slice	115	9	0.5
Diced: 1 cup, 4½ oz	530	40	2
Grated: 1 Tbsp, ¼ oz	30	2.5	0
Shredded: Cheddar, ¼ cup, 1 oz	115	9	0.5
1 cup, 4 oz	455	37	1.5
Cheddar, Red.-Fat, ¼ cup, 1 oz	80	6	1
Mozzarella, ¼ cup, 1 oz	85	6.5	0.5
Part-Skim, ¼ cup, 1 oz	70	5	1
Sliced: 1 thin (3½" sq.), ¾ oz	85	7	0.5
Rectangular (7"x 4"x ⅛"), 1½ oz	170	14	0.5
Round (3¼" diam. x ⅛"), ¾ oz	85	7	0.5
Semi-circular, 1¼ oz			
(5½" long, 3½" radius, ⅛" thick)	140	12	0.5
Fat-Free: Average all brands, 1 oz	40	0	2
Low-Fat: Average all brands, 1 oz	50	2	0.5
Reduced Fat: Avg. all brands, 1 oz	80	5	0.5

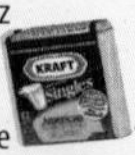

Cheese   C F Cb

Per 1 oz Unless Indicated

American:	C	F	Cb
Regular: 1 slice, 1 oz	105	9	0.5
Alpine Lace, 1 oz	90	7	2
Kraft, 0.7 oz slice	70	5	2
Shredded, ¼ cup, 1 oz	115	9	0.5
Land O'Lakes, 0.7 oz slice	70	5	2
Light: *Kraft* (2% Milk), 0.7 oz slice	50	3	1
Fat-Free: *Kraft,* 0.7 oz slice	30	0	2
Borden, Singles, 0.8 oz slice	80	0	2
Babybel (Laughing Cow), 21g	70	6	0
Light Original, 21g pce	50	3	0
Blue/Bleu, 1 oz	100	8	0.5
Bonbel (Laughing Cow), 1 pce	70	6	0
Brick (Land O'Lakes), 1" cube, 1 oz	110	8	1
Brie, 1 oz	95	8	0
Camembert, 1 oz	85	7	0
Caraway, 1 oz	105	8	1
Castello (Wegman's), avg., 1 oz	120	12	0

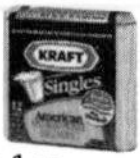

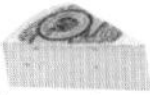

Cheddar: (Also see 'Quick Guide')	C	F	Cb
Regular: 1 oz	115	9	0.5
Alpine Lace, 1 oz	90	7	0
Reduced-Fat/Low-Fat:			
Borden, Shredded, ¼ cup, 1 oz	80	6	1
Cabot Vermont, 50% Light, 1 oz	70	4.5	0.5
Lifetime, 1oz	45	1.5	0
Fat-Free, *Kraft,* 0.7 oz slice	30	0	2
Cheese Balls (Kaukauna), 1 oz, avg.	100	7	0.5
Cheese Logs (Kaukauna), avg., 1 oz	100	7	0.5
Cheshire, 1 oz	110	9	1.5
Colby: Regular, 1 oz	110	9	0.5
Reduced-Fat (*Kraft*), 1 oz	80	6	0
Colby-Jack, regular, 1 oz	110	9	1
Cottage Cheese: *Average All Brands*			
Creamed (4% milk fat): 2 Tbsp, 1 oz	30	1	1.5
½ cup, 4 oz	120	5	6
w. fruit, ½ cup, 4 oz	130	4	15
Reduced-Fat (2%): 2 T., 1 oz	25	0.5	1
½ cup, 4 oz	100	2	4
Low-Fat (1%): 2 Tbsp, 1 oz	20	.5	1
½ cup, 4 oz	80	1	3
Fat-Free/Non-Fat: 2 Tbsp, 1 oz	20	0	1
(*Jewel*), ½ cup, 4 oz	80	0	5
Friendship: Low-Fat P'apple, 4 oz	120	1	16
Non-Fat w. Peach, ½ cup, 4 oz	110	0	15
Pot Style, ½ cup, 4 oz	90	2.5	3
Hood w. Chive/Onion, 4 oz	90	1	5
Knudsen:			
Free: Non-Fat, ½ c., 4 oz	80	0	7
2% Milk Fat, ½ c., 4 oz	100	2.5	6
Cottage Doubles, avg, 5.5 oz ctn	150	5	18
On the Go! Free, 4 oz ctn	70	0	7
Low-Fat, 4 oz ctn	90	2.5	6
Lactaid: Low-Fat, ½ cup, 4 oz	80	1	7
Light N' Lively: Fat-Free, 4.4 oz	80	0	8
Low-Fat, ½ cup, 4.4 oz	80	1.5	6
Live Active (Low-Fat 2%):			
Plain, 1/2 cup, 4 oz	90	2	10
Mixed Berry; Pineapple, avg., 4 oz	120	1.5	18
Cream Cheese: *See Page 81*			
Edam, Regular, 1 oz	100	8	0.5
Farmer (Friendship), 2 Tbsp, 1 oz	50	2.5	0
Feta: Regular, 1 oz	75	6	1
Crumbled, ½ cup, 2½ oz	190	15	3
Red.-Fat (*Athenos*), 1 oz	60	4	1
Fontina, 1 oz	110	9	0.5
Gjetost (Goat's Milk, fresh), 1 oz	130	8	12

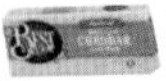

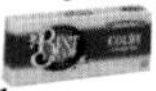

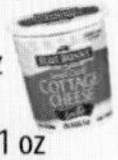

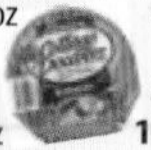

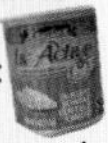

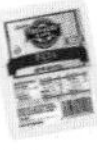

	C	F	Cb
Goat's Milk Cheese:			
Chevre, Soft, 1 oz 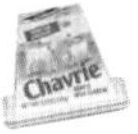	80	6	1
Chavril: 3 Tbsp, 1 oz	60	4.5	0.5
Semi-Soft, 1 oz	100	8.5	1
Hard, 1 oz	130	10	0.5
Gorgonzola, 1 oz	100	8	0.5
Galbani Dolcelatte, 1 oz	95	8	1
Gouda, 1 oz	100	8	0.5
Gruyere, 1 oz	115	9	1
Havarti *(Land O'Lakes)*, 1 oz	110	8	1
Italian Blend *(Sargento)*, 1 oz	90	7	1
Jarlsberg *(Wegman's)*, 1 oz	100	8	0
Jarlsberg Red. Fat, shredded, 1 oz	70	4	0
Kefir *(Alta Dena)*, 2 Tbsp, 1 oz	70	6	2
Labneh (Lebanese cream chse), 1.8 oz	70	4	4
Lactose Free Cheese *(Lifetime)*, 1 oz	40	0	1
Limburger, 1 oz	95	8	0
Mascarpone *(Wegman's)*, 1 oz	130	13	1
Mexican:			
Cacique: Cotija, 1 oz 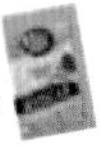	110	9	0
Queso Fresco, 1 oz	80	6	0
Queso Quesadilla, 1 oz	70	5	2
Ranchero, 1 oz	80	6	0
Chi-Chi's: Con Quéso, 2 Tbsp	90	7	4
Hot/Medium/Mild/Acante, 2 T.	10	0	2
Kraft, Taco, shredded, ¼ cup, 1 oz	100	8	2
Sargento, Shredded, ¼ cup, 1 oz	110	9	0.5
Supremo Chihuahua: Quéso Bianco	100	8	0
Quéso Fresco; Rancherito	80	6	0
Monterey, 1 oz	105	8.5	0
Monterey Jack: Regular, 1 oz	110	9	0
Kraft 2% Milk Red. Fat, 1 oz	80	6	1
Alpine Lace, Co-Jack, 1 oz 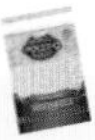	90	7	0
Weight Watchers, 1 oz	90	6	1
Mozzarella:			
Regular: 1 oz	85	6.5	0.5
Land O'Lakes/Polly-O, 1 oz, avg.	90	6	1
Shredded, ¼ cup, 1 oz	90	7	1
Light: *Polly-O Lite,* Shred., 1 oz	60	2.5	1
Kraft 2% Milk Fat, Red. Fat, 1 oz	70	4	1
Sargento Reduced Fat, ¼ c., 1 oz	80	4.5	1
Part Skim: *Alpine Lace,* 1 oz	70	5	1
Borden/Kraft, Shred., ¼ c., 1 oz	80	5	1
Polly-O, 1 oz	70	5	1
Fat-Free: *Polly-O,* 1 oz	35	0	1
Kraft, shredded, ¼ cup, 1 oz	45	0	2
Muenster: Regular, 1 oz	105	9	0.5
Low-Fat, 1 oz	85	5	1
Myzithra, grated, 4 T. 1 oz	80	4	2
Neufchatel: 1 oz 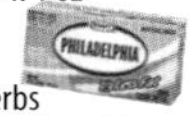	75	6	1
Philadelphia, 1 oz	70	6	1
Flavored: Fruit/Herbs	80	7	1
Chocolate *(Hickory Farms)*, 1 oz	110	8	1

	C	F	Cb
Parmesan: Fresh/Block, 1 oz	110	7.5	1
Grated (Packaged): 1 Tbsp 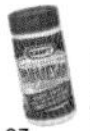	20	1.5	0
1 oz quantity	120	8	1
½ cup, 1¾ oz	215	14	2
w. Romano *(Frigo)*, grated, 1 oz	110	7	0
Kraft Reduced-Fat Topping, 1 T.	20	1	2
Pizza Cheese, shredded:			
Regular *(Kraft)* ¼ cup, 1 oz	90	7	1
Port de Salut, 1 oz 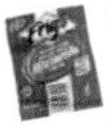	100	8	0
Port Wine *(Kaukauna)*, 1 oz	90	6	4
Pot *(Sargento)*, 1 oz	25	0	1
Provolone: Regular, 1 oz	100	7.5	0.5
Reduced-Fat: *Alpine Lace,* 1 oz	80	5	1
Sargento, 1 slice, ⅔ oz	50	3.5	0
Pub *(Rondele)*, 1 oz, avg.	95	7	1
Quark: 40% fat, 1 oz	47	3	1
20% fat, 1 oz	32	1.5	1
Skim/Non-Fat, 1 oz	22	0	1.5
Queso: Anejo/Asadero/Blanco, 1 oz	105	9	1
Chichuahua/De Papa, 1 oz	110	9	2
Ricotta Cheese:			
Whole Milk, 2 Tbsp, 1 oz 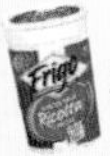	50	3.5	1
½ cup, 4½ oz	215	16	4
Part Skim, 2 Tbsp, 1 oz	40	2	1.5
½ cup, 4½ oz	170	10	6
Light/Low-Fat, 2 Tbsp, 1 oz	25	1	1.5
½ cup, 4½ oz	125	5	6
Fat-Free, ½ cup, 4½ oz	100	0	10
Baked Ricotta, 2 oz portion	130	9	3
Romano: Block/Loaf, 1 oz	110	8	1
Grated (Pkg): 1 oz	120	9	1
1 Tbsp, 5g	20	1.5	0
Roquefort, 1 oz	105	9	0.5
Sheep's Milk, 1 oz	45	3	1
Smoked: *Wegman's,* 1 oz	100	8	0
Tillamook, Smoked Cheddar, 1 oz	110	9	0
Stilton *(Wegman's)*, 1 oz	110	10	0
String *(Frigo/Kraft/Sargento)*, 1 oz	80	6	0.5
Light String-Ums *(Kraft)*, 1 oz 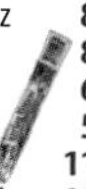	80	4.5	1
String Lite *(Frigo)*, 1 oz	60	2.5	0.5
Light *(Sargento)*, 1 stick, 0.7 oz	50	2.5	0.5
Swiss: Regular, 1 oz	110	8	1.5
Reduced-Fat: *Alpine Lace,* 1.2 oz	110	7	1
Kraft, 2% Milk, 0.7 oz slice	50	2.5	2
Taco Cheese *(Kraft)* shredded, ¼ cup	120	10	1
Tilsit, 1 oz	100	7.5	0.5
Tybo, 1 oz	100	7	0.5
Vermont *(Cabot)*, 1 oz 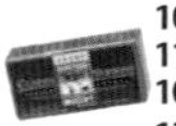	110	9	0
Wensleydale, 1 oz	100	8	0.5
Whey Cheese, 1 oz	125	8	9

Cheese Products

	C	F	Cb
Cheese Food:			
Average all flavors: ¾ oz slice	70	5	2
1 oz slice	95	7	2.5
Alouette: Sundr. Tomato, 2 T., 0.8oz	70	7	1
Light Garlic, 2 Tbsp, 0.8 oz	50	4	1
Peppercorn Cajun, 2 T., 0.8 oz	70	8	1
Savory Vegetable, 2 T., 0.8 oz	60	6	1
Cabot, Jalapeno, 1 oz	70	4.5	0
Cracker Barrel, Cheddar, 1 oz	120	10	0
Handi-Snacks: *(Kraft)*			
Breadsticks 'n Cheez, 1.1 oz	110	4.5	14
Pretzels 'n Cheez, 1 oz	90	3.5	12
Ritz Crackers 'n Cheez, 1 oz pkg	100	5	10
Mozzarella Stringchse Stick, each	80	6	0.5
Kraft: American shred., 1T.	25	2	0.5
Singles, 1 slice, ¾ oz	70	5	2
Free Singles, 1 sl., 0.7 oz	30	0	2
Pimento Spread, 2 T., 1.1 oz	80	6	3
Light String-Ums, 1 stick, 1 oz	80	4.5	1
Kraft LiveActive:			
Cheese Sticks: Cheddar,(1), 1 oz	120	10	0
Mozzarella, 1 stick, 1 oz	80	5	0
Colby Jack, Red. Fat (1), 1 oz	90	6	0
Cheese Cubes:			
Colby Jack, 7 cubes, 1 oz	110	9	0
Cheddar (Red. Fat), 7 cubes 1 oz	90	6	0
Lifetime Cholesterol Reducing,			
Slices, 1 Slice, 19g	30	1	2
Block, 1"cube, 1 oz	55	2.5	1
Lifeway Farmers Kefir, 2 Tbsp, 1 oz	75	1.5	4
Precious String Chse Stuffsters, 1 oz	70	3	1
Rondele: Soft Spread.., 2 T., 1 oz	100	9	1
Light, 2 Tbsp, 1 oz	60	5	2
Sargento Chef Style,			
Cheddar, shred., ¼ c., 1 oz	110	9	1
Mozzarella, shrd, ¼ cup	80	6	0.5
Velveeta: Regular, ⅜" slice, 1 oz	80	6	3
Light, ¾" slice, 1 oz	60	3	4
Shredded, ¼ c., 1.3 oz	130	9	3
WisPride: Port Wine,			
Ball/Cup, 2 T., 1.1 oz	90	5	5.5
Light, 2 T., 1.1 oz	80	3	5

Cheese Whiz (Sauce)

	C	F	Cb
Original, 2 Tbsp, 33g	90	7	2
Light, 2 Tbsp, 33g	80	3	6
Salsa Con Queso, 2 Tbsp, 33g	90	7	4

Cheese Substitutes

Per 1 oz Unless Indicated

	C	F	Cb
Galaxy:			
Veggie Yellow American, 1 sl., ½ oz	35	2	1
Veggie Mozz. Singles, 1 sl., ½ oz	40	2	1
Lifetime Rice Cheese, 1" cube, 1 oz	60	3	5
Mori Nu Tofu: Mozzarella, 1 oz	70	4	2
Fat-Free Mozz./Ched./Jack, 1 oz	40	0	2
Smart Beat, Fat-Free, 0.6 oz sl.	25	0	3
Soya Kaas: Regular, 1 oz	70	5	1
Fat-Free, all varieties, 1 oz	40	2	1
Soyco: Almond/Oat/Rice Slices,			
1 slice, 0.7 oz	40	2	1
Veggie Singles, 1 slice, 0.7 oz	40	2	1
Grated Parmesan, 2 tsp, 5g	15	0.5	0
Soy-Sation: Shredded Cheese, 1 oz	70	4	2
Tofu Rella, avg. all varieties, 1 oz	60	4	0
Tofutti Better Than Cream Chse, 1 oz	80	8	1
Trader Joe's: *Per Slice*			
Soy Cheese:			
Cheddar Flavor, 0.7 oz	45	2	3
Mozzarella Flavor, 1 oz	70	4	3
Sliced Yogurt Cheese, 1 oz	100	8	0
Yves, Good Slice, ¾ oz slice, avg.	35	2	1

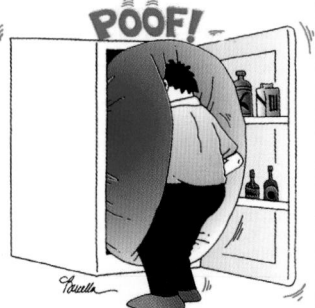

*New Diet Aid
- The Refrigerator Air Bag!*

POOF!

Cream Cheese | C | F | Cb |

Regular/Soft, average all brands:

	C	F	Cb
2 Tbsp, 1 oz	90	9	2
8 oz pkg	720	72	13
w. Chives/Herbs/Pimento, 1 oz	75	2.5	10
w. Fruit/Strawb./P'apple, 1 oz	90	8	4
Philadelphia (Kraft): Per 2 Tbsp			
Original, 2 Tbsp, 1 oz	100	10	0.5
3 oz package	300	30	2
Regular, 2 Tbsp, 1.1 oz	90	9	2
Neufchatel ⅓ Less Fat, 1 oz	70	6	1
Light: Plain, 2 Tbsp, 1.1 oz	60	4.5	2
Flavors, avg., 0.7 oz	70	4	6
Fat-Free Varieties, 1 oz	25	0	1
Flavored: Blueb./Raspberry, 1 oz	80	6	4.5
Honey Nut; Strawberry, 1 oz	80	7	4.5
Garden Vegetable, 1 oz	80	7.5	2
Jammin' Swirls, 2 Tbsp, 1.1 oz	80	6	7
Whipped: Regular, 2 Tbsp, 0.7 oz	60	6	1
Mixed Berry, 2 Tbsp, 0.7 oz	70	5	3
Snacks: Bars, avg (1), 1½ oz	180	11	20
Snack Bites (1) 1 oz	130	7	15
Bagel & Crm Chse To Go, 3.2 oz	240	9	36

Dips/Spreads

Per 2 Tbsp (1 oz), Unless Indicated
Average All Brands

	C	F	Cb
Avocado/Guacamole, 2 Tbsp, 1 oz	45	4	2
Baba Ghannoush (Eggplant/Sesame)	70	6	2
Cheese Fondue, ½ cup, 4 oz	260	15	4
French Onion Dip, 2 Tbsp	60	4.5	3
Hummus: 2 Tbsp, 1 oz	50	1	5
½ cup, 4.5 oz	220	4.5	23
Tzatziki (Cucumber/Yogurt) 2 T.	30	2.5	2
Clearman's: Original Spread, 1 oz	150	15	2
De La Casa, 5 Layer Party Dip, 2 T.	40	2.5	4
Frito Lay: Chili Cheese, 2 T.	50	3	3
Jalapeno, 2 Tbsp	50	3	3
French Onion, 2 T.	60	5	4
Bean/Jalapeno Bean, 2 T.	40	1	6
Guiltless Gourmet: Hummus, 2 T.	35	1.5	4
Other varieties	30	0	5
Heluva Good Cheese: French Onion	60	5	2
French Onion, Fat-Free	25	0	3
New England Clam	50	4.5	2
Average other flavors	60	5	3
Kaukauna: Nacho Cheese	90	7	4
Veggie Ranch	50	3	3

Dips/Spreads (Cont) | C | F | Cb |

Per 2 Tbsp (1 oz)

	C	F	Cb
Knudsen: Nacho Cheese	60	4	3
Sour Cream Bacon & Onion	60	5	2
Sour Cream French Onion	50	4	2
Kroger, The Big Dipper; all flavors	60	5	2
Kraft			
Avg. all flav., 2 T.	60	5	4
Cheez Whiz Dip:			
Original, 2 Tbsp	90	7	4.5
Light, 2 Tbsp	80	3.5	6
Lay's Dip Mix, prepared, 2 Tbsp	60	6	3
Marie's Dips, avg. all varieties	90	9	2
Nalley's,			
avg. all flavors	120	12	3
Naturally Fresh: Chocolate Dip	100	0	23
Cream Cheese Dip, 2 Tbsp	90	3.5	14
Fruit Dip, 2 Tbsp	80	4.5	10
Old Dutch French Onion, 2 Tbsp	50	2	4
Old El Paso: Black Bean, 2 Tbsp	25	0	5
Cheese 'n Salsa: Mild; Medium	40	3	4
Low-Fat, medium	30	1.5	4
Chunky Salsa varieties, avg.	15	0	3
Olys Bagel Spread: Berry	100	8	3
Garden Veg; Garlic & Herb	90	9	1
Prices: Pimiento Cheese Spread	80	7	2
Light Pimiento, 1 oz	55	3	3
Ruffles, French Onion; Ranch	60	5	3
Snyder's Mustard Pretzel	70	1	15
Stop & Shop: Veggie Dip, 2 Tbsp	110	10	3
Sour Crm French Onion, 2 T.	60	5	2
TGI Fridays: Spinach,Chse,Artichoke	45	3.5	2
Spinach Dip, 2 Tbsp	50	3.5	2
T. Marzetti: Choc Fruit, 2 Tbsp	110	2	23
Guacamole	130	13	2
Veggie: Ranch	120	12	2
Light Ranch	60	6	2
Fat-Free Ranch	30	0	6
Toby's: Tofu Pate, 2 T.	80	7	2
Other Spreads, avg., 2 T.	40	2.5	2
Tostitos Dip:			
Con Quéso Salsa	40	2.5	3
Reduced-Fat Zesty Cheese, 2 T.	40	2	4
Wise: French Onion, 2 Tbsp	60	5	3
Nacho Cheese	50	4.5	3

Condiments, Sauces | C | F | Cb

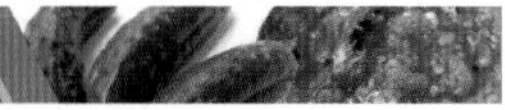

Average of Brands & Homemade

	C	F	Cb
Apple Sauce: *Also see Page 104*			
Sweetened, ¼ cup, 2½ oz	55	0	13
Unsweetened, ¼ cup, 2 oz	25	0	7
Barbecue Sauce: Avg., 2 Tbsp, 1 oz	40	0	10
Bull's Eye, Original, 1 Tbsp, ½ oz	30	0	7
Bearnaise Sauce, ¼ cup, 2½ oz	190	19	5
Buffalo Wing Sce: Honey Mustard, 1 T.	40	3	3
Average other varieties, 1 Tbsp	25	2	2
Catsup (Ketchup), regular, 1 Tbsp	15	0	4
Cheese, h/made, ¼ cup, 2½ oz	150	10	12
Chef-Mate, Hot Dog, ¼ cup	70	2.5	9
Chili Sauce: *Heinz,* 1 Tbsp, ½ oz	20	0	4.5
Del Monte, 1 Tbsp, ½ oz	20	0	5
Cocktail Sauce, ¼ cup	110	0	15
Fat-Free *(Walden Farms)* 1 Tbsp	0	0	0
Cranberry, all types, ¼ c., 2½ oz	110	0	27
Demi Glaze Gold, 2 tsp	30	0.5	3
Honey Mustard *(French's)* 1 tsp	5	0	1
Horseradish: 1 tsp	2	0	1
Kraft, 1 tsp	20	1.5	1
Ketchup: Regular, 1 Tbsp, ½ oz	15	0	4
Heinz One-Carb, 1 Tbsp	5	0	1
Mushroom Sauce, ½ cup, 2 oz	50	2	5
Mustard, average, 1 tsp	5	0	0.5
Pesto Sauce, ¼ cup, 2 oz	90	5	8
Pizza Sauce, cnd., ¼ cup, 2 oz	30	0	6
Seafood Cocktail Sce, ¼ cup	60	0	15
Soy Sauce: All types, avg., 1 Tbsp	10	0	1
Kikkoman Lite Soy, 1 Tbsp	10	0	1
Sour Cream Sce, ½ cup	250	15	22
Spaghetti Sce, ½ cup, 4½ oz	135	6	19
Steak Sauce: A1, 1 Tbsp, ½ oz	15	0	3
Lea & Perrins, 1 Tbsp, ½ oz	25	0	5
Carb Well (A1) 1 Tbsp, ½ oz	5	0	1
Str'berry Puree Sce: Unsweet., 2 T.	9	0	2
Sweet & Sour Sauce:			
Contadina, 1 Tbsp	40	1	8
Kraft, 1 Tbsp	60	0	13
La Choy, 2 Tbsp, 34g	60	0	14
Tabasco Sauce, 1 tsp	2	0	0
Taco Sauce, average, 2 Tbsp, 1 oz	10	0	1
Tartar Sauce: *Heinz,* 2 Tbsp, 1 oz	120	11	4
America's Choice, 2 Tbsp, 1 oz	160	17	1
Hellmann's, Regular, 2 Tbsp, 1 oz	80	7	4
McCormick, Fat-Free, 2 Tbsp, 1 oz	35	0	6
Teriyaki Sauce *(Kikkoman)* 1 T., ½ oz	15	0	3
Vinegar, White or Wine, 2 Tbsp	4	0	1
White Sauce, ½ cup, 5 oz	130	7	10
Worcestershire Sauce, 1 tsp	5	0	1

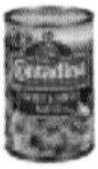

Pickles & Relish | C | F | Cb

Average All Brands

	C	F	Cb
Bread & Butter Pickles, 4 sl., 1 oz	25	0	6
Chutney, 2 Tbsp, 1¼ oz	50	0	11
Dill Pickle:			
Slices, 4 slices, 1 oz	4	0	1
1 large, (3¾"x 1¼" diam.), 2¼ oz	12	0	3
Extra lrg (4"x 1¾" diam.), 5 oz	30	0	6
Halves: Small, 1 oz	3	0	0.5
Large, 2½ oz	8	0	2
Sweet, small, ½ oz	22	0	6
Gherkins, sweet, 1 med., 1 oz	30	0	7
Green Chiles, chopped, 2 Tbsp	5	0	1
Horseradish, 1 Tbsp	10	0	2
Jalapenos, pickled (2), 2 oz	10	0.5	2
Jalapeno Relish, 1 Tbsp, ½ oz	5	0	1
Mustard, avg. all brands, 1 tsp	5	0	0.5
Peppers, Hot/Mild (1), 1.6 oz	20	0	4
Pickled: Beets, ½ cup, 4 oz	75	0	19
Onions, 1 medium, ¾ oz	10	0	2
Cocktail Onion, 1 onion	2	0	0
Red Cabbage, ½ cup, 3 oz	65	0	15
Pickles: Sweet, 2 Tbsp, 1 oz	35	0	0
Large (3"x ¾ diam.), 1¼ oz	40	0	10
Pickle in a Pouch, 1 large	12	0	3
Relishes: Sandwich Spread, 1 tsp	20	1	5
Cranberry-Orange, 1 Tbsp	30	0	7
Hot Dog *(Heinz),* 1 Tbsp, ½ oz	17	0	3
Sweet Pickle, 1 Tbsp, ½ oz	20	0	5
Sauerkraut, ½ cup, 3½ oz	25	0	5
Sweet Cauliflower, 2 Tbsp	35	0	8

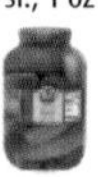

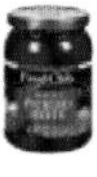

Salsa

Average all Types: Per 2 Tablespoons

	C	F	Cb
Regular, no oil, 2 Tbsp, 1 oz	15	0	3.5
Made with oil, 2 Tbsp, 1 oz	40	3	8
Kaukauna, 2 Tbsp, 1 oz	15	0	3
La Victoria, 2 Tbsp, 1 oz	10	0	2
Old El Paso, 1 Tbsp, 1 oz	10	0	3
TGI Friday's, 1.2 oz	15	0	4

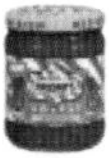

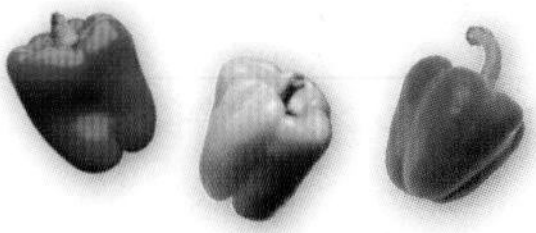

Quick Guide

	C	F	Cb
Cookies			
Average All Brands: Per Cookie			
Biscotti: Small, 0.5 oz	70	3	10
Regular, 1 oz	140	6.5	18
Chocolate Chip Cookies:			
Small/Thin 0.5 oz	70	3.5	9
Regular, 1 oz	140	7	18
Large, 2.5 oz *(Mrs Fields)*	330	16	46
Extra Large, 4 oz	555	28	73
Oatmeal/Oatmeal Raisin:			
Small/Thin 0.5 oz	65	2.5	10
Regular, 1 oz	130	5	20
Large, 2.5 oz *(Mrs Fields)*	330	14	44
Extra Large, 4 oz	510	20	78
Peanut Butter:			
Small/Thin 0.5 oz	70	3.5	9
Regular, 1 oz	135	7	17
Large, 2.5 oz *(Mrs Fields)*	330	17	41
Extra Large, 4 oz	540	27	67
Low-Fat Cookies			
Choc Chip (Low-Fat), ½ oz (1)	65	2	10
Oatmeal Raisin (Fat-Free), 1 oz (1)	95	0.5	22
Peanut Butter (Low-Fat), 1 oz (1)	105	5	15

Quick Guide

	C	F	Cb
Crackers			
Average All Brands: Per Cracker			
Cheese Crackers: Plain, 1" square	5	0	0.5
Small, octagonal	10	0	1
Round (2" diam.)	15	0	1.5
Sandwich (Peanut Butter)	35	1.5	4
Graham, 2½" square, 1 cracker	30	0.5	5
Melba Toast, plain, 1 piece	20	0	4
Oyster & Soup Crackers, ½ oz	60	2	10
(40 small oysters/20 lge hexagons)			
Rice Crackers: 1 small	9	0	1.5
Rice Snacks, Oriental-Style, 1 oz	130	2.5	23
Saltines, 5 crackers	65	2	11
Snack-type, 1 round cracker	15	0	2
Soda Crackers *(Saltine),* 2	25	1	4.5
Water Cracker *(Carr's):* Regular, 1	30	0	7
Small, 1 cracker	15	0	3
Wheat, thin, 1 cracker	9	0.5	1.5
Zweiback Toast, 1 piece	35	1	6

Brands

	C	F	Cb
All-Bran, all flavors (18), 1.1 oz	120	6	19
Annies			
Crackers: Cheddar Bunnies (50)	150	7	19
Whole Wheat Bunnies (50)	130	6	17
Sour Cream & Onion (55)	140	6	18
Grahams, Bunnies (24), avg.	130	4	22
Archway			
Classic Oatmeal (1)	110	4	18
Classic Oatmeal Raisin (1)	110	3.5	20
Original Iced Oatmeal (2)	110	4.5	17
Fruit-Filled Date Oatmeal (1)	90	3	18
Fruit & Honey Bar (1)	160	5	28
Iced Circus Animals (6)	150	7	19
Peanut Butter Creme (2)	190	8	25
Snacking Cookies (Bulk Pkg):			
Ginger Snaps (5)	150	5	23
Iced Lemonade (4)	140	7	20
Iced Molasses (3)	130	2	26
Oatmeal Raisin (4)	140	5	21
Peanut Butter Choc Chip (4)	150	8	19
Atkins, Endulge Crisps (1)	130	10	15
Austin			
Crackers: *Per Package*			
Cheese w. Cheddar Cheese, 1.38 oz	210	10	26
Cheese w. Cheddar Jack Cheese	200	11	23
Chocolatey P'nut Butter, 1.38 oz	200	10	25
Dolphins & Friends Cheddar, 2 oz	280	12	38
Mega Stuffed P'nut Butter, 1.68 oz	240	13	25
Sandwich: Cheese & Peanut Butter	200	10	23
Grilled Cheese Flavored, 1.38 oz	200	10	24
PB & J Flavored, 1.38 oz	190	9	25
Toasty Crackers w. P'nut butter, 1.3 oz	200	10	23
Wheat Crackers w. Cheddar Chse	200	10	24
Zoo Animals 2.12 oz pkg	250	4	50
Sandwich Cremes: *Per Package*			
Lemon OHs!, 1.2 oz	170	7	24
Vanilla Cremes, 1.2 oz	170	7	24
Baker's: *Per 3 oz Cookie*			
Peanut Butter	330	11	49
Peanut Butter & Jelly	320	8	52
Vegan Peanut But. Choc. Chunk	330	10	52
Other varieties, average	300	6	54
Barbara's Bakery			
Cookies: Fig Bars, avg. (1)	60	0.5	14
Animal Cookies, Vanilla (8)	110	4	17
Snackimals (10), average	120	4	19
Crackers: Rite Lite Rounds (5), avg.	60	2	11
Organic Go Go Grahams (8) avg.	130	4	22
Wheatines (4), average	60	1	11

Blue Diamond	C	F	Cb
Nut Thins: Almond, Ranch (16)	130	3.5	22
Almond, Smokehouse (16)	130	3	23
Hazelnut (16)	130	3	23
Pecan (16)	130	3.5	23

Brent & Sam's

Cookies, Oatmeal Pecan (2)	120	6	15

Cadbury

Cadbury Finger (6)	180	9	21

Carr's

Crackers: Table Water (5)	70	1.5	13
Whole Wheat (2)	80	3.5	11
Cookies: Bisc. for Tea (2)	140	6	20
Ginger Lemon Cremes (2)	130	5	20

Cheez•It ~ See Sunshine (Page 89)

Chips Ahoy! ~ See Nabisco (Page 87)

Cookies &

Cookie Bars: M&M's (1)	170	9	20
Milky Way/Snickers/Twix (1)	180	11	21
Twix w. Peanut Butter (1)	160	9	17

Country Choice

Ginger Snaps (5)	140	5	22
Sandwich Cremes (2), avg.	130	5	19
Soft Baked, avg. all varieties (1)	100	4	16
Vanilla Wafers (7)	140	5	22

Dove

Beyond Chocolate Chunk (1), ¾ oz	110	5	13
Chocolate Walnut Oasis (1)), ¾ oz	110	6	13
Chocolate Walnut Rendezvous (1)	110	6	13
Milk Chocolate Moment (3), 1.1 oz	160	9	20
Mint Chocolate Serenade (3), 1.1 oz	160	8	19
Toffee Chocolate Thrill (3), 1.1 oz	160	8	20

Dr. Knacker

Crackers: Flatbread, avg., all flav., 1 oz	110	5	11
Snacker: Kinder, Veggie Spelt (1)	40	2	8
Kribbons: Krispy Graham (5), 1 oz	120	3	20
Museli (5), 1 oz	120	4.5	15
Spelt Sunflower Cheese (8), 1 oz	100	6	12
Avg., other flavors (8), 1 oz	120	5	15

Famous Amos

Chocolate Chip (4)	150	7	20
Choc Chip & Pecan (4)	150	8	18
Choc. Creme Sandwich (3)	170	7	25
Oatmeal Choc Chip & Walnut (4)	140	7	18
Oatmeal Raisin (4)	140	6	20
Peanut Butter (4)	150	8	17
Peanut Buter Creme S'wich (3)	160	7	22
Vanilla Creme Sandwich (3)	170	7	25
Low-Fat: Gingersnaps (1 pkg)	200	3	40

Per Cookie/Cracker (Unless Indicated)

Fig Newtons ~ See Nabisco (Page 87)

Girl Scouts	C	F	Cb
Cookies: Caramel DeLites (2)	140	7	19
Peanut Butter Sandwich (2)	170	6	24

Grandma's

Peanut Butter Sandwich Creme (5)	210	10	28
Rich 'N Chewy, Choc Chip, pkg.	270	12	38
Vanilla Sandwich Creme (5)	210	9	30
Mini Vanilla Bites (9)	150	7	22
Homestyle:			
Fudge Choc. Chip (1)	170	7	27
Oatmeal Raisin (1)	160	6	27
Peanut Butter (1)	200	10	24
Chocolate Chip (1)	190	9	25

Great American Cookies

Cookies: Original; Pecan (1)	230	12	31
Chewy Pecan Supreme (1)	230	12	31
Chewy Choc. Supreme/Sugar (1)	200	9	29
Double Fudge/ Reese's (1), avg	225	11	32
Oatmeal (1)	230	10	33
Original M&M/Reese's (1)	240	12	32
Peanut Butter/M&M (1), avg	250	13	28
Snickerdoodles (1)	240	11	33
White Chunk Macadamia (1)	250	14	30
Double Doozies: Original (1)	690	34	94
M&M Big Bite (1)	340	17	46
Brownies: Cheesecake (1)	430	23	54
German Chocolate (1)	420	22	55
Iced Fudge (1)	500	23	71
Iced Fudge Nut (1)	500	27	64
Swirl Cheesecake (1)	430	23	55
Cookie Cakes: 16" Cookie (1)	460	22	67
16" M&M Cookie (1)	500	24	73
Heart Shaped (1)	440	21	64
Sliced Cookie Cake, 1 slice	580	27	83

Health Valley

Cookies

Chocolate Chip Oatmeal (1)	100	4	14
Cookie Cremes Sandwich (2) avg.	120	5	19
Oatmeal Raisin Cookie (1)	90	3.5	14
Peanut Crunch Oatmeal Cookie (1)	100	4	14
Mini: Choc. Chocolate Chip (4)	130	5	16
Other varieties (4)	120	5	16

Health Valley (Cont)	C	F	Cb
Crackers			
Original: Amaranth Graham (6)	120	3	22
Oat Bran Graham (6)	120	3	22
Rice Bran (6)	110	3	19
Cracked Pepper; Sesame (4)	70	3	10
Mediterranean Stix: Garlic Herb (8)	70	3	9
Whole Wheat (4)	70	3	9
Hershey's			
Brownies:			
Hershey's, ½ pkg	200	9	28
Reeses, ½ pkg	200	9	27
Cookies: York Cookies (2)	160	9	17
Almond Joy Cookies (2)	160	9	17
Nutter Butter, ½ pkg (2)	180	9	24
Reese's Cookies (2)	150	8	17
Choc Covered Cookie:			
Almond Joy (2)	150	9	17
Hershey's w. Caramel (2)	130	6	19
Reeses (2)	150	8	17
York (2)	160	9	17
Kisses: Confetti Sprinkles (22)	150	7	19
Double Chocolate (22)	140	6	20
Sandwich Cookies:			
Hersheys (2)	140	7	18
Reeses (2)	140	7	17
Soft Baked, Hershey's (1)	375	18	50
Jewel			
Cookies: Animal Crackers (6)	130	3.5	22
Chewy Chocolate Chip (2), 1.1 oz	130	6	18
Chunky Choc. Chip (2), 1.1 oz	160	7	20
Choc. S'wich Cremes (3), 1.2 oz	130	5	20
Double Filled (3), 1½ oz	195	7.5	30
Vanilla Wafers (9), 1.1 oz	160	4.5	24
Graham Crackers: Cinnamon (2)	130	3	25
Honey (2), 1.1 oz	140	3	24
Low-Fat Honey (2), 1 oz	110	1	22
Joseph's Cookies			
Sugar Free Cookies			
Brownies: Original, 1½ oz bag	150	7	26
Pecan Walnut (9 brownies)	100	5	15
Crispy Bite Size: *Per 4 Cookies*			
Chocolate Peanut Butter	95	5	13
Pecan Chocolate Chip	95	5	13
Almond; Chocolate Chip	100	5	13
Chocolate Walnut; Oatmeal Choc	100	6	14
Lemon; Peanut Butter, avg.	95	4	15
Oatmeal; Pecan Shortbread, avg.	100	5	15

Per Cookie/Cracker (Unless indicated)	C	F	Cb
Kashi TLC			
Cookies	130	5	21
Crackers:			
Mini: Vegetable (15)	130	3.5	21
Honey Sesame (15)	130	3.5	21
Large: Bruschetta (4)	120	4	18
Garlic & Thyme (4)	130	4.5	18
Stoneground 7 Grain (4)	130	5	17
Keebler			
Crackers:			
Club: Original (4)	70	3	9
Reduced Fat (5)	70	2.5	12
Grahams: Original (8), 1 oz	130	3.5	22
Low-Fat varieties (8), 1 oz	110	1.5	22
Town House: Original (5)	80	4.5	10
Reduced Fat (6)	60	1.5	11
Wheatables: Reduced Fat (19)	140	4	22
Other varieties, average (17)	140	6	20
Cookies: Chips Deluxe			
Chocolate Lovers; Coconut (1)	80	4.5	10
Original, 2 oz	300	16	37
Rainbow (1)	80	4	10
Rainbow Mini's 1.4 oz pkg	200	10	27
Soft & Chewy (1)	80	3.5	11
Country Style Oatmeal (2)	130	6	18
Danish Wedding (4)	130	6	18
Dippin Delights Choc. S'wich (1)	90	4	13
Dunkin Delights Chsecake S'wich (1)	90	3.5	13
E.L. Fudge: Original (1)	90	3.5	13
Double Stuffed (2)	180	9	24
Fudge Shoppe:			
Deluxe Grahams, regular (3)	140	7	17
Fudge Sticks (3), avg.	150	8	20
Fudge Stripes: Regular, avg. (3)	150	7	21
Mini's, 1 pkg	200	9	27
Grasshopper (4)	140	7	19
Gripz, avg., 1 pouch	125	5	17
Iced Animal (6)	140	5	22
Mint Creme Filled (2)	160	9	20
Sandies Cookies: Reduced-Fat (1)	80	3.5	11
Cookies (1) avg. all flavors	90	5	9
100 Calorie Right Bites	100	3	17
Soft Batch (1)	80	3.5	11
Vienna Fingers: Regular (2)	150	6	23
Reduced Fat (2)	140	4.5	24
Wafers: Golden Vanilla Wafers (8)	140	6	21
Golden Vanilla Minis (18)	150	6	21

Per Cookie/Cracker (Unless indicated)

Kroger	C	F	Cb
Cookies: Chip Mates			
Original, 2 cookies, 1 oz	120	8	16
Chewy, 1 cookie, 0.7 oz	100	4.5	13
Chunky, 2 cookies, 1 oz	150	7	20
Olde Southern Pecan Shortbread, 1 oz	150	9	15
Sugar Wafer, 3 wafers, 1.1 oz	160	9	20
Vanilla Wafers, 7 wafers, 1.1 oz	130	3.5	23
Crackers:			
Grahams: Original /Honey (4)	120	3	20
Saltines, Original, 5 crackers, 0.5 oz	60	1.5	10

Lance	C	F	Cb
Nekot, Peanut Butter, 1 pkg	240	11	30
O Lunch, 1 pkg, avg.	230	10	34
Strawberry Cookies (5)	190	8	27
Crackers: Toasty, 1 pkg	180	9	16
Nipchee, 1 pkg	190	11	22
Toastchee: Original, 1 pkg	220	11	23
Reduced-Fat, 1 pkg	180	7	23
Malt Crackers, 1 pkg	190	10	18

Little Debbie	C	F	Cb
Fig Bars (1)	160	3	31
Marshmallow Pies, avg. (1)	180	7	28
Marshmallow Treats (1)	160	4	31
Oatmeal Creme Pies (1)	170	7	26
Nutty Bars: Twin Pack, 2 oz	310	18	33
100 Calories Singles, 1 oz	100	6	11
Crackers: Chse w. P'nut Butter (4)	140	7	15
Toasty w. P'nut Butter (4)	140	7	15

Lu	C	F	Cb
Marie Lu (3)	160	6	24
Le Fondant Wafers (4)	170	10	19
Le Petit Beurre (4)	140	4	26
Le Petit Ecolier, avg. (2)	130	6	17
Pim's, Orange (2)	100	3	17
Shortbread (2)	140	8	16

Manischewitz	C	F	Cb
Matzo Boards: See Page 105			
Chocolate Macaroons, each	45	2	8
Matzo Cracker, Miniatures, each	9	0	2
Tam Tam Crackers: Everything (10)	130	5	19
Original (10)	130	4	22

Miss Meringue	C	F	Cb
Chocolettes (10) average	110	3.5	23
Madeleines (2) average	160	9	19
Classiques:	110	0	27
Choc. Chip/Mint Choc. Chip (4)	120	1.5	25
Cappuccino/Rainbow Vanilla (4)	110	0	27
Meringue Minis: Chocolate (13)	110	0	26
Chocolate Chip (12)	130	1.5	27
Other varieties (13)	110	0	27
Meringue Minis, Sugar Free (13) avg.	40	0	8

Mrs Fields Cookies: See Fast-Foods Section

Mother's	C	F	Cb
Butter Cookies (6)	160	8	21
Checkerboard Wafers (4)	150	9	17
Chocolate Chip: Cookies (5)	160	7	21
Chocolate Chip Parade (4)	140	7	19
Chocolate Peanut Butter Creme (2)	180	8	25
Chocolate Vanilla Creme (2)	190	9	26
Chocolate Sandwich Creme (2)	190	9	26
Cocodas Coconut (2)	160	8	21
Coconut Fudge Creme (2)	190	9	26
Cookie Parade: Animal (4)	150	7	19
Circus Animal (14)	130	4.5	22
Iced Circus (6)	150	7	21
Double Fudge (2)	190	9	26
English Tea/Taffy S'wich (2)	185	7	28
Fudge Flaky Flix (3)	160	8	21
Fudge Vanilla Creme (2)	190	10	25
Ginger Snaps (5)	150	5	23
Peanut Butter Gaucho (2)	190	8	25
Iced Raisin (2)	170	6	24
Oatmeal Cookies: Regular (2)	130	5	19
Chocolate Chip (2)	160	8	22
Striped Shortbread Cookies (3)	160	7	24
Vanilla Cremes (2)	180	7	23
Vanilla Fudge Creme (2)	190	8	27
Bakery Wagon: Macaroons(1)	170	11	17
Iced Oatmeal/Lemon (2)	140	4.5	23
Sugar Free: Chocolate Chip (4)	130	6	23
Checkerboard Wafers (6)	140	9	18
Pecan Shortbread (4)	170	11	17
Peanut Butter (4)	150	9	19
Oatmeal (4)	120	5	19

Murray SugarFree Cookies	C	F	Cb
Choc Chip with Pecans (3)	160	9	20
Double Fudge (3)	160	8	21
Fudge-Dipped: Grahams (4)	150	8	19
Mint Cookies (4)	130	7	16
Shortbread (5)	130	5	19
Vanilla Wafers (4)	150	10	19
Gingersnaps (7)	130	5	23
Lemon/Choc Cremes (3)	130	6	20
Lemon Wafers (4)	130	8	19
Oatmeal (4)	140	7	21
Peanut Butter (3)	150	9	16
Shortbread (8)	130	5	21
Shortbread Pecan (3)	170	11	18
Vanilla Sugar Wafers (4)	140	8	20

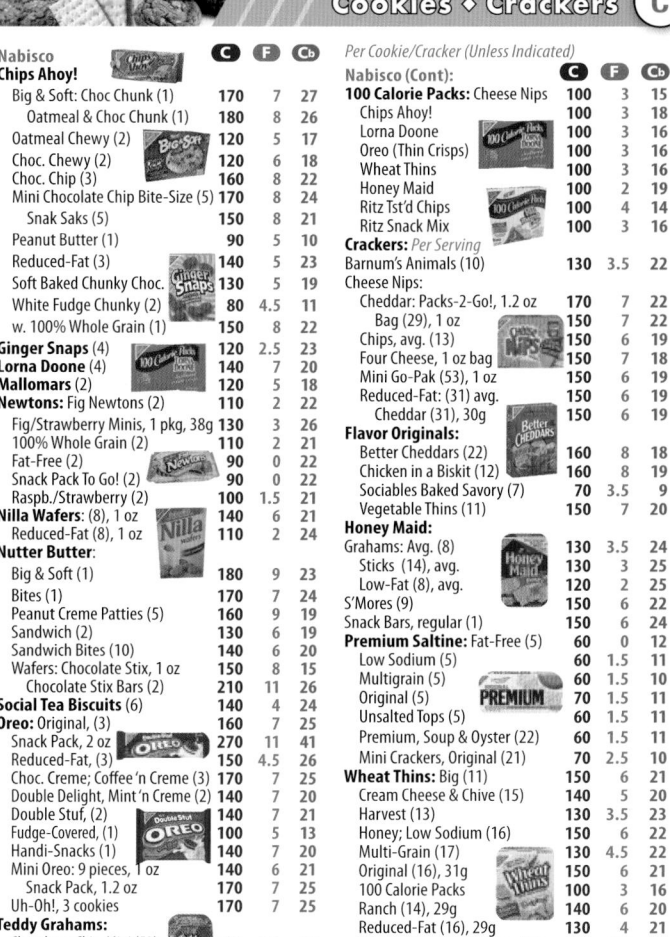

Nabisco

Per Cookie/Cracker (Unless Indicated)

Chips Ahoy!

	C	F	Cb
Big & Soft: Choc Chunk (1)	170	7	27
Oatmeal & Choc Chunk (1)	180	8	26
Oatmeal Chewy (2)	120	5	17
Choc. Chewy (2)	120	6	18
Choc. Chip (3)	160	8	22
Mini Chocolate Chip Bite-Size (5)	170	8	24
Snak Saks (5)	150	8	21
Peanut Butter (1)	90	5	10
Reduced-Fat (3)	140	5	23
Soft Baked Chunky Choc. (1)	130	5	19
White Fudge Chunky (2)	80	4.5	11
w. 100% Whole Grain (1)	150	8	22
Ginger Snaps (4)	120	2.5	23
Lorna Doone (4)	140	7	20
Mallomars (2)	120	5	18
Newtons: Fig Newtons (2)	110	2	22
Fig/Strawberry Minis, 1 pkg, 38g	130	3	26
100% Whole Grain (2)	110	2	21
Fat-Free (2)	90	0	22
Snack Pack To Go! (2)	90	0	22
Raspb./Strawberry (2)	100	1.5	21
Nilla Wafers: (8), 1 oz	140	6	21
Reduced-Fat (8), 1 oz	110	2	24
Nutter Butter:			
Big & Soft (1)	180	9	23
Bites (1)	170	7	24
Peanut Creme Patties (5)	160	9	19
Sandwich (2)	130	6	19
Sandwich Bites (10)	140	6	20
Wafers: Chocolate Stix, 1 oz	150	8	15
Chocolate Stix Bars (2)	210	11	26
Social Tea Biscuits (6)	140	4	24
Oreo: Original, (3)	160	7	25
Snack Pack, 2 oz	270	11	41
Reduced-Fat, (3)	150	4.5	26
Choc. Creme; Coffee 'n Creme (3)	170	7	25
Double Delight, Mint 'n Creme (2)	140	7	20
Double Stuf, (2)	140	7	21
Fudge-Covered, (1)	100	5	13
Handi-Snacks (1)	140	7	20
Mini Oreo: 9 pieces, 1 oz	140	6	21
Snack Pack, 1.2 oz	170	7	25
Uh-Oh!, 3 cookies	170	7	25
Teddy Grahams:			
Chocolatey Chip, Mini (53)	130	4.5	23
Cinnamon Snacks (24)	130	4	23
Honey Mini, Snak Saks (30)	130	4	23
Chocolate; Honey Snack (24), avg.	130	4	23

Nabisco (Cont):

	C	F	Cb
100 Calorie Packs: Cheese Nips	100	3	15
Chips Ahoy!	100	3	18
Lorna Doone	100	3	16
Oreo (Thin Crisps)	100	3	16
Wheat Thins	100	3	16
Honey Maid	100	2	19
Ritz Tst'd Chips	100	4	14
Ritz Snack Mix	100	3	16
Crackers: *Per Serving*			
Barnum's Animals (10)	130	3.5	22
Cheese Nips:			
Cheddar: Packs-2-Go!, 1.2 oz	170	7	22
Bag (29), 1 oz	150	7	22
Chips, avg. (13)	150	6	19
Four Cheese, 1 oz bag	150	7	18
Mini Go-Pak (53), 1 oz	150	6	19
Reduced-Fat: (31) avg.	150	6	19
Cheddar (31), 30g	150	6	19
Flavor Originals:			
Better Cheddars (22)	160	8	18
Chicken in a Biskit (12)	160	8	19
Sociables Baked Savory (7)	70	3.5	9
Vegetable Thins (11)	150	7	19
Honey Maid:			
Grahams: Avg. (8)	130	3.5	24
Sticks (14), avg.	130	3	25
Low-Fat (8), avg.	120	2	25
S'Mores (9)	150	6	24
Snack Bars, regular (1)	150	6	24
Premium Saltine: Fat-Free (5)	60	0	12
Low Sodium (5)	60	1.5	11
Multigrain (5)	60	1.5	10
Original (5)	70	1.5	11
Unsalted Tops (5)	60	1.5	11
Premium, Soup & Oyster (22)	60	1.5	11
Mini Crackers, Original (21)	70	2.5	10
Wheat Thins: Big (11)	150	6	21
Cream Cheese & Chive (15)	140	5	20
Harvest (9)	130	3.5	23
Honey; Low Sodium (16)	150	6	22
Multi-Grain (17)	130	4.5	23
Original (16), 31g	150	6	21
100 Calorie Packs	100	3	16
Ranch (14), 29g	140	6	20
Reduced-Fat (16), 29g	130	4	21
Toasted Chip, Multi-Grain (15)	140	4.5	22
Vegetable Thins (21)	150	7	21
Wheatsworth, Stone Ground Wheat (5)	80	3.5	10
Zwieback, 8g	35	1	6

Per Cookie/Cracker (Unless Indicated)

Newman's Own Organics	C	F	Cb
Alphabet Cookies (10) avg.	120	3	22
Champion Chip: Chocolate Chip (4)	160	7	21
Expresso Chocolate Chip (4)	150	7	21
Wheat-Free & Dairy-Free (4)	160	8	21
Other varieties, avg.	160	8	21
Fig Newman's: Fat-Free, 2 bars	120	0	28
Low-Fat, 2 bars	140	2	28
Wheat/Dairy-Free, 2 bars	120	1.5	26
Newman-O's: Original (2)	130	4.5	20
Choc. Creme (2); Mint Creme (2)	130	4.5	20
Ginger-O's (2)	120	4.5	19
Tops & Bottoms (6)	120	3	21
Wheat-Free & Dairy-Free (2)	130	4.5	21

Peek Freans			
Assorted Creme (2)	140	6	19
Nice Biscuits (2)	160	6	21
Shortcake (2)	140	7	18

Pepperidge Farm			
Cookies			
Choc Chunk: Double (1)	140	7	18
Chocolate Dipped Nantucket (1)	140	7	18
Dark Choc. Pecan Chesapeake (1)	140	8	15
Milk Choc.: Cashew Stowe (1)	130	6	17
Macadamia Nut Sausalito (1)	140	8	16
White Choc. Macadamia (1)	130	6	17
Other varieties, avg. (1)	140	7	18
Chocolate Delight, avg. all varieties	180	9	21
Collection: Ginger Family (4)	160	5	26
Other varieties, avg. (2)	135	7	17
Distinctive Milano: Milk Choc. (3)	170	9	21
Other varieties, avg. (2)	130	7	16
Distinctive: Brussels (3)	150	7	20
Brussels Mint (3)	190	10	22
Chessman (3)	120	5	19
Geneva (3)	160	9	19
Lido (1)	90	5	10
Raspberry Chantilly (2)	120	3	23
Other varieties, avg. (3)	140	6	20
Homestyle: Gingerman (4)	130	4	20
Shortbread (2)	140	7	16
Sugar (3)	140	6	20
Mini: Chessmen (9)	140	6	21
Brussels (3)	190	10	22
Milano (6); Mint Milano (6) avg.	165	85	19
Soft Baked Cookies (1) avg.	150	7	20
Sugar-Free Cookies (3) avg.	170	9	21

Per Cookie/Cracker (Unless Indicated)

Pepperidge Farm (Cont)	C	F	Cb
Crackers			
Entertaining Collection (4)	70	2.5	10
Goldfish Flavor Blasted (51) avg.	150	7	19
Goldfish, Original (55)	150	6	20
Snack Sticks: Three Cheese (25)	150	6	20
Pumpernickel (15)	120	1.5	24
Sesame (12)	130	5	18

President's Choice			
Milk Choc Chunk Pecan (2), 1.1 oz	170	10	19
Peanut Butter Persuasion (2), 1 oz	150	8	17
The Decadent: Choc Chip (2), 1.1 oz	160	8	21
Chocolate Chunk (2), 1.1 oz	160	8	21
White Chocolate Chip (2), 1.1 oz	160	8	19
Vanilla Wafers (6), 1.1 oz	140	5	22

Ritz			
Crackers: Original, ½ oz	80	4	10
Reduced-Fat, ½ oz	70	2	11
Assortment, ½ oz	80	4	10
Dinosaurs, 1 oz	130	3.5	22
Garlic Butter, ½ oz	80	4	10
Honey Butter (5)	80	4	10
Peanut Butter, 1.4 oz pkg	190	9	24
Real Cheese, 1.4 oz pkg	200	11	22
Whole Wheat, ½ oz	70	2.5	11
100 Calorie Snack Mix, 1 pkg, 22g	100	3	16
Ritz Bits Sandwiches: Cheese, 1 oz	150	9	16
Cheese Go-Pak (12) 1 oz	175	9	16
Cheese Packs 2 Go!, 1.5 oz	220	13	24
Graham S'mores, 1 oz	150	6	22
Peanut Butter/& Jelly, 1 oz	140	8	16
Peanut Butter Packs 2 Go!, 1.2 oz	170	10	20
Real Cheese, 1 oz	150	9	16
Ritz Chips: Original, 1 oz	130	4.5	21
Cheddar; Sour Crm & Onion, 1 oz	130	6	19

Safeway Select			
Crunchy Peanut Butter	130	6	17
Double Chocolate Chunk	130	7	18
Oatmeal Raisin	130	6	18
Pecan Choc Chunk	140	9	16
White Choc Macadamia	140	8	17
Vanilla Wafers (9), 1.1 oz	140	4.5	24
Healthy Advantage			
Oatmeal & Raisin (2)	120	2	24

Salerno			
Butter Cookies (6), 1.1 oz	160	8	21
Coconut Bar (2), 0.9 oz	120	5	17

Snackwell's	C	F	Cb
Creme s'wich (2) 1 oz	110	3	20
Creme Sandwich, Packs To Go! (1) pkg	210	5	38
Devil's Food Cake, Fat-Free (1) ½ oz	50	0	12
Lemon Creme Sandwich Sugar Free (3)	130	6	20
Shortbread Sugar Free (3) 1 oz	130	6	21
Sorbee			
Sugar Free: Animal (10)	100	3	21
Chocolate Chip; Choc. Fudge (1)	110	6	15
Oatmeal (1)	110	4	16
Peanut Butter (1)	110	7	13
Snicker Cookies,			
1.15 oz pkg	150	5	22
South Beach Diet (Kraft)			
Cookies: Peanut Butter, 1 pkg	100	5	15
Oatmeal Chocolate Chip, 1 pkg	100	5	16
Crackers, Woven Wheat, 1 pkg	100	3.5	16
Stella D'Oro			
Almond Toast (3)	115	2.5	21
Anginetti, 1 oz	130	3.5	22
Anisette Sponge Low-Fat (2)	95	1	19
Anisette Toast Low-Fat (3)	125	1	27
Biscotti, average, ¾ oz	95	4	13
Breakfast Treats: Chocolate Cookie (1)	90	3	15
Original (1)	90	3	15
Original Mini, 1 oz	120	3.5	21
Viennese Cinnamon (1)	90	2.5	16
Coffee Treats: Almond Toast (2)	110	2.5	19
Angel Wings, 1 oz	170	12	14
Anisette Sponge (2)	90	1	18
Anisette Toast, 1.1 oz	130	1	27
Banana Walnut Toast, 1 oz	100	2	19
Blueberry; Cinn. Toast, 1 oz	100	1	20
Roman Egg Biscuits, 1.1 oz	130	4	21
Continental Cookie Collection, 1 oz	130	4.5	20
Egg Jumbo, 1.1 oz	120	1.5	26
Lady Stella Assortment, 1 oz	130	4.5	20
Margherite (2)	130	4.5	20
Margherite Mini, 1.1 oz	150	5	24
Swiss Fudge (2) 1.1 oz	170	9	22
Streit's			
Wafers: Chocolate (3)	160	9	19
Vanilla (3)	170	11	18
Kedem Tea Biscuits, all flavors (2)	32	1	6
Sunshine			
Krispy: Original; Whole Wheat (5)	60	1.5	11
Oyster & Soup, 16 crackers	60	1	11
Unsalted Tops (1)	10	0.1	1
Cheez-It Crackers: Orig. (26), 1 oz	150	7.5	17
Reduced-Fat (24), 1 oz	130	3.5	20

Per Cookie/Cracker (Unless Indicated)	C	F	Cb
Trader Joe's			
100 Calorie Packs, avg	100	3	18
All Butter Shortbread w. Filling (2)	145	8	17
Almond Crisps (6), 1 oz	140	7	14
Brownie Bites (3)	135	6	19
Cherry Granola (2), 1 oz	110	4	18
Chocolate Almond Laceys (2)	170	12	18
Chocolate Chip: Small (1), 1.1 oz	130	6	18
Large, Singles (1), 1.7 oz	280	14	35
Cinnamon Grahams (2 squares)	100	3	14
Coconut Macaroon (3)	160	10	18
Dark Choc Chunks w. Almonds (3)	140	7	17
Dunkers: Chip (2)	160	7	21
Coated Choc. Chip (2)	190	9	24
Ginger Snaps (5)	140	6	21
Joe Joe's S'wich Cremes,			
Choc./ Vanilla (2), 1 oz	130	6	19
Lemon Crisps (5)	120	4	19
Meringues: Chocolate (4)	120	1.5	25
Fat Free (5)	110	0	27
Mini Meringues, vanilla (10)	100	0	24
Oatmeal Raisin (1), 1.8 oz	270	12	35
Triple Choc Chunk (1), 1 oz	140	7	20
Water Crackers (4)	60	1	12
Triscuit			
Baked Whole Wheat Crackers: *Per Serving*			
Original (15) 1 oz	120	4.5	19
Thin Crisps, Original (15) 1 oz	130	5	21
Cheddar (6); Rstd Garlic (8)	120	4.5	20
Garden Herb; Rosemary (6) 1 oz	120	4	20
Voortman			
Shortbread Cookies (2), 1.3 oz	180	10	20
Sugar Free Cookies:			
Fudge Chocolate Chip (2), 1.4 oz	180	10	26
Iced Almonette (2), 1.1 oz	150	8	17
Peanut Butter Wafers (4), 1 oz	150	7	17
Vanilla Wafers: Regular (3), 1.1 oz	140	7	20
Sugar Free (3), 1.1 oz	130	8	17
Zesta			
Crackers: Whole Wheat (5)	60	1.5	11
Fat Free, 5 crackers	60	0	13
Original, 5 crackers	60	1.5	11
Red. Sodium; Unsalted Tops (5)	60	1.5	11
Soup & Oyster, 51 crackers	70	3	10
365 (Whole Foods):			
Choc Chip (5), 1 oz	130	6	19
Fig Bars (2), 1.3 oz	130	2	27
Lady Fingers (5), 1.1 oz	120	1.5	25
Lemon Wafers (5), 0.9 oz	120	5	17
Oatmeal (6), 1 oz	130	4.5	20
Sandwich Cremes (2)	130	5	20
Sugar (5), 1.1 oz	130	4	22

Thaw, Bake & Serve   C   F   Cb

	C	F	Cb
Grands! Biscuits (Pillsbury): *Per Biscuit*			
Extra Rich	210	10	26
Butter Tastin'; Buttermilk, avg.	185	9	24
Reduced Fat	170	6	26
Flaky; Homestyle; Southern Style	190	9	24
Pillsbury Cookies: *Per 1 oz*			
Refrigerated Cookie Dough			
Big Deluxe Classics:			
Oatmeal Raisin (1)	170	7	26
Peanut Butter Cup (1)	190	9	24
White Chunk Macadamia Nut (1)	200	11	24
Other varieties (1)	200	10	25
Ready To Bake: Sugar Cookie (1)	100	5	12
Chocolate Chip w. Walnuts (1)	100	5	12
Chocolate Chunk Chip (1)	100	5	12
Peanut Butter w. Reese's Pces (1)	100	4.5	13
S'mores (1); Choc. Candy (1)	100	4.5	13
Shape Sugar Cookie (2)	120	6	15
Create n Bake: Peanut Butter	130	6	16
Chocolate Chip/Chunk /Dble Choc	130	7	17
Oatmeal Choc. Chip; Sugar, avg.	130	6	18
Refrigerated Dough:			
Cinnamon Roll	150	5	23
Cinnamon Twists	180	9	22
Flaky Supreme w. Cinnabon (1)	380	18	48
Grands Cinnamon Rolls (1)	310	9	54
Simply Bake Bars:			
P.B. Choc.; Turtle Supreme, ¹⁄₁₀ pkg	180	9	24
Spread & Bake Brownies:			
Choc. Fudge, ¹⁄₁₂ pkg	150	6	24
Triple Choc Chunk, ¹⁄₁₂ pkg	160	6	24
Toll House *(Nestlé)*			
Refrigerated Dough			
Chocolate Chip (1)	120	6	15
Chocolate Chunk/Chunk (1)	120	6	15
Fudgy Brownie (1)	190	9	26
Jumbo Chocolate Chip (1)	200	10	26
Mini Chocolate Chip (2)	120	6	15
Walnut Chocolate Chip (1)	70	6	15
Other varieties, avg. (1)	110	5	15
Ultimates Refrigerated Dough			
Chocolate Chip Lovers (1)	180	9	23
Choc. Chips & Chunks w. Pecans (1)	190	10	22
P. Butter Chips & Choc Chunks (1)	180	9	23
Triple Chocolate Decadence (1)	170	8	23
Turtle (1)	180	9	23
White Choc. Macadamia Nut (1)	190	10	22

Crispbreads   C   F   Cb

Per Crispbread/Cracker

	C	F	Cb
Finn Crisp: Original, rye,1	35	0	7
Other types,1 crispbread	19	0	3
Kavli Norwegian: Thin (3)	50	0	11
Thick, 2 crispbreads	60	0.5	12
Malsovit Meal Wafers,1	75	4	7
New York Flatbread Crisps, 1	35	0	7
Ry-Krisp: Natural, 1 crispbread	25	0	5
Seasoned,1 crispbread	30	0	5
Sesame,1 crispbread	25	1	5
Ryvita: Dark/Light, 1 piece	26	0	4
WASA: Delikatess (1)	25	0	5.5
Fiber (1); Sesame (1)	30	1	5
Original (1)	35	0.2	7.5
Runda (1)	55	1.5	9
Wheat Dore (1)	50	1	9
Westbrae Rice Wafers (7), 15g	50	0	11

Matzos

	C	F	Cb
Manischewitz			
Egg 'n Onion Matzo, 1 oz	100	1	23
Mandelin (9)	35	2	4
Matzo Meal, ½ cup	130	0	28
Matzo Farfel, 1 cup, 2.7 oz	180	0.5	60
Passover Egg Matzos, 1.1 oz	120	0	28
Tam Tam Crackers (10)	130	4	22
Thin Salted Tea Matzos, 0.9 oz	100	0	22
Unsalted; Whole Wheat, 1 oz	110	0	24
Crackers: Miniatures (12)	110	0.5	25
Passover Egg Matzo (11)	110	0	20
Streit's			
Whole Wheat Matzos,			
1 Matzo, 1 oz	110	0.5	23
Unsalted Matzos,			
1 Matzo, 1 oz	100	0	23

There are 1440 minutes in every day...

Schedule 30 of them for exercise!

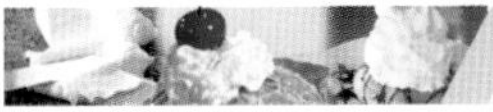

Quick Guide

Cream
Average All Brands

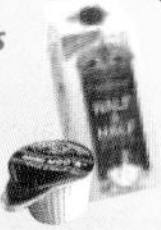

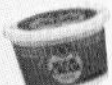

	C	**F**	**Cb**
Half & Half Cream:			
1 Tbsp, 0.5 oz	20	1.5	0.5
2 Tbsp, 1 oz	40	3	1
¼ cup, 2 oz	80	6	2
Single Serve Cup, ⅜ fl.oz	15	1.5	0.5
Light: Coffee/table (20% fat): 1 T.	30	3	0.5
2 Tbsp, 1 oz	60	6	1

Sour Cream:

	C	**F**	**Cb**
Regular: 1 Tbsp, 0.5 oz	25	2.5	1
1 cup, 8 oz	490	48	10
Low-Fat/Light: 1 Tbsp, 0.5 oz	20	1.5	1
2 Tbsp, 1 oz	40	3	2
Fat-Free: Average, 2 Tbsp, 1 oz	25	0	4
Hood, 2 Tbsp, 1 oz	25	0	4
Kroger, 2 Tbsp, 1 oz	20	0	3
Naturally Yours; Oak Farm, 2 T.	20	0	3
Knudsen, 2 Tbsp, 1 oz	30	0	5
Sour Cream Substitute:			
Albertson's, 2 Tbsp, 1 oz	60	5	2
Tofutti Sour Supreme, 2 T., 1 oz	85	7	9

Whipping Cream:

	C	**F**	**Cb**
Heavy (37% fat):			
1 T. fluid/2 T. whipped	50	5.5	0.5
¼ cup whipped	100	11	1
½ cup fluid/1 c. whipped	400	44	3.5
Light (30% fat):			
1 Tbsp fluid/2 Tbsp whipped	45	4.5	0.5
½ cup fluid/1 cup whipped	350	37	4

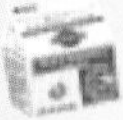

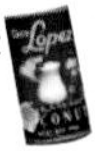

Coconut Cream/Milk

	C	**F**	**Cb**
Coconut Cream (Canned),			
Plain/unsweetened: 2 Tbsp, 1 oz	75	6.5	3
½ cup, 4 oz	285	26	12
Sweetened: *Coco Lopez*, 1 oz	130	5	21
½ cup, 4 oz	520	20	84
Coconut Milk (Canned):			
Natural Value: Reg., ¼ c., 2 fl.oz	105	10	2
Lite, ¼ cup, 2 fl.oz	55	5	1
Thai Kitchen: Lite, ¼ cup, 2 fl.oz	45	4	1
Premium, 2 fl.oz	120	10	4
Coconut Water (Center), 1 cup	45	0.5	9

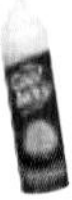

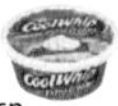

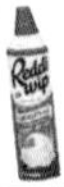

Whipped Toppings C F Cb
Average All Brands

	C	**F**	**Cb**
Cream (Pressurized): 2 T.	20	1	1
¼ cup	45	4	2
½ cup	90	8	4
Cream Topping: Lite, 2 Tbsp	20	1	3
Cool Whip: Extra Creamy, 2 T.	25	2	2
Lite, 2 Tbsp, 9g	20	1	3
Free, 2 Tbsp, 9g	15	0	3
Kraft: Dream Whip, 2 Tbsp	15	0	2
Reddi-Wip: Original, 2 T., 8g	15	1	0.5
Chocolate, 2 Tbsp, 8g	15	1	1
Extra Creamy, 2 Tbsp, 8g	15	1.5	0.5
Fat-Free, 2 Tbsp, 8g	5	0	1

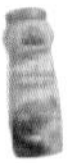

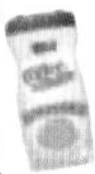

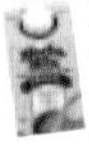

Creamers (Non-Dairy)

	C	**F**	**Cb**
Powder:			
Coffee-Mate/Cremora/N-Rich			
Original, 1 tsp	10	0.5	1
1 heaping tsp	25	2	2
Lite, 1 tsp	10	1.5	2
Flavors: 4 tsp	60	3	8
Fat-Free: Average, 4 tsp	50	0	11
Liquid/Refrigerated: *Per Tablespoon*			
Coffee-Mate			
Plain: Original/Plain, 1 Tbsp	20	1	2
Fat-Free, 1 Tbsp	15	0	2
Low-Fat, 1 Tbsp	10	0.5	1
Flavors: All flavors, 1 Tbsp	35	1.5	5
Fat-Free, all flavors, 1 Tbsp	25	0	5
Hood (Non-Dairy), 1 Tbsp	20	1.5	2
International Delight:			
1 Tbsp	35	1.5	6
Fat-Free flavors, 1 Tbsp	30	0	7
Kroger			
Coffee, Fat-Free & Lactose Free:			
French Vanilla, 1 Tbsp	35	1.5	6
Hazelnut, 1 Tbsp	35	1.5	6
Mocha Mix: Original, 1 Tbsp	20	1.5	1
Fat-Free, 1 Tbsp	10	0	1
Lite, 1 Tbsp	10	0.5	1
Silk: Original, 1Tbsp	15	1	1
French Vanilla; Hazelnut, 1 Tbsp	20	1	3

D Desserts ~ Puddings • Gelatin

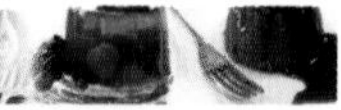

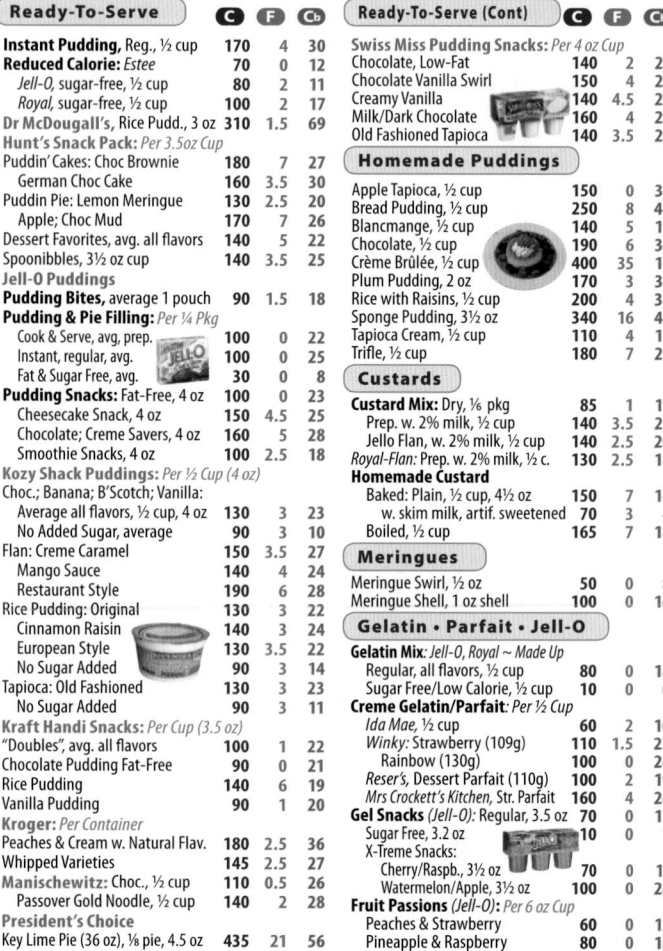

Ready-To-Serve

	C	F	Cb
Instant Pudding, Reg., ½ cup	170	4	30
Reduced Calorie: *Estee*	70	0	12
Jell-O, sugar-free, ½ cup	80	2	11
Royal, sugar-free, ½ cup	100	2	17
Dr McDougall's, Rice Pudd., 3 oz	310	1.5	69
Hunt's Snack Pack: *Per 3.5oz Cup*			
Puddin' Cakes: Choc Brownie	180	7	27
German Choc Cake	160	3.5	30
Puddin Pie: Lemon Meringue	130	2.5	20
Apple; Choc Mud	170	7	26
Dessert Favorites, avg. all flavors	140	5	22
Spoonibbles, 3½ oz cup	140	3.5	25
Jell-O Puddings			
Pudding Bites, average 1 pouch	90	1.5	18
Pudding & Pie Filling: *Per ¼ Pkg*			
Cook & Serve, avg, prep.	100	0	22
Instant, regular, avg.	100	0	25
Fat & Sugar Free, avg.	30	0	8
Pudding Snacks: Fat-Free, 4 oz	100	0	23
Cheesecake Snack, 4 oz	150	4.5	25
Chocolate; Creme Savers, 4 oz	160	5	28
Smoothie Snacks, 4 oz	100	2.5	18
Kozy Shack Puddings: *Per ½ Cup (4 oz)*			
Choc.; Banana; B'Scotch; Vanilla:			
Average all flavors, ½ cup, 4 oz	130	3	23
No Added Sugar, average	90	3	10
Flan: Creme Caramel	150	3.5	27
Mango Sauce	140	4	24
Restaurant Style	190	6	28
Rice Pudding: Original	130	3	22
Cinnamon Raisin	140	3	24
European Style	130	3.5	22
No Sugar Added	90	3	14
Tapioca: Old Fashioned	130	3	23
No Sugar Added	90	3	11
Kraft Handi Snacks: *Per Cup (3.5 oz)*			
"Doubles", avg. all flavors	100	1	22
Chocolate Pudding Fat-Free	90	0	21
Rice Pudding	140	6	19
Vanilla Pudding	90	1	20
Kroger: *Per Container*			
Peaches & Cream w. Natural Flav.	180	2.5	36
Whipped Varieties	145	2.5	27
Manischewitz: Choc., ½ cup	110	0.5	26
Passover Gold Noodle, ½ cup	140	2	28
President's Choice			
Key Lime Pie (36 oz), ⅛ pie, 4.5 oz	435	21	56
Mississippi Mud Pie (36 oz), ⅑, 4 oz	405	22	49

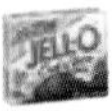

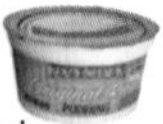

Ready-To-Serve (Cont)

	C	F	Cb
Swiss Miss Pudding Snacks: *Per 4 oz Cup*			
Chocolate, Low-Fat	140	2	27
Chocolate Vanilla Swirl	150	4	26
Creamy Vanilla	140	4.5	23
Milk/Dark Chocolate	160	4	28
Old Fashioned Tapioca	140	3.5	24

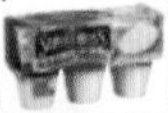

Homemade Puddings

	C	F	Cb
Apple Tapioca, ½ cup	150	0	32
Bread Pudding, ½ cup	250	8	40
Blancmange, ½ cup	140	5	19
Chocolate, ½ cup	190	6	30
Crème Brûlée, ½ cup	400	35	16
Plum Pudding, 2 oz	170	3	32
Rice with Raisins, ½ cup	200	4	38
Sponge Pudding, 3½ oz	340	16	45
Tapioca Cream, ½ cup	110	4	15
Trifle, ½ cup	180	7	26

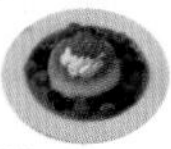

Custards

	C	F	Cb
Custard Mix: Dry, ⅙ pkg	85	1	17
Prep. w. 2% milk, ½ cup	140	3.5	21
Jello Flan, w. 2% milk, ½ cup	140	2.5	20
Royal-Flan: Prep. w. 2% milk, ½ c.	130	2.5	18
Homemade Custard			
Baked: Plain, ½ cup, 4½ oz	150	7	16
w. skim milk, artif. sweetened	70	3	4
Boiled, ½ cup	165	7	18

Meringues

	C	F	Cb
Meringue Swirl, ½ oz	50	0	8
Meringue Shell, 1 oz shell	100	0	16

Gelatin • Parfait • Jell-O

	C	F	Cb
Gelatin Mix: *Jell-O, Royal ~ Made Up*			
Regular, all flavors, ½ cup	80	0	18
Sugar Free/Low Calorie, ½ cup	10	0	0
Creme Gelatin/Parfait: *Per ½ Cup*			
Ida Mae, ½ cup	60	2	10
Winky: Strawberry (109g)	110	1.5	22
Rainbow (130g)	100	0	24
Reser's, Dessert Parfait (110g)	100	2	19
Mrs Crockett's Kitchen, Str. Parfait	160	4	26
Gel Snacks *(Jell-O):* Regular, 3.5 oz	70	0	17
Sugar Free, 3.2 oz	10	0	1
X-Treme Snacks:			
Cherry/Raspb., 3½ oz	70	0	17
Watermelon/Apple, 3½ oz	100	0	24
Fruit Passions *(Jell-O)*: *Per 6 oz Cup*			
Peaches & Strawberry	60	0	13
Pineapple & Raspberry	80	0	18
Tropical Fruit & Peach	70	0	15

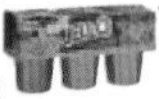

Chicken Eggs

Fresh Eggs	C	F	Cb
Raw (weight with shell):			
Small, 40g	65	4	0
Medium, 44g	70	4	0
Large, 50g	75	4.5	0
Extra Large, 56g	80	5	0
Jumbo, 63g	90	5.5	0
Egg Yolk, 1 extra large	63	5	0
Egg White, 1 extra large	16	0	0
Dried Egg Powder			
Whole Egg: ¼ cup, 1 oz	170	12	0
1 Tbsp	30	2	0
Egg White, ¼ cup, 1 oz	105	0	0
Egg Yolk, ¼ cup, 1 oz	195	18	0

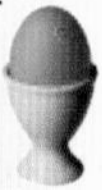

Egg Substitutes

¼ Cup (Equivalent to 1 Egg) ~ Zero Cholesterol.

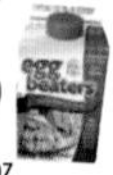

	C	F	Cb
Better 'n Eggs (Papetti), ¼ cup, 2 oz	30	0	1
EggBeaters (Fleischmann's) Frozen/Liquid, Regular/Flavors, ¼ c., 2.2 oz	30	0	1
Egg Watchers (Tofutti), ¼ c., 2 oz	30	0	1
Ener-G, Egg Replacer, 1½ tsp, 4 g	15	0	4
Egg Substitute (Jewel), ¼ cup	30	0	1
Egg Whites, 4 Tbsp, ¼ cup, 2 oz	30	0	0
Nature Egg, Simply Egg White, ¼ c., 2 oz	25	0	0
Scramblers (Morning Star), ¼ cup	35	0	0
Second Nature, Fat-Free, ¼ c., 2 fl.oz	35	0	1

Other Eggs

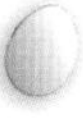

	C	F	Cb
Duck, 1 large, 2½ oz	130	9.5	0
Goose, 1 large, 5 oz	280	19	0
Quail, 3 eggs, 2 oz	42	3	0
Turkey, 1 large, 3 oz	135	9.5	0
Turtle, 1 egg, 1¾ oz	75	5	0

Omega-3 Fat Enriched

	C	F	Cb
Eggland's Best, 1 large	70	4	0
Eggs Plus (Pilgrim's Pride), 1 large	70	4.5	1

Note: Cholesterol content same as regular eggs, but Omega-3 fats inhibit blood cholesterol increase. (Extra Notes ~ See Page 271)

Cooked Eggs

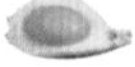

	C	F	Cb
Boiled Egg: Same as raw egg			
Hard-Cooked (Egg-Lands), Peeled	60	3.5	0
Fried Egg:			
With fat: 1 large egg	105	9	0.5
2 small eggs	175	13	1
No fat/nonstick pan, 1 large	75	5	0.5
Deviled Egg, 2 halves	145	13	0.5
Eggs Benedict (2) on toast or English muffin	860	56	25
Eggs Florentine (2) on toast or English Muffin	890	59	25
Pickled Egg, 1 large	80	5.5	0
Poached Egg, 1 large	65	4	0
Quiche (Home-Made):			
Egg & Bacon, 1 slice, 5.3 oz	580	43	27
Ham & Cheese, 1 slice, 5.3 oz	475	33	29
Scotch Egg, 1 egg	300	21	16
Scrambled Eggs: 1 large egg:			
w. 1 Tbsp milk + 1 tsp fat	120	9	1
w. 1 Tbsp skim milk/no fat	85	5.5	1
2 large eggs:			
w. 2 Tbsp milk + 2 tsp fat	260	20	2
w. 2 Tbsp skim milk/no fat	180	11	2

Omelets

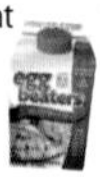

	C	F	Cb
1 Egg: Plain (w. 1 tsp fat)	125	10	0.5
with ½ oz cheese	175	15	0.5
w. ½ oz cheese + ½ oz ham	200	16	0.5
2 Eggs: Plain (w. 2 tsp fat)	250	20	1
with 1 oz cheese	360	29	2
w. 1 oz cheese + 1 oz ham	410	32	2
3 Eggs: Plain (w. 1 Tbsp fat)	360	29	1.5
w. 2 oz cheese	580	47	2.5
w. 2 oz cheese + 2 oz ham	680	53	2.5
Extras: Tomato/Onion/Veggies	20	0	4.5
Egg Substitute (EggBeaters):			
2 eggs (½ cup) + 1 tsp fat	100	4	2
3 eggs (¾ cup) + 2 tsp fat	160	8	3
Extras: 1 oz cheese	110	9	1
1 oz ham	50	3	1
Tom./Onion/Veges	20	0	4.5

Egg Nog

~ Per ½ Cup (4 fl.oz)

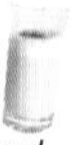

	C	F	Cb
Average all Brands, ½ cup	170	9.5	17
Regular: Borden	160	9	17
Hood (Golden)	180	9	22
Light/Low-Fat: Horizon; Hood	140	4	22

93

Breakfast Sides

	C	F	Cb
Toast: Plain, 1 thick slice	85	1	13
with 2 tsp butter/marg.	155	9	13
with 3 tsp/1 Tbsp fat	190	13	13
English Muffin: Plain, 2 oz	130	1	26
with 3 tsp fat	230	12	26
Bacon, 2 strips	70	5	0
Ham, Lean, 2 oz	100	3	0
Hash Browns:			
½ cup, 3 oz	125	6.5	14
1 cup serving, 6 oz	250	13	28
Sausages, 2 links (1 oz ea.)	180	16	1.5

Frozen Egg Breakfasts

Aunt Jemima Great Starts: *Per Package*

	C	F	Cb
French Toast & Sausage Bkfst	440	27	35
Griddle Cake w. Ham, Egg, Cheese	240	8	33
Pancakes & Sausage Breakfast	470	25	50
Sausage, Egg & Chse Biscuit	340	21	27
Sausage, Egg & Chse Croissant	350	23	22
Scrambled Eggs & Saus. Bkfst	370	24	18

Jimmy Dean

	C	F	Cb
Bacon, Egg, Cheese Muffin (1)	230	9	27
Croissant: Egg & Cheese (1)	310	20	24
Egg, Sausage, Cheese (1)	450	33	24
Egg, Sausage, Cheese Biscuit (1)	430	30	28
Omelet: 3 Cheese (1)	290	23	5
Ham Cheese (1)	280	17	5

Pillsbury: Toaster Scrambles,

	C	F	Cb
Cheese, Egg & Bacon	180	12	15
Cheese, Egg & Sausage	180	11	15

Red Baron

	C	F	Cb
Scrambles: Ham (1), 5 oz	330	15	33
Bacon (1), 5 oz	400	22	35
Minis, 4 pieces, 5½ oz	390	17	45

Swanson Great Starts

	C	F	Cb
Hungry-Man Hearty Breakfast	1170	61	125
Frozen Pancake/Waffles: *See Page 122*			

Frozen Egg Rolls

Chun King/La Choy: *Average All Brands*

	C	F	Cb
Chicken Egg Rolls, Mini, 6 rolls	210	9	25
Pork & Shrimp Egg Rolls:			
Mini, 6 rolls, 3 oz	210	9	27
Shrimp Egg Rolls, Mini, 6 rolls	190	6	28
Lotus: Pork, 3.8 oz	180	7	18
Vegetable, 3.8 oz	70	1.5	13
Kahiki: Pork, 3 oz	140	3.5	20
Chicken, 3 oz	160	6	19
Vegetable Egg Roll, 3 oz	130	3.5	21

Fast-Foods/Restaurants

	C	F	Cb
Arby's: Bacon & Egg Croissant	335	22	23
Au Bon Pain: Egg on a Bagel	360	4	59
w. Bacon & Cheese	500	15	59
Bob Evans:			
Farmers Market Omelette	780	60	13
Ham & Cheddar Omelette	635	48	3
Three Cheese Omelette	645	52	4
Western Omelette	655	48	8
Bojangles: Egg Biscuit	400	30	26
Bacon, Egg & Cheese Biscuit	550	42	27
Bruegger's Bagels: Breakfast Sandwiches,			
Egg & Cheese	420	18	71
Egg & Cheese & Sausage	640	38	72
Burger King: Croissan'wich			
Bacon Egg & Cheese	340	20	26
Ham Egg & Cheese	340	18	26
Sausage & Cheese	370	25	23
Carl's Jr: Bacon & Egg Burrito	570	33	37
Chick-Fil-A			
Chicken, Egg & Cheese Bagel	500	20	49
Denny's: Two Eggs & More B'Fast	630	47	21
All American Slam, no toast	950	75	21
Heartland Scramble, no syrup/marg.	1080	63	93
Ultimate Omelette w. Hash Browns	830	62	26
Del Taco, Egg & cheese Burrito	450	24	39
Dunkin Donuts			
Bacon, Egg & Cheese Croissant	440	25	33
Ham, Egg & Cheese Bagel S/wich	510	16	65
Eat 'N Park: Cheese Omelette	390	30	2.5
Supreme Omelette	420	30	9
Hardee's: Bacon Platter	980	56	90
Loaded Omelet	640	44	37
IHOP: T-Bone Steak & Eggs	1310	86	63
Colorado Omelette	790	68	5
Jack in the Box			
Bacon, Egg & Cheese Biscuit	430	25	34
McDonald's: Egg McMuffin	300	12	30
Bacon, Egg & Cheese Bisc., Reg.	450	25	36
Scrambled Eggs (2)	170	11	1
Whataburger			
Breakfast Platter w. Bacon (2 sl.)	740	45	53

Quick Guide — **C** **F** **Cb**

Butter & Margarine
Average All Brands

Regular: 1 tsp (5g) — 35 4 0
- 1 Pat/Single Portion, 5g — 35 4 0
- 1 Tbsp, approx. ½ oz — 100 11 0
- 2 Tbsp, 1 oz — 205 23 0
- 1 Stick, ½ cup, 4 oz — 815 92 0
- 1 Pound, 2 cups, 16 oz — 3260 368 0

Light (Regular) 40% Fat:
- 1 tsp (5g) — 25 3 0
- 1 Tbsp, ½ oz — 75 8.5 0
- 2 Tbsp, 1 oz — 150 16 0

Whipped Butter (Regular):
- 1 tsp (4 g) — 30 3 0
- 1 Tbsp (10g) — 70 7.5 0
- 1 Stick, ½ cup, 2 ⅔ oz — 545 62 0

Whipped Light Butter (40% Fat):
- 1 tsp, 5g — 25 3 0.5
- 1 Tbsp, 9g — 45 5 1
- 2 Tbsp, 18g — 90 10 2

Unsalted: Same as Regular

Flavored Butter/Spreads
Average All Brands

Honey Butter (60% Fat):
- 1 Tbsp, ½ oz — 90 8 4
- *Downey's*, 1 Tbsp, ½ oz — 60 1 11

Garlic Butter (80% Fat):
- 1 Tbsp, ½ oz — 100 11 0

Sweet Cream Butter:
- Regular, 1 Tbsp — 100 11 0
- Stick (*Parkay*), 70% Fat, 1 Tbsp — 90 10 0
- Tub (*Land O'Lakes*), 60% Fat, 1 T. — 80 8 0

Ghee (Clarified Butter)
(Example: *Purity Farms*)
Note: Ghee is 100% fat compared to regular butter (80% fat + 20% water)
- 1 tsp (5g) — 45 5 0
- 1 Tbsp, ½ oz — 120 14 0
- 2¼ Tbsp, 1 oz — 250 28 0

Light & Reduced Fat Spreads
Per 1 Tbsp, ½ oz (Unless Stated) — **C** **F** **Cb**

- **Albertson's:** Country (48%), 1 T. — 60 7 0
- Butter Blend, 1 Tbsp — 80 9 0
- **Benecol:** Spread, 1 T., 14g — 70 8 0
- Light, Spread, 1 T., 14g — 50 5 0
- **Blue Bonnet,** Homestyle (48% Veg Oil) — 60 7 0
- **Brummel & Brown,** Spread, 1 T. — 45 5 0
- **Country Crock** (*Shedd's*): Regular — 60 7 0
- Light; Calcium & Vitamins — 50 5 0
- Spreadable Butter, 1 Tbsp — 80 9 0
- **Downey's,** Honey Butter, 1 Tbsp — 60 1 11
- **Fleischmann's:** Soft Spread — 70 8 0
- Original Stick, 1 Tbsp — 100 11 0
- Light Spread, 1 Tbsp — 40 4.5 0
- **'I Can't Believe It's Not Butter':** Reg. — 80 8 0
- Light; Sweet Cream — 50 6 0
- **Imperial:** Stick, 1 Tbsp — 80 9 0
- Tub, 1 Tbsp — 60 7 0
- **Land O'Lakes:** Buttery Taste, 1 T. — 80 8 0
- Honey Butter, 1 Tbsp — 90 8 4
- Light Butter Whipped — 45 5 0
- Light Butter, 1 Tbsp — 50 6 0
- **Parkay:** Squeeze, 1 Tbsp — 70 8 0
- Light Spread, 1 Tbsp — 50 5 0
- Original Stick, 1 Tbsp — 80 9 0
- Original Spread, 1 Tbsp — 60 7 0
- **Promise:** Buttery, 1 Tbsp — 80 8 0
- Fat-Free, 1 Tbsp — 5 0 0
- Buttery Light, 1 Tbsp — 45 5 0
- **Smart Balance:** 67% Buttery, 1 T. — 80 9 0
- Light (37%), 1 Tbsp — 45 5 0
- Omega Plus, 1 Tbsp — 80 9 0
- **Take Control:**
- Regular, 1 Tbsp — 80 8 0
- Light Spread, 1 Tbsp — 45 5 0
- **Smart Beat,** Fat-Free, 1 Tbsp — 50 0 1
- **Smart Squeeze,** 1 Tbsp — 5 0 1

Butter Substitutes
- **Apple Butter,** average, 1 Tbsp, 19g — 20 0 4
- **Butter Buds:** 1 serving, ½ tsp — 5 0 2
- Sprinkles, 1 tsp — 5 0 0
- **Earth Balance,** Non GMO,1 Tbsp — 100 11 0
- **Molly McButter,** ½ tsp — 5 0 1
- **Shedd's Willow Run,** Soy, 1 T. — 100 1 0
- **Sunsweet,** Lighter Bake, 1Tbsp, 19g — 35 0 9
(Butter/Oil Replacement)

Spreads Comparison

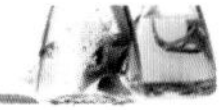

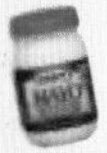

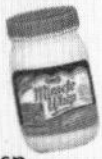

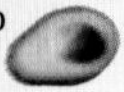

	C	F	Cb
Mayonnaise: Regular, 1 T.	100	11	0
Light, average, 1 Tbsp	50	5	1
Fat-Free, 1 Tbsp	10	0	2
Miracle Whip *(Kraft):*			
Regular, 1 Tbsp	40	3.5	2
Light, 1 Tbsp	25	1.5	3
Free, 1 Tbsp	15	0	3
Smart Beat Dressing: 1 Tbsp	10	0	2.5

Extra Listings for Mayonnaise & Dressings
~ See Page 89 ~

	C	F	Cb
Avocado, mashed, 1 Tbsp	45	4	2.5
Peanut Butter, 1 Tbsp	100	8	3.5
Nutella, 1 Tbsp	100	5.5	12

Animal Fats/Lards

	C	F	Cb

Average All Types
Beef Tallow/Drippings, Lard (Pork),
Chicken, Duck, Goose, Turkey.

	C	F	Cb
1 Tbsp (13g)	115	13	0
2¼ Tbsp, 1 oz	255	28	0
1 cup, 7¼ oz	1850	205	0
½ pound, 8 oz	2040	227	0
Ghee/Butter Oil: 1 Tbsp, ½ oz	120	14	0
2¼ Tbsp, 1 oz	250	28	0

Vegetable Shortening

Average All Types (example: Crisco)

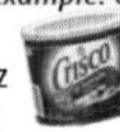

	C	F	Cb
1 Tbsp, 13g	115	13	0
2¼ Tbsp, 1 oz	250	28	0
1 cup, 7¼ oz	1810	205	0

Vegetable Oils

Includes almond, avocado, canola, corn, coconut, flaxseed, grapeseed, linseed, mustard, olive, palm, peanut, rice-bran, safflower, sesame, sunflower, soybean, wheat germ. Note: Oil is 100% fat.

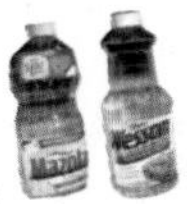

	C	F	Cb
1 tsp, 5g	45	5	0
1 Tbsp, ½ oz	120	14	0
2 Tbsp, 1 oz	250	28	0
1 cup, 7¾ oz	1930	205	0

Fish Oils

Average All Types (Includes cod liver, herring, salmon, sardine): 1 Tbsp, ½ oz **125 14 0**

Cooking Sprays/Squeezes

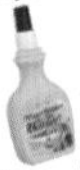

Cooking Sprays *(Pam, Mazola, I Can't Believe It's Not Butter, Weight Watchers, Wesson):*

	C	F	Cb
Per serving	2	0	0
1-3 second spray	6	1	0
I Can't Believe It's Not Butter	0	0	0
Parkay Buttery Spray	0	0	0
Squeeze (Parkay), 1 Tbsp, ½ oz	70	8	0

Olestra (Olean)

Olestra *(Olean)* **0 0 0**

Note: *Olean is Proctor & Gamble's brand name for olestra – a no-calorie cooking oil that gives snacks (like potato chips, tortilla chips and crackers) taste and texture without adding fat or calories.*

Examples:
- *Frito-Lay Light Products*
  (Lays, Ruffles, Tostitos, Doritos)
- *Pringles Fat-Free Potato Crisps*

Quick Guide

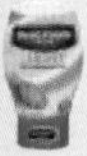

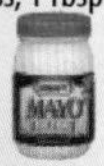

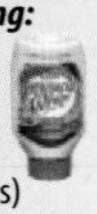

Mayonnaise	C	F	Cb
Regular			
Average All Brands, 1 Tbsp	100	11	0
Best Foods, Kraft, 1 Tbsp	100	11	0
½ cup, 4 oz	800	88	0
Light/Reduced Fat			
Kraft, 1 Tbsp	45	3.5	2
Best Foods, 1 Tbsp	45	4.5	0.5
½ cup, 4 oz	360	36	7
Hain, Safflower Oil, 1 Tbsp	100	11	0
Hellman's, 1 Tbsp	45	4.5	0.5
Spectrum: Canola Mayo, 1 Tbsp	100	11	0
Light Canola Mayo Eggless, 1 Tbsp	35	3.5	
Fat Free			
Kraft: 1 Tbsp	10	0	2
½ cup, 4 oz	80	0	16
Smart Beat, 1 Tbsp	10	0	3
Sugar Free: Dukes Mayo, 1 Tbsp	100	12	0
Mayonnaise Style Dressing			
BAMA Dressing, 1 Tbsp, ½ oz	50	4	3
Best Foods Sandwich Spread, 1 T.	60	5	2
Gourmayo (French's), 1 Tbsp, ½ oz	50	5	2
Miracle Whip Salad Dressing:			
Regular, 1 Tbsp, ½ oz	40	3.5	2
Light, 1 Tbsp, ½ oz	30	2	3
Free, 1 Tbsp, ½ oz	15	0	2
Nayonaise *(Nasoya)*			
(Tofu Base/Dairy Free/Eggless)			
Regular, 1 Tbsp, ½ oz	35	3.5	1
Fat-Free, 1 Tbsp, ½ oz	10	0	2

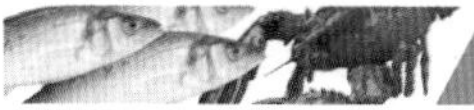

Quick Guide

Fresh Fish   C   F   Cb

Low Oil (Less than 2.5% fat)

White/pale colored flesh. Examples:
Cod, Flounder, Haddock, Halibut, Mahi Mahi, Perch, Pike, Pollock, Snapper, Sole, Whiting.

Per 4 oz Edible Portion

	C	F	Cb
Raw, 4 oz (no bones)	90	1	0
Steamed, Broiled, Baked	130	1	0
Fried: Lightly Floured	210	8	3.5
Breaded	260	12	8
In Batter	320	16	27

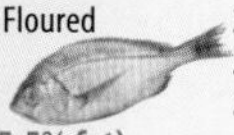

Medium Oil (2.5-5% fat)   C   F   Cb

Pale colored flesh. Examples:
Bluefin Tuna, Catfish, Kingfish, Orange Roughy, Salmon (Pink), Swordfish, Rainbow Trout, Yellowtail.

	C	F	Cb
Raw, 4 oz (no bones)	140	5	0
Baked, Broiled, 4 oz	175	6	0
Fried, 4 oz	230	11	8

High Oil (Over 5% fat)   C   F   Cb

Darker colored flesh. Examples:
Albacore Tuna, Bluefish, Herring, Mackerel, Salmon (Atl./Chinook/Sockeye), Sardines, Trout, Whitefish.

	C	F	Cb
Raw, 4 oz (no bones)	230	16	0
Baked, Broiled, 4 oz	275	17	0
Fried, 4 oz	340	23	12

Cooking Yields (Fin Fish):
4 oz Raw wt. = 3½ oz Cooked wt.
4 oz Cooked wt. = 5 oz Raw wt.

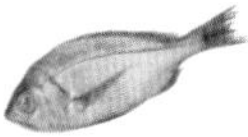

Calorie & Fat Variations
The amount of fat/oil in fish varies with the species, season and locality. Within the same fish, fat/oil content is generally higher towards the head.

Get Moving!
Take a computer
break every hour.

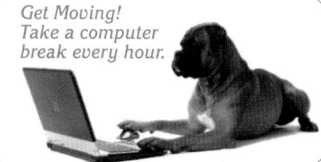

Fish & Shellfish   C   F   Cb

Edible Weights: (no bones/shell)

	C	F	Cb
Abalone, Raw, 3 oz	90	0.5	5
Ahi Tuna, grilled, 6 oz fillet (no fat)	220	2	0
Anchovy: Paste, 1 Tbsp, ¼ oz	15	1	0.5
Cnd. in oil, drnd., 5 only, ¾ oz	40	2	0
Pickled, 1 oz	50	3	0
Barracuda (Pacific), raw, 4 oz	130	3	0
Bass: Sea, raw, 4.6 oz fillet	125	2.5	0
Striped: Raw, 1 fillet, 5½ oz	150	3.5	0
Baked, 3 oz	105	3	0
Blue Fish: Raw, 1 fillet, 5¼ oz	185	6.5	0
Baked, 3 oz	130	5	0
Butterfish, raw, 3 oz	125	7	0
Cajun & Creole Dishes: See Page 176			
Calamari, breaded/fried, 1 serve	360	21	10
Carp, raw, 3 oz	110	5	0
Catfish: Raw, 4 oz	115	6.5	0
Fried, breaded, 1 fillet, 3 oz	200	12	7
Baked, 3 oz	130	7	0
Caviar, black/red, 1 Tbsp, 16g	40	3	0.5
Clams: Raw, 3 oz (4 lge/9 small)	65	1	2
Fried, breaded, 6.6 oz (20 small)	380	21	20
Canned, drained, ½ cup, 2½ oz	105	1.5	3.5
Minced, ¼ cup, 2 oz	25	0	2
Clam Juice: (Snow's) 1 Tbsp	0	0	0
Cod, Atlantic/Pacific: Raw, 4 oz	95	1	0
Baked/Broiled, 1 fillet, 6¼ oz	190	2	0
Canned, 3 oz	90	1	0
Minced, ¼ cup, 2 oz	25	0	0
Smoked/Dry Heat, 3 oz	95	1	0
Crab: Alaska King, raw, 1 leg, 6 oz	145	1	0
1 leg, cooked, 4¾ oz	130	2	0
Blue: Raw, 1 crab			
(⅓ lb whole crab, ¾ oz flesh)	20	0.2	0
Steamed, 3 oz	85	1	0
Canned, drained, ½ cup, 2½ oz	65	1	0
Dungeness, 1 crab, 5¾ oz edible			
(from 1½ lb whole crab)	180	2	2
Imitation Crab Legs/Stix, 3oz	85	1	8.5
Crab Cakes (Low-fat), (1), 2 oz	95	4.5	0.5
Regular (1), 3 oz	130	6.5	0.5
Crab Legs, restaurant (Red Lobster)	260	4.5	0
Crayfish, raw, 4 oz (edible)	100	1	0
Croaker, raw, 3 oz	90	3	0
Cuttlefish, raw, 3 oz	70	1	1
Dolphinfish, raw, 1 fillet, 7 oz	175	1.5	0
Eel: Raw, 3 oz	155	10	0
Smoked/Dry Heat, 3 oz	200	13	0
Fish & Chips: Arthur Treacher	1540	101	132
Denny's, no condiments	960	54	83
Fish S'wich w. Tartar Sce, 5½ oz	430	23	41
Fish Sticks (1), frozen, breaded, 1 oz	70	3.5	6

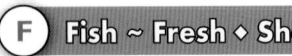

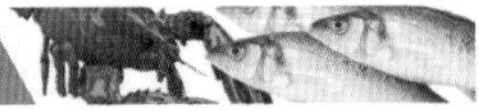

Fish & Shellfish (Cont)

Edible Weights: (no bones/shell)	C	F	Cb
Fish Oil, 1 Tbsp, ½ oz	125	14	0
Flounder/Sole: Raw, 4 oz	105	1.5	0
Baked, 1 fillet, 4½ oz	150	2	0
Frozen Fish & Entrees: See Page 60			
Gefilte Fish: See Kosher/Deli Foods, Page 179			
Grouper, raw, 4 oz	105	1	0
Haddock: Raw, 4 oz	100	1	0
Broiled, 1 fillet, 5¼ oz	170	1.5	0
Smoked, 3 oz	100	1	0
Baked, 3 oz	90	1	0
Halibut: Raw, 4 oz	125	3	0
Baked, ½ fillet, 2¾ oz	225	5	0
Herring: Atlantic, raw, 4 oz	180	10	0
Pickled, 2 pieces, 1 oz	80	5	3
In Sour Cream, 1 oz	55	3	5
Party Snacks, ¼ cup, dr., 2 oz	120	5	0
Rollmops, 1½ oz	110	8	6
Canned: Plain, drained, 3 oz	130	8	0
in Tomato Sauce, 3.5 oz	140	8	2
Smoked, kippered, 4 oz	245	14	0
Jellyfish: Raw, 4 oz	30	0	0
Dried, Salted, 1 cup, 2 oz	20	1	0
King Fish, raw, 4 oz	120	2.5	0
Ling, raw, 4 oz	100	0.5	0
Lobster, Northern: Raw, 4 oz	105	1	0.5
1 Lobster, 6¼ oz			
(from 1½ lb whole lobster)	160	1.5	1
Cooked, 1 cup, 5 oz	140	1	2
Lobster Newberg, ¾ cup	360	20	9
Lobster Thermidor, 1 serving	370	22	15
Lobster Salads, ½ cup	220	13	5
Lobster Tail, restaurant (Red Lobster)	260	3	0
Lomi Salmon, ¼ cup, 2 oz	20	1	3
Lox, Regular/Nova, 2 oz	65	2.5	0
Mackerel: Atlantic, raw, 4 oz	230	16	0
Broiled, 3 oz fillet	230	16	0
Jack, canned, ½ c., 3⅓ oz	150	6	0
King, raw, 4 oz	120	2	0
Pacific/Jack: Raw, 4 oz	180	9	0
Broiled, 3 oz	170	9	0
Spanish, raw, 4 oz	160	7	0
Mahi-Mahi, raw, 4 oz	125	1	0
Milkfish, raw, 4 oz	170	7.5	0
Monkfish: Raw, 4 oz	85	1.5	0
Baked, 3 oz	80	2	0
Mullet, striped, raw, 4 oz	135	4.5	0
Mussels: Raw, 4 oz (edible wt.)	100	2.5	4
1 cup, 5¼ oz (edible wt.)	130	3.5	5
Cooked, moist heat, 3 oz	150	4	6

	C	F	Cb
Ocean Perch: Raw, 4 oz	105	1	0
Baked, 3 oz	100	1	0
Octopus, common, raw, 4 oz	95	1	2.5
Orange Roughy, raw, 4 oz	85	1	0
Oysters: Common, raw, 3 oz	70	2	4
Eastern raw: 6 medium, 3 oz	50	1.5	4.5
1 cup, 8¾ oz	150	4	14
Fried/breaded, 6 med., 3 oz	170	11	10
Pacific, raw, 1 med., 1¾ oz	40	1	2
Oysters Rockerfeller, 3 oysters	220	13	12
Perch, average, raw, 4 oz	105	1	0
Pike: Northern, raw, 4 oz	100	1	0
Walleye, raw, 4 oz	105	1.5	0
Pollock, raw, 4 oz	105	1	0
Pout (Ocean), raw, 4 oz	90	1	0
Pompano, Florida, raw, 4 oz	190	10	0
Porgy/Scup, raw, 4 oz	150	4	0
Quahogs ~ See Clams			
Red-Snapper, raw, 4 oz	115	1.5	0
Rockfish, Pacific, raw, 4 oz	110	2	0
Roe, raw, 2 Tbsp, 1 oz	40	2	0.5
Sablefish: Raw, 4 oz	220	17	0
Smoked, 3 oz	220	17	0
Salmon:			
Raw: Chinook, 4 oz	205	12	0
Atlantic; Coho/Silver, 4 oz	210	12	0
Chum; Pink, 4 oz	135	4	0
Red/Sockeye, 4 oz	190	10	0
Baked: Atlantic/Coho, 3 oz	150	7	0
Smoked Salmon: Chinook, 3 oz	100	4	0
Pacific Supreme, 2 oz	100	4	0
Canned Salmon: Average All Brands			
Pink: 1 oz	40	2	0
¼ cup, 63g (2.2 oz)	90	5	0
3¾ oz can, whole	155	8.5	0
7½ oz can, whole	300	17	0
Skinless/boneless, ¼ c., 2 oz	70	2	0
Red Sockeye: 1 oz	50	3	0
¼ cup, 63g (2.2 oz)	110	7	0
3¾ oz can, whole	190	12	0
Atlantic, ½ cup, 3½ oz	230	14	0
Chinook/King, ½ cup	210	14	0
Chum, ½ cup, 3½ oz	140	5	0
Coho/Silver, ½ cup	155	5	0
Atlantic Steaks: Small, 8 oz	320	14	0
Medium, 12 oz	480	21	0
Large, 16 oz	640	28	0
Salmon Cake, take-out, 3 oz	240	15	6

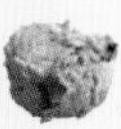

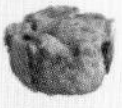

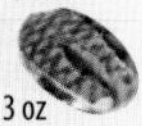

Fish (Cont)

	C	F	Cb
Sardines (Canned): *Average All Brands*			
In Oil, undrained, 1 oz	85	7	0
Drained of oil, 1 oz	60	3	0
3¾ oz can, drained, (3¼ oz)	190	11	0
1 lge/2 med. ³/₅ " small, 0.8 oz	50	3	0
In Tom./ Mustard Sce, 1 oz	45	3	0
3¾ oz can (3 sardines)	210	12	1
Sashimi: *See Japanese Foods, Page 178*			
Scallop: Raw, 6 lge/15 small, 3 oz	80	0.5	2
Breaded/fried, 6 pces, 3½ oz	200	10	10
Sea Bass, raw, 4 oz	110	2	0
Seafood Salad, (Deli Style),			
½ cup, 3.5 oz	250	21	11
Shark: Raw, 4 oz	150	5	0
Batter-dipped, fried, 4 oz	260	16	7
Baked, 4 oz	185	7	0
Shark Fin, dried, 1 oz	30	0	0
Shrimp: Raw, in shell, ½ lb	140	2	1.5
Raw, shelled, 3 oz (12 lge)	90	1.5	0.5
Breaded/fried, 3 oz (11 lge)	210	11	10
Canned, 1 oz (10 shrimp)	65	1	0
Tiger, cooked, 1 shrimp, ½ oz	15	0.5	0
Battered, fried, 1 shrimp	60	4	3
Shrimp Cocktail, restaurant-style	140	2	1
Smelt, Rainbow, raw, 4 oz	110	3	0
Snapper: Raw, 3 oz	85	1	0
Cooked, 1 fillet, 6 oz	215	3	0
Sole, Raw, 4 oz	105	1.5	0
Squid: Raw, 4 oz	105	1.5	3.5
Fried, 3 oz	150	6	7
Surimi (Imitation Crab), 4 oz	115	1.5	11
Sweet & Sour Fish, ½ dish, 10 oz	580	29	53
Swordfish raw:			
Small Steak, 4 oz	135	4.5	0
Medium Steak, 6 oz	205	7	0
Tilapia, Rain Forest Fillets, 4 oz	110	2	0
Trout, Rainbow: Raw, 4 oz	135	4	0
Broiled, 3 oz	125	5	0
Smoked, 2 oz	110	6	0
Tuna: *Average All Brands*			
Raw: Albacore, 4 oz	190	8	0
Bluefin, 4 oz	165	5.5	0
Skipjack, Yellowfin, 4 oz	125	1	0
Broiled, 3 oz	115	1	0
Canned:			
In Water, drained:			
Chunk/Solid: 2 oz can	75	1.5	0
3 oz can	110	2.5	0
6 oz can	220	5	0
In Oil, drained:			
Chunk Light: 2 oz	110	5	0
6 oz can, drained	340	14	0

Tuna (Cont)	C	F	Cb
Solid White, 2 oz	105	4.5	0
6.3 oz can, drained	330	14	0
Tuna Salad: Deli Style, ½ c., 4oz	300	24	15
Lower fat, 4 oz	210	10	11
Whitefish: Raw, 4 oz	150	6.5	0
Baked, 3 oz	145	6.5	1
Smoked, 3 oz	90	1	0
Whiting: Raw, 4 oz	100	1.5	0
Baked, 3 oz	85	1	0
Yellowtail: Raw, 4 oz	165	6	0
Grilled, 3 oz (from 4 oz raw)	160	6	0

Other Canned/Packaged Fish

	C	F	Cb
Bumble Bee: *Incl. Mayo & Crackers*			
Tuna Salad Kit: Original	280	20	18
Fat-Free Kit	150	1.5	24
w. Mayonnaise Kit	420	22	24
Seafood Salad w. Crab Kit	180	5.5	27
Sensations Bowls: Spring Thai Chili Kit	250	12	20
Other varieties, average	200	8.5	13
Lunch on the Run, Tuna Salad Kit	320	14	19
Chicken of the Sea			
Albacore Tuna, 3 oz pouch	100	1.5	0
Light Tuna, 3 oz pouch	90	1	0
Shrimp, 2.5 oz pouch	55	0.5	1
Smoked Pacific Salmon, 3 oz pouch	120	3.5	1
Starkist			
Pouch: *Per 3 oz Pouch (Drained)*			
Tuna Chunk Light, in water, 2 oz	90	1	0
Albacore Tuna, in water, 2 oz	105	1.5	0
Lunch-To-Go Kit: Chunk Light Tuna			
w. Mayo/Crackers, 4.5 oz	210	9	27
Tuna Creations, all varieties, 2 oz	60	0	0

Frozen Fish Products

Gorton's: *Page 120*
Kroger: *Page 121*
Van De Kamp's: *Page 124*
Restaurant Chains: *Page 182*
Captain D's Seafood: *Page 94*
Long John Silver's: *Page 221*
Shoney's: *Page 249*
Southern Tsunami: *Page 253*
Wahoo's Fish Taco: *Page 265*

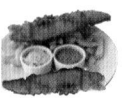

Flours & Grains	C	F	Cb
Amaranth Flour, ½ cup, 3½ oz	365	6.5	65
Arrowroot Flour, ½ cup, 2¼ oz	230	0	56
Barley: Regular, ½ cup, 2.6 oz	255	1	55
Pearled, raw, 3½ oz	350	1	78
Buckwheat: Regular, ½ c., 3 oz	290	3	61
Groats: Roasted, dry, ½ c., 2.9 oz	285	2	62
Roasted, cooked, 3½ oz	80	0.5	17
Flour, whole-groat, ½ cup, 2 oz	200	2	42
Bulgur: Dry, ½ cup, 2½ oz	240	1	53
Cooked, ½ cup, 3.2 oz	75	0.5	17
Carob Flour, ½ cup, 1.8 oz	115	0.5	46
Corn Kernels avg., cooked, ½ cup	80	0.5	18
Corn Bran, ½ cup, 1.3 oz	85	0.5	33
Corn Flour/Masa, ½ cup, 2 oz	215	2.5	43
Corn Grits: Dry, ½ cup, 2¾ oz	290	1	62
Cooked, ½ cup, 4¼ oz	70	0.5	15
Corn Germ, toasted, ½ cup, 4 oz	100	1.5	22
Cornmeal: Average all Types,			
3 Tbsp, 1 oz	105	0.5	22
½ cup, 2½ oz	255	1	54
Mixes: same as above	230	1	48
Made Up, ½ cup, 4.8 oz	95	0.5	20
Cornstarch: 1 Tbsp, 8g	30	0	8
½ cup, 2¼ oz	245	0	58
Couscous: Dry, 1 oz (yield 3 oz ckd)	110	0	22
1 cup cooked, 5½ oz	175	0	37
Farina: Dry, ½ cup, 3.1 oz	325	0.5	69
Cooked, ½ cup, 4.1 oz	55	0	12
Flaxseed: Seeds, 1 Tbsp, 8g	45	3.5	2
Ground, 2 Tbsp, 8g	60	4.5	4
Garbanzo (Chick Pea), ½ c., 1.6 oz	180	3	27
Kuzu Root Starch, 1 Tbsp, 10g	35	0	9
Matzo Meal, ½ cup, 2.2 oz	230	0.5	48
Millet: Raw, ½ cup, 3½ oz	380	4	73
Cooked, ½ cup, 3 oz	105	1	21
Oat Bran: Raw, ⅓ cup, 1.1 oz	75	2	21
Cooked, ½ cup, 3¾ oz	45	1	13
Oats, rolled/oatmeal:			
Dry/Groats, ½ cup, 1.5 oz	160	3	28
Cooked, ½ cup, 4.2 oz	75	1	13
Polenta: *See Cornmeal*			
Potato Flour, ½ cup, 2.8 oz	285	0.5	66
Psyllium Husks, 1 Tbsp (5g)	20	0	4
Quinoa: Dry ½ cup, 3 oz	320	5	59
Cooked, ½ cup, 3¾ oz	130	2	24
Rice Bran, ½ cup, 2 oz	180	12	28
Rice Flour, ½ cup, 2¾ oz	290	1	63

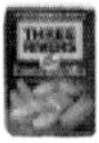

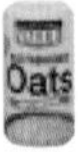

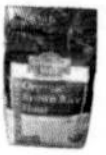

Flours & Grains (Cont)	C	F	Cb
Rice Polish, ½ cup, 3½ oz	360	0.5	80
Rye Flour: Dark, ½ cup, 2.3 oz	210	2	44
Medium, ½ cup, 1.8 oz	180	1	40
Light, ½ cup, 1.8 oz	190	1	41
Rye Grain: ½ cup, 3 oz	280	2	59
Flakes, ¼ cup, 1 oz	100	0.5	21
Semolina, ½ cup, 3 oz	300	1	61
Sorghum, ½ cup, 3.4 oz	325	3	72
Soy Flour:			
Defatted, 1 cup, 3½ oz	330	1	38
Low-Fat, 1 cup, 3 oz	325	6	33
Full-Fat, 1 cup, 3 oz	365	17	29
Soy Meal, defatted, 1 cup, 4.3 oz	415	3	49
Spelt Flour, ½ cup, 2 oz	190	1	41
Tapioca, Pearl:			
Dry, ½ cup, 2.7 oz	270	0	67
3 Tbsp, 1 oz	100	0	25
Teff (Seed) Flour, 2 oz	215	2	42
Tortilla Flour Mix, ½ cup, 2 oz	220	6	37
Triticale: ½ cup, 3.4 oz	325	2	70
Flour, whole-grain, ½ c., 2.3 oz	220	1	48
Wheat Bran, unproc., ½ c., 1 oz	65	1	19
Wheat Flakes, ½ cup, 1½ oz	160	1	35
Wheat Germ: Raw, ¼ cup, 1 oz	105	3	15
Toasted, ¼ cup, 1 oz	110	3	14
Wheat Flour:			
White, All Purpose/Self-Rising,			
1 level Tbsp, 0.6 oz	60	0	13
½ cup, 2.2 oz	230	0.5	48
1 cup, 4.4 oz	455	1.5	95
Whole Wheat, 1 cup, 4.2 oz	405	2	87

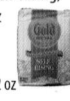

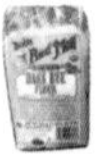

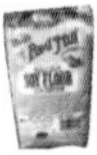

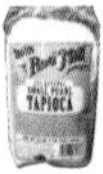

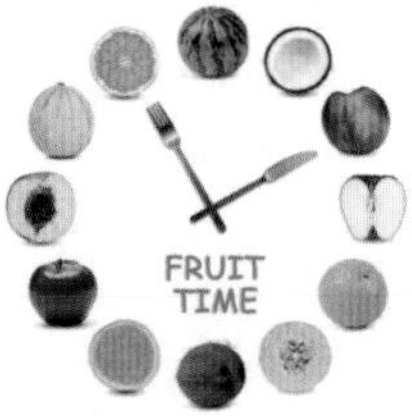

FRUIT TIME

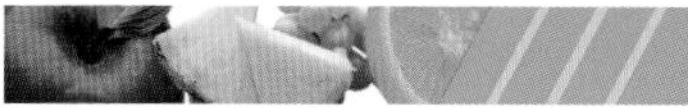

Weights As Purchased	C	F	Cb
Acerola, 1 cup, 20 pcs, 3½ oz	30	0	7.5
Apples: Whole, average all varieties,			
1 small (4 per lb), 4 oz	55	0	13
1 medium (3 per lb), 5½ oz	70	0	17
1 large (2 per lb), 8 oz	110	0	26
1 extra large, 11 oz	150	0	36
without skin: 1 medium, 4½ oz	60	0	14
1 cup slices, 4 oz	55	0	13
Candy/Caramel Apple, 1 med., 6½ oz	245	4	54
Nut Coated, 1 medium, 7 oz	325	11	56
Chiquita Apple Bites, 10 sl., 3½ oz	50	0	12
Apricots: 1 small (12 per lb)	17	0	4
1 medium (8 per lb), 2 oz	25	0	6
1 large (5-6 per lb), 3 oz	40	0	10
Asian Pear (Nashi Fruit)**,** 1 med., 7 oz	85	0	21
Avocado (w/out seed/skin):			
Avg., ½ medium, 3½ oz	160	15	8
1 salad slice, ½ oz	25	2	1
Mashed/Puree, 2 Tbsp, 1 oz	50	4.5	2
¼ cup, 2 oz	90	9	5
Californian, ½ medium, 3 oz	160	14	8
Mashed/Puree, ½ c., 4 oz	190	18	10
Florida, ½ medium, 5½ oz	180	15	12
Mashed/Puree, ½ c., 4 oz	140	11	9
½ cup cubed, 3 oz	105	8	7
Banana, (weight with skin):			
1 small (6", 4 per lb), 4 oz	90	0	23
1 medium (7", 3 per lb), 5 oz	105	0	27
1 large (8"), 7 oz	120	0	30
1 extra large (9"), 9 oz	135	0	35
w/out skin, 1 oz	25	0	6
Berries: (Blueberries/Black/Boysenberries)			
½ cup, 2.5 oz	40	0	10
1 pint, 14 oz	230	1.5	58
Breadfruit, ½ cup, 4 oz	115	0	30
Cactus Pear, 1 fruit, 3½ oz	40	0	9
Cantaloupe: Flesh (no rind), 1 oz	10	0	2
1 cup pieces/balls, 5.5 oz	55	0	13
½ Circle Slices (no rind):			
1 thin (¼"), 1 oz	10	0	2
1 medium (½"), 2 oz	20	0	5
1 thick (¾"), 3 oz	30	0	7
Wedges (Length cut, no rind):			
1 thin, 1/16 medium, 2 oz	20	0	5
1 thick, ⅛ medium, 4 oz	40	0	9
Whole (Weights with seeds and rind):			
½ small, 20 oz	195	1	46
½ medium, 28 oz	270	1.5	65
½ large, 2½ lb	370	2	90
Carambola (Starfruit), 1 med, 3 oz	30	0	6
Cassava, ⅓ cup, 2½ oz	115	0	27
Cherimoya, 1 cup, 5.5 oz	115	1	27

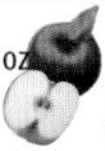
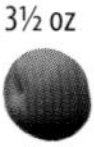
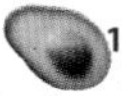
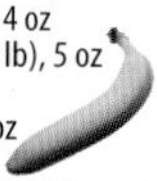
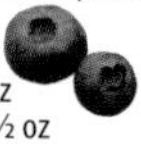
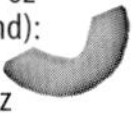
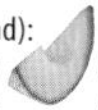

Weights As Purchased	C	F	Cb
Cherries: Sweet (Red/White), raw,			
8 cherries, 2 oz	30	0	8
1 cup, 4½ oz	75	0	19
½ lb (30 cherries)	130	0.5	32
Sour, red, raw, 1 cup, 4 oz	50	0	12
Clementine, 1 med., 2.6 oz	35	0	9
Coconut: Fresh,			
1 piece, 2"x2"x ½", 1 oz	100	10	4.5
Shredded, fresh, ½ cup, 1.4 oz	140	13	6
Sweetened, dried, ½ cup, 1.6 oz	235	16	22
Crabapples, ½ cup slices, 2 oz	40	0	11
Cranberries, ¼ cup, 1 oz	25	0	6.5
Currants, raw, ½ cup, 2 oz	35	0	8
Custard Apple, 4 oz, edible	115	1	28
(from 7 oz with skin/seeds)			
Dates*: See Dried Fruits*			
Dragon Pearl Fruit,			
1 medium, 11½ oz	330	1.5	76
Durian, flesh, 4 oz	165	6	31
Elderberries, ½ cup, 2½ oz	55	0.5	13
Feijoa (Pineapple Guava),			
1 medium, 2 oz	30	0.5	5.5
Figs, green/black:			
1 medium, 2 oz	40	0	10
1 large, 3 oz	60	0	15
Gooseberries, raw, ½ c., 2½ oz	35	0	7
Grapefruit: Average all types,			
½ fruit, 10 oz (6 oz flesh)	55	0	13
1 cup sections w. juice, 8 oz	75	0	18
Grapes: Average, 1 cup, 5½ oz	105	0	28
1 small bunch, 4 oz	80	0	20
1 medium bunch, 7 oz	140	0	36
1 large bunch, 16 oz	315	0	82
Granadilla, flesh, 3½ oz	95	0	23
Guava: 1 medium, 4 oz	80	1	16
Honeydew: 1 slice, ¾" thick, 3 oz	30	0	7
1 wedge (⅛ of 7" diam.),			
12 oz (with rind)	80	0	20
1 cup cubes/balls, 6 oz	60	0	14
½ small (4½ lb whole)	180	0.5	42
½ medium (6lb whole)	230	1	56
Honey Murcots, 1 only, 5 oz	45	0	11
Jaboticaba, flesh, 4 oz	75	2	15
Jackfruit, flesh, ⅛ average, 4 oz	105	0	27
Java-Plum, 4 plums, ½ oz	10	0	2
Jujube, 3 oz	65	0	17
Kiwifruit, 1 medium, 2.7 oz	45	0	11
1 large, 3.2 oz	55	0.5	13
Kumquats, 5 medium, 3½ oz	65	1	15
Kiwano, ½ medium, 5 oz	35	0	8
Langsat, Duku, 1 medium, 2 oz	25	0	5
Lemon: 1 medium, 3 oz	25	0	8
1 wedge, 1 oz	5	0	1.5
Peel, grated, 1 Tbsp	5	0	1

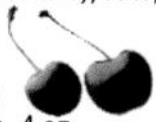
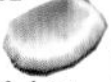
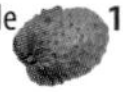
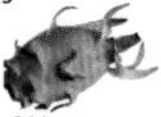
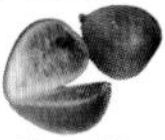
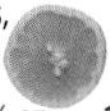
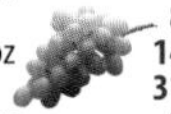
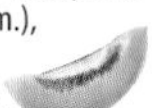

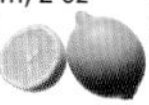

Weights As Purchased	C	F	Cb
Limes, 1 med. (2" diam.), 2.4 oz	20	0	7
Loganberries, froz., ½ cup, 2½ oz	40	0	9
Longans, 5 fruit, ½ oz	10	0	2.5
Loquats, 4 fruit, 2¼ oz	30	0	8
Lychees, 4 fruit, 2¼ oz	30	0	7
Mamey Apple: 1 whole, 3 lb	430	4	106
¼ fruit (1 cup flesh), 7 oz	100	1	25
Mandarin: 1 small, 3 oz	35	0	9
1 medium, 4 oz	45	0	11
1 large, 6 oz	50	0	13
Mango: Flesh, ½ cup slices. 3 oz	55	0	14
1 small mango, 7 oz	90	0.5	24
1 medium, 10 oz	130	0.5	34
1 cheek, 4 oz	60	0	14
1 large, 17 oz	220	1	58
1 extra large mango, 24 oz	310	1.5	82
Melon, avg, 1 cup, cubes/balls, 6 oz	60	0	14
Monstera Deliciosa (Taxonia), Edible part, 4 oz	50	0	11
Mulberries, 20 fruit, 1 oz	15	0	3
Nashi Fruit (Asian Pear), 1 med., 7 oz	85	0	21
Nectarines, 1 medium, 4 oz	50	0	12
1 large, 5½ oz	70	0	16
Oheloberries, ½ cup, 2½ oz	20	0	7
Olives (Pickled): Green, 10 lrg, 1½ oz	60	6.5	1.5
Ripe, Greek Style, 10 oz, 1 oz	70	6	4
Ripe (Black) Californian:			
1 small/medium	5	0	0.2
1 large/extra large	6	0.5	0.5
1 jumbo	7	0.5	0.5
1 colossal	11	1	0.5
Oranges: Avg. all varieties (wts with skin)			
1 small, 5 oz	45	0	11
1 medium (3" diam.), 7 oz	85	0	21
1 large, 10 oz	130	0	33
Californian Valencia, 1 medium (2¾" diam.), 6 oz	60	0	14
Calif. Navels (3" diam.), 7 oz	70	0	17
Sunkist Navel, large, 14 oz	130	0	30
Florida Orange, 1 med, 7 oz	70	0	17
Flesh only, 1 cup, 6 oz	85	0	21
Peel, 1 Tbsp	0	0	0
Papaya: ½ cup, cubed, 2½ oz	30	0	7
1 medium, (5"x3" diam.), 16 oz	120	0	30
Green (unripe), ½ cup, 3½ oz	20	0	5
Passionfruit, 1 medium, 1¼ oz	35	0	8
PawPaw (see Papaya)			
Peaches: 1 small/donut, 3 oz	30	0	7.5
1 medium (4 per lb), 4 oz	45	0	11
1 large, 6 oz	65	0	16
1 extra large, 10 oz	110	0	27

Weights As Purchased	C	F	Cb
Pears, Average all types:			
1 mini, 2½ oz	35	0	8
1 small, 5 oz	75	0	18
1 medium, 7 oz	105	0	25
1 large, 9 oz	135	0	33
1 extra large, 12 oz	175	0	42
Pepino, ½ medium, 4 oz	20	0	4
Persimmons: Native, 1 oz	35	0	9
Japanese (2½"d. x 2½"h), 7 oz	120	0	30
Seedless (Maui), 1 med., 5 oz	100	0	25
Pineapple (wts without skin):			
1 thin slice (½"), 2 oz	25	0	6
1 thick slice (¾"), 3 oz	40	0	10
1 cup, diced, 5½ oz	75	0	19
1 medium, 1½ lb (peeled)	325	0	86
Wedges *(Del Monte),* 12 oz pkg	195	0	47
Canned: *See Page 104*			
Pitanga, (Surinam-Cherry) (5), 1.2 oz	10	0	2
Plaintains, ½ cup slices, 2½ oz	90	0	22
Plums: Average all types:			
Mini/Damson, (1" diam.), ½ oz	7	0	1.5
Small (2" diam.), 2¼ oz	30	0	7
Med. (2½" diam.), 3½ oz	45	0	10
Large (3" diam.), 4 oz	60	0	14
Pluot (plum-apricot), 1 med., 5 oz	80	0	19
Pomegranate, 1 medium, 10 oz	105	0.5	25
Pummelo, flesh, ½ cup, 3½ oz	35	0	9
Prickly Pear, (Nopal):			
1 small, 2½ oz	20	0	5
1 medium, 5 oz	40	0	10
Quince, 1 medium, 3½ oz	55	0	14
Rambutan (Rambotang), Red/Yellow, 1 med., 2 oz	15	0	4
Raspberries, ½ cup, 2 oz	30	0	7
10 Raspberries, ¾ oz	10	0	2
1 Cup, 4¼ oz	65	1	15
1 Pint, 11 oz	160	2	37
Sapodilla (Chico), 1 med., 7½ oz	140	2	34
Sapote, ½ medium, 8 oz	150	0.5	38
Satsuma Tangerine, 1 med., 3 oz	45	0	11
Soursop, 1 cup pulp, 8 oz	150	0.5	38
Starfruit, 1 medium, 3 oz	30	0	6
Strawberries: 1 cup, 5½ oz	50	0.5	12
6 medium/3 large, 2 oz	20	0	4
1 pint, 14 oz	115	1	27
Chocolate Dipped, 1 large	45	2.5	6
Sugar Apple (Custard Apple) ½ cup pulp, 4 oz	120	0	30
Tamarillo, 1 medium, 3 oz	20	0	3
Tamarind: 1 fruit (3"x1")	5	0	1.5
Pulp, ½ cup, 2 oz	140	0.5	37

Weights as Purchased

	C	F	Cb
Tangelo: 1 small, 4 oz	55	0	13
1 medium, 5 oz	70	0	17
1 large, 7 oz	95	0	23
Tangerine, 1 medium, (2½" diam.), 4 oz	50	0	13
Tangor, 1 medium, 4 oz	35	0	7
Tomatillos (3), 3½ oz	35	1	6
Tomatoes:			
1 small (2¼" diam.), 3 oz	15	0	3
1 medium (2¾" diam.), 5 oz	25	0	5
1 large (3½" diam.), 8 oz	40	0.5	9
1 extra large (3" diam.), 12 oz	60	0.5	14
Grape, 1 cup, 2 oz	10	0	2
Yellow Tear Drop, 3 medium, 1 oz	5	0	2
Cherry: 4 medium, 2 oz	10	0	2
1 cup, 5 oz	25	0	6
Slices (Medium Tomato):			
2 thin slices, 1 oz	5	0	1
2 thick (⅜"), 2 oz	10	0	2
Wedge, ¼ medium tomato, 1¼ oz	6	0	1
Chopped, 1 cup, 6½ oz	35	0.5	7
Fried Green Tomato, 2 slices, 2½ oz	140	11	9
Canned Tomatoes/Products: See Page 168			
Tree Tomato (Tamarillo), 3 oz	20	0	5
Ugli Fruit, Tangelo type, 5 oz	40	0	8
Watermelon: Flesh only-no rind, 1 oz	8	0	2
1 thin slice, (¼ circle, ⅜"), 2 oz	15	0	4
1 Extra			
1 cup cubes or balls, 5½ oz	45	0	11
10 balls, 4.3 oz	35	0	9
Buffet Slice, thin, 1 oz	8	0	2
Regular (Long Shape):			
1 thick (1") slice (¼ circle, 4½" radius)			
9 oz w. skin (5½ oz no rind)	50	0	12
1 thin (½") slice (¼ circle)			
18 oz with rind	25	0	6
1 thick (1") slice (½ circle)			
18 oz with rind	100	1	22
1 whole melon (15" long, 7½"diam.)			
20 lb w. rind, (10 lb no rind)	1360	7	330
Seedless (Round Shape):			
Medium size (13 lb, 8¼" diam.)			
1 whole, 8½ lb (no rind)	1160	5	280
Wedge, (⅛ whole melon),			
26 oz (with rind)	145	1	35
Flesh only (no rind), 8 oz	70	0.5	17
Mini size (6 lb, 6½" diam.),			
1 whole, 3½ lb (no rind)	480	2.5	110
Wedge (⅛ whole),			
1½ lb (with rind)	60	0.5	14
Xoconostle: *see Prickly Pear*			

FRUIT & VEGETABLE JUICES
~ *See Beverages Page 41*

Dried Fruit

	C	F	Cb
Apples, 5 rings, 1 oz	80	0	19
Apricots, 8 halves, 1 oz	65	0	16
Banana Chips, ½ cup, 1½ oz	220	14	25
Banana Flakes, 4 Tbsp, 1 oz	80	0	20
Cranberries *(Craisins):*			
Sweetened, ¼ cup, 1 oz	100	0	24
Unsweetened, ¼ cup, 1 oz	80	0	19
Choc-coated, 1 oz	135	7.5	18
Currants, ¼ cup, 1¼ oz	100	0	25
Dates: 5 medium dates, 1½ oz	120	0	29
Large Calif.: 1 date, 0.7 oz	55	0	13
3 dates, 2 oz	170	0	39
½ cup, chopped, 3 oz	240	0	58
Pecan Date Rolls, 1 oz	100	2.5	19
Date Crumbles *(Bob's Redmill),*			
1 oz, ¼ cup	90	0	22
Figs, 3 medium figs, 1 oz	90	0	23
Goji Berries, 3 Tbsp, 1 oz	100	1	20
Longans; Lychees, 1 oz	80	0	20
Mango Slices, 5 pieces, 1.4 oz	25	0	6
Papaya Spears, 2 pieces, 1.4 oz	120	0	30
Peaches, 2 halves, 1 oz	60	0	15
Pears, 3 halves, 2 oz	140	0.5	34
Plums *(Sunsweet)* (5), 1.4 oz	100	0	24
Prunes (dried Plums): w. pits, 1 oz	70	0	17
1 medium (60/lb)	16	0	4
1 large (50/lb)	22	0	5
1 extra large (40/lb)	25	0	6
Without pits, 4 med., 1 oz	70	0	17
Cooked: w. sugar, ½ cup, 5 oz	155	0	38
w/out sugar, ½ cup, 4½ oz	135	0	33
Raisins: 2 Tbsp, 1 oz pkg	85	0	22
½ cup, 2.8 oz	220	0.5	56

Candied/Glazed Fruit

	C	F	Cb
Apricot, 1 medium, 1 oz	70	0	17
Cherry, (Maraschino) (1)	8	0	2
Citron/Fruit Peel, 1 oz	85	0	20
Ginger, 1 oz	90	0	21
Pineapple, 1 slice, 1¼ oz	120	0	29

Fruit Leather/Rolls

	C	F	Cb
Average All Brands, 1 oz	105	1	24
Fruit By The Foot, (Betty Crocker)			
1 roll, ¾ oz	80	0	17
Fruit Gushers, (Betty Crocker), 1 oz	90	1	20
Fruit Roll-Ups, (Betty Crocker) 1 roll	50	1	12
Stretch Island, Leathers, 2 pces, 1 oz	90	0	24

Canned/Bottled Fruit

Solids & Liquids:

Per ½ Cup (Approx. 4½ oz)

	C	F	Cb
Apricots: In water/diet	35	0	8
In juice/lite	60	0	15
In syrup	105	0	28
Black/Blueberries: Heavy syrup	120	0	30
In light syrup	110	0	26
Cherries, pitted: in water	55	0	15
In light syrup	85	0	22
In heavy syrup	105	0	27
In extra heavy syrup	135	0	34
Maraschino, 1 oz	50	0	12
Pie Cherries, ⅔ cup, 5 oz	90	0	23
Fruit Salad: In water/diet	35	0	10
In juice/Light	60	0	16
In heavy syrup	95	0	25
Gooseberries, Light syrup	90	0	24
Grapefruit: Juice pack	45	0	12
In light syrup	75	0	18
Lychees, ½ cup, 4.5 oz	105	0	26
Mixed Fruit: In water/diet	40	0	10
In fruit juices/light syrup	70	0	18
In heavy syrup	90	0	24
Peaches (halves/slices): In water/diet	30	0	7
In juice/light	55	0	14
In light syrup	70	0	18
drained, ½ peach	55	0	14
In heavy syrup	100	0	26
Pears: In water/diet	35	0	10
In juice/light	60	0	16
In heavy syrup	100	0	26
Pineapple: All types			
In own juice	75	0	18
In heavy syrup	100	0	26
1 slice (ring), drained, 1½ oz	15	0	4
Prunes: In heavy syrup	125	0	33
In Liqueur, ½ cup, 125g	280	0	70
Stewed in Water, ½ cup	135	0	35
Tropical Fruit Salad: In light syrup	80	0	21
In heavy syrup	110	0	29

Fruit Snack Cups

	C	F	Cb
Deli/Take-Out: Small, 6 oz	70	0	16
Large, 12 oz	140	0	32
Yogurt & Fruit Cup, 15 oz	380	4.5	75
Del Monte Fruit Cups			
Fruit Cups: *Per 4 oz Cup*			
Strawberry Banana	70	0	17
Mandarin Or. Segments	70	0	17
Pineapple Tidbits	70	0	18
Tropical Fruit	70	0	18
Fruit Naturals: *Per 8 oz Cup*			
Cherry Mixed Fruit	140	0	35
Peach Chunks	140	0	35
Pineapple Chunks	140	0	35
Red Grapefruit	120	0	30
Fruit-n-Gel Cups: *Per 4½ oz Cup*			
Mixed Fruit/Peaches in Fruit Gel	90	0	22
Lite varieties in Gel, avg.	60	0	14
Carb Clever: *Per ½ Cup (4.2 oz)*			
Fruit Cocktail/Pears (chunks/slices)	40	0	10
Peaches (chunks/slices)	30	0	7
Pull Top Cans: in 100% Juice, 4 oz	80	0	20
Lite varieties, 4 oz	50	0	13
Dole Fruit Bowls			
4 oz Bowls: Peaches	70	0	18
Mixed Fruit; Tropical Fruit	80	0	19
Pineapple	60	0	16
Fruit-n-Gel Bowls (4.3 oz): Regular	90	0	23
Reduced Sugar	60	0	16
Mott's: Healthy Harvest, 4 oz cup	50	0	13
Vons: Mixed Fruit,			
In heavy syrup, 1 cup, 4.5 oz	100	0	25
In lite syrup, 1 cup	60	0	14

Apple & Fruit Sauces

	C	F	Cb
Apple Sauce:			
Regular/sweetened, 2 Tbsp, 1 oz	20	0	6
4 oz package	85	0	22
¼ cup	50	0	13
Fruit Sauces & Purees:			
Average all fruit types, 2 Tbsp, 1 oz	25	0	6
½ cup, 4 oz	100	0	24
Mott's:			
Classics, avg. 4 oz	100	0	24
Apple Sauce: Original, 4 oz	100	0	24
Fruit Flavored, avg., 4 oz	90	0	23
No Sugar Added, 4 oz	50	0	12
Ocean Spray: *Per ¼ Cup (2½ oz)*			
Jellied Cranberry Sauce	110	0	25
Whole Berry Cranberry Sauce	110	0	27
Pie Fillings ~ See Page 136			

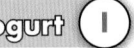
Quick Guide   C F Cb

Ice Cream

Vanilla: *Average All Brands*
Other flavors ~ See Brand Listings.
Regular Ice Cream (10% fat):
Examples: Borden/Hood

	C	F	Cb
3 fl.oz scoop	105	5	12
½ cup, 4 fl.oz	140	7	17
1 Pint, 16 fl.oz	560	28	68
½ Gallon (4 Pints)	2240	112	272

Rich (16% fat):
Example: Hood (Red Sox)

	C	F	Cb
3 fl.oz scoop	135	7.5	15
½ cup, 4 fl.oz	180	10	20
1 Pint	720	40	80

Super-Rich (20% fat): Haagen-Dazs/Ben & Jerry's

	C	F	Cb
3 fl.oz scoop	200	13	18
½ cup, 4 fl.oz	270	17	24
1 Pint	1080	68	96

Reduced-Fat/Light (6% fat):
Breyer's Light/Hood Light

	C	F	Cb
3 fl.oz scoop	95	3	15
½ cup, 4 fl.oz	125	4	20
1 Pint	500	16	80

Fat-Free: Baskin-Robbins FF/Borden FF/
Breyers FF/Dreyers FF/Hood FF

	C	F	Cb
3 fl.oz scoop	70	0	16
½ cup, 4 fl.oz	90	0	21
1 Pint	360	0	84

Soft Serve: Regular, ½ cup

	C	F	Cb
Soft Serve: Regular, ½ cup	190	11	19
1 cup	380	22	38
Light, ½ cup	110	2	19
1 cup	220	4	38

Quick Guide   C F Cb

Frozen Yogurt
Average All Brands

	C	F	Cb
Hard: Low-Fat, ½ cup	110	3	19
Non-Fat, ½ cup	110	0	24
Soft: Low-Fat, ½ cup	120	4	17
Non-Fat, ½ cup	100	0	30

Brands: See Ice Cream & Ices Section

Quick Guide   C F Cb

Gelato/Ices/Frozen Custard

Gelato: Per ½ Cup

	C	F	Cb
Milk base: Vanilla	160	6	25
Choc. Hazelnut	230	15	21
Water base, ½ cup	100	0	26

Frozen Custard: Per ½ Cup

	C	F	Cb
Chocolate	140	6	18
Orange Sherbet	105	2	21
Vanilla	130	6	16

Ice (Milk base): Average all flavors

	C	F	Cb
Hard (4% fat), ½ cup	100	3	15
Soft Serve (3% fat), ½ cup	110	2	19
Shaved Ice: Average, 12 fl. oz	160	0	40
Sherbet: Avg., ½ cup	110	1.5	22
Sorbet: Fruit (no fat), ½ cup	70	0	19
Fruit Ice Pops	80	0	20

Tofu Frozen Desserts: See Page 35

Sundaes   C F Cb

Baskin Robbins:

	C	F	Cb
2 Scoop Hot Fudge	530	29	62
Banana Royale	630	27	91
Banana Split	1030	39	168
Heath Banana Sundae	1210	59	160
Oreo Layered Sundae	1030	47	146
Reeses Peanut Butter Cup	1400	90	124

Denny's: Banana Split

	C	F	Cb
Denny's: Banana Split	895	43	121
Single Scoop, no topping	190	14	14
Double Scoop, no topping	380	27	29
Chocolate, Topping, 2 oz	135	0.5	34
Other Toppings ~ See Page 203			

McDonald's:

	C	F	Cb
Hot Caramel Sundae	340	8	60
Hot Fudge Sundae	330	10	54
Strawberry Sundae	280	6	49
Toppings: Peanuts, ¼ oz	45	3.5	2

Ice Cream, Cones & Cups

Average All Brands   C F Cb

	C	F	Cb
Wafer Cone/Cup, average	20	0	4
Sugar Cone, average	50	0	14
Waffle Cone:			
Small	50	1	10
Large	90	0.5	19
Brands:			
Oreo Chocolate Cone	50	1	10
Comet Sugar Cone	50	0	11
Keebler Sugar Cone	50	0	10

Brands

	C	F	Cb
Baskin-Robbins: *See Fast-Foods Section*			
Ben & Jerry's: *Per ½ Cup*			
Singles: *Per Container (3.6 oz)*			
Cherry Garcia	220	13	22
Chocolate Fudge Brownie	230	11	28
Cookie Dough	240	13	26
Vanilla	200	13	17
Original: Butter Pecan	280	21	20
Cherry Garcia	250	14	26
Chocolate	260	16	25
Chocolate Chip Cookie Dough	270	15	32
Chocolate Fudge Brownie	260	13	32
Chubby Hubby	330	20	31
Chunky Monkey	300	18	30
Coffee	240	15	21
Coffee Heath Bar Crunch	290	18	29
Everything But The...	310	19	30
Half Baked	280	14	34
Karamel Sutra	280	15	32
Mint Choc Chunk	270	17	26
New York Super Fudge Chunk	310	20	29
Oatmeal Cookie Chunk	270	15	31
Peanut Butter Cup	360	26	27
Phish Food: ½ Cup	280	13	37
Light	210	6	37
Pistachio Pistachio	260	17	21
Smores	290	16	36
Turtle Soup	280	15	30
Vanilla	240	16	21
Vanilla Heath Bar Crunch	290	18	29
Vermonty Python	310	19	30
Frozen Yogurt: *Per ½ Cup*			
Phish Food	220	4.5	41
Ligten-Up!: Black Raspberry	140	1.5	28
Cherry Garcia	170	3	32
Choc. Fudge Brownie	190	2.5	35
Half Baked	190	3	35
Sorbet: Avg. all flavors	115	0	30
Blue Bunny			
Fat-Free, No Added Sugar: *Per ½ Cup*			
Brownie Sundae	90	0	23
Average other flavors	80	0	19
Reduced-Fat, No Added Sugar: *Per ½ Cup*			
Banana Split	120	5	20
Butter Pecan	130	6	16
Rocky Road	130	6	19
Turtle Sundae	140	7	20

	C	F	Cb
Blue Bunny (Cont)			
Hi Lite: Butter Pecan	120	4.5	17
Caramel Pecan	130	4	21
Cookies & Cream	130	4	21
Personals (Light): Bunny Tracks	130	5	21
Chocolate Raspb. Cheesecake	100	2.5	18
Super Fudge Brownie	120	3	22
Frozen Yogurt			
Brownie Fudge Fantasy	110	0	24
Homemade Chocolate	100	0	19
Strawberry Cheesecake,	100	0	21
Frozen Yogurt, ½ cup	100	0	21
Bars/Pops: *See Page 110*			
Breyers: *Per ½ Cup:*			
CarbSmart: Rocky Road	130	10	12
Chocolate	120	10	8
Vanilla	110	8	10
All Natural: Butter Pecan, avg.	160	10	14
Cherry Vanilla	140	8	17
Cookies & Cream; Rocky Road	160	8	19
Fried Ice Cream	140	4.5	22
Fruit Sherbet	130	1.5	26
Lactose Free Vanilla	130	7	14
Vanilla, Choc., Strawberry	130	7	16
Other flavors, average	160	8	17
Double Churn Fat-Free:			
Chocolate; Vanilla,	90	0	22
Cappuccino Choc Chunk	110	0	26
Caramel Swirl	120	0	29
Fun & Indulgent:			
Peanut Butter Tracks	170	9	19
Very Chocolate Cherry	140	4.5	21
Other flavors, average	160	8	20
Light: Butter Pecan, ½ cup	120	5	16
Choc. Mocha Silk; Mint Choc. Chip	130	5	19
Rocky Road	130	4.5	22
Vanilla, Chocolate, Strawberry	100	3.5	16
Other flavors, average	120	4	19
Natural:			
Chocolate Caramel Brownie	150	4.5	23
Cookies & Cream	140	5	21
Creamy Vanilla	120	4	18
Extra Creamy Choc.	120	4	18
No Sugar Added: Butter Pecan	110	6	14
Chocolate Fudge Brownie	90	1.5	20
Peanut Butter; Triple Choc., avg.	115	6	17
Other flavors, average	85	4	14

Brands (Cont)

	C	F	Cb
Brigham's: *Per ½ Cup*			
Ice Cream: Big Dig	210	12	24
Choc. Chip; Vanilla, avg.	200	13	19
Coffee	190	12	17
Mocha Almond	210	15	18
Raspberry Lime Rickey Sherbert	130	2	27
Bruster's			
Frozen Yogurt: Chocolate, ½ cup	150	4.5	24
Vanilla, ½ cup	220	6.5	34
No Added Sugar Ice Cream: *Per ½ Cup*			
Chocolate; Vanilla, avg.	210	12	24
Choc. Caramel Swirl/Fudge Ripple	120	0	31
Cinnamon; Coffee	100	0	24
Other varieties, average	110	0	30
Carvel Ice Cream: *See Fast-Foods Section*			
Coldstone Creamery: *See Fast-Foods Section*			
Colombo: *Per ½ Cup*			
Frozen, Soft Serve: Non-Fat, avg.	105	0	22
Slender Sensations, average	60	0	15
Low-Fat, Old Worlde; Cookies	120	2	21
Sorbet, all varieties	100	0	25
Costco: Frozen Yogurt, 12 oz	270	0	57
CremaLita (Soft Serve)			

Calories will vary with density (air in product) and serving size. Best to weigh product and calculate on 25 cals per 1 oz weight.

	C	F	Cb
Vanilla: Small (4 fl.oz cup),			
If 4 oz weight*	100	0.5	23
If 6 oz weight*	150	1	35
(*) Most common weights			
Medium (8 fl.oz cup), 11 oz wt	275	1.5	63
Chocolate: Small, 6 oz weight	160	1	36
Dairy Queen/Brazier: *See Fast-Foods Section*			
Dippin' Dots			
Dots 'n Cream: *Per ½ Cup*			
Banana Split; Vanilla	170	10	16
Butter Pecan	180	10	14
Chocolate	165	10	15
Mint Chocolate Chip	200	9	25
Dove: *Per ½ Cup*			
Beyond Vanilla	240	15	23
Caramel Pecan Perfection	300	18	30
Chocolate & Brownie Affair	300	19	30
Irresistibly Raspberry	240	13	29
Unconditional Chocolate	290	17	21
Other varieties, avg.	300	19	30

	C	F	Cb
Dreyers/Edys: *Per ½ Cup*			
Grand: Real Strawberry	130	6	16
Chocolate; Vanilla Bean, avg.	150	8	17
Coffee; Neapolitan, avg.	140	8	15
Fudge Tracks; Peanut Butter Cup	180	11	18
Nestle Drumstick Sundae Cone	180	10	19
Toffee Bar Crunch	160	8	21
Vanilla	150	10	14
Other flavors, avg.	160	9	18
Loaded, Chocolate Fudge Brownie	120	4	19
Light, Slow Churned: Neopolitan	100	3	15
Cherry Choc Chip	120	4	18
Other varieties, average	110	4	18
Yogurt Blends, average	110	3	17
Sherbet, avg. all flavors	130	1.5	28
Friendly's: *Per ½ Cup Unless Indicated*			
Ice Cream: Butter Crunch	150	7	19
Chocolate Alm. Chip	160	10	17
Forbidden Chocolate	160	9	17
Hunka Chunka PB Fudge	240	16	21
Vanilla Choc. Strawberry	140	7	16
Vienna Mocha Chunk	180	9	20
Light, Purely Pistachio	120	5	16
Frozen Yogurt: *Per ½ Cup*			
Fudge Berry Swirl	150	4	24
Sundaes: *Per 3 Scoops*			
Royal Banana Split	940	37	136
Jim Dandy	1130	48	159
Reese's Peanut Butter Cup	930	54	90
Friend-Z's: Oreo Cookies, 12 fl.oz	750	23	120
Frostline (Soft Serve): Chocolate	90	1	19
Vanilla, ½ cup	100	1	20
Gelati-da			
Gelato: *Per ½ Cup (4 oz)*			
Amaretto Chocolate	150	4.5	23
Choc Mint Milano	120	2.5	22
Coffee Fudge Latte	130	2	22
Red Raspberry	130	1.5	25
Vanilla Marsala	120	2	21

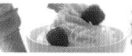

Brands (Cont)

	C	**F**	**Cb**

Haagen-Dazs

Ice Cream, Sorbet, Frozen Yogurt: *See Fast-Foods Section*

Bars: *See Page 111*

Hola Fruta!: *Per ½ cup*

	C	F	Cb
Pure Fruit Sherbert: Margarita	140	1	30
Peach; Strawberry	130	1	31
Pina Colada	140	1.5	31
Pomegranate; Raspberry	140	1	32
Pomegranate & Blueberry	150	1	34

Hood: *Per ½ Cup*

	C	F	Cb
Frozen Yogurt: Mocha Fudge	120	0	27
Old Fashioned Vanilla	110	0	24
Fat-Free, Double Raspberry	110	0	25
Ice Cream: Birthday Party	150	8	19
Chippedy Chocolaty	150	9	19
Chocolate	140	7	17
Cookie Dough Delight	160	8	20
Cookies 'N Cream	160	8	19
Fudge Twister	150	7	20
Golden Vanilla	140	7	17
Maple Walnut	150	9	17
Red Sox, Fenway Fudge	180	10	20

New England Creamery ~ www.CalorieKing.com

Bars: *See Page 111*

I Can't Believe It's Yogurt: *See Fast-Foods Section*

Jerseymaid (Vons): *Per ½ Cup*

	C	F	Cb
Cookies & Cream	160	8	18
Choc Chip; Mint Choc Chip	150	9	16
Heavenly Hash; Nut Chunky Choc.	170	10	17
Mocha Almd Fudge; Rocky Road	155	9	17
Neopolitan; Vanilla	145	7	16
Strawberry	130	6	17

Oberweis: *Per ½ Cup*

Super Premium:

	C	F	Cb
Chocolate	230	15	21
Choc.Peanut Butter	280	19	21
Cookie Dough	230	13	26
Vanilla	210	14	18

Per Serving

	C	**F**	**Cb**

Rice Dream (Non-Dairy):

Per ½ Cup, 2½ oz

Supreme:

	C	F	Cb
Average all flavors	150	7	22

Bars: *See Page 112*

Soy Delicious: *Per ½ Cup*

	C	F	Cb
It's Soy Delicious: Choc Almond	140	4.5	23
Choc Peanut Butter	135	3.5	24
Pistachio Almond	130	4.5	23
Other flavors, avg.	110	1.5	25
So Delicious Organic: Butter Pecan	160	7	22
Cookies 'N Cream	150	4	26
Chocolate Velvet	130	3	24
Creamy Vanilla; Mocha Fudge	130	3	24
Neapolitan; Strawberry	120	3	23
Peanut Butter	150	6	23
Other varieties, avg	140	4	25
Purely Decadent: PB Zig Zag	230	13	32
Other flavors, avg.	200	8.5	32

Soy Dream (Non-Dairy): *Per ½ Cup*

	C	F	Cb
Butter Pecan	150	9	19
Chocolate	120	6	17
Chocolate Fudge Brownie	130	7	18
Mocha Fudge	140	7	21
Green Tea	140	8	18
French Vanilla; Vanilla	140	8	17

Starbucks: *Per ½ Cup*

	C	F	Cb
Caramel Cappuccino	240	12	30
Classic Coffee	230	12	26
Coffee Almond Fudge; Java Chip	250	13	29
Coffee Fudge Brownie	190	11	25
Mud Pie	240	11	32
Low-Fat Latte	170	3	30

Bars: *See Page 112*

Stonyfield Farm (Organic)

Premium Ice Cream: *Per ½ Cup*

	C	F	Cb
Chocolate Raspberry Swirl	230	13	25
Cookies 'n Dream	270	16	27
Creme Caramel	250	14	29
Gotta Have Java	250	16	22
Gotta Have Vanilla	240	16	21
Vanilla Chai	240	16	21

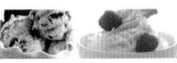
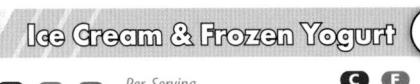
Brands (Cont)

	C	F	Cb
Stop & Shop: *Per ½ Cup*			
Butterscotch Ripple	140	7	19
Chocolate	140	8	18
Chocolate Chip (Reg./Chunky)	150	9	17
Country Club	130	6	19
Heavenly Hash	170	8	22
Neopolitan; Vanilla	140	8	18
Vanilla Fudge Swirl	150	8	18

Tasti D-Lite (Soft Serve)
Calories will vary with density (air in product) and serving size
Best to weigh product and calculate on 25 cals per 1 oz weight.

	C	F	Cb
Vanilla: Small (4 fl.oz cup), 6 oz wt	180	4	35
Medium (8 fl.oz cup), 11 oz wt	330	7	64

TCBY

	C	F	Cb
Soft Serve Frozen Yogurt: *Average all Flavors*			
96% Fat-Free: Kids Cup	110	2	18
Small Cup	280	6	46
Regular Cup	360	8	60
Large Cup	460	10	76
Non-Fat: Small Cup	220	0	48
Regular Cup	290	0	62
Large Cup	360	0	79
No Sugar Added/Non-Fat: Small	180	0	48
Regular Cup	230	0	62
Large Cup	300	0	79
Hand-Scooped Frozen Yogurt: *Average all Flavors*			
Kids Cup	105	6.5	16
Small Cup	215	7	32
Regular Cup	320	11	49
Large Cup	425	14	64
No Added Sugar:			
Chocolate Chocolate Swirl			
Small Cup	130	0.5	32
Regular Cup	200	1	49
Large Cup	270	1.5	65

Tofutti, Non-Dairy Dessert: *Per ½ Cup*

	C	F	Cb
Premium Pints: Better Pecan	210	13	21
Chocolate Cookie Crunch	210	11	26
Chocolate Supreme	180	11	18
Vanilla	210	13	21
Vanilla Almond Bark	240	15	24
Vanilla Fudge; Wildberry, avg.	190	9	25

Trader Joe's

	C	F	Cb
Trader Giotto's Gelato: Choc.	220	8	30
Vanilla	160	6	25

Per Serving

	C	F	Cb
Turkey Hill: *Per ½ Cup*			
Premium: Black Cherry	130	6	18
Butter Pecan	160	10	15
Choc Mint Chip	160	9	17
Choc. Peanut Butter	180	11	18
Cookies 'n Crm	150	8	19
French Vanilla	140	7	16
Rocky Road	170	8	23
Tin Roof Sundae	150	8	19
Lite: Moose Tracks	130	6	19
Peanut Butter Mania	130	5	19
Vanilla Bean	100	2.5	16
Other flavors, average	120	4	19
All Natural: Avg. all flavors	140	8	17
No Sugar Added: *Per ½ Cup*			
Cherry Fudge Ripple	80	0	22
Dutch Chocolate; Vanilla	70	0	20
Peanut Brittle	120	0	16
Frozen Yogurt:			
Choc. Chip Cookie Dough	130	3.5	21
Low-Fat: Mint Cookies 'n Cream	110	1.5	21
Vanilla Bean	100	2	17
Fat-Free: Choc. Marshmallow	110	0	24
Other flavors, average	100	0	21
Smoothie, all flavors, average	100	0	21
Sherbet	120	1	26

Walgreens

	C	F	Cb
Premium One Pint Container: *Per ½ Cup*			
Banana Split	130	5	20
Creme de Menthe	160	9	19
Homemade Vanilla	130	7	16
New York Cherry	130	6	17
Rocky Road	150	7	18
Strawberries 'n Cream	130	6	14
Toasted Butter Pecan	170	10	18
Waffle Cone	150	7	19
Scoops Orange Sherbert	120	1	26
Premium 1.75 Quarts Container: *Per ½ Cup*			
Banana Split	150	6	22
Homemade Vanilla	150	8	17
New York Cherry	150	7	20
Old Fashioned1.75 Quarts (Square)			
Avg., all flavors, ½ cup	140	7	16
Whole Soy Frozen Yogurt			
Average all flavors,			
½ cup, 2½ oz	120	1	25

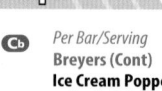

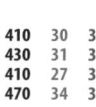

Bars & Pops

C F Cb

Per Bar/Serving

	C	F	Cb
Barq's Root Beer & Ice Cream Float, 4 fl.oz cup	120	3	22
Ben & Jerry's			
Peace Pops: Cherry Garcia (1)	270	19	29
Vanilla Almond	340	23	30
Half Baked (1)	340	16	46
Vanilla (1)	300	20	26
The Cone	360	19	44
Novelties: 'Wich Ice Cream, Cookie Sandwich	350	18	45
Big Bear: *See Klondike*			
Big Ed's Super Saucer, 10 fl.oz	590	29	75
Blue Bunny: Ice Pops, avg.	120	0	24
Bomb Pops, avg.	50	0	11
Chocolate Cup, 1.7 oz	100	5	12
Choc Raspberry	270	18	25
Cookies and Cream	250	15	28
Fudge Bar, 2.7 oz	110	1.5	21
Health Smart, 2.2 oz	60	0	15
Hot Fudge Bar	370	25	33
Milk Choc Bar	300	21	25
Milk Choc with Almonds	320	23	25
Sweet Freedom S'wich, avg.	140	1.5	32
Turtle Bar	360	24	33
Twin Pops	70	0	18
Vanilla Brownie Cone, King Size	440	22	56
Vanilla Nutty Cone, 3 oz	250	11	34
FrozFruit:			
Banana; Strawb. Crm Bar, avg.	160	6	27
Fruit Bars: Pina Colada	180	10	21
Coconut	150	10	14
Superfruit Bar: Acacia	60	0	15
Cherry	80	0	19
Personals: Banana Split	170	8	22
Turtle Sundae	180	10	21
Premium: Bunny Tracks	220	14	22
Peanut Butter Panic	230	16	19
Super Fudge Brownie	200	12	23
Breyers			
Berry Swirls; Fruit Variety	40	0	10
Strawberry Tropical Raspb	25	0	5
Pomegranate Blends	40	0	10

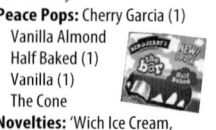

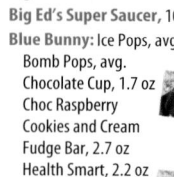
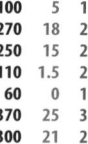

Per Bar/Serving

C F Cb

	C	F	Cb
Breyers (Cont)			
Ice Cream Poppers:			
Heath (27)	410	30	32
Hershey's (27)	430	31	31
Oreo (27)	410	27	38
Reese's (27)	470	34	35
Dble Churn Extra Crmy Bars Light			
Creamy Vanilla	160	8	21
Vanilla & Almd, 1 bar, 3 fl.oz	170	9	21
No Sugar Added: Creamy Vanilla	150	9	18
Krunch	150	9	18
Blisscotti: Coffee & Milk Chocolate	280	15	34
Raspberry & Dark Chocolate	270	15	28
Vanilla & Chocolate	290	15	33
Butterfinger *(Nestle):* 52g Bar	180	13	16
King Size, 112g	310	22	26
California Natural: Mango Sorbet	130	0	33
Lemon & Strawberry Sorbet Cups	120	0	31
Carnation *(Nestle):*			
Ice Cream Sandwich, avg.	200	8	28
Sundae Cups, avg	205	10	28
Chiquita: Swirls, all flavors	80	3	12
Cool Creations			
Cool Classics: Pops, average	35	0	9
Mini Sandwich	110	4	16
Vanilla Sandwich	170	6	28
Toffee/Chocolate Bar, avg.	155	11	14
Cream Pops, 61g	100	2.5	18
Fudge Pops	100	1	21
Sundae Cones	300	18	30
Creamsicle: Sugar-Free Pops (2)	40	2	10
Orange, 2.7 oz	110	2	21
Orange, 1.65 oz	70	1	13
Crunch *(Nestle):*			
Caramel	210	14	19
Vanilla Flavored	210	14	18
Reduced-Fat	140	8	15
Dove: Original Dove	320	21	32
Milk Chocolate	330	21	31
Miniatures, 5 pces	300	20	30
Dreyers/Edys			
Dibs: With Chocolaty Coating (26 Pieces)			
Caramel	440	32	35
Chocolate; Mint; Vanilla	420	32	29
Coffee	400	29	31
Peanut Butter	510	39	32
Real Fruit Bars	80	0	20
Van. w. Nestle Crunch/Drumstick	390	29	29

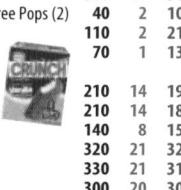
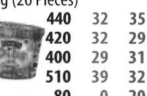

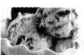

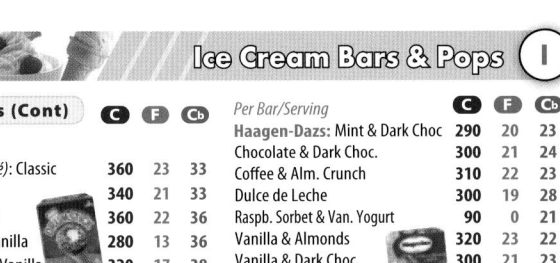

Bars & Pops (Cont)

	C	F	Cb

Per Bar/Serving

	C	F	Cb
Drumstick (*Nestlé*): Classic	360	23	33
Original Vanilla	340	21	33
Vanilla Caramel	360	22	36
Reduced Fat, Vanilla	280	13	36
Simply Dipped: Vanilla	320	17	38
Cookies & Cream	330	17	40
Edy's, Slow Churned Bars:			
Cookies & Cream	150	8	20
Creamy Vanilla	160	8	19
Vanilla Almond	150	9	19
Fat Boy: Ice Cream Sandwich	220	10	30
Cookies N Cream Sandwich	240	10	34
Ice Cream Sandwich Jr., 49g	120	5	17
Nut Sundae on a Stick	310	24	21
Raspberry Cheesecake Sandwich	220	8	33
Fruit A Freeze: Coconut	160	9	20
Lime	70	0	17
Banana; Strawberry	120	4	19
Cappuccino	140	6	21
Dark Choc-Dipped Strawberry	210	12	26
Mango	70	0	16
Fudge Bar (*Nestlé*)	110	1	23
Fudgesicle: Fudge Bar	100	2	21
Fat-Free	70	0	14
No Added Sugar	40	0	10
Good Humor: Oreo Bar	250	15	28
Candy Center Crunch	310	23	24
Chocolate Eclair	220	11	30
Premium Vanilla	260	17	24
Reese's P'nut Butter Cups	310	21	27
Toasted Almond	235	12	30
Cones: Giant King	390	21	44
King	250	13	30
Premium Sundae	260	15	29
Strawberry Shortcake	230	12	30
Sandwiches: Premium Vanilla	160	5	26
Giant Neapolitan/Van., 6 oz	250	9	38
Swirlwind Cup, 6 oz	160	2.5	31

Per Bar/Serving

	C	F	Cb
Haagen-Dazs: Mint & Dark Choc	290	20	23
Chocolate & Dark Choc.	300	21	24
Coffee & Alm. Crunch	310	22	23
Dulce de Leche	300	19	28
Raspb. Sorbet & Van. Yogurt	90	0	21
Vanilla & Almonds	320	23	22
Vanilla & Dark Choc.	300	21	23
Vanilla & Milk Choc.	290	21	22
Healthy Choice: Fudge Bar	80	1	13
Caramel Swirl Sandwich	150	2	30
Swirls, average	90	1.5	17
Vanilla Sandwich	130	3	25
Hood: Chocolate Eclair, 1 bar	150	10	14
Fudge Bar: Chocolate	90	0.5	20
Fudge Stix	90	0	20
Nutty Royal Cone	220	12	26
Vanilla Sandwich	180	6	29
Light Sandwich	160	3	29
Hoodsie Cup Van./Choc.	100	5	12
Hoodsie Pops	60	0	16
Orange Cream Bar	90	1.5	19
Sport Sundae Bar	250	16	26
Ice Cream Sandwich (*Nestle*)	240	10	34
Icee Freeze, 2.25 oz	70	0	17
Klondike			
Heath	240	15	24
Krunch	260	17	24
Nascar	300	14	40
Strawberry Cheesecake	290	18	29
The Original Vanilla	250	17	22
Triple Chocolate	240	14	27
Whitehouse Cherry	250	17	24
Single Serve Cup, Sundae	270	17	26
Single Serve Sandwiches			
Choco Taco	290	15	36
Oreo	230	9	35
Vanilla	260	5	50
Slim-a-Bear Bars			
Krunch	170	10	22
Vanilla	170	9	21
Slim-a-Bear Sandwich			
100 Calorie, Vanilla	100	1.5	21

Bars & Pops (Cont)	C	F	Cb
Per Bar/Serving			
Luigi's Real Italian Ice: *Per 6 fl.oz Cup*			
Cups, all flavors, average, 6 fl.oz	130	0	33
Squeeze Tubes, 4 oz	70	0	18
M&M's			
Cookie Ice Cream Sandwich:			
Single, 2.6 oz	260	12	64
6 pack, 1 sandwich, 2.3 oz	220	10	29
Cone, 2.7 oz	250	12	33
Minute Maid: Fruit Juice Pops	60	0	15
Soft Frozen Lemonade	70	0	19
Molli Coolz!: *Per 2.5 oz Cup*			
Strawberry	90	10	7
Cookies N' Cream	155	10	14
Sour Cherry & Blue Raz Sorbet	70	1	13
Nestlé: Push Up Pop, average	80	1	18
Crunch Vanilla, 3 oz bar	210	14	18
Mini Wiches	90	3	14
Rolo King Size, 4 oz	300	19	30
Drumstick: Cookies n Cream	350	19	40
Vanilla w. Choc Layers	440	24	50
Oreo: Sandwich	260	11	38
Popsicles: Cups, Snow Cone (1)	30	0	7
Creamsicle			
Bars, Orange, 1 bar, 2.7 fl.oz	110	2	21
Pops: Orange & Raspb. Low-Fat	70	1	13
NSA Fat-Free, 2 pops, 3.3 fl.oz	45	0.5	10
Fudgsicle			
Bars: Orig. Fudge (1), 2.5 fl.oz	100	2	17
NSA Bar (1)	40	1	10
Low-Fat Bar (1)	60	1.5	12
Pops: Triple Chocolate	60	1.5	12
Pops: Big Stick Cherry Pineapple	60	0	15
Mighty Magic Minis (3)	40	0	10
Rainbow (1)	40	0	10
Scribblers, avg all, 2 pops	60	0	15
Shots: Cookie Dough, ½ cup	130	3	18
Cookies & Cream, ½ cup	110	4.5	16
Sugar Free Pops			
Creamsicle: 2 pops, 3.3 fl.oz	40	2	10
Variety, 2 pops, 3.4 oz	40	2	10
Reese's Peanut Butter Ice Cream	270	17	18
Rice Dream Supreme, all flav., 3 fl.oz	240	15	28
Safeway Select Coffee Almd Bar	270	17	26
Skinny Cow			
Ice Cream Cones, avg.	150	3	28
Fudge Bars, Low-Fat	100	1	22
Minis Fudge Pops	100	2	19
Sandwiches, average	145	2	30
Slim A Bear ~ *See Klondike*			

Per Bar/Serving	C	F	Cb
Snickers: Ice Cream Bar, 50g	180	11	18
Cone	280	15	33
Snack Bar (1)	90	6	9
SnoCone *(Wonder):* 7 fl.oz Cone	60	0	15
So Delicious Sugar Free: Fudge Bar	80	5	12
Vanilla Bar	150	14	15
Soy Dream (Non-Dairy):			
Lil' Dreamers, all flavors	100	4	15
Starbucks Frappuccino Bars, avg.	120	2	22
Mud Pies Bars	320	19	32
Sweet Nothings: Fudge Bar	100	0	23
Mango Raspberry	100	0	23
Other flavors, 3 oz, average	120	1	28
Tofutti (Non-Dairy):			
Cuties: Peanut Butter	165	8	20
Other varieties, avg.	125	5	17
Sticks: Fudge Treats Pops	30	0	6
Hooray! (No Sugar Added)	150	9	10
Marry Me Bar	170	8	22
Totally Fudge Pops	95	1.5	19
Trader Joe's Fruit Floes: Cafe Latte	130	0	26
Caribbean	80	0	21
Lime Juice	60	0	16
Mocha Fudge	140	1.5	27
Strawberry	110	0	31
Trix: Pops, regular	40	0	10
Sugar Free	15	0	4
Turkey Hill: Cookie S'wich, avg.	320	16	43
Ice Cream Sandwich	190	7	30
Light Sandwich	160	3	32
Sundae Cone	320	18	33
Twix Bar	170	10	19
Walgreens			
Choc Nut Sundae Cones	220	12	25
Ice Cream S'wiches	170	5	28
Turbo Tubes, 3 fl.oz	120	1	26
Weight Watchers			
Bars: English Toffee Crunch	220	12	26
Giant: Chocolate Cookies & Crm	130	4.5	24
Choc. Fudge/Fudge Bar	110	1	25
Cookies & Cream	140	5	26
Latte Bar	90	1	21
Cones: Avg. all flavors	140	4	30
Cups: Choc. Chip Cookie Dough	140	2.5	31
Chocolate Fudge Brownie	140	1.5	35
Giant Choc./Van. Fudge Sundae	160	1	37
Mint Chocolate Chip	140	3.5	29
Sandwiches: Choc./Van. Round	140	2	33
Vanilla Ice Cream	120	2	28

Canned & Packaged Meals

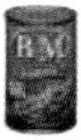

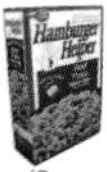

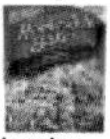

	C	F	Cb
B & M: *Per ½ Cup (4½ oz)*			
Baked Beans: Original	170	2	31
Barbeque	190	0.5	39
Vegetarian	160	1	28
Brown Raisin Bread, ½" slice, 2 oz	130	0.5	29
Banquet			
Homestyle Bakes: *Per Serving (Prepared)*			
Asian Style Fried Rice	250	1.5	49
Beef Stew & Biscuits	300	8	43
Chicken & Dumplings	230	4.5	33
Creamy Chsy Chkn Alfredo	400	22	36
Country Chicken, Potato, Biscuits	250	11	31
Creamy Chicken & Biscuits	350	18	39
Lasagna	290	11	36
Pasta & Meatballs	310	10	41
Betty Crocker			
Complete Meals: *Per Serving (⅓ Pkg)*			
Cheesy Beef Taco	250	5	43
Chicken & Buttermilk Biscuits	280	11	37
Chicken Fettuccini Alfredo	240	9	31
Stroganoff	200	4.5	30
Three Cheese Chicken	260	10	33
Hamburger Helper: *Per Cup (Prep. as Directed)*			
Bacon Cheeseburger	380	15	38
Beef Pasta	270	11	24
Cheeseburger Macaroni	300	13	27
Cheesy Enchilada; Quesadilla	350	13	40
Cheesy Hashbrown	400	19	39
Cheesy Italian Shells	350	13	37
Chili Macaroni	290	11	29
Crunchy Taco	300	14	27
Salisbury	280	11	26
Tuna Helper: *Per Serving (Prep. as Directed)*			
Creamy Parmesan	290	9	37
Other varieties, average	310	12	37
Chicken Helper: *Per Cup (Prep. as Directed)*			
Cheesy Chicken Enchilada	320	7	40
Chicken Fried Rice	260	9	25
Fettuccini Alfredo	300	9	29
Mashed Potatoes: *Per Serving (Prepared)*			
Potato Buds, ⅓ cup	160	8	19
Other varieties, average, ½ cup	170	7	22
Side Dishes/Casseroles: *Per Serving (Prepared)*			
Au Gratin; Cheesy Scalloped, ½ cup	150	5	22
Cheddar & Bacon; Cheesy Scallops	120	3	22
Roasted Garlic	120	4	20
Scalloped Potatoes, ⅔ cup	130	4	22
Other varieties, ⅔ cup	120	3.5	22
Deluxe Potatoes: *Per ½ Cup (Prepared)*			
Cheesy Cheddar Au Gratin	170	8	23
Loaded Au Gratin	140	4	23
Three Cheese Mashed Pot. Bake	190	9	24

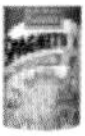

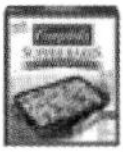

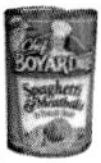

Betty Crocker (Cont)	C	F	Cb
Microwaveable Mashed Potato:			
Creamy Butter; Rstd Garlic, ⅔ cup	90	1	18
Seasoned Skillets:			
Hash Brown, ½ cup	120	4	19
Roasted Garlic & Herb, ⅔ cup	170	9	22
Traditional, ½ cup	180	9	22
Bowl Appetit: *Per Bowl*			
Cheddar Broccoli Rice	290	7	51
Homestyle Chicken Pasta	260	6	42
Pasta Alfredo	360	11	53
Teriyaki Rice	260	3	54
Three Cheese Rotini	360	10	55
Bush's Best: *Per ½ Cup*			
Chili Beans	120	1	20
Dark Red Kidney Beans, ½ cup	105	2	22
Frijoles Negras, ½ cup	110	0.5	23
Garbanzo Beans/Chick Peas, ½ c.	105	2	20
Refried Beans: Traditional	150	3	24
Fat Free	130	0	24
Baked Beans: Vegetarian	130	0	29
Other flavors, average	150	1	32
Campbell's: *Per Cup (8 fl.oz)*			
Chunky Chili: Roadhouse; Firehouse	230	8	25
Tantalizin Turkey	190	2.5	29
Pork & Beans in Tom. Sce	140	1.5	25
Spaghetti O's Original	180	1	37
Spaghetti O's Meatballs	240	8	32
Supper Bakes: *Per ⅙ Box (Prepared as Directed)*			
Cheesy Chicken	170	4	27
Creamy Stroganoff	190	4	31
Garlic Chicken w. Pasta	230	1	44
Herb Chicken w. Rice	190	1	40
Lemon Chicken w. Rice	200	1	43
Southwestern Style Chicken	150	1	32
Chef Boyardee			
Beefaroni, all types, 1 cup	260	9	32
Mini Bites (15 oz Can): *Per Cup*			
Mini Beef Ravioli w. Meatballs	280	13	31
Mini Pasta Shells w. Meatballs	260	10	32
Mini Spaghetti w. Meatballs	250	10	30
Jumbo (15 oz Can): *Per Cup*			
99% Fat Free:			
Beef Ravioli	170	1.5	33
Cheese Ravioli	240	2.5	45
Lasagna	270	10	36
Spaghetti w. Meatballs	270	12	28
Overstuffed Ital. Sausage Ravioli	240	4.5	40
Microwaveable Cups: *Per Cup*			
Beef Ravioli	190	5	29
Macaroni & Cheese	190	8	22
Mini Bites Spaghetti Rings	220	8	29
Spaghetti & Meatballs	200	8	23
Rice w. Chicken/Vegetables	230	9	30

Chef Boyardee (Cont)	**C**	**F**	**Cb**
Microwaveable Big Bowls: Per ½ Bowl			
Beefaroni	250	9	31
Mini Ravioli	240	8	33
Ravioli	220	7	32
Twistaroni: Cheesy Nacho, 1 cup	220	7	32
Chili Cheese Dog, 1 cup	220	6	32
Tomato & Beef, 1 cup	250	6	40
Dinner Kits: Per Serving			
Cheese Pizza	250	4	45
Lasagna	340	8	54
Spaghetti & Meatballs	300	8	45
Dennison's Chili (15 oz Can): Per Cup			
Chili Con Carne With Beans:			
Original; Hot, 1 cup, avg.	360	14	37
Chunky	300	10	32
99% Fat Free: Beef Chili w. Beans	210	2	29
Turkey Chili w. Beans	210	3	29
Dinty Moore (Hormel Foods)			
1½ lb Can: Beef Stew, 1 cup	180	8	17
7½ oz Can: Beef Stew, 1 cup	180	8	17
American Classics: Per Microwave Bowl			
Beef Stew, 10 oz	250	11	22
Noodles & Chicken, 7.5 oz	250	8	28
Microwave Cup: Beef Stew, 7.5 oz	150	6	15
Chicken & Dumplings, 7.5 oz	200	6	26
Other varieties, average	180	8	17
Dr. McDougall's: Per 10 oz			
Ramen Noodles	150	0.5	29
Rice Pilaf, average	260	2	52
Eden Soy (Vegetarian): Per ½ Cup (4½ oz)			
Baked Beans w. Sorghum, Mustard	150	0	27
Black Eyed Peas	90	1	16
Black Soybeans	120	6	8
Refried Black/Pinto/Kid. Beans, avg.	85	1	17
Other varieties, average	125	0	21
Fantastic: Per Cup			
Bean Chili	160	2	33
Black Bean Chipotle	130	0.5	31
Sesame Miso, 1.8 oz	140	2	27
Spicy Thai	150	0.5	32
Tuscan Tomato & Shells	140	1	31
Farmhouse			
Pasta: Per ¾ Cup			
Chicken Pasta	370	15	49
Creamy Garlic	420	20	49
Herb & Butter	430	20	48
White Cheddar Pasta	380	14	50
Rice: Per ⅓ Cup (Prepared as Directed)			
Chicken Rice	230	4	43
Long Grain & Wild Herb Butter	250	7	43
Other varieties, average	230	5	41

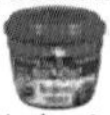

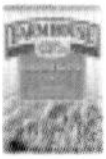

French's Fried Onions	**C**	**F**	**Cb**
Regular: 2 Tbsp, ¼ oz	45	3.5	3
¼ cup, ½ oz	90	7	6
1 cup, 2 oz	360	28	24
Cheddar: 2 Tbsp, ¼ oz	40	3	3
¼ cup, ½ oz	80	6	6
1 cup, 2 oz	320	24	24
Health Valley (Vegetarian)			
Fat Free Beans & Chili:			
Vegetarian/Chili, 1 cup	160	1	30
Other varieties, ½ cup	80	0	15
Meal Cups, average all varieties	140	1	27
Heinz			
Vegetarian Beans, ½ cup	140	0.5	27
Hormel: Per Cup			
Compleats: Per 10 oz Serving			
Beef & Beans in BBQ Sauce	390	11	43
Beef Pot Roast	230	3	27
Beef Steak Tips	280	9	29
Chicken & Dumplings	260	8	34
Chicken & Noodles	250	8	28
Chicken & Rice	260	10	30
Chicken Alfredo	360	20	28
Chicken Breast w. Mash Potatoes	210	3	24
Chicken Breast w. Dressing	280	5	35
Lasagne	280	7	42
Meatloaf	310	11	34
Roast Beef w. Mashed Potato	230	3	27
Salisbury Steak	280	11	30
Spaghetti & Meatballs	280	8	36
Teriyaki Chicken	270	1.5	57
Turkey & Hearty Vegetables	180	3.5	24
Turkey w. Dressing	280	8	31
Healthy Lifestyle Meals: Per 10 oz Serving			
Homestyle Beef	220	6	30
Santa Fe Style Chicken	280	4	41
Sesame Chicken	320	8	41
Kid's Kitchen: Beans & Wieners	320	13	37
Cheesy Mac 'N Cheese	280	16	24
Mini Beef Ravioli	250	6	38
Noodle Rings & Chicken	140	4	18
Chili (15 oz Can): Per ½ Can			
With Beans: Homestyle Chili	270	7	34
Reg./Hot/Chunky, average	270	7	34
Turkey (99% Fat Free)	200	3	26
Vegetarian (99% Fat Free)	200	1	38
Less Sodium Without Beans:			
Hot/Chili, 1 cup	210	9	17
Chunky No Beans	210	8	19
Turkey No Beans	190	3	17
Tamales (15 oz Can), 2 Tamales	140	7	15
Hungry Jack Potatoes			
Instant Potato Flakes, ⅓ cup	80	0	19

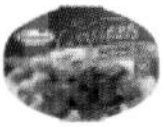

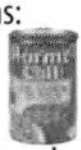

Hunt's	C	F	Cb
Manwich Sloppy Joe, ¼ cup	30	0	7

Knorr Lipton

Asian Sides: *Per Cup, Prepared*

	C	F	Cb
Beef Lo Mein; Thai Sesame, avg.	280	9	42
Chicken Fried/Teriyaki Rice, avg.	280	7.5	48
Teriyaki Noodles	300	8	49

Cajun Sides: *Per Cup, Prepared*

Garlic Butter Rice	300	8	48
New Orleans Style Chicken	290	5.5	50
Dirty Rice	300	6.5	50
Red Beans & Rice	330	5.5	61

Fiesta Sides: *Per Cup, Prepared*

Taco Rice	290	7	51
Nacho Pasta	280	7.5	44

Pasta Sides: *Per Cup, Prepared*

Alfredo; Parmesan	320	12	43
Butter	290	11	46
Creamy Garlic Shells	350	12	50
Stroganoff	290	9	42

Rice Sides: *Per Cup, Prepared*

Cheddar Broccoli	260	5.5	47
Creamy Chicken	320	10	49
Herb & Butter	300	9	46
Other varieites, avg.	310	10	49

Sides Plus: *Per Cup, Prepared*

Alfredo Pasta Primavera	310	12	42
Roasted Chicken Rice	320	6.5	56
Southwestern Style Rice	310	7.5	51
Teriyaki Noodles	340	8	56

Whole Grain Sides: *Per ⅔ Cup*

Alfredo	300	4	39
Sesame Chicken	300	4	51
Other varieties, avg.	270	7	45

Kraft

It's Pasta Anytime Meals: *Per Package*

Fettuccine w. Classic Alfredo Sce	580	22	74

Bistro Deluxe: Sundried Tom. Parm

Sundried Tom. Parm	300	11	40
Other varieties, average	310	11	40

Dinners: *Per Serving (Prepared as Directed)*

Macaroni & Cheese: Orig., ⅓ box	320	16	48
Scooby-Doo Spirals	410	19	47
Mac & Chse: Crazy Noodles, ½ box	410	18	48
Thick'n Creamy, ⅓ box	380	16	50
Easy Mac, avg. all varieties.., 1 pch	230	4	42
Deluxe: Orig.; Sharp Chedd., ¼ box	320	10	45
Rotini White Cheese Sce, ½ box	390	15	48
Velveeta Shells & Cheese, ⅓ box	360	12	49

Velveeta Cheesy Potatoes: *Per ½ Cup (Prepared)*

Au Gratin Potatoes	190	7	26
Bacon Scalloped Potatoes	200	8	26
Mashed Potatoes	200	12	21

La Choy	C	F	Cb
Beef Chow Mein, 1 cup	90	2	11
Chicken Chow Mein, 1 cup	100	3	10
Beef Pepper Oriental, 1 cup	100	2.5	12
Chop Suey Vegetables, ½ cup	15	0	3
Chow Mein Noodles, ½ cup	130	5	19

Lightlife

Tempeh: Flax; Soy, avg., 4 oz	225	9	16
Fakin' Bacon Strips, 3 sl., 2 oz	100	3	10
Garden Veggie, 4 oz	250	10	17
Three Grain; Wild Rice, avg., 4 oz	230	9	21

Smart Stuffers: *Per 4 oz*

Light Burgers Patty (1) 3 oz	120	1.5	11
Smart Bacon, 2 slices, 22g	45	2	1
Smart Deli: Baked Ham	80	0	6
Country Ham Style, 4 slices	90	0	5
Old World Bologna Style, 4 sl., 2 oz	70	0	4
Pepperoni Slices, 13 slices, 1 oz	40	0	3
Roast Turkey Style, 4 slices, 2 oz	80	0	6

Lunchables *(Oscar Mayer): Per Package*

Cracker Stackers Ham & Cheddar	420	23	37
Nachos Chse & Salsa, 4.4 oz	380	21	39
Pizza varieties, avg., 4.5 oz	300	13	28
Taco Bell Beef Tacos, 5.35 oz	310	11	34

Fun Fuel: Ham Bagels, 5.6 oz

Ham Bagels, 5.6 oz	410	10	64
Chicken/Ham Wraps, 5.5 oz	435	13	64
Peanut Butter Soft White Bread	600	19	85
Turkey Bagels, 5.6 oz	420	10	64
Pizza Dunks Soft Breadsticks	500	13	84
Beef Taco, 5.7 oz	495	15	69
Waffles & Sausage, 4.8 oz	460	16	66

Mega Pack: Combo Ham & Ched.

Combo Ham & Ched.	765	32	101
Combo Turkey & Cheddar, 5.4 oz	750	31	101
Pizza: Pepperoni, 6.85 oz	760	28	105
Extra Cheesy, 6.8 oz	700	25	104
Pizza Stix, 7.15 oz	680	16	118

Ultimate Nachos Cheese & Salsa	780	32	113

Lunch Bucket *(Armour)*

Beans 'n Weiners, 7.5 oz	290	10	37
Chili w. Beans, 7.5 oz	235	9	25
Hearty Beef Stew, 7.5 oz	155	8	15
Rings 'n Franks, 7.5 oz	225	9	30

Lunchmakers *(Armour)*

Loco Nachos	370	13	59
Cheese Pizza	310	13	36

Maruchan	**C**	**F**	**Cb**
Ramen Noodles: Beef/Chicken/Shrimp Flavors,			
½ block, 1½ oz	190	7	26
Noodles: Instant Wonton,			
Hot & Sour, 1 pkg	200	12	20
Chicken, 1 pkg	210	13	18
Roast Beef Cup O Noodles	290	12	38
Minute Rice: *Individual Servings*			
Brown Rice	170	4.5	28
Chicken Rice Mix	190	4	35
White Rice	190	4	34
Morningstar Farms			
Asian Veggie Patties, 1 patty	100	4	10
Cheddar Burger, 4 pieces	150	7	10
Chick'n Nuggets, 4 pieces	190	7	18
Italian Herb Chicken, 1 patty	170	5	22
Philly Cheesesteak	120	6	6
Nissin			
Choice Ramen: *Per Cup*			
All flavors	140	1	28
Top Ramen: *Per ½ Dry Noodle Block, w. Seasoning*			
Beef/Chicken Flavor	190	7	27
Chow Mein: Per ½ Pkg, 56.7g			
w. Shrimp	280	14	32
Chicken Flavor	240	9	34
Chinese Chicken Vegetable	260	11	34
Teriyaki Beef/Thai Peanut	270	12	36
Noodle Cups: *Per Cup*			
Beef/Shrimp Flavor	300	13	38
Beef Flavor Minestrone	270	11	37
Chicken Flavor	300	13	33
Shrimp w. Tom. & Garlic, ½ cup	280	12	37
Old El Paso			
Dinner Kits: *Per Serving (Prepared)*			
Chicken Soft Taco (2)	310	10	32
Enchilada Bake, ¼ pkg	370	13	33
Fajita (2), 84g	320	12	34
Hard Taco (2)	290	16	18
Shells, Taco Sce, Seasoning (2)	160	6	23
Soft Taco, 82g	380	10	33
Taco Dinner (2)	260	14	18
Side Dishes: Spanish Rice, ⅓ pkt	280	4.5	55
Cheesy Mexican Rice, ⅓ pkt	290	6	55
Refried Beans: Regular, ½ cup	100	0.5	17
w. Green Chiles, ½ cup	100	0.5	19
Vegetarian, ½ cup	100	1	17
Fat Free varieties, ½ cup	100	0	19

Pasta Roni: *Per Cup (Prepared)*	**C**	**F**	**Cb**
Angel Hair Pasta varieties, avg.	310	14	39
Asian Garlic Chicken	280	11	39
Butter Herb Italiana	300	12	40
Chicken & Broccoli	360	15	49
Chicken (flavor)	300	12	39
Chicken; Shells & Cheddar	290	12	38
Chicken Quesadilla	310	13	40
Fettuccine Alfredo	450	25	47
Four Cheese	370	16	49
Parmesan	310	14	39
Nature's Way: Creamy Parmesan	280	9	41
Mushroom in Sauce	280	10	39
Olive Oil & Italian Herb	250	8	38
Rice-A-Roni: *Per Cup (Prepared)*			
Beef; Herb & Butter; Rice Pilaf, avg.	310	9	51
Broccoli Au Gratin	360	17	46
Chicken	310	9	51
⅓ Less Salt	270	5	51
Chicken & Broccoli	230	5	40
Chicken & Garlic	260	8	41
Fried Rice	320	11	49
Spanish Rice	260	7	44
(Reduced Fat Recipe: If only 1 Tbsp fat is used instead			
of 2 Tbsp, deduct 35 calories and 4g fat.)			
Nature's Way: Parmesan & Romano	280	9	42
Italian Cheese & Herb	340	12	52
Long Grain & Wild Rice	250	7	43
Savory Whole Grains: *Per Cup (Prepared)*			
Chicken & Herb	260	8	41
Roasted Garlic Italiano	270	9	41
Spanish	250	8	42
Ronzoni Bistro: *Per 8 oz*			
Penne with Chicken & Broccoli	210	7	23
Rotini with tomato & Basil	260	10	34
Rosarita			
Refried Beans: *Per ½ Cup*			
Traditional; Vegetarian; Spicy	120	2	19
Low-Fat Black Bean	110	0	19
Fat-Free varieties	100	0	19
Shedd's			
Country Crock Side Dishes			
Garlic, ⅔ cup, 5 oz	170	7	23
Cheddar Mashed Potato, ⅔ cup	200	10	24
Chunky Tomato pasta, 1 cup	320	13	40
Deluxe, 1 cup	370	17	40
Elbow Macaroni & Cheese, 1 cup	380	17	40
Four Cheese Pasta, 1 cup	380	17	41
Southwestern Rice, 1 cup	250	6	44
Deluxe: Cheddar Broccoli Rice, 1 cup	270	11	35
Loaded Mashed Potatoes, ⅔ cup	200	11	23
Scalloped Potatoes, ⅔ cup	210	11	22

Simply Asia

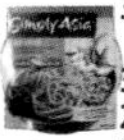

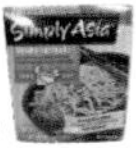

	C	F	Cb
Noodle & Sauce Meal Kits: *Per Cup (Prepared)*			
Chili Garlic	**330**	5	62
Roasted Peanut	**385**	14	55
Sesame Teriyaki	**285**	1	60
Other varieties, average	**305**	5	58
Noodle Bowls: *Per 4 oz*			
Roasted Peanut	**340**	6	60
Sesame Teriyaki	**200**	2	40
Soy Ginger; Spicy Kung Pao, avg.	**330**	5	51
Quick Noodles: *Per Tray*			
Pad Thai	**660**	9	133
Szechwan Garlic Chow Mein	**650**	12	121
Other varieties, average	**630**	8	126
Take Out Noodle Boxes: *Per ½ Box (5.3 oz)*			
Honey Teriyaki	**380**	3	73
Pad Thai	**390**	3	79
Sweet & Sour	**370**	2	75
Other varieties, average	**390**	5	71

South Beach Diet *(Kraft)*

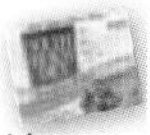

	C	F	Cb
Wraps: *Per Package*			
Deli Ham & Turkey	**220**	10	24
Grilled Chicken Caesar	**230**	10	24
Southwestern Style Chicken	**240**	10	26
Turkey & Bacon Club	**250**	12	25

Stagg Chili

	C	F	Cb
14.3 oz Box: *Per Cup (8.7 oz)*			
Chili w. Beans: Classic/Dynamite	**335**	17	29
Country/Laredo	**320**	16	29
Ranch House Chicken	**240**	8	26
White Chili	**260**	12	20
No Beans: Steakhouse/Double	**320**	22	14
Fat Free: Veg. Gdn/4 Bean	**200**	1	37
Turkey Ranchero	**240**	3	31
Silverado	**250**	7	30

S & W: *Per ½ Cup*

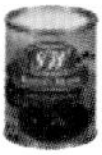

	C	F	Cb
Baked Beans, avg. all types	**140**	0.5	28
Caribbean Black Beans	**90**	0	18
Kidney Beans	**100**	0.5	23
San Antonio; Santa Fe Beans, avg.	**90**	0.5	21
White Beans	**80**	0.5	19

Taco Bell

	C	F	Cb
Home Originals: *Per Serving*			
Dinner Kits: Taco, ⅙ pkg	**240**	11	19
Cheesy Dbl Decker Taco, ⅙ pkg	**350**	14	30
Soft Taco, ⅕ pkg	**370**	13	40
Ultimate Nachos, ¼ pkg	**280**	14	31
Refried Beans (16 oz Can): *Per ½ Cup Serving*			
Fat-Free (w. Green Chilies), 4.6 oz	**100**	0	18
Vege Blend, 4.6 oz	**120**	1	20
Bowlz (9 oz): Santa Fe Beef	**360**	7	49
Salsa Chicken; Fiesta Steak, average	**270**	6	43

Tasty Bite

	C	F	Cb
Vegetarian Entrees: *Per ½ Package*			
Agra Peas & Greens	**140**	10	9
Bengal Lentils	**160**	8	16
Bombay Potatoes	**105**	4	13
Jaipur Vegetables	**170**	11	10
Jodhpur Lentils	**105**	4	12
Madras Lentils	**125**	5	14
Punjab Eggplant	**145**	9	13
Ready Meals: *Per Package (w. Rice)*			
Peas Paneer	**425**	15	54
Spinach Dal	**370**	9	62
Vegetable Supreme	**315**	6	55

Thai Kitchen

	C	F	Cb
Bowls, avg. all types, 1.7 oz	**120**	2	24
Stir Fry: *Per Serving*			
Curry Stir Fry, 1 cup	**280**	4	55
Lemongrass & Chili Stir Fry, 1 cup	**270**	2.5	55
Pad Thai varieties, ½ pkg, 4.5 oz	**360**	1	80
Savory Garlic, ½ package	**230**	2.5	47
Thai Peanut, 1 pkg, 2.25 oz	**280**	6	51
Thin/Stir Fry/Wide, 2 oz	**180**	0.5	40
Toasted Sesame Stir Fry, 1 cup	**260**	2.5	55

The Spice Hunter: *Per Cup Meal*

	C	F	Cb
Stuffed Potato: Creamy Butter	**140**	3.5	25
Broccoli & Cheddar	**170**	3	31
Sour Cream & Chives	**160**	2	31
Risotto: 3 Cheese Wild Mushroom	**260**	3	47
Spinach & Garlic	**240**	1.5	47

Tofurky

	C	F	Cb
Deli Slices, average, 5 pces	**100**	3	6
Holiday: Dumplings (2), 4 oz	**210**	1	45
Tofurky Roast, 4 oz	**190**	5	10
Jurky, 4 pieces	**100**	2	9
Sausages: Beer Brats (1), 3.5 oz	**280**	16	8
Kielbasa (1), 3.5 oz	**240**	12	12
Sweet Italian Sausages (1), 3.5 oz	**280**	13	12

Trader Joe's

	C	F	Cb
Turkey Chili w. Beans, 1 cup	**230**	3	30
Chicken Chili w. Beans, 1 cup	**290**	9	32
Pasta, Shells & White Cheddar, 1 cup	**280**	6	48
Refried Beans, avg., ½ cup	**110**	0.5	20
Organic Beans, avg., ½ cup	**140**	0	29
Black Beans: Regular, ½ cup	**110**	0	19
Cuban Style, ½ cup	**100**	0.5	19
Potatoes: Garlic Mashed, ½ cup	**150**	7	19
Cheddar Cheese Au Gratin, ½ cup	**140**	5	21
Premium: Beef Stew, 1 cup	**230**	11	19
Chicken Stew, 1 cup	**230**	14	16

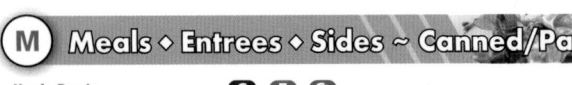
Uncle Ben's	C	F	Cb
Flavorful Rice: *Per Cup (Prepared w. Margarine)*			
Average all varieties	280	10	44
Country Inn: *Per Cup (Prepared w/out Margarine)*			
Broccoli Rice Au Gratin	200	2	43
Other varieties, avg.	200	1	43
Ready Rice: *Per ½ Pouch (Prepared)*			
Butter & Garlic Flavored Rice	190	4.5	47
Roasted Chicken	230	4	41
Teriyaki	260	3.5	51
Whole Grain Brown	220	4	41
Valley Fresh			
Chicken: *Per 2 oz*			
White & Dark Chunk	80	2	0
Premium Chunk White	70	1	0
Turkey, Premium Chunk White, ¼ can	80	1.5	0
Van Camps			
Pork & Beans, ½ cup	110	1.5	23
Original Baked Beans, ½ cup	160	1	30
Beanie Weanie Original, 7¾ oz	240	8	29
White Wave (Vegetarian)			
Seitan: Chicken w. Broth, 5 oz	110	2	4
Traditional, 3 oz	90	1	3
Tofu Town: *Per ½ Container*			
Grilled Tenders: Havana Black Bean	210	8	18
Light Tamari, 5 oz	120	7	15
Mediterranean Tahini, 5 oz	240	13	16
Sesame Ginger Teriyaki, 5 oz	240	9	24
Soy Milks & Yogurts: *See Pages 27, 30*			
Tofu: *See Page 77*			
Worthington/Loma Linda (Vegetarian)			
Big Franks: 1 link, 1.8 oz	110	6	3
Low-fat, 1 link, 1.8 oz	80	2.5	3
Chili, 1 cup, 8 oz	280	10	25
Choplets, 2 slices, 3.2 oz	90	1	4
Diced Chik, 2 oz	50	0	2
Dinner Cuts, 2 slices, 3.2 oz	90	1	4
FriChik, 2 pces, 3.1 oz	140	8	3
Linketts, (1), 1¼ oz	70	4	1
Little Links, 2 links, 1.6 oz	90	5	8
Low-Fat Veja-Links (1), 1 oz	45	1.5	3
Multigrain Cutlets, 2 sl., 2¾ oz	100	1	5
Prime Stakes (1) 3.2 oz	120	6	7
Redi-Burger, ⅝" slice, 3 oz	120	2.5	7

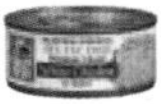

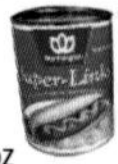

Worthington/Loma Linda (Cont)	C	F	Cb
Saucettes, 4 pces, 3 oz	90	6	1
Super Links (1) 1.6 oz	110	8	2
Tender Bits, 6 pieces, 3 oz	120	4	7
Tender Rounds (8), 2¾ oz	120	4.5	6
Vega-Links (1), 1 oz	50	3	1
Veg.-Burger, ¼ cup, 2 oz	60	0.5	2
Vegetable Skallops, ½ cup, 3 oz	90	1	4
Vegetarian Burger, ¼ cup, 1.9 oz	70	1.5	3
Yves Veggie Cuisine (Vegetarian)			
Breakfast: Brkfast Links (2) 1.8 oz	70	2	3
Breakfast Patties (1) 2 oz	80	0.5	2
Canadian Veg. Bacon, 3 slices	80	0.5	1
Burgers: Meatless Beef Burger	110	4	8
Lentil & Veggie Burger (1) 2.6 oz	100	3	5
Deli: Roast Beef, 4 slices	110	2.5	4
Smoked Chicken, 4 slices	100	1.5	5
Dogs & Brats: Jumbo Dog (1) 2.6 oz	110	3	5
Brat Zesty Italian (1), 3.3 oz	150	5	9
Good Dog (1) 1.8 oz	70	3.5	2
Hot Dog (1)	50	0.5	2
Thai Lemongrass Veggie Chicken	330	9	49
Tofu Dog, avg. (1), 1.3 oz	45	1	2
Veggie Brats Classic (1), 3.3 oz	160	5	9
Veggie Penne, 10.5 oz	210	1.5	36
Entree: Chili, 10.5 oz	240	1	37
Lasagne, 10.5 oz	300	3	51
Santa Fe Beef, 10½ oz	360	9	57
Mac n Soy Cheese, 10½ oz	340	9	52
Skewers: BBQ Beef, 2.8 oz	100	0.5	10
Lemon Herb Chicken, 2.8 oz	100	1	7
Veggie Deli Slices: Bologna, 2 oz	80	2.5	2
Ham, 2 oz	100	2	5
Pizza Pepperoni, 1.7 oz	60	1	4
Salami, 2 oz	80	0	4
Veggie Turkey, 2 oz	100	1.5	5
Veggie Ground Round: Orig., ⅓ c.	60	0.5	5
Ground Turkey, ⅓ cup	60	1	4
Taco Stuffers, ⅓ cup, 1.93 oz	90	2.5	5
Zatarain's			
Black Beans & Rice, 1 cup, 2.3 oz	235	1	48
Caribbean Rice Mix, 1 cup, 1.6 oz	160	1.5	34
Dirty Rice Mix, 1 cup, 1.3 oz	130	0	29
Fire, Rstd Vegetables & Rice Mix	190	0	43
Garlic & Herb Rice Mix, 1 c., 1.6 oz	160	1.5	34
Gumbo Mix w. Rice, 1 cup, 0.8 oz	70	0	16
New Orleans Style:			
Caribbean Rice, 1 cup	320	6	61
Dirty Rice Mix, 1.3 oz	130	0	29
Jambalaya Mix, 1.3 oz	130	0	29
Red Beans & Rice, 2 oz	190	0	40

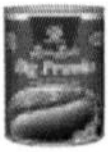

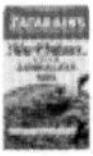

Amy's (Vegetarian) | C | F | Cb

Per Serving

	C	F	Cb
Bowls: Brown Rice & Vegs, 10 oz	260	9	36
Santa Fe Enchilada, 10 oz	350	11	47
(Other Varieties ~ www.CalorieKing.com)			
Asian Meals: Thai Stir Fry, 9.5 oz	310	11	45
Asian Noodle Stir Fry, 10 oz	290	7	50
Entrees: Chse Enchilada, 4.7 oz	240	14	18
Cheese Lasagna, 10.3 oz	380	14	44
Macaroni & Cheese, 9 oz	410	16	47
Macaroni & Soy Cheeze, 9 oz	370	15	42
Whole Meals: Chse Enchilada, 9 oz	350	15	38
Black Bean Enchilada	330	8	53
Veggie Loaf	290	8	47
Pot Pies: Country Vegge	370	16	47
Mex. Tamale; Shepherd's Pie,	155	4	27
Vegetable (Non Dairy)	360	13	50
Burgers: Californian Veggie, 2½ oz	140	5	19
Other varieties (1), avg., 2½ oz	120	2.5	14
Burritos: Bean & Rice, 6 oz	280	6	48
Bean & Cheese	300	9	43
Breakfast Burrito	250	7	38
Snacks: Nacho, 5-6 pieces	210	8	26
Cheese Pizza, 5-6 pieces	190	7	22

Extra Product Listings ~ www.CalorieKing.com

Bagel Bites

	C	F	Cb
Three Cheese, 4 pieces, 3 oz	200	6	29
Cheese Sausage, Pepperoni, 4 pcs	200	6	29

Banquet

	C	F	Cb
Pot Pies: Beef, 7 oz	450	27	36
Chicken/Turkey, average, 7 oz	375	21	35
Chicken: Breast Patties (1)	230	17	12
Chicken Breast Nuggets (5)	270	19	15
Crispy Chicken, Skinless, 4.2 oz	340	19	16
Popcorn Chicken, 11 pieces	180	9	14
Wings: Hot & Spicy, 3 oz	260	17	8
Honey Barbecue, 3 oz	270	17	12
Crock Pot Classics			
Chicken & Dumplings, ⅔ cup	200	8	21
Chicken & Red Potatoes, ⅔ cup	170	9	15
Meatballs in Stroganoff	300	14	29
Hearty Beef & Veggies, 5½ cup	140	6	14
Herb Chicken & Rice, ⅔ cup	200	3	34
Homestyle Pork, ⅔ cup	140	3	16
Hearty One Dinners: Turkey, 16 oz	430	14	43
Boneless Pork Rib, 16 oz	590	27	59
Chicken Fried Beef Steak, 16 oz	750	42	66
Fried Chicken, 16 oz	810	41	71
Salisbury, 16 oz	630	38	40

Banquet (Cont) | C | F | Cb

	C	F	Cb
Meals: BBQ Chicken	250	6	31
Boneless Pork Rib, 10 oz	370	18	37
Cheese Enchilada Meal, 11 oz	430	15	62
Chicken Fingers, 7.1 oz	460	15	69
Corn Dog Meal, 7.5 oz	470	18	68
Fettuccine Alfredo	370	15	44
Fried Chicken, 9 oz	420	26	26
Fried Rice w. Chicken & Egg Roll	310	10	45
Homestyle Noodles & Chicken	300	11	36
Lasagna w. Meat Sauce, 11 oz	340	9	50
Mac & Cheese, 12 oz	390	11	58
Macaroni & Beef	330	8	56
Meatloaf Meal	300	14	27
Mexican Style Enchilada Combo	400	15	60
Our Original Fried Chicken	420	26	26
Pepperoni Pizza, 6.75	550	29	57
Salisbury Steak Meal, 9.5 oz	290	14	27
Spaghetti & Meatballs, 10.5 oz	400	17	40
Swedish Meatballs, 10.25 oz	430	23	35
Sweet & Sour Chicken, 10 oz	430	16	60
Turkey Mostly White Meat	240	6	27

Birds Eye ~ Voila!

Per Cup, Cooked (2 Cups Frozen)

	C	F	Cb
Chicken Voila!: Garlic Chicken	240	8	21
Other varieties, average	220	7	28
Steak Voila! Beef Sirloin/Potato	190	7	22
Be Well Viola:			
Garden Ravioli Meatless Meal, 1½ cup	190	8	23
Six Cheese Pasta, 1½ cup	190	7	22
Teriyaki Beef & Vegetables, 1 cup	160	4	15

Boca (Vegetarian)

	C	F	Cb
Burger: Cheeseburger, 1 patty	100	5	5
All American Flame Grilled	90	3	4
Vegan, Original, 1 patty	70	0.5	6
Organic Burgers: Vegan, Orig.	100	2.5	9
Roasted Garlic/Onion	130	3	10
Chik'n: Nuggets (4), 3 oz	180	7	17
Hot & Spicy Buffalo Wings	160	7	14
Patties (1), 2.5 oz	160	6	15
Sausages: Bratwurst	140	7	6
Italian, 2.5 oz	130	6	6

Boston Market

	C	F	Cb
Beef Sirloin & Noodles	470	12	59
Chicken Parmesan, 16 oz	610	23	67
Chicken Pot Pie, ½ box	560	36	43
Meatloaf	670	39	50
Salisbury Steak	720	39	57
Swedish Meatballs	860	49	70
Turkey Breast Medallions	420	14	42

Claim Jumper

	C	F	Cb
Baby Back Pork Ribs (3)	210	14	8
Beef Pot Roast, 1 box	480	20	46
Buffalo Wings (2)	160	9	5
Chicken Alfredo, 1 box	600	26	52
Chicken Fried Beef Steak, 16¼ oz	660	36	68
Chicken Pot Pie, ½ pie, 9 oz	550	37	39
Chicken Tenderloins, 2 pieces	160	6	12
Country Fried Chicken, 19 oz	610	26	72
Country Fried Pork Chop, 15 oz	620	32	49
Lasagna w. Meat Sauce, 8 oz	280	13	26
Meatloaf Dinner, 15¼ oz	480	29	35
Rst Turkey Brst w. Gravy & Dressing	520	24	53
Spaghetti & Meatballs, 1 box	725	27	80
Spicy Chicken Tenderloins, 3 oz	210	8	20
Turkey Pot Pie, ½ pie, 9 oz	550	38	38
Sauce: Hot Sauce, ½ Tbsp	0	0	0
Original Barbecue, 4 T., 2 oz	100	1.5	22

Contessa

	C	F	Cb
Meals: *Per Serving*			
Beef Goulash, 8 oz	250	5	34
Burgandy Beef Stew, 8 oz	240	11	22
Chicken Cacciatore, 8 oz	240	7	28
Chicken Chow Mein, 8 oz	340	4	53
Chicken Tandoori, 1⅓ cups, 8 oz	200	3.5	27
Kung Pao Shrimp, 8 oz	200	3.5	30
Shrimp Mediteranean, 1¾ cups	400	5	63
Shrimp Stir Fry, 1¾ cups	150	2	14
Sweet n Sour Shrimp, 1½ cups	200	0	34

Croissant Pockets

	C	F	Cb
Five Cheese Pizza	390	20	40
Ham & Cheddar	340	16	39
Pepperoni Pizza	390	20	42
Philly Steak & Chse	360	19	36
Other varieties, avg.	320	15	39

Essensia (Albertson's)

	C	F	Cb
Entrees: Mac & Cheese, 1 cup	300	10	36
2 Meat Lasagna, 1 cup	280	11	29
6 Cheese Cannelloni (1)	180	7	18
7 Cheese Lasagna, 5 oz	280	19	35
Chicken Fettuccini Alfredo, 1 cup	210	6	26
Chicken Enchilada (1)	200	9	23
Eggplant Parmesan, 1 cup	310	18	26
Striped Ravioli, 1 cup	360	20	31
Tamale Bake, 1 cup	370	16	37
Vegetable Lasagna, 1 cup	220	5	31

GardenBurger

	C	F	Cb
Meals: Chicken n Grill, 1 patty	100	2.5	5
Herb Crusted Chicken Cutlet (1)	150	9	11
Mamma Mia Meatballs (6)	110	4.5	7
Riblets, 1 riblet + sauce	240	4.5	33
Burgers: *Per 2½ oz Patty*			
Original Burger; Black Bean, avg	90	3	13
Flame Grilled, Homestyle Classic, avg.	100	5	6
Garden Vegan	100	1	12
Other varieties, average	100	3	15
Wraps: Margherita Pizza	240	8	34
Black Bean Chipotle	240	8	32

Gorton's

	C	F	Cb
Fish Fillets: Beer Batter	115	7	9
Crispy Battered	130	8.5	9
Crunchy Golden	120	6	12
Grilled, avg. all flav.	100	3	1
Grilled Salmon, avg.	100	3.5	1
Fish Sticks, Breaded (6), 3.7 oz	250	14	20
Grilled Fillet	100	3	1
Lemmon Butter Fillet	100	3	1
Popcorn Shrimp, 3.2 oz	240	12	24
Shrimp Bowl: Alfredo, 1 bowl	250	5	39
Fried Rice, 1 bowl	350	2.5	68
Garlic Butter, 1 bowl	260	6	38
Teriyaki, 1 bowl	320	6	57
Tenders: Extra Crunchy, 3½ pieces	260	12	29
Original, 3½ pieces, 4 oz	270	15	25

Healthy Choice

	C	F	Cb
Simple Selections: *Per Meal*			
Cheesy Rice & Chicken	220	6	24
Chicken Enchilada	270	5	45
Lasagna Bake	240	4.5	38
Macaroni & Cheese	210	4	32
Roast Turkey Breast	200	3.5	27
Complete Selections:			
Beef Pot Roast	310	7	45
Chicken Enchilada	310	7	46
Chicken Teriyaki	280	4	44
Lemon Pepper Fish	310	4.5	53
Rstd Chicken Breast	290	7	39
Salisbury Steak	360	9	46
Sweet & Sour Chicken	430	9	69
Cafe Steamers: Beef Merlot	220	6	22
Chicken Tuscany	300	8	34
Chicken Margherita	340	8	43
Whiskey Steak	250	4	34

Home Bistro

Dinners: Per Package

Beef, Filet Mignon & Shrimp Duet	990	72	33
Crab Stuffed Omelette w. Cheddar	690	50	44
Pork Loin in Thai Red Curry Sauce	530	23	30
Poultry: Cherry Duck Confit	700	37	35
Maple Dijon Chicken	390	17	19
Seafood: Down East Brunch	580	40	31
Grilled Swordfish in Sauce	370	7	50
Salmon Fillet & Shrimp in Sauce	510	26	34
Low-Carb: Beef Stir Fry	400	17	15
Blackened Chicken Breast	560	32	8
Chicken Stir Fry	310	7	15
Filet Mignon w. Bernaise Sauce	870	73	14
French Toast Breakfast	670	55	26
Poached Salmon Fillet in Sauce	580	44	10
Pork Loin in Red Curry Sauce	340	39	13
Rstd Crab Cakes with Lobster Sce	540	43	10
Roasted Rack of Lamb with Sce	700	41	16
Rstd Turkey Breast with Stuffing	440	20	19
Sea Scallops in Sauce	590	31	51

Hot Pockets

Calzones: Per ½ Calzone, 4.2 oz

4 Meat & 4 Cheese	300	13	35
Pepperoni & 3 Cheese	330	15	39
Supreme	300	13	25
Pizza Minis: Per 3 oz			
Double Cheese; Saus & Pepperoni	240	11	30
Pepperoni	280	14	32
Pot Pie Express, average 1 pie	350	17	40
Stuffed Sandwiches: Per 4½ oz Sandwich			
Barbecue Sauce w. Beef Steak	340	12	50
Beef Taco	320	13	37
Cheeseburger	340	14	43
Four Cheese Pizza	390	20	44
Four Meat & Four Cheese Pizza	360	19	38
Meatballs & Mozzarella	390	14	45
Sausage & Pepperoni Pizza	380	20	41
Subs: Ham 'N Cheese	360	10	49
Meatballs & Mozzarella	390	14	45
Pepperoni Pizza; Philly Steak & Chse	410	16	49
Twisted Stix, average1 pce	130	4.5	18

José Olé

	C	**F**	**Cb**
Breakfast Burrito			
Egg, Sausage & Cheese, 4 oz	270	11	34
Egg, Ham & Cheese, 4 oz	260	9	34
Taquitos, average, 3 pieces	190	7	25
Mexi-Minis: Beef & Chse Tacos (4)	200	11	19
Chimichangas, 3 pces	250	12	29
Taquitos, 4 pces	190	9	24
Quesadillas, 3 pces	240	8	32
Burrito: Beef & Cheese	300	10	39
Chicken Monterey (1)	270	6	40
Chimichanga: Beef, 1 pce	340	15	40
Chicken , 1 pce	330	12	43
Skillet Meals: Per ½ Package			
Chicken Fajitas	310	9	40
Chicken Monterey Pasta	540	30	47
Southwest Style Chicken Pasta	400	8	62
Steak Fajitas	300	9	37
Fire Grilled Fiesta: Per Single			
Chicken & 3 Cheese Quesidillas	250	8	32
Chicken Fajitas	370	10	52
Steak & Monterey Jack Quesidillas	260	8	33
Steak Fajitas	380	11	53

Kid Cuisine

Meals: Cheese Pizza Painter	440	17	53
All American Fried Chicken	470	20	47
Cheeseburger Builder	390	12	56
Chicken Nuggets	440	17	53
Fiesta Beef Taco Dippers	400	18	48
Macaroni & Cheese	380	11	58
Pepperoni Pizza	390	7	69

Kroger

	C	**F**	**Cb**
Beef Stir Fry, 1¾ cups	180	4	26
Chicken Alfredo, 1¾ cups	270	9	30
Chicken Stir Fry, 1½ cups	200	2	30
Coconut Shrimp, 5 shrimp	320	19	27
Coconut Shrimp Sauce, ¾ Tbsp	40	3	3
Crab Cakes, 1 patty	190	13	7
Gr. Fillet Cajun Topper Fish, 1 piece	100	3.5	1
Gr. Fillet Lemon Pepper, 1 piece	100	3.5	1
Haddock Fillet, 1 fillet	120	5	4
Shrimp Fried Rice, 1¼ cups, 8 oz	190	0.5	36
Shrimp Linguini, 1½ cups, 8 oz	340	8	51
Swedish Style Meatballs, 6 balls	250	18	7

Lean Cuisine

Cafe Classics Entrees: *Per Meal*

	C	F	Cb
Beef Portabello	220	6	25
Bow Tie Pasta & Chicken	240	4.5	33
Sweet & Sour Chicken	300	3	51
Thai Style Chicken	220	4	30

Cafe Classics Bowls: *Per Bowl*

Chicken Teriyaki	250	2	44
Grilled Chicken Caesar	230	6	24
Three Cheese Stuffed Rigatoni	240	6	35

One Dish Favorites: Rstd Chicken

Rstd Chicken	230	6	30
Angel Hair Pasta	260	4	48
Chicken Enchilada	270	4.5	47
Lasagna w. Meat Sauce	320	7	44
Macaroni & Cheese	290	7	41
Santa Fe Rice & Beans	290	6	49

Panini: *Per Panini*

Chicken Club/Stk Cheddar	320	9	34
Chicken, Spinach & Mushrooms	280	8	32
Chicken Tuscan; Philly-Style Steak	350	9	46
Southwest-style Chicken Panini	280	7	32

Skillets: Chicken Alfredo

Chicken Alfredo	190	4.5	25
Chicken Primavera	180	2.5	28
Garlic Chicken	240	4	40
Herb Chicken & Roasted Veggies	160	3.5	22

Lean Pockets

Chicken Fajita	260	7	39
Crispy Cheesy Crust: Cheeseburger	280	7	43
Chicken, Broccoli & Cheddar	260	7	40
Four Chse Pizza; Meatballs & Mozz.	290	7	45
Steak Fajita	260	7	40
Three Chse & Chkn Quesadilla	280	7	42
Whole Grain: Chkn Broccoli & Cheddar	250	7	38
Garlic Chkn White Pizza	290	8	40
Grilled Chicken Mushr. & Spinach	260	7	38
Ham & Cheese	240	7	33
Supreme Pizza	220	7	30
Three Chse & Broccoli	250	7	38
Turkey, Broccoli/Ham & Cheese	260	7	39

Marie Callender's

Complete Dinners: *Per Serving*

Beef Pot Roast	330	10	32
Beef Tips in Mushroom Sce, 13.6 oz	360	12	35
Country Fried Chick. & Gvy, 1 din.	670	37	58
Golden Battered Fish Fillet, 12 oz	450	16	53
Grilled Chicken Alfredo Bake, 13 oz	630	39	40
Grilled Chkn & Mashed Pot., 15 oz	450	17	39
Honey Roasted Chicken, 14 oz	340	12	37
Honey Roasted Turkey, 13 oz	310	10	32
Meatloaf & Gravy w. Mashed Pot.	480	22	39
Pork Chop, 1 dinner	510	23	53

Marie Callender's (Cont)

Complete Dinners (Cont): *Per Serving*

	C	F	Cb
Salisbury Steak & Gravy, 14 oz	400	16	38
Spaghetti w. Meat Sauce, 17 oz	630	19	91
Swedish Meatballs	450	22	42

One Dish Classics:

Cheesy Chicken Breast & Rice	440	15	44
Fettucini Alfredo, 14 oz	770	46	69
Fettuccini w. Chicken/Broc., 13 oz	670	43	39
Meat Lasagna, 8 oz	240	9	24

Pot Pies: Grilled Chicken Alfredo

Grilled Chicken Alfredo	680	39	60
Savory herb Turkey, 10 oz	660	36	64

Michael Angelo's *Per Single Serve Package*

Baked Ziti & Meatballs, 12 oz Tray	480	15	60
Chicken Alfredo, 12 oz	470	14	57
Chicken Parmesan, 12 oz	480	15	60
Chicken Marsala, 10 oz	390	9	55
Chicken Piccata, 10 oz	510	24	52
Chicken Milano, 10 oz tray	410	21	29
Chicken Toscana, 12 oz	490	15	58
Eggplant & Chicken, 12 oz	360	16	28
Eggplant Parmesan, ½ pkg, 6 oz	240	14	16
Four Cheese Lasagna, 12 oz	600	33	42
Lasagna with Meat Sauce, 12 oz	450	16	45
Lasagna with Sausage, 12 oz	525	25	46
Manicotti with Sauce, ½ pkg, 6 oz	230	12	11
Pepperoni Mini-Calzones (1), 1 oz	80	3.5	8
Ravioli Florentine, 12 oz	360	16	43
Sausage, Peppers & Onions, 12 oz	450	17	57
Shrimp Scampi, 10 oz	570	30	53
Vegetable Lasagna, 12 oz	345	11	35

Morningstar Farms

Breakfast Pattie, 1 patty	80	3	4
Burgers: Made with Organic Soy			
Classic/Cheddar Burger	150	7	10
Mushroom Lovers	110	6	8
Philly Cheesesteak Burger	120	6	6
Spicy Black Bean	140	4.5	13
Tex Mex Burger	110	1	17
Thai Burger	100	3.5	7
Grillers: Original Veggie Burger	130	6	5
Prime Veggie Burger	170	9	4
Vegan	100	2.5	7
Patties: Parmesan Ranch	170	7	17
Breaded Original Veggie Patties	150	6	16
Poultry: Buffalo Wings (5)	200	9	19
Chik'n Nuggets (4)	190	7	18
Okara Pattie	120	5	6
Roasted Herb Chicken	110	2.5	9
Veggie Corn Dogs (1)	150	4	22

Safeway Select

	C	F	Cb
Gourmet Club Meals: *Per Serving*			
Cha Siu Bao, 1 bau, 3 oz	210	4.5	34
Chicken Enchiladas	210	8	25
Meat Lasagna, 1 cup	310	11	34
St. Louis Ribs (2), 125g	370	23	17
Stir Fry: Chicken Fajita	130	3	14
Shrimp & Vegetable	120	0	20
Teriyaki Beef	170	4	24

South Beach Diet (Kraft)

	C	F	Cb
Beef & Broccoli w. Asian Noodles	330	11	32
Caprese Style Chicken w. Broccoli	260	7	12
Garlic Herb Chicken w. Beans, 10 oz	270	11	13
Garlic Parmesan Chicken w. Penne	290	11	24
Orange Beef Slices & Rice in Sauce	260	8	27
Wraps: Chicken Monterey, 8.3 oz	220	7	26
Herb Chicken, 8.3 oz	210	7	22
Teriyaki Steak, 8.3 oz	190	6	24

Stouffer's

	C	F	Cb
Homestyle Dinners: *Per Serving*			
Chicken Fettucini, 10.5 oz	370	14	37
Country Fried Beef Steak, 16 oz	520	33	52
Meatloaf, 17 oz	560	29	40
Monterey Chicken, 14.25 oz	500	17	58
Roast Turkey Breast, 16 oz	390	13	48
Slow Roasted Beef, 14 oz	320	15	27
Entrees: Stroganoff, 9.75 oz	380	17	34
Breaded Boneless Pork Cutlet	370	21	31
Creamed Chipped Beef, 5.5 oz	140	7	9
Grilled Teriyaki Chicken	300	3.5	45
Chicken a la King, 11.5 oz	360	12	44
Fish Fillet w. Mac Cheese, 9 oz	400	16	36
Lasagna w. Meat Sce, 11½ oz	380	13	47
Macaroni & Beef w. Tomatoes	330	11	38
Macaroni & Cheese, 1 cup, 6 oz	350	17	34
Salisbury Steak, 16 oz	470	24	44
Spaghetti w. Meat Sauce, 12 oz	350	12	44
Stuffed Pepper, 10 oz	220	10	22
Entrees (Cont): Swedish Meatball	560	27	47
Tuna Noodle Casserole, 10 oz	350	15	35
Turkey Tetrazzini, 10 oz	380	20	32
Skillets: *Per Bowl*			
Broccoli & Beef; Garlic Chkn, avg.	320	6	42
Chicken Alfredo, 8.3 oz	410	11	49
Chicken & Pasta, 8.3 oz	340	7	42
Chicken & Veggies	360	9	43
Homestyle Beef	300	11	32
Teriyaki Chicken, 12.5 oz	310	4.5	44
Steak Teriyaki	310	5	49
Yankee Pot Roast, 8 oz	300	9	39

Swanson

	C	F	Cb
Hungry-Man Dinners: Meatloaf	680	37	61
Boneless Pork Rib	930	49	106
Boneless White Meat Fried Chkn	710	29	86
Buffalo Chicken Strips	920	35	71
Classic Fried Chicken	960	45	91
Mexican Style Fiesta	870	38	113
Roasted Carved Turkey, 18.7 oz	550	18	72
Rotisserie Chicken	690	35	48
Salisbury Steak	580	34	41
Hungry-Man XXL: Backyard BBQ	860	48	62
Roasted Carved Turkey Dinner	1360	70	114
Southern Fried Boneless Chicken	760	16	84
Classics: Salisbury Steak	500	26	48
Boneless White Meat Fried Chkn	230	11	23
Breaded Fish Fillet, 7.3 oz	370	14	45
Chicken Strips w. Fries, 6¾ oz	300	10	39
Classic Fried Chicken, 11½ oz	770	37	72
Meatloaf 9¼ oz	270	13	22
Turkey Breast w. Stuffing & Gravy	380	17	40

TGI Friday's

	C	F	Cb
Buffalo Wings (3)	150	10	2
Chicken Egg Rolls (1)	150	5	19
Chicken Quesadilla, 4½ oz	290	13	26
Honey BBQ Wings (3)	150	9	6
Mozzarella Sticks & Sce, 1 Serve	110	6	8
Popcorn Chicken, 3 pces, 2.6 oz	250	8	29
Potato Skins, Ched. & Bacon, 3 pces	210	12	20
Quesadilla Rolls: Chicken (2)	250	12	26
Steak (2)	250	11	21

Trader Joe's

	C	F	Cb
Meals: *Per Serving*			
Asian Style Chkn Stir Fry w. Sce, 8 oz	190	1	30
BBQ Chicken Teriyaki, 1 cup	150	3.5	13
Chicken Chow Mein, ⅓ pkg, 6.75 oz	240	2	45
Chicken Fried Rice, 1 cup, 5 oz	200	3.5	33
Chicken Marsala, 1 pkg, 11 oz	320	6	34
Citrus Glazed Chicken, 8 oz	270	5	40
Rice Bowls, average, 11 oz bowl	390	3.5	55
Shrimp Stir Fry, 6.4 oz	70	0.5	6
Turkey Saus. Stromboli, ¼ loaf, 4.5 oz	250	7	31
Pies: Shepherds Pie, ½ pie, 8 oz	190	3.5	23
Spinach Pie, ¼ pie, 6 oz	240	4	37
Quiche: Broccoli & Cheddar, 6 oz	460	30	32
Mexicaine, 6 oz	500	34	31
Spinach & Mushroom, 6 oz	460	26	38

Tyson

	C	F	Cb
Meal Kits: Beef Fajita (1)	140	4	17
Chicken Fajita (1)	130	3.5	17
Chicken Fried Rice, 2½ cups	440	6	69
Chicken Quesadilla (1)	250	10	26
Meals: Buffalo Hot Wings, 4 pieces	220	15	1
Chicken Bites, 13 pieces	270	18	15
Chicken Brst Fillets, breaded (1)	240	9	20
Meals: Chkn Brst Nuggets, 5 pces	280	18	16
Chicken Breast Strips, 3 oz	120	3.5	1
Chicken Breast Tenderloins, 1 pce	150	7	12
Country Fried Steak, 1 piece	310	23	15
Crispy Chicken Strips, 2 pces	200	10	13
Fajita Style Chicken Strips, 3 oz	110	4	1
Fun Nuggets, 5 pieces	280	18	16
Honey Barbecue Wings, 4 pces	220	14	19
Honey Chicken Brst Tenders, 5 pce	220	13	13
Popcorn Chicken, 6 pces	250	12	22
Southern Style Chkn Brst Patties (1)	240	18	14
Steak Fingers, 2 pces	250	18	14
Any'tizers: Chicken Fries, 7 pces	230	11	19
Buffalo Style Chicken Wings, 3 pces	150	7	8
Cheddar & Bacon Chse Bites, 4 pces	240	14	12

Van De Kamp's

	C	F	Cb
Butterfly Shrimp, 7 pces, 4 oz	270	13	26
Crispy Battered Halibut, 3 fillets	230	11	22
Crispy Fish Tenders, 4 pces, 4 oz	210	10	22
Popcorn Shrimp, 20 pces, 4 oz	260	11	30
Fish Sticks, Breaded, 6 stix, 4 oz	230	11	23
Battered Fillets, 2.6 oz fillet	120	6	12
Crunchy Fish Fillets, 1 pce, 2.6 oz	230	13	21
Crisp & Healthy, Breaded (2), 1.8 oz	170	2.5	25

Weight Watchers

	C	F	Cb
Smart Ones Bistro Selections: Per Meal			
Chicken Fettucini	340	8	42
Chicken Parmesan	290	5	35
Fajita Chicken Supreme	260	7	32
Grilled Mandarin Chicken	230	4.5	42
Homestyle Chicken	230	9	12
Meatloaf w. Mashed Potatoes	260	8	22
Picante Chicken & Pasta	260	4	32
Roasted Chicken w. Sour Cream	180	4	20
Sirloin Beef Asian Veggies	160	4	13
Southwest Style Adobo Chicken	310	10	36
Stuffed Turkey Breast	290	6	42
Sweet & Sour Chicken	140	3	13
Teriyaki Chicken & Vegetables	230	2.5	39
Thai Style Chicken & Rice Noodles	260	4	43

Weight Watchers (Cont)

	C	F	Cb
Morning Express, Breakfast: Per Meal			
English Muffin Sandwich	210	5	27
Canadian Style Bacon Eng. Muffin	210	6	27
Breakfast Quesadilla,	220	6	28
Stuffed Breakfast Sandwich	240	7	24
Smart Ones Entrees: Per Meal			
Angel Hair Marinara	230	1.5	41
Broccoli & Cheddar Roasted Pot.	220	6	34
Chicken Enchiladas Suiza	310	8	45
Honey Dijon Chicken	220	3.5	38
Lasagna Bolognese	270	4	43
Lemon Herb Chicken Piccata	250	5	36
Macaroni & Cheese	270	2	52
Pasta Primavera	280	6	44
Rst Turkey Medallions	220	1.5	38
Salisbury Steak	260	7	26
Santa Fe Style Rice & Beans	310	7	51
Shrimp Marinara	180	1.5	31
Spaghetti Bolognese; 3 Chse Mac, avg.	305	6	48
Spaghetti Marinara	300	4.5	54
Spicy Szechuan Style Vege & Chkn	240	5	36
Traditional Lasagna w. Meat Sce	300	6	43
Tuna Noodle Gratin	250	4.5	37
Smartwiches, avg. all, 127g	270	6	40
Smart Ones Fruit Inspirations: Per Meal			
Cranberry Turkey Medallions	350	4.5	59
Honey Mango BBQ Chkn	240	3.5	34
Orange Sesame Chicken	320	8	48
Pineapple Beef Teriyaki	260	4.5	38

Worthington/Loma Linda

	C	F	Cb
Bolono, 3 slices, 2 oz	80	3	3
Chicken Roll, ⅜ slice, 1.9 oz	90	4.5	2
Chicken Slices, 3 slices, 2 oz	90	4.5	2
Corned Beef Slices, 3 slices, 2 oz	140	9	5
Dinner Roast, ¾" slice	180	11	6
Fried Chik'n w. Gravy, 2 pieces	150	10	5
FriPats, 1 pattie, 2¼ oz	130	6	5
Leanies, 1 link, 1.4 oz	100	7	2
Prosage, Links, 2 links, 1.6 oz	80	3	3
Smkd Turkey Slices, 3 slices	140	9	4
Stakelets, 2.5 oz pce	150	7	7
Stripples, 2 slices	60	4.5	2
Swiss Steak, 1 piece	130	6	9
Tuno (tuna substitute), ½ cup	90	6	3
Wham Veggie Slices, 2 slices	110	7	3

Zatarains

	C	F	Cb
Blackened Chicken Alfredo	535	30	44
Jambalaya seasoned with Chicken	360	8	53
Jambalaya seasoned with Sausage	390	12	58
Red Beans & Rice with Sausage,	565	19	76

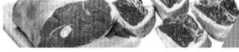
Note: Cooking reduces weight of meat by 20-45% due to water and fat losses. Average weight loss is 30%. Actual loss depends on cooking method and cooking time. Examples:

4 oz raw wt. = approx. 3 oz cooked wt.

4 oz cooked wt. = approx. 5½ oz raw wt.

What 3 oz Cooked Meat Looks Like
- Half the size of this book (4¼" x 3" x ⅜" thick)
- Rectangular piece (4" x 2½" x ½" thick)
- Deck of cards (3½" x 2½" x ⅝" thick)

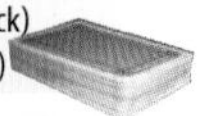

STEAK QUICK GUIDE

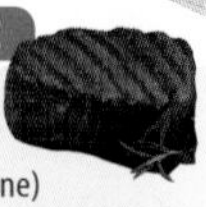

Sirloin (Choice Grade)
External fat trimmed to ¼"
Broiled, Edible Portion (no bone)

	C	F	Cb
Small/Regular Serving, 3 oz (cooked)			
(from 4-4½ oz raw)			
Lean + external fat (¼"), 3 oz	225	13	0
Lean + marbling, 3 oz	195	10	0
Lean only, 3 oz	160	6	0
(No external fat or marbling)			
Medium Serving, 5 oz (cooked wt)			
(from approx. 7 oz raw)			
Lean + external fat (¼"), 5 oz	350	21	0
Lean + marbling, 5 oz	325	17	0
Lean only, 5 oz	265	10	0
Large Serving, 8 oz (cooked wt)			
(from 11-12 oz raw)			
Lean + external fat, 8 oz	600	36	0
Lean + marbling, 8 oz	520	27	0
Lean only, 8 oz	425	15	0
Extra Large Serving, 12 oz (cooked wt)			
(from approx. 16-17 oz raw)			
Lean + external fat (¼"), 12 oz	900	52	0
Lean + marbling, 12 oz	740	40	0
Lean only, 12 oz	640	23	0
Pan Fried			
Sirloin (choice), medium serving:			
Lean + external fat (¼"), 5 oz	460	33	0
Lean only, 5 oz	340	16	0

Other Steaks

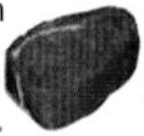

	C	F	Cb
Filet Mignon (Tenderloin):			
1 Medium steak (6 oz raw wt.)			
Broiled, with ¼" fat trim			
Lean + fat (¼"), 4 oz	360	27	0
Lean only, 3½ oz	230	12	0
New York/Club Steak:			
Top Loin/Short Loin			
1 steak, regular (9¼ oz raw, ¼" fat)			
Broiled: Lean + fat (¼"), 6¼ oz	580	43	0
Lean + marbling, 5½ oz	400	25	0
Lean only, 5¼ oz	360	20	0
Porterhouse Steak:			
1 Medium, (6 oz raw wt. no bone), broiled			
Lean + fat (¼"), 4¼ oz	410	33	0
Lean only, 3½ oz	210	11	0
1 Large (12 oz raw wt. no bone), broiled			
Lean + fat (¼") 8½ oz cooked	820	66	0
Lean only, 7 oz cooked	420	22	0
T-Bone Steak: Broiled or Grilled			
Medium Size: 8 oz raw weight			
(Approx. 6 oz cooked)			
Lean + Fat (¼"), 5 oz, no bone	400	28	0
Lean only, 4 oz (no bone)	265	12	0
Large Size: 12 oz raw weight			
(Approx. 9 oz cooked)			
Lean + fat (¼"), 7 oz (no bone)	560	39	0
Lean only, 6 oz (no bone)	400	18	0
Extra Large Size: 20 oz raw weight			
(Approx. 16 oz cooked)			
Lean + Fat (¼"), 12 oz (no bone)	960	66	0
Lean Only, 10 oz (no bone)	660	30	0

Also See Fast-Foods & Restaurants Section ~
Lone Star Steakhouse
Outback Steakhouse

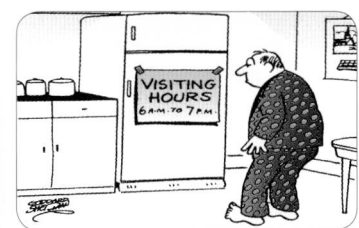

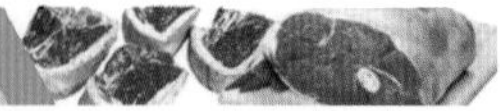

Beef – Individual Cuts

	C	**F**	**Cb**
Average All Grades			
Edible Weight (no bone)			
Brisket, whole, braised:			
Lean + fat (¼" trim), 3 oz	330	27	0
Lean + marbling, 3 oz	250	17	0
Lean only, 3 oz	185	9	0
Chuck blade, braised:			
Lean + fat (¼"), 3 oz	310	24	0
Lean + marbling, 3 oz	295	22	0
Lean only, 3 oz	245	13	0
Flank: Raw, 4 oz	175	8	0
Braised, 3 oz	225	14	0
Broiled, 3 oz	155	6	0
Round, bottom, braised:			
Lean + marbling, 3 oz	190	7.5	0
Lean only, 3 oz	185	6.5	0
Round, eye/tip, roasted:			
Lean + fat (¼"), 3 oz	205	11	0
Lean (with marbling), 3 oz	150	5	0
Round, top: *Per 3 oz (cooked wt)*			
Braised, Lean + fat	210	10	0
Lean only	170	4	0
Broiled, Lean + fat	180	8	0
Lean only	160	5	0
Pan-fried, Lean + fat	235	13	0
Lean only	195	7	0

Beef Ribs

	C	**F**	**Cb**
Back Ribs (7" long, visible fat trimmed to ¼")			
10.3 oz raw (with bone) or 3½ oz cooked (braised, no bone)			
1 average rib	410	34	0
3 ribs	1230	102	0
Short Ribs (2½" long, visible fat trimmed to ¼")			
6 oz raw (with bone) or 2½ oz cooked (braised, no bone)			
1 average rib	320	28	0
3 ribs	960	85	0

Ground Beef

	C	**F**	**Cb**
Ground Beef, Raw: *Per 4 oz*			
70% lean (30% fat)	380	34	0
75% lean (25% fat)	335	29	0
80% lean (20% fat)	290	23	0
85% lean (15% fat)	245	17	0
90% lean (10% fat)	200	12	0
95% lean (5% fat)	155	6	0
Baked/Broiled: Reg. (70%), 3 oz	230	16	0
Lean (80%), 3 oz	215	14	0
Extra lean (90%), 3 oz	185	14	0
Pan-Broiled: Reg. (70%), 3 oz	230	15	0
Lean (80%), 3 oz	210	14	0
Extra lean (90%), 3 oz	195	10	0
Ground Beef Patties: Average (23% Fat)			
Raw, 4 oz	330	25	0
Broiled, 3 oz (from 4 oz raw)	250	19	0

Quick Guide

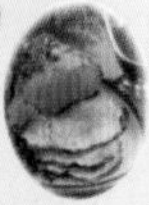

Roast Beef (Roasted)	**C**	**F**	**Cb**
Round (Eye/Tip, average) Average All Cuts			
Small/Regular Serving, 3 oz			
(2 thin slices/1 thick slice)			
Lean + fat (¼"), 3 oz	200	11	0
Lean only, 3 oz	150	5	0
Medium Serving, 5 oz			
(3–4 thin slices)			
Lean + fat, 5 oz	330	19	0
Lean only, 5 oz	245	9	0
Large Serving, 8 oz (3 thick slices)			
Lean + fat, 8 oz	525	30	0
Lean only, 8 oz	390	14	0

Roast Dinner Extras

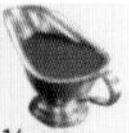

	C	**F**	**Cb**
Gravy: Thin, 2 Tbsp	20	0.5	3.5
Thick, 2 Tbsp	50	2	0.5
1 Ladle/4 Tbsp	100	4	1
Veggies: Beans, green, ½ cup	20	0	5
Cauliflower w. cheese sce, 4 oz	135	9	15
Corn, kernels, ¼ cup	35	0	9
Carrots, ¼ cup	20	0	3
Peas, ¼ cup	35	0	6
Potato: Roasted w. fat, 1 small	155	8	30
Baked in Jacket, 1 large	280	0	63
with 1 Tbsp whipped butter	350	8	63
with Sour Cream, 2 Tbsp	270	5	64
Sweet Potato/Yam, 1 medium	105	1	24

Beef Kabobs (Cooked):			
Beef & Veggies, 2 oz	160	10	4
If very lean meat	100	4	4

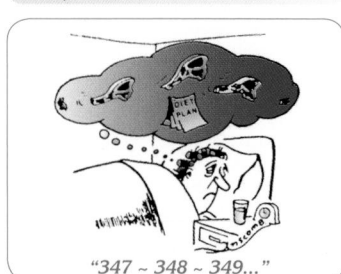

"347 ~ 348 ~ 349..."

Lamb

	C	F	Cb
Choice Grade			
Leg (Whole), roasted:			
Lean + fat, 3 oz	220	14	0
Lean only, 3 oz	160	7	0
Leg (Sirloin Half), roasted:			
Lean + fat, 3 oz	250	18	0
Lean only, 3 oz	175	8	0
Leg (Shank Half), roasted:			
Lean + fat, 3 oz	190	11	0
Lean only, 3 oz	155	6	0
Loin Chop, broiled:			
1 chop (raw wt., 4¼ oz):	250	17	0
Lean + fat (2¼ oz edible)	180	12	0
Lean only (1.6 oz edible)	85	3.5	0
Rib Chop, broiled/roasted:			
1 chop (raw wt., 3½ oz)			
Lean + fat (2½ oz edible)	255	21	0
Lean only (1¾ oz edible)	105	6	0
Shoulder (Arm/Blade):			
Braised: Lean + fat, 3 oz	295	21	0
Lean only, 3 oz	240	12	0
Broiled: Lean + fat, 3 oz	240	17	0
Lean only, 3 oz	170	8	0
Roasted: Similar to Broiled			
Cubed Lamb (Leg/Shoulder):			
For stew or kabob			
Braised, lean only, 3 oz	190	8	0
Broiled, lean only, 3 oz	160	6	0

Veal

	C	F	Cb
Edible Weights			
Leg (Top Round):			
Braised: Lean + fat, 3 oz	180	6	0
Lean only, 3 oz	175	5	0
Pan-fried, breaded:			
Lean + fat, 3 oz	195	8	9
Lean only, 3 oz	185	6	9
Pan-fried, not breaded:			
Lean + fat, 3 oz	180	7	0
Lean only, 3 oz	155	4	0
Roasted: Lean + fat, 3 oz	135	4	0
Lean only, 3 oz	130	3	0

Veal (Cont)

	C	F	Cb
Loin Chop: 1 chop, 7 oz raw wt.			
Braised: Lean + fat, 3 oz	240	15	0
Lean only, 3 oz	190	8	0
Roasted: Lean + fat, 3 oz	185	11	0
Lean only, 3 oz	150	6	0
Rib, roasted: Lean + fat, 3 oz	195	12	0
Lean only, 3 oz	150	7	0
Shoulder, Arm/Blade, roasted:			
Lean + fat, 3 oz	155	7	0
Lean only, 3 oz	140	5	0
Sirloin, roasted:			
Lean + fat, 3 oz	170	9	0
Lean only, 3 oz	145	6	0
Cubed for Stew, braised:			
Leg/Shoulder, lean only, 3 oz	160	4	0
(1 lb raw yields approx. 9¼ oz cooked)			

Pork

	C	F	Cb
Fresh Pork (Cooked Wt., no bone)			
(4 oz raw wt. = approx. 3 oz cooked wt.)			
Blade Steak, broiled:			
Lean + fat, 3 oz	220	15	0
Lean only, 3 oz	190	11	0
Country Style Ribs, broiled/roasted:			
Lean + fat, 3 oz	280	22	0
Lean only, 3 oz	210	13	0
Spareribs, **braised:** lean & fat, 6 oz			
(from 1 lb raw wt)	675	52	0
Leg (Ham), whole, roasted:			
Lean + fat, 3 oz	230	15	0
Lean only, 3 oz	180	8	0
(Ham, cured ~ See Cold Meats)			
Loin Chops, broiled: Average			
(From 1 chop: 5 oz raw wt. w. bone			
or 4 oz raw wt., no bone)			
Lean + fat, 3 oz	200	11	0
Lean only, 3 oz	165	7	0
Loin Roast, roasted:			
Lean + fat, 3 oz	210	13	0
Lean only, 3 oz	180	8	0
Rib Chops, (Boneless), broiled:			
Lean + fat, 3 oz	220	14	0
Lean only, 3 oz	185	9	0
Rib Roast, roasted:			
Lean + fat, 3 oz	215	13	0
Lean only, 3 oz	180	9	0

Pork (Cont)

	C	F	Cb
Sirloin Chop, broiled:			
Lean + fat, 3 oz	180	8	0
Lean only, 3 oz	165	6	0
Sirloin Roast, roasted:			
Lean + fat, 3 oz	175	8	0
Lean only, 3 oz	170	7	0
Tenderloin (Boneless), roasted:			
Lean + fat, 3 oz	125	4	0
Lean only, 3 oz	120	3	0
Ground Pork			
Raw: Average, ¼ lb, 4 oz	300	24	0
Broiled, 3 oz	250	18	0
Pan-fried, drained, 3 oz	260	19	0

Bacon

Raw: 1 med. slice (20 lb), ¾ oz	95	9	0
1 thick slice (12 lb), 1⅓ oz	175	17	0
(1 lb raw yields approx. 5 oz cooked)			
Broiled/Pan-Fried: 1 med. sl., 8g	40	3	0
3 medium slices, 24g	125	10	0
2 thin slices, ½ oz	75	6	0
1 thick slice, 12g	65	5	0
Canadian Bacon: Cooked, 1 slice, 1 oz	45	2	0.5
Packaged, 3 slices, 2 oz	90	4	1
Bacon Bits, 1 Tbsp, ¼ oz	35	2	0
Breakfast Strips, Broil., 1 sl., 12 g	50	4	0

Ham

	C	F	Cb
Boneless Ham, cooked:			
Regular, (approx. 13% fat):			
Roasted, 3 oz	150	8	0
Extra Lean (5% fat):			
Roasted, 3 oz	125	5	0
Whole Ham, cooked:			
Lean + fat (as purchased)			
Roasted, 3 oz	210	15	0
Lean only, Roasted, 3 oz	135	5	0
Canned Ham: Similar to boneless ham			
Chopped, canned, 3 oz	200	16	0
Ham Patties, cooked, 1 patty, 2¼ oz	220	20	1
Ham Steak, extra lean, 2 oz	70	2.5	0
Lunch Slices: See Deli Meats, Page 131			

Game & Other Meats

	C	F	Cb
Bison Steak,			
lean, 6 oz (raw)	205	4	0
Boar (wild), roasted, 3 oz	140	4	0
Buffalo Steak: New West Foods, 4 oz	70	3	0
Trader Joe's, 1 patty	430	30	1
Caribou, roasted, 3 oz	140	4	0
Deer/Venison, roasted 3 oz	135	3	0
Goat (Capretto): Raw, 3 oz	95	2	0
Roasted, 3 oz	120	2.5	0
Ostrich: Blackwing Ostrich Meats,			
Sport Jerky, ½ pce	25	0	0
Sausage Patties (2) 2 oz	60	0.5	0
New West Foods:			
Ground Ostrich, 4 oz	165	7	0
Ostrich Steak, 4 oz steak	130	2.5	0
Rabbit: Roasted, 3 oz	165	7	0
Stewed, 1 cup, diced, 5 oz	290	12	0

Variety & Organ Meats

Brain (Lamb): Braised, 3 oz	125	9	0
Pan-fried, 3 oz	230	19	0
Chitterlings, pork, simmered, 3 oz	260	25	0
Ears, pork, simmered, 1 ear, 4 oz	185	12	0
Feet, pork: Simmered, 3 oz	200	14	0
Cured, pickled, 3 oz	170	14	0
Hormel, 2 oz	80	6	0
Head Cheese (Pork Snouts/Ears/Vinegar/Spices):			
1 oz slice	50	4	0
Heart, Beef, braised, 3 oz	140	4	24
Jowl, pork, raw, 4 oz	750	80	0
Kidneys, braised, 3 oz	140	5	0
Liver (beef): Raw, 4 oz	150	4	4
Braised, 3 oz	140	4	3
Pan-fried, 3 oz	185	7	7
Pancreas, pork, braised, 3 oz	185	8	0
Pork Cracklins, 0.5 oz	80	6	0
Pork Hocks, 1 piece, 6 oz	340	23	0
Scrapple, pork, 2 oz	120	8	8
Spleen, pork, braised, 3 oz	130	3	0
Stomach, pork, raw, 4 oz	185	12	0
Sweetbreads: Beef, ckd., 3 oz	125	9	0
Lamb, cooked, 3 oz	125	9	0
Tail, pork, simmered, 3 oz	340	31	0
Tongue: braised: Veal, 3 oz	170	9	0
Beef/Lamb/Pork, average, 3 oz	235	17	0
Tripe, beef, raw, 3 oz	85	3.5	0

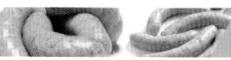

Quick Guide

Franks & Weiners
Average All Brands

	C	**F**	**Cb**
Regular/Smoked: *Per Frank*			
Regular, 1.5oz (10/16 oz pkg)	140	13	1
Jumbo, 2 oz (8/16 oz pkg)	170	16	0
Bun Length, 2 oz	180	17	2
Extra Long, 2.75 oz	240	21	2
Small/Cocktail (50/lb) each	30	3	0.5
Beef Franks: *Per Frank*			
Regular, 1.6 oz (10/16 oz pkg)	140	13	1
Jumbo, 2 oz (8/16 oz pkg)	170	15	2
Bun Length, 2 oz	180	16	2
¼ lb Dog, 4 oz	300	24	4

Franks & Weiners

	C	**F**	**Cb**
Ball Park			
Franks & Weiners: *Per Frank*			
Angus Beef Franks	170	15	3
Cheese	160	15	2.5
Turkey Franks	120	7	6
GrillMaster: Deli Style Beef; Beef	250	23	4
Hot 'N Spicy; Smokehouse	260	24	4
Lite: Franks; Beef	100	7	3
Beef Kosher			
Beef: 2 oz link	180	14	4
2.6 oz link (6/16 oz)	230	19	6
Foster Farms			
Chicken Franks, 2 oz (8/16 oz)	140	12	1
Healthy Choice			
Turkey Franks, 1.76 oz link	70	2.5	6
Hebrew National			
Beef: 1.72 oz link	150	14	1
4 oz link	340	32	1
97% Fat-Free, 1.72 oz link	50	1.5	2
Jennie-O			
Turkey Franks:			
1.2 oz link	70	5	2
2 oz link	120	10	2
Scooby-Doo, 1.6 oz	110	9	1
Oscar Mayer			
Reg./Smoked, Fat-Free, 1.76 oz	40	0	3
Beef, Reduced-Fat, 2 oz	110	8	2
Cheese Franks, 1.6 oz	140	13	1
Turkey Frank: 1.6 oz	100	8	2
2 oz link	120	10	3
Shelton's			
Chicken Franks, 1.2 oz link	70	6	0
Turkey Franks, 1.2 oz link	60	4.5	1
Zacky Farms			
Chicken Frank, 2 oz link	160	12	1

Quick Guide

Fresh Sausages

	C	**F**	**Cb**
Pork/Beef: *Average All Types*			
Small: Raw, 4" link, 1 oz	85	7.5	0
Broiled/Pan-fried	80	7	0
Medium: Raw, 2 oz	170	15	0
Broiled/Pan-fried	165	14	0
Large: Raw, 3 oz	255	22	0
Broiled/Pan-fried	245	21	0
Italian: Raw, 3.2 oz	315	28	0.5
Cooked, 2.4 oz	230	18	3
Chorizo: Beef Chorizo, 2.5 oz pce	250	23	5
Pork Chorizo, 2 oz piece	250	23	5

Note: Fat is lost in broiling/pan frying.
(Cooked wt. = approx. 60-70% raw wt.)

Smoked Sausage

	C	**F**	**Cb**
Average All Brands: 2 oz link	170	15	0
3 oz link	255	22	0
Ball Park, Bun Size, 2 oz	180	17	2
Butterball			
(w. Turkey), 2 oz	100	6	4
Eckrich, 2 oz	180	16	2
Healthy Choice, Beef/Polska, 2 oz	80	2.5	6

Breakfast Sausages/Patties

	C	**F**	**Cb**
Armour Brown 'n Serve			
Pork/Turkey, 3 links, 2.1 oz	210	19	2
Lite Original, 3 links	120	8	2
Beef Sausage, 3 links, 2 oz	230	22	1
Butterball: Turkey Brkfast Pats (2)	120	7	2
Turkey Breakfast Links (3)	120	8	2
Healthy Choice, Patties/Links (3), 2 oz	70	3	3
Jennie-O, Italian Turkey Saus. (2)	160	10	0
Jimmy Dean: Pork Saus. Patties (2)	260	24	0
Pork Sausage Links: Original (3)	290	28	0
Country Maple (3)	230	20	3
Breakfast Sandwiches: See Page 94			
Jones/Golden Brown:			
Pork Sausage Patties: Original	75	7	0.5
All Natural	95	9	0
Sandwich Patties	170	16	1
Pork Sausage Links:			
2 links	180	18	2
Light, 2 links	110	8	1
Vegetarian Patties:			
Boca: *See Page 119*			
Garden Burger: *See Page 120*			

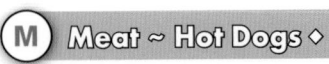

Bagel, Corn & Hot Dogs

Hot Dogs, Ready-To-Go

(Includes Ketchup/Relish; no Mayo)

	C	F	Cb
Regular (1.5 oz frank, 1.5 oz bun)	260	15	22
Bun Length (2 oz frank, 1.5 oz bun)	290	18	21
Jumbo Dog (2 oz frank, 2 oz bun)	360	20	36
¼ lb Beef Dog (¼ lb dog, 2 oz bun)	480	15	36
Mile Long Dog (2.6 oz dog, 1.5 oz bun)	360	24	23

Weinerschnitzel: *See Fast-Foods*

Corn Dogs

Beef/Pork Frank: Avg., 2.6 oz	170	10	16
Foster Farms Chicken Franks:			
1 dog, 2.6 oz (75g)	180	10	15
Chili Cheese, 1 dog, 2.6 oz (75g)	200	9	24
Mini Corn Dogs (4), 2.68 oz	210	12	18
Oscar Mayer			
Turkey & Pork, 3.2 oz	260	15	25
State Fair w. Ball Park Franks,			
Corn Dogs 1 dog, 2.7 oz (76g)	210	12	23
Mini Corn Dogs (4)	230	13	22

Bagel Dogs

Vienna Beef: 1 piece, 1 oz	85	3.5	7
Mini, 1 piece, 0.8 oz	60	2	8

Hot Dog Toppings/Extras:

American Chse, 1 slice, 1 oz	110	9	1
Catsup, 1 Tbsp	16	0	4
Chili (w. Beans), ¼ cup	70	3.5	9
Ketchup, 1 Tbsp	15	0	4
Mustard, 1 Tbsp	20	0	1
Onions, Chopped, 1 Tbsp	5	0	1
Pickle Relish, 1 Tbsp	20	0	5
Sauerkraut, ½ cup	20	0	5

Deli & Lunch Meats

	C	F	Cb
Beef Jerky/Meat Snacks:			
Bridgeford Beef Jerky, 1 oz	100	0.5	5
Beef Stick (5.5 oz stick), 1 oz	150	13	2
Beef Steak, 1 oz	70	0.5	2
Beef & Cheese (Giant Size),			
½ pkg, 1.5 oz	170	14	1
Pepperoni Sticks (2), 1 oz	160	13	2
Pepperoni (1" diam.), 1 oz	130	12	0
Teriyaki, 1 oz pkg	80	0.5	4
Original; Hot 'n Spicy	70	1	5
Berliner (pork/beef), 1 oz	65	5	1
Beerwurst (Beef)			
Small (2.75"diam.), ¹⁄₁₆" slice	20	2	0

Large (4"diam), ⅛" slice	75	7	0.5

Deli & Lunch Meats

	C	F	Cb
Beerwurst (Pork):			
Small (2.75"diam), ¹⁄₁₆" slice	15	1	0
Large (4"diam), ⅛" Slice	55	4	0.5
Bologna: 1 Slice, 1 oz	65	6	1
Fat-Free, 1 slice, 1 oz	20	0	2
Beef Bologna: 1 slice, 1 oz	90	8	1
Light, 1 slice, 1 oz	60	4	2
Light *(Oscar Mayer)*, 1 sl., 1 oz	60	4	2
Fat Free *(Osc. M.)*, 2 sl., 1.6 oz	40	0	1
Ring *(Boar's Head)*, 2 oz	150	13	1
Turkey, average, 1 oz	60	5	0.5
Blood Sausage, 1 oz	100	9	0.5
Bratwurst: Average, 1 oz	80	7	1
Boar's Head, cook., 1 wurst, 4 oz	300	25	0
Bob Evan's, 2.6 oz link	270	21	1
Braunschweiger (Pork/Liver/Sausage),			
Oscar Mayer, 1 oz slice	110	10	1
Chicken, *Average All Brands*			
1 thick or 2 thin slices, 1 oz	30	1	1
Chicken Roll, 1 slice, 2 oz	90	4	1.5
Corned Beef: Average, full fat, 1 oz	60	5	0.5
Hillshire Farm, 1oz	30	1	0
Loaf, jellied, 1 oz	45	2	0
Hash, canned, average, 1 oz	50	3	3
Dutch Brand Loaf, average, 1 oz	70	5	1.5
Ham, Sliced:			
Baked/Boiled, sliced, 1 oz	30	1	0.5
Chopped: *Eckrich* (97% FF), 1 oz	25	1	1
Armour: Canned, 1 oz	35	1.5	0.5
97% Fat Free, 1 oz	25	1	1.5
Healthy Choice, 2 sl., 2 oz	60	1.5	1
Oscar Mayer, 1 oz slice	60	2	0.5
Honey/Brown Sugar: Avg., 1 oz	30	1	1
Healthy Choice Deli Traditions:			
Hearty Slices, 2 slices, 2 oz	60	1.5	2
Prosciutto, average, 1 oz	70	5	0
Ham & Cheese Loaf, avg., 1 oz	70	5	1
Italian Sausage, 2.6 oz	250	20	3
Kielbasa (Polish Sausage), 1 oz	65	5	1
Beef, 2 oz link	190	17	1
Boar's Head, 1 oz	60	5	0

	C	F	Cb
Kippered Beefsteak:			
Hickory Farms, 3 slices, 0.75 oz	50	1	1
Knockwurst, 1 oz	90	8	0.5
Linguica (*Gaspar's*), 2 oz	180	8	1
Liverwurst, 1 oz	65	5	1
Liver Pate, fresh, average, 1 oz	90	8	1
Luncheon Loaf (*Foods Co*), 1 oz	65	5	2
Mortadella, 1 oz	105	9	0
Olive Loaf: Average, 1 oz	70	5	3
Oscar Mayer, 1 oz slice	75	6	2
Pastrami (Beef): Average, 1 oz	45	3	1
Healthy Deli, 1 oz	34	1	0.5
Hillshire (DeliSelect), 6 sl., 2 oz	60	1	0
Boar's Head, 2 oz	70	4	2
Peppered Beef, 1 oz slice	40	2	1
Pepperoni, 5 slices, 1 oz	140	13	0
Pickle Loaf, 1 oz	70	5	5
Pickle & Pimento Loaf			
Oscar Mayer, 1 oz	75	6	3
Polish Sausage: *See Kielbasa*			
Proscuitto/Proscuitti: Avg., 1 oz	70	5	1
Hormel, 1 oz	90	7	1
Roast Beef: Lean, 1 oz	40	2	0
Healthy Choice, all types, 2 oz	60	1.5	1
Salami: Beef, average, 1 oz	80	7	1
Beer Salami, average, 1 oz	50	4	0.5
Cotto: *Oscar Mayer*, 1 sl., 1 oz	70	6	1
Dry: Hard, avg., 4 slices, 1 oz	110	10	3
Oscar Mayer, 2 slices, 1.6 oz	100	8	1
Genoa: Average, 1 oz	120	9	1
Stick (*Best's Kosher*), 2, 1.75 oz	180	15	2
Italian (*Bridgeford*), 1 oz	120	11	0
Turkey, average, 1 oz	55	4	1
Spam (*Hormel*): *Per 2 oz Serving*			
Classic	180	16	1
Spam Lite	110	8	1
Hot & Spicy	180	16	2
Oven Rstd Turkey	80	4	1
Smoked	170	15	2
Spam w. Bacon	180	16	1
Spam w. Cheese	170	15	1
25% Less Sodium	180	16	1
Spam Single Lite, 3 oz pkg	160	11	2
Summer Sausage:			
Bridgeford, 1 oz	100	9	1
Oscar Mayer, 1 slice, 0.8 oz	70	7	0.5
Treet (*Armour*), canned, 1 oz	100	9	1.5
Turkey: Average, 1 oz slice	30	1	0.5
¾ oz slice	22	0.5	0.5

	C	F	Cb
Turkey Breast:			
Butterball Fat Free, 3 sl., 2 oz	60	0	4
Deli Thin Smoked, 2 sl., 1 oz	50	0.5	2
Hillshire Deli Select, 6 sl., 2 oz	50	0.5	2
Louis Rich Carvery Board,			
2 slices, 1.8 oz (52g)	50	0	2
Free, 2 slices, 2 oz	50	0	2
Healthy Choice: Deli Thin: *Per 4 Slices, 52g (1.8 oz)*			
Oven-Roasted	60	1.5	2
Smoked/Rotisserie Seasoned	60	1.5	3
Honey Roasted & Smoked	60	1.5	4
Hearty Deli Sliced:			
Oven Rstd Turkey Brst. 1 sl., 1 oz	30	1	1
Turkey Ham, 1 slice, 1 oz	35	1.5	0.5
Turkey Pastrami, 1 oz	35	1.5	1
Turkey Roll, 1 oz	40	2	0.5
Turkey Loaf, 1 oz	30	1	1
Vegetarian Deli (Worthington, Yves): *See Page 76*			

Meat Spreads

	C	F	Cb
Average All Brands: *Per 1/4 Cup (2 oz)*			
Chicken	90	10	2
Ham, Deviled	140	11	0
Liverwurst	190	16	2
Roast Beef	130	10	2
Sandwich Spread	140	10	9
Turkey	110	7	2

Paté

	C	F	Cb
Canned: *Average All Brands*			
Chicken Liver, 2 Tbsp, 1 oz	60	4	2
Paté de Foie Gras, goose liver, 1 oz	130	12	2
Fresh (Refrigerated):			
Average all types, 1 oz	110	10	1
Boar's Head Liverwurst Pate, 2 oz	145	12	0
Marcel Henri			
Pate de Champagne	210	18	2
Chicken Liver w. Port Wine, 2 oz	210	18	2
Duck Truffle w. Port Wine, 2 oz	240	24	2
Old Wisconsin Pate			
All types, 1 oz	105	9	1.5
Vegetable Pate; Spin/Mushr., 2 oz	105	7	10
Trois Petit Cochons			
Mediterranean, 2 oz	130	11	3
Smoked Salmon, 2 oz	115	9	2
Wegmans			
Alexian Wild, 2 oz	270	27	1
Cognac; Black Peppercorn, 2 oz	160	17	4

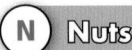

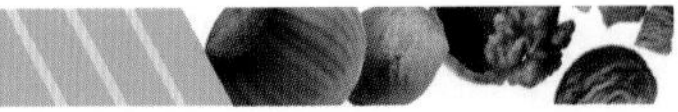

Nuts

Per 1 oz Unless Indicated — **C** **F** **Cb**

	C	F	Cb
Acorns, raw 1 oz	110	7	12
Almonds, Dried/Dry Roasted:			
Whole, 24-28 med., 1 oz	170	15	5.5
½ cup, 2½ oz	420	37	13
Chopped,½ cup, 2¼ oz	380	34	12
Sliced, ½ cup, 1⅔ oz	280	25	9
Choc. coated (5-6), 1 oz	150	10	15
Oil Rstd *(Blue Diamond)*, 1 oz	170	16	5
Honey Roasted, 1 oz	170	14	8
Almond Meal (partially defattened)			
1 cup (not packed), 2¼ oz	260	11	11
Brazil Nuts, 8 medium, 1 oz	185	19	3.5
Cashews, Dry or Oil Roasted:			
14 large/18 med./26 small, 1 oz	165	14	9
½ cup, 2.4 oz	375	31	20
Honey Roasted, 1 oz	165	13	10
Chestnuts, avg. all: Dried, 1 oz	105	1	22
Raw/Fresh, 5-6 nuts, 1 oz	60	0	13
Canned, water chestnuts,			
sliced/whole/drained, 1 oz	30	0	7
Coconut: Fresh,			
1 piece, 2"x2"x ½", 1 oz	100	10	4.5
Shredded, fresh, ½ cup, 1.4 oz	140	13	6
Dried (Desiccated):			
Unsweetened, 1 oz	185	18	7
Sweetened: Shredded, 1 oz	140	10	13
Grated, ½ cup, 1.3 oz	185	12	18
Cream (canned), ½ cup, 5.2 oz	285	26	12
Milk (canned), ½ cup, 4 oz	225	24	3
Water (center liq.), ½ c., 4¼ oz	25	0	4.5
Filberts or Hazelnuts:			
Shelled, 18-20 nuts	180	17	4.5
Chopped, ¼ cup, 1 oz	180	18	5
Ground, ¼ cup, 0.6 oz	120	12	3
Ginkgo Nuts, can., 14 med., 1 oz	32	0.5	6.5
Hickory, 30 small nuts, 1 oz	200	18	5
Macadamia Nuts, shelled:			
Raw, 7 med./14 small, 1 oz	200	21	4
½ cup, 2.3 oz	480	51	10
Dry Roasted, 1 oz	205	22	4
½ cup, 2.4 oz	480	51	9
Choc. coated, 2-3 pces, 1 oz	170	12	14
Mixed Nuts: 18-22 nuts, 1 oz	170	15	7
Planters: Dry Roasted/Honey	160	12	9
Oil Roasted, all types	170	16	6
Sweet Roasts, 26 pces, 1 oz	160	12	10
Nut Toppings: Chopped, 1 T., ¼ oz	40	4	1.5

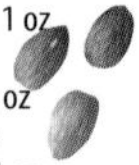

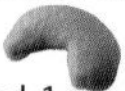

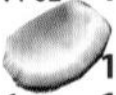

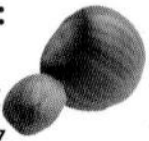

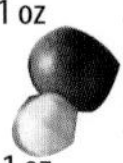

Per 1 oz Unless Indicated — **C** **F** **Cb**

	C	F	Cb
Peanuts:			
Raw/Dried:			
In shell, 1 oz	117	10	3
Shelled, 1 oz	160	14	4.5
Boiled, shelled, ½ cup, 3.1 oz	285	20	19
Roasted: 30 lge./60 sml., 1 oz	165	14	6
1 cup, 5.1 oz	860	76	22
Chopped, 3 Tbsp, 1 oz	165	14	6
Planters: Cocktail, 1 oz	170	14	6
Rich Roasted in Choc., 2½ oz	220	14	19
Roasted in Shell, Salted, 1 oz	160	14	5
Dry Roasted, 1oz	160	13	6
Honey/ & Dry Roasted, 1 oz	160	13	8
Spanish Raw, 1 oz	150	13	6
Spanish Redskin, 1 oz	180	14	5
Sweet N' Crunchy, 1 oz	140	7	16
Pecans: Kernel halves, 1 oz	195	20	4
(20 Jumbo or 31 large halves)			
1 cup halves, 3.8 oz	755	78	15
Chopped, ½ cup, 2 oz	380	39	7.5
Oil Roasted, 15 halves, 1 oz	205	20	4
Honey Roasted, 1 oz	200	21	4
Pilinuts, dried, ¼ cup, 1 oz	215	24	1
Pine Nuts, dried, 1 Tbsp, 10g	70	7	1.5
Pistachios: Unshelled, ½ cup, 2 oz	165	14	7
Shelled, ¼ cup, 45 nuts, 1 oz	170	14	8.5
Lance, 1.1 oz package	95	7	4
Sesame Nut Mix: *Planters,* 1 oz	160	13	9
Soy Nuts: Dry Roasted, 1 oz	130	6	9
½ cup, 3 oz	390	18	28
Dr Soy: Choc coated, 1 oz pkg	140	7	13
Flavors, average, 1 oz	150	8	8
Trail Mix *(Planters):* Fruit & Nut, 1 oz	140	9	14
Golden Nut Crunch, 1 oz	160	11	12
Honey Nut & Caramel, 1 oz	160	10	16
Mixed Nuts & Raisins, 1 oz	150	11	10
Nut & Chocolate, 1 oz	160	10	16
Nuts, Seeds & Raisins, 1 oz	160	12	11
Spicy Nuts & Cajun Sticks, 1 oz	150	11	13
Sweet & Nutty, 1 oz	150	10	14
Walnuts:			
Black: 15-20 halves, 1 oz	175	17	3
Chopped, ¼ cup, 1.1 oz	195	18	3
English/Persian:			
14 halves, 1 oz	185	18	4
Chopped, ¼ cup, 1 oz	190	19	4
Ground, ¼ cup, 0.7 oz	130	13	3

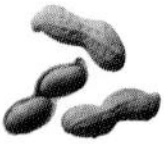

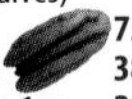

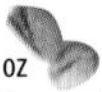

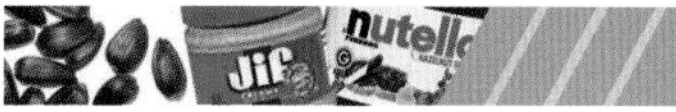

Quick Guide

Peanut Butter: *Average All Brands*	C	F	Cb
1 level tsp, 6g	**35**	3	1.5
1 level Tbsp, 0.6 oz	**105**	8.5	3.5
2 level Tbsp, 1.2 oz	**210**	17	7
1 oz Quantity	**170**	14	6
½ cup, 5 oz	**850**	70	30
Jif: Reduced Fat, 2 Tbsp	**190**	12	15
Creamy; Crunchy; Simply, 2 Tbsp	**190**	16	7
Peanut Butter & Honey, 2 Tbsp	**190**	15	11
Laura Scudder's: Reg./Org., 2 T, 1.1 oz	**210**	16	6
Reduced-Fat, 2 T, 1¼ oz	**200**	12	12
Peter Pan: Plus (Vits/Mins) 2 T., 1.2 oz	**190**	16	6
Honey Roast, 2 Tbsp, 1.2 oz	**190**	14	12
Peanut Wonder, 2 Tbsp	**100**	2.5	13
Smucker's: Honey Swtnd., 2 Tbsp	**200**	16	9
Goober Grape/Strawb., 2 Tbsp	**160**	9	16
Skippy: Reduced Fat, 2 Tbsp	**190**	12	15
Squeeze Stix, 1 Tube, 0.9 oz	**140**	12	5

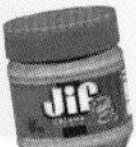

Peanut Butter & Jelly Sandwich

1 sandwich, with 2 oz Bread:

	C	F	Cb
Lightly spread: (1 Tbsp. P'nut Butter + 1 Tbsp Jelly)	**310**	10	48
Thickly spread: (2 Tbsp. P'nut Butter + 2 Tbsp Jelly)	**480**	19	67

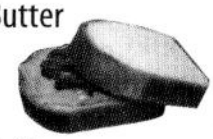

Nutella

Nut & Chocolate Spread	C	F	Cb
1 Tbsp, ½ oz	**50**	3	6
2 Tbsp, 1 oz	**100**	5.5	12

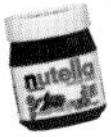

Note: *Nutella* contains approximately 50% sugar and only 13% hazelnuts

Other Nut & Seed Butters

	C	F	Cb
Almond Butter, 1 Tbsp, ½ oz	**100**	10	3.5
Almond Butter Honey Rstd, 1 T.	**90**	7	5.5
Beanut Butter, 1 Tbsp, ½ oz	**90**	5.5	7
Cashew Butter, 1 Tbsp, ½ oz	**95**	8	4.5
Hazelnut Butter, 1 Tbsp, ½ oz	**105**	10	2.5
Pecan Butter, 1 Tbsp, ½ oz	**110**	10	2
Pistachio Butter, 1 Tbsp, ½ oz	**90**	6.5	4.5
Sesame Butter (Tahini), 1 T., ½ oz	**90**	8	3
Soy Nut Butter, 1 Tbsp, ½ oz	**75**	5	4

Tahini ~ *See Sesame Butter*

Seeds

	C	F	Cb
Alfalfa Seeds, sprouted, ½ c., ½ oz	**5**	0	1
Caraway, Fennel, 1 tsp	**7**	0.5	1
Cottonseed Kernels, roasted, 1 Tbsp	**50**	3.5	2
Flax Seeds, 3 Tbsp, 1 oz	**140**	9	9
Lotus Seeds, dried, ½ cup, ½ oz	**55**	0.5	10
Poppy Seeds, 1 tsp	**15**	1	1
Pumpkin & Squash Seeds, whole:			
Roasted/Tamari, 1 oz	**150**	12	4
½ cup, 4 oz	**590**	48	15
Dried, (hulled), ¼ cup, 1 oz	**155**	13	5
Safflower Kernels, dried, 1 oz	**150**	11	10
Sesame Seeds:			
Dried, 1 Tbsp, 9g	**50**	4.5	2
Roasted/Toasted, 1 oz	**160**	14	7.5
Sunflower Kernels/Seed:			
Dried, ¼ cup without hulls, ¼ oz	**200**	18	7
Dry Roasted, 1 Tbsp, 8g	**45**	4	2
¼ cup, 1 oz	**165**	14	7
Oil Roasted, ⅕ cup, 1 oz	**170**	14	6.5
Watermelon Seeds, dried, ¼ cup, 1 oz	**150**	13	4

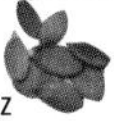

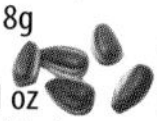

Nut eaters are healthier and live longer, say scientists.

Nuts are a nutritious source of protein, vitamins, minerals, fiber, healthy fats, and antioxidants.

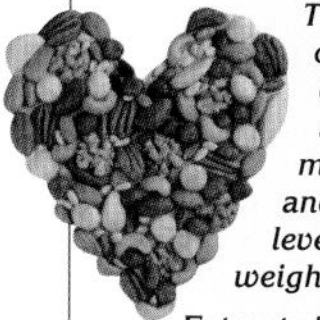

The fat and fiber of nuts can help reduce blood cholesterol. Their protein and fiber also promotes meal satiety (fullness) and reduces hunger levels – of benefit in weight control.

Eat nuts instead of high-sugar snacks, candy and soft drinks. Add chopped nuts to breakfast cereals.

Quick Guide C F Cb

Pancakes

Plain: *Average All Types*

	C	F	Cb
Small (3" diam.), ¾ oz	50	2	6
Medium (4" diam.), 1¼ oz	85	3.5	11
Large (5" diam.), 2½ oz	175	7.5	22

Add Extra for Syrups/Butter

	C	F	Cb
Pancake Syrup: Regular, 1 Tbsp	50	0	13
¼ cup, 4 Tbsp	210	0	52
Lite, 1 Tbsp	25	0	6
¼ cup, 4 Tbsp	100	0	26
Butter/Margarine: Regular, 1 T.	100	11	0
Whipped, 1 Tbsp	70	7.5	0

Waffles

	C	F	Cb
Homemade: 7" waffle, 2½ oz	245	13	26
From Mix: 7" waffle, 2½ oz	205	8	28

Frozen Breakfasts

Aunt Jemima

	C	F	Cb
Pancakes: Buttermilk (3)	200	3.5	37
Homestyle (3)	200	3.5	37
Low-Fat (3)	190	2.5	35
Whole Grain (3)	230	6	38
Mini Pancakes (11)	240	4	46
Frozen Breakfasts:			
French Toast, Cinnamon, 2 slices	220	6	34
French Toast, Homestyle, 2 slices	240	6	39
French Toast, Sticks, 5 sticks	330	11	54

Eggo *(Kellog's)*

	C	F	Cb
French Toast: Toaster Swirlz, set of 4	120	3	20
French Toaster Sticks, avg., (2)	220	6	38
Stuffed French Toaster Sticks (2)	310	7	55
Pancakes: Buttermilk, 3 pancakes	280	9	44
Jungle, 3 pancakes	280	8	46
Nutri-Grain, 3 pancakes	240	7	40

Pillsbury

	C	F	Cb
Pancakes: Mini, average, (14)	425	7	88
Chocolate Chip (3)	270	5	50
French Toast Sticks (6)	360	7	69
Dunkables Cinn. Bites/Icing (3)	140	4.5	23
Toaster Strudel, avg. (1)	190	9	26

Krusteaz

	C	F	Cb
Pancakes: Mini (12)	220	2.5	43
Buttermilk (3)	280	4	52
French Toast: Average, 1 slice	115	2.5	18
Sticks, 4 sticks	230	5	41

Weight Watchers

	C	F	Cb
Breakfast Quesadilla	220	6	28
English Muffin S'wich, avg.	210	6	27
Stuffed Breakfast S/wich	240	7	28

Pancake Brands C F Cb

	C	F	Cb
Atkins: All-Purpose, 2 tsp. dry mix	30	0	5
Bake Mix, ¼ cup dry mix	80	0.5	8
Aunt Jemima			
Buckwheat, 4 x 4"	170	6	26
Buttermilk, 4 x 4"	180	6	25
Original Complete, 2 x 4"	160	1.5	32
Original, 4 x 4" pancakes	250	8	37
Whole Wheat Blend, 3 x 4" pancakes	200	6	29
Betty Crocker Pancake Mixes			
Complete Original/Buttermilk, 3	200	2.5	40
Bisquick (Shake 'N Pour), 3	200	3	38
CarbSense: 2 pancakes prep.	320	15	9
Hungry Jack Pancakes			
Mixes: *Per ⅓ Cup (Prepared)*			
Buttermilk: Complete, 3 x 4"	150	1.5	31
Original, w. 2% Milk, Oil, Egg	250	8	37
w. Skim Milk, Oil, Egg Whites	180	1	37
Extra Lights: Complete (3)	150	2	30
Potato Pancakes, 2 Tbsp mix	70	0	15
Microwave (frozen): Pancakes (3)	270	4.5	51
Krusteaz: No Sugar, prepared,			
3 x 4" pancakes	180	5	23
Northern Pines: 3 x 4" pancakes	380	7	71

Frozen Waffles

	C	F	Cb
Aunt Jemima: Buttermilk (2)	200	5	33
Homestyle (2); Blueberry (2)	190	5	32
Low-Fat (2)	160	2.5	30
Eggo *(Kellog's)*: Minis, avg. (3)	250	8	39
Original: Chocolate Chip (2)	210	7	32
Cinnamon Toast (3)	290	10	46
French Vanilla (2)	200	8	27
Other varieties, avg. (2)	190	6	30
Flip Flops, avg. (2)	190	6	29
Homestyle: Original (2)	180	6	27
Lego (2)	190	6	30
Nutri-Grain: Average (2)	170	4.5	29
Low-Fat (2)	140	2.5	28
Special K, 99% Fat-Free (3)	190	1	37
Waf-Fulls (1)	150	5	27
GO-LEAN *(Kashi)*: Average (1)	90	1.5	16
Hungry Jack: Blueberry, 1 waffle	105	4	17
Buttermilk; Homestyle (1)	95	3	15
Nature's Path: Average (1)	120	4	18
Lifestream: Gorilla; Koala, avg.	105	3.5	16
Other varieties, avg. (1)	120	4	17
Pillsbury: Waffles, avg. (2)	90	2.5	15
Waffle Sticks (6) & syrup	340	7	64
Van's: Belgian Original (1)	85	2	15
97% Fat Free (1)	90	1	15
Mini Homestyle (8), avg.	120	4	20

Updated Nutrition Data ~ www.CalorieKing.com
Persons with Diabetes ~ See Disclaimer (Page 24)

- Pasta includes all shapes and sizes; (e.g. spaghetti, fettuccini, elbows, shells, twists, sheets, cannelloni, tubes, ziti,).
- All regular pasta products have the same cals/fat/carb. on a weight basis.
- 1 oz Dry = approx. 2½ -3 oz cooked.

Dry Spaghetti/Pasta

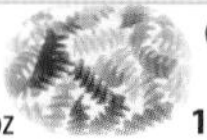

	C	F	Cb
1 oz quantity	105	0.5	21
1lb box/pkg., 16 oz	1685	7	339
Elbows, 1 cup, 3¾ oz	380	2	80
Shells, small, 1 cup, 3¼ oz	330	1.5	69
Spirals, 1 cup, 3 oz	305	1.5	64

Cooked Spaghetti/Pasta

	C	F	Cb
Plain, All Types (no added fat):			
Firm/Al Dente (8-10 mins.), 1 oz	42	0.5	8.5
Medium (11-13 mins.), 1 oz	37	0.5	7.5
Tender (14-20 mins.), 1 oz	32	0.5	7
(Longer cooking increases water absorbed)			
Spaghetti, ½ cup, 2 ½ oz	90	0.5	18
Medium serving, 1 cup, 5 oz	225	1.5	44
Large Serving, 2 cups, 10 oz	450	3	88
Extra Large, 3 cups, 15 oz	675	5	132
Elbows/Spirals, 1 cup, 5 oz	220	1.5	43
Small Shells, 1 cup, 4 oz	180	1	36
Protein-fortified: Dry, 1 c., 3⅓ oz	350	2	63
Cooked, 1 cup, 5 oz	230	0.5	45
Spinach/Vegetable: Dry, 1 c., 3 oz	310	1	61
Cooked, 1 cup, 5 oz	180	0.5	38
Whole-wheat: Dry, 1 c., 3¾ oz	365	1.5	79
Cooked, 1 cup, 5 oz	175	1	37

Fresh Pasta (Refrigerated)

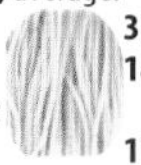

	C	F	Cb
Plain/Spinach/Tomato, average:			
As purchased, 4.5 oz	370	3	70
Cooked, 1 cup, 5 oz	185	1.5	35
Home-made, without egg:			
Cooked, 1 cup, 5 oz	175	1	35
Buitoni			
Cut Pasta: *Per ⅓ of 9 oz Pkg*			
Angel Hair	230	2.5	43
Fettuccine	260	3	46
Linguine	240	2.5	45
Spinach Fettuccine	260	3	46
Ravioletti, Three Cheese, 1 c., 90g	270	5	43

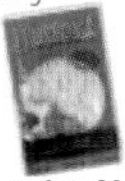

Buitoni (Cont):	C	F	Cb
Ravioli: Chkn & Rstd Garlic, 1¼ cup	330	10	47
Classic Beef, 1¼ cup	350	10	49
Four Cheese, 1¼ cups	330	10	45
Light Four Cheese, 1¼ cups	260	4.5	41
Whole Wheat Four Chse, 1¼ cups	320	11	40
Tortellini: Herb Chkn, 1 cup, 4 oz	350	10	52
Spinach Cheese, 1 cup, 3.7 oz	320	7	49
Three Cheese, 1 cup, 3.7 oz	320	7	50
Tortelloni: Chse & Rstd Garlic, 1 c.	270	8	37
Portabello Mushr. & Chse, 1 cup	290	6	49
Other varieties, avg., 1 cup	330	10	47

Pasta Sauces: *See Page 148*

Macaroni & Cheese

	C	F	Cb
Packaged: *Kraft/Hormel ~ See Page 114-115*			
Restaurant, average: Side, 9 oz	265	13	26
Medium serving, 16 oz	350	17	34
Large serving, 2 cups, 18 oz	700	34	68

Noodles

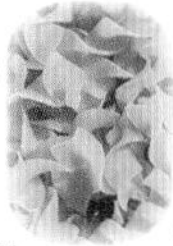

	C	F	Cb
Plain/Egg: Dry, 1 oz	110	1.5	20
1 cup, 1⅓ oz	145	1.5	27
Cooked: 1 oz	40	0.5	7
½ cup, 2¾ oz	110	1.5	20
1 cup, 5½ oz	220	3.5	40
Stir-Fried: 1 cup, 5½ oz	270	9	40
2 cup serving, 11 oz	540	18	80
Yolk Free (Cooked): *Per Cup*			
'No Yolks' (Foulds), 2 oz	210	0.5	41
Passover Gold (Manischewitz)	200	0	41
Chinese: Cellophane/Rice, dry, 1 oz	100	0	25
Chow Mein/hard, dry, 1 oz	150	9	16
Japanese: Soba, dry, 1 oz	95	0.5	21
cooked, 1 cup, 4 oz	115	0.5	24
Somen, dry, 1 oz	100	0.5	21
cooked, 1 cup, 6 oz	230	0.5	49
Japanese Style Pan Fried:			
Maruchan's Yaki-Sobu, 5.6 oz cup	260	3	50
Ramen Noodles (Maruchan/Nissin): *See Page 116*			
Rice Noodles: Dry, 3.5 oz	365	0.5	83
Cooked, 1 cup, 6.2 oz	190	0.5	44
Stir Fry (Yakisoba), 3.5 oz serving	430	6	52
Udon (Chikara), avg., 7.5 oz pkt	250	1	52
Simply Asia/Thai Kitchen ~ *Page 117*			

Egg Roll/Won Ton Wrappers

	C	F	Cb
Egg/Spring Roll (1), 0.8 oz	65	0	15
Won Ton Wrapper (1), ¼ oz	20	0	4

Quick Guide

Fruit Pies: Average All Brands (9")

Apple; Blueberry; Cherry:	C	F	Cb
Small, 1/8 pie, 4¾ oz	320	15	46
Medium, 1/6 pie, 6⅓ oz	425	20	61
Large, 1/4 pie, 9½ oz	640	30	92
Whole Pie (9"), 38oz	2560	120	368

Other Pies: Per Serving (1/6 of 8" Pie)

	C	F	Cb
Chocolate Cream Pie	345	22	38
Custard; Coconut Custard	270	14	31
Lemon Chiffon Pie	360	14	50
Lemon Meringue	360	13	57
Pecan Pie	440	23	57
Pumpkin Pie	300	12	42
Strawberry Pie	230	9	37

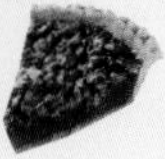

Brands ~ Per Serving

	C	F	Cb
Denny's: Apple Pie, 7 oz	470	21	68
French Silk, 7 oz	737	56	68
Hostess: Fruit; Cherry, 4.5 oz	480	20	68
Lemon, 4.5 oz	490	22	69
Long John Silver's: Pecan Pie	370	15	23
Chocolate Cream Pie	310	22	34
Pineapple Cream Pie	290	13	39
Marie Callender's			
Cobbler, avg., ¼ pkg, 4 oz	290	15	36
Mrs Smith's: Peach Cobbler, 1/8 pie	240	8	41
Deep Dish Apple, 1/12 pie	290	14	40
Slices: Apple; Peach, 1 pce	270	13	36
Dutch Apple, 1 piece	250	10	40
Sara Lee			
Pies: Choc Dream Pie, 1/8 pie	420	24	47
Choc Mint Creme Pie, 1/8 pie	420	27	44
Key West Lime Pie, 1/8 pie	380	18	50
Peach Pie, 1/8 pie	310	15	42
Southern Pecan Pie, 1/8 pie	470	23	62
Oven Fresh Pies (9", 37 oz Box): *Per Slice (4.6 oz)*			
Apple Pie, 1/8	340	16	47
Cherry Pie, 1/8	340	16	45
Mince Pie; Blueberry Pie, 1/8, avg.	380	17	53
Pumpkin Pie, 1/8	260	10	39
Southern Sweet Potato Pie, 1/8	280	9	45
Simple Sweets: Apple Pie, ¼ pie	290	15	45
Cherry Pie, ¼ pie	330	16	45
Tastykake: Fruit Pie, average	390	19	47
French Apple Pie	330	12	55
Coconut Cream Pie	370	20	40
Lemon Pie	300	14	45

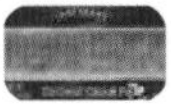

Croissants

	C	F	Cb
Average all Brands			
Plain/Butter/Cheese: Mini, 1 oz	115	6	13
Small, 1½ oz	170	9	19
Medium, 2 oz	230	12	26
Large, 2½ oz	290	15	32
Extra Large, 3 oz	330	19	37
Sweet Croissants:			
Almond Filled, 3 oz	330	18	39
Chocolate Filled, 3 oz	360	19	43
Dunkin' Donuts: Plain Croissant	330	18	37
Sara Lee: French Style Petite, 2 oz	230	11	26
French Style Original, 1½ oz	170	8	20
Croissant Sandwiches: See Page 172			

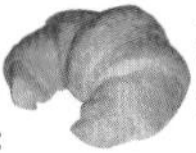

Pastry & Pie Crust

	C	F	Cb
Pie Crust: Baked, 9" diameter shell			
1 Pie Shell, 6½ oz	970	64	87
2-crust Pie, 9", 11¼ oz	1660	109	150
Filo Pastry: 4 sheets, 2½ oz	210	2.5	40
Athens: 5 sheets, 2 oz	180	1	37
Pepp. Farm, 2 sheets, 1½ oz	120	1	25
Puff *(Pepp.Farm)*, ½ sheet, 4.5 oz	510	33	42
1/6 sheet, 1½ oz	170	11	14
Bake & Fill Shell, 1.7 oz	190	13	16
Arrowhead Mills, Pie Crust, 1/8, avg.	110	6	14
Bisquick: Baking Mix,			
Original, ⅓ cup, 1½ oz	160	5	26
Heart Smart, ⅓ cup, 1½ oz	140	2.5	27
Hershey's *(Keebler)*, Choc Crust, 1/8	100	4.5	14
Keebler: Graham Cracker, 1/8 of 9"	110	5	14
Reduced Fat, 1/8	100	3.5	15
Shortbread Crust, 1/8	110	5	14
Graham Crackers Minis (1)	110	5	15
Marie Callendars Deep Dish Pie Shell,			
1/8 pie, 1 oz	140	10	11
Mrs Smith's			
Deep Dish, 9" (1/8)	130	7	14
Nabisco Oreo, 1/8 of 9" crust	100	5	14
Honey Maid Graham, 1/8, 1 oz	220	5	14
Nilla Pie Crust, 1/8, 1 oz	110	6	13
Pillsbury (All Ready), 1/8 pie, 1 oz	110	7	12
Trader Joe's, Pie Crust, 1/8 pie	190	13	17

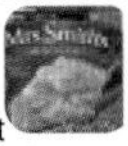

Pie Fillings (Canned)

	C	F	Cb
Fruit: *Average all Fruits*			
(Apple/Blueberry/Cherry/Strawberry)			
Sweetened: ⅓ cup, 3.2oz	90	0	22
1 cup, 9½ oz	270	0	66
1 can, 21 oz	600	0	150
Light/Lite, ⅓ c., 3.2 oz	60	0	15
Unsweetened, ⅓ c., 3.2 oz	35	0	9
Lemon Cream/Creme, ⅓ c., 3.2 oz	130	1.5	28

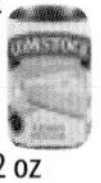

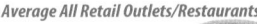

Pizzas ~ Ready-To-Eat **C** **F** **Cb**

Average All Retail Outlets/Restaurants

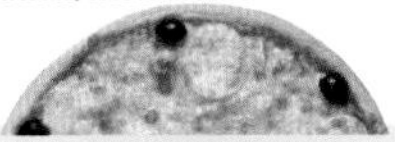

Cheese Pizza
Medium Size (12"):

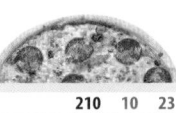

	C	F	Cb
Thin Crust:			
⅛ Pizza (1 slice)	200	8	22
½ Pizza (4 slices)	800	32	88
Whole Pizza (8 slices)	1600	64	172
Deep Dish/Pan:			
⅛ Pizza (1 slice)	270	13	27
½ Pizza (4 slices)	1080	52	108
Whole Pizza (8 slices)	2160	104	216

Pepperoni
Medium Size (12"):

	C	F	Cb
Thin Crust:			
⅛ Pizza (1 slice)	210	10	23
½ Pizza (4 slices)	840	40	84
Whole Pizza (8 slices)	1680	80	168
Deep Dish/Pan:			
⅛ Pizza (1 slice)	280	15	27
½ Pizza (4 slices)	1120	60	108
Whole Pizza (8 slices)	2240	120	216

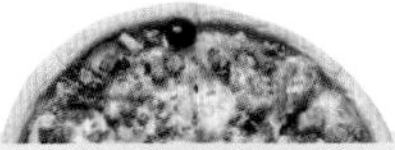

Supreme:
Medium Size (12"):

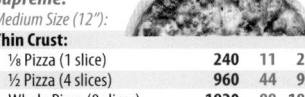

	C	F	Cb
Thin Crust:			
⅛ Pizza (1 slice)	240	11	23
½ Pizza (4 slices)	960	44	92
Whole Pizza (8 slices)	1920	88	184
Deep Dish/Pan:			
⅛ Pizza (1 slice)	310	16	28
½ Pizza (4 slices)	1240	64	112
Whole Pizza (8 slices)	2480	128	224

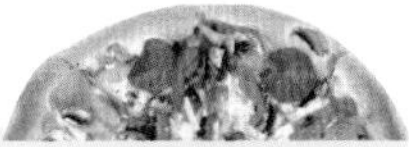

Meat Deluxe
Medium Size (12"):

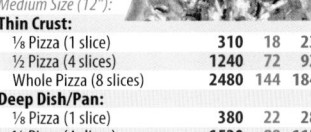

	C	F	Cb
Thin Crust:			
⅛ Pizza (1 slice)	310	18	23
½ Pizza (4 slices)	1240	72	92
Whole Pizza (8 slices)	2480	144	184
Deep Dish/Pan:			
⅛ Pizza (1 slice)	380	22	28
½ Pizza (4 slices)	1520	88	112
Whole Pizza (8 slices)	3040	176	224

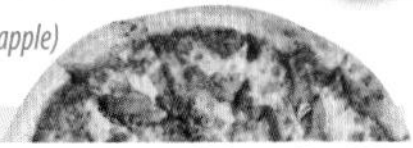

Hawaiian (Ham & Pineapple)
Medium Size (12"):

	C	F	Cb
Thin Crust:			
⅛ Pizza (1 slice)	190	7	23
½ Pizza (4 slices)	760	28	92
Whole Pizza (8 slices)	1520	56	184
Deep Dish/Pan:			
⅛ Pizza (1 slice)	250	11	28
½ Pizza (4 slices)	1000	44	112
Whole Pizza (8 slices)	2000	88	224

Veggie:
Similar to Hawaiian

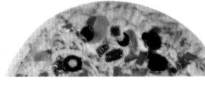

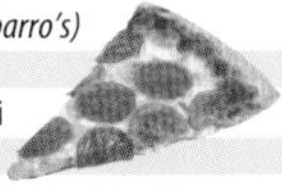

Single Slices
(Extra Large):
(Example: Sbarro's)

	C	F	Cb
Cheese	460	13	60
Pepperoni	730	37	61
Sausage	670	31	60
Supreme	630	27	63

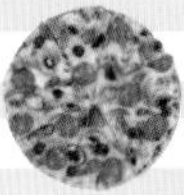

Individual Pizza (6")
Deep Dish/Pan
(Approx. 9 oz weight):

	C	F	Cb
Cheese	600	24	69
Hawaiian	570	21	70
Meat Deluxe	900	50	70
Pepperoni	650	30	67
Veggie	560	22	70

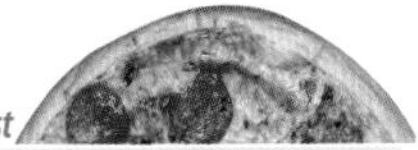

Large (14") Thin Crust

	C	F	Cb
Cheese: ⅛ Pizza	290	12	30
½ Pizza	1160	48	120
Hawaiian: ⅛ pizza	260	9	33
½ Pizza	1040	36	132
Pepperoni: ⅛ Pizza	310	15	30
½ Pizza	1240	60	120
Supreme: ⅛ Pizza	340	17	32
½ Pizza	1360	68	128
Meat Deluxe: ⅛ Pizza	440	26	31
½ Pizza	1760	104	124
Veggie: ⅛ Pizza	260	10	32
½ Pizza	1040	40	128

Frozen Pizzas   C   F   Cb

	C	F	Cb
Amy's: Per 1/3 pizza			
Cheese; Spinach; Pesto, avg.	310	12	38
Cheese Pesto	360	18	37
Cheese Pizza	300	14	31
Mushroom & Olive	250	9	33
Roasted Vegetable	270	9	42
California Pizza Kitchen			
BBQ Chicken, Small, 1/3 pizza, 4.3 oz	270	9	33
Five Cheese & Tomato, small, 1/3 pizza	320	15	29
Thai Chicken, small, 1/3 pizza, 4.3 oz	280	10	34
Crispy Thin Crust: Per 1/3 Pizza			
Garlic Chicken; Margherita	290	13	31
Sicilian Recipe, 1/3 pizza, 4.2 oz	310	14	30
Swt & Spicy Ital. Sausage; White	290	12	31
Individual Pizza: Four Cheese, 6.9 oz	510	17	69
Margherita, 6 oz	420	18	45
Sicilian, 5.5 oz	450	22	42
Celeste			
Pizza For One: Original, 1 pizza	350	17	39
Deluxe; Pepperoni, Chseburger	410	21	44
Original/Zesty 4 Cheese, avg.	360	16	48
Sausage & Pepperoni; Suprema	470	26	44
Zesty Chicken Supreme	340	15	39
DiGiorno			
Deep Dish: Per 1/6 Pizza			
Pepperoni	340	18	32
Supreme; Three Meat, avg.	320	15	33
For One: Per 1/3 Pizza			
Garlic Bread Crust: Pepperoni	840	44	81
Supreme	850	44	82
Traditional Crust: Pepperoni	770	35	83
Supreme	790	36	85
Microwave: Per 1/2 Pizza			
Four Cheese	370	15	44
Pepperoni; Supreme, avg.	390	18	44
Three Meat	420	19	44
Rising Crust: Per 1/6 Pizza			
Four Cheese	310	11	40
Pepperoni; Supreme, avg.	360	16	40
Thin Crispy Crust: Per 1/3 Pizza			
Four Meat	320	13	37
Grilled Chicken Tomato & Spinach	260	8	33
Ultimate Focaccia: Per 1/6 Pizza			
Four Cheese	380	18	43
Meat Trio; Supreme; Pepperoni	390	19	43
Ultimate Thin Crust: Per 1/3 Pizza			
Four Cheese	330	14	33
Four Meat; Pepperoni, avg.	390	20	33
Supreme	360	17	34

	C	F	Cb
Freschetta			
Brick Oven Singles:			
5-Italian Cheese, 1 single, 6 oz	420	18	50
Classic Supreme, 1 single, 6.7 oz	440	18	50
Italian Pepperoni, 1 single, 6.7 oz	480	22	50
Naturally Rising (Large):			
4 Cheese, 1/5 pizza	380	14	46
4 Meat, 1/6 pizza	350	15	40
Pepperoni, 1/6 pizza	340	14	40
Can. Bacon P'apple, 1/5	340	9	49
Supreme, 1/6 pizza	350	14	41
PizzAmore:			
6 Cheese, medium, 2 pces	330	13	40
6 Cheese, large, 1 piece	240	9	29
Meat; Pepperoni; Supreme, avg.,			
Medium, 2 pieces	380	16	41
Large, 1 piece	270	11	29
Stuffed Breadsticks: Garlic (1)	110	3.5	18
Cinnamon w. Cream Cheese (1)	140	4.5	23
12" Ultra Thin: Supreme, 3 slices	350	19	27
5 Cheese; Pepperoni, 3 slices	330	17	25
Healthy Choice: Per Pizza (6 oz)			
French Bread Pizza, Average	350	4.5	54
Cafe Selections Pizza, Average	370	4	58
Jeno's: Per Pizza (7 oz)			
Crispy 'N Tasty: Cheese	440	20	50
Sausage; Pepperoni, average	490	25	50
Heaven's Bistro: Per 1/3 Pizza			
Chicken w. BBQ Sauce, 5 oz	270	2	48
Grilled Vegetable, 5.1 oz	230	1	42
Pepperoni; Sausage, avg., 4½ oz	250	3	42
Three Cheese, 4.3 oz	250	3	42
Home Run Inn (Chicago):			
Large: Cheese, 1/6, 5.3 oz	400	21	39
Sausage/Supreme, avg., 1/6, 6 oz	430	22	38
Sausage & Pepperoni, 1/6, 6 oz	450	24	38
Deep Dish, Sausage, 1/5, 5½ oz	390	20	37
Kashi, average, 1/3 pizza	300	9	39
Lean Cuisine			
French Bread Pizza: Cheese, 6 oz	370	7	50
Deluxe; Pepperoni, average	310	9	44
Casual Eating: Deluxe, 6 oz	370	9	55
Four Cheese, 6 oz	400	9	59
Rstd Garlic; Mushroom, avg., 6 oz	330	7	39
Roasted Vegetable, 6 oz	330	5	58
Flatbread Melt: Chkn Philly, 6.4 oz	330	8	41
Other varieties, average 6.4 oz	330	9	41
Lean Pockets Pizza, average (1)	280	7	39

Updated Nutrition Data ~ www.CalorieKing.com
Persons with Diabetes ~ See Disclaimer (Page 24)

Frozen Pizzas (Cont) C F Cb

Private Selection

	C	F	Cb
Thin Crust: BBQ Chicken, ⅓	350	14	41
Extra Pepperoni, ⅓ pizza	410	23	29
Sliced Provolone Cheese, ⅓	340	14	38
Gourmet Class: Dble Pepperoni, ⅛	350	16	36
Italian Style Supreme, ⅛ pizza	340	15	37

Red Baron

Classic (Large):

	C	F	Cb
4 Cheese, ¼ pizza	440	18	43
Pepperoni, ⅕ pizza	330	16	32
Supreme, ⅕ pizza	330	15	36
Special Deluxe, ⅕ pizza	330	15	35

Deep Dish Pan Style:

4 Cheese, ⅓ pizza	380	17	41
Meat Trio, ⅓ pizza	410	20	41
Pepperoni, ⅓ pizza	400	20	41
Supreme, ⅓ pizza	420	20	43

Deep Dish Singles:

4 Cheese (1)	430	20	44
Pepperoni (1)	440	22	44
Supreme	420	20	43
Mini Pizzas, Pepperoni (4)	470	26	43
French Bread Pizzas: Supreme (1)	360	15	42
5 Cheese & Garlic (1)	410	22	39
Pepperoni; 3 Meat, average (1)	360	15	42
Pizzeria Style: Per ⅙ Pizza			
4 Cheese; Pepperoni, average	350	14	40
Special Deluxe; Supreme, average	370	16	41
Singles (Thin & Crispy): 4 Cheese	300	16	24
Pepperoni	300	15	27
Stone Hearth: Per ¼ Pizza			
4 Cheese	360	15	40
Pepperoni; Supreme	380	17	40
Thin Crust: Per ¼ of 12" Pizza			
5 Cheese	290	13	32
Pepperoni	320	16	32
Supreme	340	17	33

Reggio's

Individual Pizza: Cheese (1)	250	8	33
Pepperoni, 1 pizza	290	13	33
Sausage & Mushroom (1)	280	10	34
Dinner Size: Cheese, ¼ pizza	330	12	41
Pepperoni & Sausage, ¼ pizza	400	18	41
Sausage; Supreme, average, ¼	380	16	41

Stouffer's: Per ½ Pkg

French Bread Pizzas: Deluxe

Deluxe	430	21	44
Cheese	360	15	43
Extra Cheese	400	18	44
Pepperoni	410	20	43
Sausage & Pepperoni	460	24	43

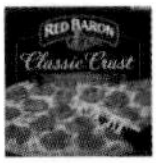

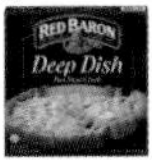

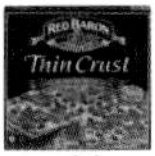

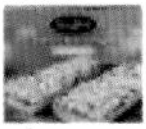

Tombstone

Original: Per ¼ of Large 12" Pizza

	C	F	Cb
4 Meat	390	18	38
Canadian Style Bacon	320	12	37
Deluxe	360	15	39
Extra Cheese	350	15	37
Pepperoni	390	20	37
Pepperoni & Sausage	370	17	37
Sausage/& Mushroom	360	17	38
Supreme	375	18	39
Double Top: Sausage, ⅙ pizza	310	16	27
Sausage & Pepperoni, ⅙ pizza	330	18	26

Harvest Wheat Thin Crust:

Cheese, ¼ pizza	225	7.5	27
Pepperoni, ¼ pizza	260	10	29
Supreme, ¼ pizza	260	10	29
Light Veg., ⅕ pizza	230	6	31
Thin Crust: 3 Cheese, ¼ pizza	310	15	28
Pepperoni; Sausage, avg., ¼	320	18	29
Brick Oven Style: Cheese, ¼ pizza	260	12	29
Other varieties, average, ¼ pizza	320	16	29

Tony's

Original: Cheese, ⅓ pizza	360	14	44
Pepperoni, ⅓ pizza	390	17	43
Saus.; Pepperoni; Supreme, avg. ⅓	410	20	44
Deep Dish (Individual): Cheese (1)	390	16	47
Pepperoni (1)	480	24	49

Totino's

Crisp Crust Party Pizza: Per ½ Pizza

Cheese	310	15	33
Pepperoni	370	20	35
Pizza Rolls: Cheese (6), 3 oz	200	8	26
Pepperoni (6), 3 oz	220	10	24

Trader Joe's: Per ⅓ Pizza

4 Cheese	350	14	42
Vegetarian	330	11	43

Verdi (Safeway Select)

Small (8"): Per ⅓ Pizza

BBQ Style Chicken	250	8	34
Margherita	360	12	48
Roasted Murshr.; Vegetables, avg.	250	7	35

Weight Watchers (Smart Ones): Per Pizza

Deluxe	360	9	52
Four Cheese	390	10	56
Pepperoni	390	11	50
Veggie Ultimate	330	6	54

Wolfgang Puck

All Natural Pizzas: Per ⅓ Pizza

BBQ Chicken	360	15	40
Cheese	340	16	33
Four Cheese; Tomato & Pesto	330	17	30
Margherita	330	16	33
Uncured Pepperoni	360	19	32

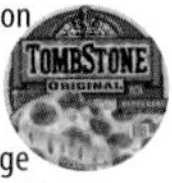

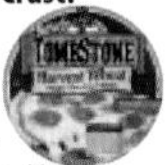

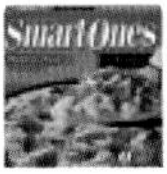

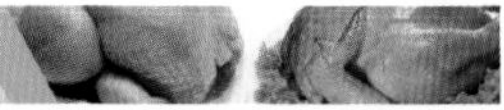

Quick Guide

Chicken	C	F	Cb
From 3lb ready-to-cook chicken			
Breast/Wing Quarter			
Roasted: With skin	300	15	0
Without skin	185	5	0
Fried, batter dipped	530	30	17
Leg Quarter:			
Thigh & Drumstick			
Roasted: With skin, 4 oz	265	15	0
Without skin, 3.35 oz	180	8	0
Fried, batter dipped	430	25	14
(KFC: See Fast-Foods Section)			

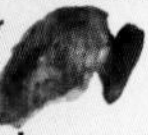

Per 4 oz Edible Portion

	C	F	Cb
Average of Light Meat: Per 4 oz (no bone)			
Roasted: with skin	250	12	0
without skin	175	4.5	0
Stewed: with skin	230	12	0
without skin	180	4.5	0
Fried: Batter-dipped, 4 oz	315	17	11
Flour-coated, 4 oz	280	14	2
Average of Dark Meat: Per 4 oz (no bone)			
Roasted: with skin	290	18	0
without skin	235	11	0
Stewed: with skin	265	17	0
without skin	220	10	0
Fried: Batter-dipped, 4 oz	340	21	11
Flour-coated, 4 oz	325	19	5

Chicken Parts

	C	F	Cb
Broilers or Fryers: Edible Weights (no bone)			
Breast: Per ½ Breast			
Raw: With skin, 5 oz	250	14	0
Without skin, 4¼ oz	130	1.5	0
Roasted: With skin, 3½ oz	195	8	0
Without skin, 3 oz	140	3	0
Stewed: With skin, 4 oz	200	8	0
Without skin, 3¼ oz	145	3	0
Fried: Batter-dipped, 5 oz	365	19	13
Flour-coated, w. skin, 3½ oz	220	9	2
Drumstick: Per Drumstick			
Roasted: With skin, 2 oz	115	6	0
Without skin, 1½ oz	75	2.5	0
Fried: Batter-dipped, 2½ oz	195	11	6
Flour-coated, 1¾ oz	120	7	1
Stewed: With skin, 2 oz	115	6	0
Without skin, 1½ oz	80	3	0

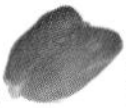

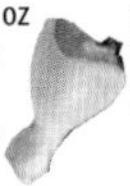

Thigh Portion: Edible Wt. (no bone)	C	F	Cb
Raw: With skin, 3.3 oz	200	14	0
(4¼ oz with bone)			
Without skin, 2.4 oz	80	3	0
Roasted: With skin, 2¼ oz	155	10	0
Without skin, 2 oz	110	6	0
Stewed: With skin, 2½ oz	160	10	0
Without skin, 2 oz	105	5	0
Fried: Batter-dipped, 3 oz	240	14	8
Flour-coated, 2¼ oz	165	9	2
Wing: Per Wing			
Raw Weight 3.2 oz (with bone)			
Raw: With skin	110	8	0
Without skin	35	1	0
Roasted: With skin	100	7	0
Without skin	45	2	0
Fried: Batter-dipped	160	11	5
Flour-coated	105	7	1
Stewed: With skin, 4 oz	100	7	0
Buffalo Wings: See Fast-Foods Section			
Neck: Simmered, with skin	95	7	0
Without skin	30	2	0
Skin Only: Skin from ½ Chicken			
Raw skin, 2¾ oz	275	26	0
Roasted skin, 2 oz	255	23	0
Stewed skin, 2½ oz	260	24	0
Fried, Flour-coated, 2 oz	280	24	5
Fried, Batter-dipped, 6¾ oz	750	55	44
Roasters			
Average of Light & Dark Meat:			
Roasted: With skin, 4 oz	250	15	0
Without skin, 4 oz	190	8	0
Light Meat: Without skin, roasted	175	5	0
Dark Meat: Without skin, roasted	200	10	0
Stewing Chicken			
Average of Light & Dark Meat: Per 4 oz Stewed			
With skin	325	22	0
Without skin	270	14	0
Light Meat: Without skin	240	9	0
Dark Meat: Without skin	290	17	0
Capon Chicken			
Roasted: With skin, 4 oz	260	13	0
½ Chicken, with skin	1460	74	0

Chicken Offal & Stuffing	C	F	Cb
Giblets: Simmered, 1 cup	230	7	0.5
Fried, flour-coated, 1 cup	400	20	6
Gizzard, simmered, 1 cup	210	4	0
Heart, simmered, 1 cup	270	12	0.2
Liver: Raw, 4 oz	130	5.5	0
Simmered, 1 cup	215	8.5	1
Liver Pate Fresh, 1 Tbsp, ½ oz	30	2	1
Stuffing: Average, ½ cup	180	9	22

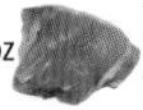

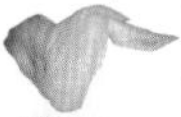

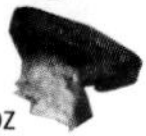

Updated Nutrition Data ~ www.CalorieKing.com
Persons with Diabetes ~ See Disclaimer (Page 24)

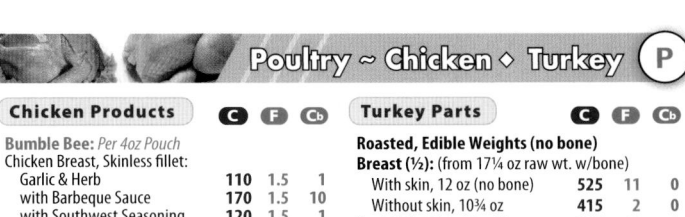

Chicken Products   C F Cb

Bumble Bee: *Per 4oz Pouch*
Chicken Breast, Skinless fillet:

Garlic & Herb	110	1.5	1
with Barbeque Sauce	170	1.5	10
with Southwest Seasoning	120	1.5	1

Foster Farms

Breast, Boneless Skinless (1), 4.7 oz	140	1	0
Chicken Breast Strips, 3 oz	110	2.5	2
Drumsticks (1), 2.8 oz	130	7	0
Wings: Chipotle, 4 wings, 2.9 oz	190	14	1
Honey BBQ, 4 wings, 2.9 oz	170	10	5
Hot & Spice, 4 wings, 2.9 oz	170	13	1
Tyson: Breaded Nuggets (5)	280	18	16
Breast Nuggets (5)	280	16	21
Southern Style Nuggets (6)	270	21	11
Breast Patties: Regular, 2.6 oz	180	11	12
Southern Style (1), 2.6 oz	240	18	10
Wings: Flavored, average (4)	220	15	1
BBQ Style (4), 3½ oz	220	14	9

Duck, Goose, Quail

Duck: Roasted, with skin, 3 oz	290	24	0
Without skin, 3 oz	170	10	0
½ whole duck, with skin	1290	108	0
Goose: Roast, with skin, 3 oz	260	19	0
Without skin, 3 oz	200	11	0
Pheasant, cooked, 3 oz	210	10	0
Quail, cooked, 1 whole, 6 oz	400	24	0

Turkey

Fryer-Roasters: *Per 3 oz Serving*

Roasted: Light Meat, with skin	140	4	0
without skin	120	1	0
Dark Meat: with skin	155	6	0
without skin	140	4	0

½ of Whole Turkey: (Approx. 3¼ lbs raw wt.
w/out neck and giblets; 1.8 lbs cooked wt.)

Roasted: with skin	1650	74	0
without skin	1125	31	0

Ground Turkey, Raw: (4 oz raw wt. = 3 oz ckd wt.)

Regular (85% lean), 4 oz	170	10	0
Lean (93% lean), avg., 4 oz	160	8	0
Foster Farms (94% lean), 4 oz	150	7	0
Jennie-O (93% lean), 4 oz	170	8	0
Trader Joe's (93% lean), 4 oz	150	8	0
Breast, no skin, 4 oz	115	1	0
Patties: Small, 3 oz	130	7	0
Medium, 4 oz	170	10	0
Large, 5.3 oz	225	13	0

Turkey Parts   C F Cb

Roasted, Edible Weights (no bone)
Breast (½): (from 17¼ oz raw wt. w/bone)

With skin, 12 oz (no bone)	525	11	0
Without skin, 10¾ oz	415	2	0

Back (½): With skin, 4½ oz

	265	13	0
Without skin, 3½ oz	165	6	0

Leg (Thigh & Drumstick):
(from 1 lb raw wt. w/bone)

With skin, 8½ oz (no bone)	410	13	0
Without skin, 7¾ oz	355	8.5	0

Wing: (from 7¼ oz raw wt. w/bone)

With skin, 3 oz (no bone)	185	9	0
Without skin, 2 oz	100	2	0
Neck: Simmered, 1 neck, (9 oz w. bone)	275	11	0
Giblets, simm., 1 cup, 5 oz	240	7	3

Young Hens (Roasted)

Light Meat: With skin, 3 oz	175	8	0
Without skin, 3 oz	135	3	0
Dark Meat: With skin, 3 oz	200	11	0
Without skin, 3 oz	165	7	0

Young Toms — Similar to Young Hens

Turkey Products

Banquet: *See Frozen Meals, Page 119*
Foster Farms: Meatballs (3) **150 7 8**
Hormel: Turkey Ham & Chunks (canned), ckd:

Breast & White Turkey, 2 oz	60	1	2
Pastrami, 2 oz	70	3	1
Turkey Ham, 2 oz	70	3	1
Jennie-O, Turkey Bacon, 2 slices	35	3	0
Turkey Bratwurst, 4 oz	170	10	2

John Morrell, Off the Bone,

Roasted Turkey Breast, 4 oz	160	4	12

Louis Rich: 98% Fat Free,
Breast of Turkey

Rotiss'd/Smoked/Rstd, 2 oz, 3 sl.	60	0	0
Franks: Medium, 1½ oz	100	8	2
Large, 2 oz	120	10	3
Turkey Bacon, 2 oz	140	10	0

Lunch Slices: *See Deli Meats, Page 131*
Spam, Oven Roasted Turkey, 2 oz **80 4 2**
Swanson: *Frozen Meals, Page 123*
Trader Joe's, Turkey Meatloaf, 3 oz **140 8 5**

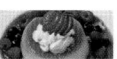
See CalorieKing.com for All Recipes & Serving Sizes

Starters/Appetizers:

Cheesy Grape Balls (1)	20	1.5	1
Shiitake Summer Rolls (1)	120	1	24
Spring Rolls (1)	135	4.5	15

Soups:

Beef Stew	435	8	35
Cheesy Broccoli Potato Soup, 1 cup	150	5	16
Chicken Soup with Rice Dumplings	110	1	22
Chili Con Carne	360	15	25
Creamy Butternut Squash Soup	115	3	22
Spicy Pumpkin Soup	205	5	29
Sweet Potato Soup	120	4	16

Salads:

Apple Raspberry Salad	95	2.5	11
Cherry and Smoked Turkey Salad	265	9	31
Citrus Fruit Salad	125	0.5	30
Green Bean Potato Salad	185	5	32
Hot Rosemary Potato Salad	205	0.5	29
Watermelon Salad	40	0	10

Meat Entrees:

Beef and Mushroom Burgers (2)	450	14	51
Gr. Marinated Lamb Filet, 3½ oz	150	7	1
Lamb and Rosemary Kebobs (1)	230	11	6
Mustard Steak with Tuscan Salad	200	8	4
Veal and Mushrooms	250	10	8

CALORIE KING TIPS
TO REDUCE CALORIES:

- Use non-fat milk in place of whole or 2% milk
- Use low-fat yogurt in place of sour cream
- Skim fat from surface of soups and casseroles after cooling
- Add extra vegetables to soups and hot entrees
- Cakes/cookies/muffins: Replace most or all the fat/oil with applesauce and/or prune puree (Example: *Sunsweet Lighter Bake*)
- Drinks: Replace sugar with no-calorie sweeteners such as *Equal, Stevia, Splenda* and *Sweet 'N Low*

Chicken Entrees:

Baked Chicken with Mushrooms	155	2	4
Baked Rosemary Drumsticks (2)	320	11	22
Basil & Lemon Chicken Thighs (1)	150	9.5	3
Chicken Cacciatore	400	8	33
Chicken Kiev	205	9	9
Easy Chicken Pot Pie	275	12	23
Lemon Chicken with Olives	200	9	8
Mushroom & Chicken Coq au Vin	360	9	9

Fish Entrees:

Fish Cutlets in Herb Tomato Coulis	300	4.5	5
Grilled Fish with Corn & Leek, 4 oz	245	10	12
Stir-Fry Mixed Seafood & Noodles	250	4	28
Thai Fish Cakes	260	4	36
Tuna-Mayo Wrap	250	3.5	26

Vegetarian:

Avocado Tacos (1)	100	3	17
Coconut Vegetable Curry	200	11	12
Eggplant Stuffed with Tofu	320	6	50
Fettuccini w/Tomato & Basil Sauce	340	8	56
Gourmet Vegetable Pizza	170	5	24
Nutty Soy 'n Rice Burgers (1)	140	3.5	23
Veggie Lasagna	185	8.5	14
Veg. Burgers (1)	220	11	13
Zucchini Moussaka	260	5	36

Desserts:

Angel Food Cake	85	0	18
Apple and Rice Pudding	110	0.5	25
Brandy Pumpkin Flan	145	5	17
Fruit Salad Dessert Cake	175	8.5	23
Low-Fat Carrot Cake	185	2	39
Melon Sorbet	100	2	21
Non-Fat Brownies (1)	115	0	26
Non-Fat Chocolate Cupcakes (1)	105	0	22
Non-Fat Vanilla Ice Cream	60	0	11
Watermelon Blueb. Banana Split	175	1	42

Drinks: Per 1 Cup, 8 fl.oz

Apple and Fruit Frappe	135	0	33
Banana Daiquiri	190	2	44
Fruity Iced Tea	50	0	12
Mocha Shake	95	0	14
Pineapple Float	185	6	30
Watermelon Coconut Margarita	235	6	34
Watermelon Kiwi Smoothie	115	0	24

Updated Nutrition Data ~ www.CalorieKing.com
Persons with Diabetes ~ See Disclaimer (Page 24)

White Rice	C	F	Cb
Raw: Short/Med. Grain, 1 c., 7 oz	715	1	158
Long Grain, 1 cup, 6½ oz	675	1	148
Glutinous, 1 cup, 6½ oz	685	1	151
Cooked Rice (Boiled/Steamed):			
Short/Medium Grain:			
½ cup, 3¼ oz	135	0	30
1 cup (½ Pint), 7.2 oz	270	0.5	59
2 cups (1 Pint), 13 oz	480	1	106
Long Grain: ½ cup, 2¾ oz	105	0	22
1 cup, 5½ oz	205	0.5	44
Glutinous/Sticky, ckd 1 c., 6 oz	170	0.5	37
Parboiled, cooked, ½ cup, 3 oz	105	0.5	22
Precook./Instant: Dry,½ c., 3½ oz	370	0	80
Cooked, ½ cup, 3 oz	90	0	20
Wild Rice: Raw, 1 cup, 5½ oz	570	2	120
Cooked, 1 cup, 5¾ oz	165	0.5	35

Brown Rice	C	F	Cb
Average of Short or Long Grain			
Raw/Dry: ½ cup, 3¼ oz	340	2.5	71
1 cup, 6½ oz	685	5.5	143
Cooked: ½ cup, 3½ oz	110	1	22
1 cup, 7 oz	220	2	46

Rice Dishes	C	F	Cb
Chinese Fried Rice:			
½ cup, 2½ oz	140	4.5	21
1 cup, (½ Pint), 5 oz	280	9	42
2 cups, (1 Pint), 10 oz	565	18	84
Mexican Rice: 1 cup	500	12	90
Taco John's, 1 serving (6 oz)	250	5	45
Taco Time, 1 serving (4 oz)	160	2	30
Rice-A-Roni: *See Page 116*			
Rice w. Raisins/Pinenuts, 1 cup	400	11	60
Rice Pilaf: Restaurant, 1 cup	275	7.5	46
O'Charley's, 1 order	200	5	31
Rice Pudding *(Kozy Shack),*			
Original, ½ cup	130	3	22
Risotto, 1 cup	420	12	70
Saffron Rice, 4 oz	175	7	25
Spanish Rice: 1 cup	390	9	72
El Pollo Loco, small, 5 oz	160	1	35
Taco Cabana, 4 oz	180	5	30
Sticky Rice, 5 oz	155	0.5	34
Sushi Rice: 1 Tbsp	25	0	5
1 cup, 5.2 oz	390	0	77

Other Packaged Rice Products:
Rice-A-Roni: See Page 116
Uncle Ben's / Zatarain's: See Page 118

Nutrition & Exercise Manager

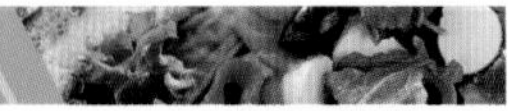

Deli Salads

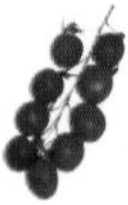

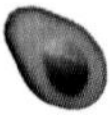

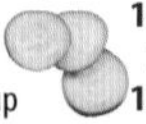

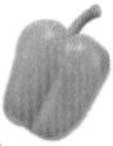

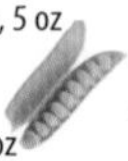

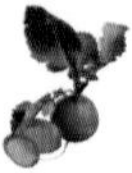

	C	F	Cb
General Average, All Outlets			
Antipasto Salad, ½ c,	135	8	13
3-Bean Salad, ½ cup	110	4	17
Bulgur Salad, ½ cup	70	2	12
Caesar Salad, Classic, 1 c.	200	14	15
Side Salad, no Dress,	25	0	6
Carrot Raisin: No Dressing, ½ cup	20	0	5
with Dressing, ½ cup	135	12	6
Chef's Salad: Regular, no Dress.	620	37	8
w. 2 oz 1000 Island	860	61	8
Chicken Salad, ½ cup/scoop, 4 oz	280	21	2
Coleslaw: Traditional, ½ c.	150	8	18
w. Low Cal Dressing, ½ c.	50	2	8
Corn, Mexican, ½ cup	240	12	33
Cucumber: Non-Oil Dressing, ½ c.	60	0	14
w. Oil Dressing, ½ c.	140	12	8
Eggplant Salad, ½ cup	75	5	7
Fettucini w. veges, ½ cup	135	6	16
Garden Salad, no Dress., 1 c.	10	0	2
Greek Salad, 1 cup	105	8	7
Greek Vegetables, 1 c.	110	8	6
Lettuce, hearts, ½ head	15	0	2.5
Lobster Salad, ½ c., 4 oz	250	21	11
Macaroni Salad, ½ cup, 5 oz	360	26	26
Nicoise, 1 cup	450	32	18
Pasta Salad, ½ cup	200	11	19
Potato Salad: Dijon, 3 oz	120	7	13
w. Mayonnaise, ½ cup, 4 oz	215	15	17
Lowfat, ½ cup	110	1.5	21
Rice Salad, ½ cup	150	10	13
Saffron Rice, 4 oz	175	7	25
Spinach Salad, 1 cup	180	13	13
Tabouli, ½ cup	125	7	13
Three Bean Salad, ½ cup	90	4.5	12
Tomato & Mozzarella, ½ cup	180	14	10
Tortellini w. Basil Pesto, ½ cup	150	9	15
Waldorf w. Mayo, ½ cup	110	7	12
Signature Salads: Per 6 oz Serving			
(Supplied to Deli's and Institutions)			
Antipasto Salad, 6 oz	510	50	4
Artichoke Salad, marinated	400	41	8
California Medley	120	7	15
Cheese Agnolotti	250	8	23
Chicken Salad	420	33	11
Crabmeat Flavored	450	38	20

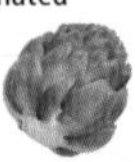

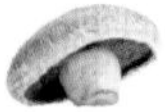

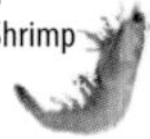

Signature Salads (Cont): *Per 6 oz Serving*	C	F	Cb
Egg Salad	300	23	14
Fresh Button Mushroom	190	16	6
Garden Olive	630	67	3
Ham Salad	400	32	14
Prima Pasta Salad	360	30	18
Seafood Pasta Del Mar	170	10	21
Seafood with Crab & Shrimp	420	34	20
Shrimp Salad	360	32	8
Tuna Salad	450	36	14
Fast-Food Restaurants: *See Page 182*			

Fresh Salad Packs

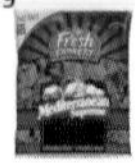

	C	F	Cb
Pre-Packaged (Supermarkets)			
Dole: Caesar Kit, 3½ oz	170	15	8
Asian Crunch Kit, 3½ oz	120	6	12
Bacon Lettuce Kit, 3 oz	130	9	8
Regular Salad Packs *(no added dressing):*			
Classic Coleslaw, 3 oz	25	0	5
Classic Iceberg, 3 oz	15	0	4
Fresh Mates: *Per ¼ Container*			
Broccoli ranch, 1½ cups	230	13	25
Cheddar Bacon Ranch, 1½ c.	370	22	35
Garden Vegetable, 1½ cups	240	14	25
Italian Herb, 1½ cups	270	12	33
Fresh Express			
Complete Salad Kits: *Per Serving, Prepared*			
Asian Supreme, ¼ bag	170	10	17
B.L.T. Caesar, ⅓ bag	170	14	8
Caesar: ⅓ bag	150	13	8
Lite, ⅓ bag	100	7	8
Supreme, ⅓ bag	170	14	8
Mediterranean Supreme, ⅓ bag	150	10	16
Pacifica! Veggie Supreme	220	15	18
Salsa! Ensalada Supreme, ¼ bag	120	8	10

Salad Toppings

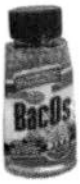

	C	F	Cb
Bacon Bits: Bacos, 1 Tbsp	30	1.5	2
Hormel, 1 Tbsp	25	1.5	0
Chow Mein Noodles, dry, ½ c.	120	7	13
Croutons, 2 Tbsp, 10g	40	1	7
Olives, 5 medium	25	2	0
Sunflower Seeds, 1 Tbsp, 8 g	45	4	1.5
Toasted sliced Almonds, 2 T., ½ oz	85	7	3
Tortilla Chips, 12 chips, 1 oz	140	7	19

Updated Nutrition Data ~ www.CalorieKing.com
Persons with Diabetes ~ See Disclaimer (Page 24)

Quick Guide

Salad Dressings
Average All Brands
Per 2 Tbsp (Approx 1 fl.oz)

	C	F	Cb
Balsamic Vinaigrette: Regular	90	9	3
Light, 2 Tbsp	45	4	2
Fat Free, 2 Tbsp	25	0	6
Blue Cheese: Regular, 2 Tbsp	150	16	2
Regular, ¼ cup, 2 oz	300	32	4
Light, 2 Tbsp	30	1	4
Caesar: Regular, 2 Tbsp	155	17	1
Regular, ¼ cup, 2 oz	310	34	2
Light, 2 Tbsp	70	8	5
Coleslaw: Regular, 2 Tbsp	125	11	8
Regular, ¼ cup, 2 oz	245	21	15
Light, 2 Tbsp	110	7	14
French/Italian: Regular	150	14	5
Regular, ¼ cup, 2 oz	290	28	10
Light, 2 Tbsp	65	4	9
Fat/Oil-Free, 2 Tbsp	40	0	10
Ranch: Regular, 2 Tbsp	145	16	2
Regular, ¼ cup, 2 oz	290	31	4
Light, 2 Tbsp	80	3	7
Fat-Free, 2 Tbsp	50	0.5	11
Thousand Island: Regular	120	11	5
Regular, ¼ cup, 2 oz	230	22	9
Light, 2 Tbsp	60	4	7
Fat-Free, 2 Tbsp	40	0.5	10

Brands ~ Salad Dressings

	C	F	Cb
Annie's Naturals: *Per 2 Tbsp*			
Cowgirl Ranch	120	11	3
Goddess	130	13	1
Roasted Red Pepper	70	6	3
Shiitake & Sesame	120	13	1
Tuscany Italian	80	7	5
Vinaigrette: Balsamic	100	10	3
Lite, Honey Mustard	45	2	6
Organic: Buttermilk	70	7	1
Creamy Asiago Cheese	60	9	0
Cucumber Yogurt	60	5	2
Red Wine & Olive Oil	160	17	1
Thousand Island	90	7	5
Bernstein's: *Per 2 Tbsp*			
Creamy Caesar	120	13	1
Herb Garden French	130	12	6
Italian	110	12	1
Restaurant Recipe Italian	120	12	1
Other varieties, average	110	11	2
Fat-Free Cheese & Garlic Italian	10	0	2
Light Fantastic: Cheese Fantastico	25	1.5	3
Roasted Garlic Balsamic	45	3.5	3
Best Foods			
Dijonnaise Mustard, 1 tsp	5	0	1
Mayonnaise: *Per 1 Tbsp*			
Canola	45	4.5	0
Low-Fat	15	1	2
Light	45	0	1
Real Mayonnaise	90	10	0
Tartar Sauce, 2 Tbsp	80	7	4
Bob's Famous: *Per 2 Tbsp*			
Bleu Cheese	140	15	1
Lite	80	8	1
Ranch Country	150	16	1
Roquefort	140	15	1
Thousand Island	140	14	4
Bolthouse			
Creamy Yogurt Dressings: *Per 2 Tbsp*			
Caesar Parmigiano	80	6.5	3
Chunky Blue Cheese	70	6.5	2
Classic Ranch	80	7.5	3
Brianna's: *Per 2 Tbsp*			
Blue Cheese	120	11	5
Blush Vintage	120	7	14
French Vinaigrette	130	13	0
New American	160	17	6
Rich Santa Fe Blend	25	0	5
Zesty French	150	15	4
Other varieties, average	155	14	8

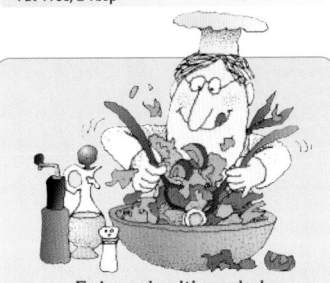

*Enjoy a healthy salad
but don't drown it
in high-fat salad dressings.
Use 'light' dressings to halve
the fat and calories.*

Brands ~ Salad Dressings (Cont)

Per 2 Tbsp (Approx 1 fl.oz)

	C	F	Cb
Carb Options: Italian	70	8	1
Ranch	150	17	0
Cardini's			
Caesar, 2 Tbsp	160	17	1
Fat-Free Caesar	40	0	9
Light Caesar	80	7	5
Honey Mustard	140	13	5
Parmesan Ranch	150	15	2
Poppyseed w. Shallots	160	14	8
Southwest Caesar	140	14	3
Vintage White Wine	110	12	1
Other varieties, avg.	125	13	1
Vinaigrette Dressing: Balsamic	50	3	5
Greek	50	4.5	3
Caesar	60	5	2
El Torito: Cilantro Pepita Caesar	140	14	1
Emeril's: *Per 2 Tbsp*			
House Herb Viniagrette	100	10	1
Kicked Up French	80	5	8
Girard's: *Per 2 Tbsp*			
Blue Cheese Vinaigrette	100	10	3
Caesar	140	15	1
Light Caesar	90	8	5
Champagne	150	16	1
Light Champagne	60	5	2
Olde Venice Italian	130	13	2
Fat-Free: Balsamic/Red Wine, avg.	25	0	6
Caesar	40	0	9
Raspberry	60	0	14
Hidden Valley: *Per 2 Tbsp*			
Regular Ranch: Italian Ranch	140	14	2
Old-Fashioned Buttermilk Ranch	140	14	2
Bacon Ranch	140	14	1
Cracked Peppercorn Ranch	120	12	2
Cole Slaw	150	15	5
Light, Original Ranch	70	5	3
Fat-Free, Original Ranch	30	0	6
Ken's Steak House Dressings: *Per 2 Tbsp*			
Balsamic & Basil Vinaigrette	110	12	1
Chunky Blue Cheese	150	16	1
Country French	150	12	10
Creamy Caesar	160	18	0
Peppercorn Ranch	180	19	1
Ranch	140	15	2
Italian w. Aged Romano	110	12	1
Thousand Island	140	13	4
Lite: Caesar/Olive Oil Vinaigrette, avg.	70	6	2
Ranch	80	6	3

Kraft

	C	F	Cb
Regular Dressings: *Per 2 Tbsp*			
Honey Dijon	110	10	6
Classic Caesar	110	11	1
Coleslaw	110	9	7
Creamy Italian	110	11	2
Creamy French	160	15	5
Light Raspb. Vinaigrette	60	4	5
Ranch	150	16	2
Roka Brand Blue Cheese	130	13	2
Thousand Island w. Bacon	100	8	7
Tuscan House Italian	120	12	3
Kraft Free (Fat-Free): Italian	20	0	4
Caesar Italian	50	0	10
Honey Dijon	50	0	12
Light Done Right!:			
Caesar	60	4.5	3
Creamy Ranch	80	5	10
Other flavors, avg.	80	4.5	9
Special Collection: Caesar Italian	100	10	2
Balsamic Vinaigrette	90	8	4
Sundried Tomato	60	5	4
Sweet Honey Catalina	130	10	8
Other varieties, avg.	60	5	1
Seven Seas: Viva Robust lt.	90	9	2
Red Wine Vinaigrette	90	0	2
Kroger: *Per 2 Tbsp*			
3 Cheese Ranch/Creamy Ranch	130	14	2
Balsamic Vinaigrette	90	9	2
California Honey French	140	12	9
Chunky Bleu Chse; Crmy Cucumber	150	16	3
Creamy Italian	120	13	3
Italian Fat Free	20	0	4
Lite Ranch	70	6	3
Lite Zesty Italian	35	2	4
Peppercorn Ranch	130	14	2
Poppy Seed	160	14	8
Ranch w. Bacon	120	13	1
Thousand Island	90	8	5
Zesty Italian	90	9	3
French Fat-Free	35	0	9
Honey Dijon Fat-Free	30	0	7
Ranch Fat-Free	30	0	7
Thousand Island Fat-Free	45	0	10
Zesty Italian Fat-Free	15	0	4
Litehouse: Caesar	130	13	2
Chunky Bleu Cheese	150	16	1
Coleslaw	100	8	8
Jalapeno Ranch	120	12	1
Lite Bleu Cheese	70	6	2
Other varieties, avg.	120	12	2

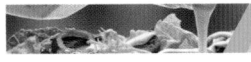

Brands ~ Salad Dressings (Cont)

Per 2 Tbsp (Approx 1 fl.oz)

	C	F	Cb
Maple Grove: *Per 2 Tbsp (1 fl.oz)*			
Regular: Honey Mustard	120	9	9
Sweet & Sour	110	7	12
Fat Free: Balsamic Vinaigrette	35	0	9
Caesar Vinaigrette; Greek, avg.	10	0	3
Dijon; Poppyseed, avg.	40	0	10
Other varieties, avg.	25	0	6
Low Carb: Dijon	70	8	1
Balsamic; Raspberry Vinaigrette	5	0	1
Lite: Caesar	60	4.5	5
Honey Mustard	80	5	9
Marie's: *Per 2 Tbsp*			
1000 Island	150	15	4
Blue Cheese Chunky	160	17	0
Caesar	170	19	1
Honey Dijon	130	12	5
Poppy Seed	150	13	8
Ranch (15.5 fl.oz ctn), 2 Tbsp	170	19	1
Premium: Spinach Salad, 2 Tbsp	70	1.5	13
Italian Cheese Blend	170	18	1
Nasoya: *Per 2 Tbsp*			
Vegi-Dressing (Tofu Base/Dairy Free):			
Thousand Island	60	5	2
Other flavors	60	7	1
Nayonaise: Reg., 2 T., 1 oz	70	7	2
Fat-Free, 2 Tbsp, 1 oz	20	0	4
Newman's Own: *Per 2 Tbsp*			
Balsamic Vinaigrette, 2 Tbsp	90	9	3
Creamy Caesar	170	18	1
Family Recipe Italian	120	13	1
Olive Oil & Vinegar	150	16	1
Parmesan Roasted Garlic	110	11	2
Ranch	140	15	2
Two Thousand Island	140	14	4
Lighten Up: Light Italian	60	6	0
Light Raspberry & Walnut	70	5	7
Light Balsamic Vinaigrette	45	4	1
San-J: *Per 2 Tbsp*			
Tamari Peanut, 2 Tbsp	70	2	9
Tamari Sesame	45	2.5	4
Fat-Free: Tamari Ginger	25	0	5
Tamari Mustard	25	0	5
S & W: *Per 2 Tbsp, 1 oz*			
Light: Italian	35	0	8
Red/White Wine; Raspberry Blush	40	0	10
Seven Seas, avg., 2 Tbsp	90	9	2

	C	F	Cb
Spectrum: *Per 2 Tbsp*			
Fat Free: Creamy Dill/Garlic	25	0	4
Sweet On. & Garlic; Tstd Sesame	15	0	3
Low-Fat: Honey Dijon	35	2	4
Zesty Italian	30	2	1
Organic Omega-3:			
Asian Ginger	140	14	3
Creamy Garlic Ranch	120	13	1
Golden Balsamic Vin.	110	11	3
Lemon Sesame	120	12	2
Pomegranate Chipotle	130	13	2
Shititake Sesame	110	11	1
Vegan Caesar	80	9	2
T. Marzetti's			
Asiago Peppercorn	160	16	1
Asian Ginger	120	12	4
Baja Ranch	150	15	2
Buffalo Blue Cheese	140	15	1
Chunky Blue Cheese	150	15	2
Honey Balsamic	120	11	4
Original Slaw	160	16	6
Ranch	160	17	1
Wishbone			
Regular: 5 Cheese Italian	120	10	6
Chunky Blue Cheese	150	15	2
Creamy Caesar	170	18	1
French: Deluxe French	120	11	5
Sweet 'N Spicy	100	12	6
Italian: Regular	90	8	3
House Italian	100	10	3
Robusto Italian	90	8	3
Ranch: Original	120	13	2
w. Garlic	140	15	2
Spring Onion	130	14	2
Balsamic Vinaigrette	50	5	3
Red Wine Vinaigrette	80	5	9
Russian, regular	120	6	14
Thousand Island	130	12	5
Dressing & Marinades: Asian	70	5	6
Balsamic Olive Oil & Herbs	50	5	3
Lemon Garlic & Herb	70	5	5
Tangy Honey Mustard	80	6	7
Ranch Up!	140	15	2
Fat-Free:			
Chunky Blue Cheese	35	0	7
Italian	20	0	4
Ranch	30	0	7
Light: Blue Cheese	50	2	6
Classic/Creamy Caesar; Ranch	50	2	7
Country Italian; Italian	30	1.5	4
Parmesan Peppercorn Ranch	50	2	7
Thousand Island	50	2	9
Salad Spritzers: All flavors, 10 sprays (¼ fl.oz) for 1 cup salad	10	1	1

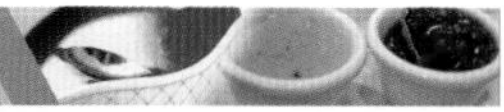

Gravy

	C	F	Cb
Homemade Gravy, avg:			
Thin, little fat, 2 Tbsp, 1 oz	20	1	3
Thick, 2 Tbsp, 1¼ oz	50	2	9
¼ cup, 2½ oz	100	4	18
Franco·American (Canned)			
Beef; Turkey Gravy, 2 oz	25	0.5	3
Chicken Gravy, ¼ cup, 2 oz	40	4	4
Pillsbury (Gravy Mixes): *Prepared*			
Brown; Homestyle, ¼ cup, 2 oz	15	0	3
Chicken, as prep., ¼ cup, 2 oz	20	0	4

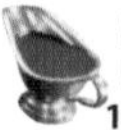

Gravy-In-Jars-Homestyle

	C	F	Cb
Boston Market, ¼ c., 2 oz	40	2.5	3
Franco-American (In Jars):			
99% Fat Free, ¼ cup, 2 oz	20	0	4
Heinz, reg., all types, ¼ c., 2 oz	25	1	3
Fat Free Roast Turkey, ¼ c., 2 oz	10	0	2
Vons, all types, ¼ c., 2 oz	20	0.5	4

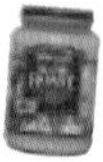

Tomato Products

	C	F	Cb
Whole/Chopped/Crushed/Diced			
1 cup, 8½ oz	50	0	10
In Aspic, ½ cup	50	0	10
w. Green Chili, 1 c., 8½ oz	60	0	16
Stewed, ½ cup, 1.7 oz	40	1.5	6.5
Wedges in Tom Juice, 1 cup	70	0.5	18
Salsa, average, 1 Tbsp	15	0	3.5
Tomato Ketchup:			
Regular: 1 Tbsp, ½ oz	15	0	4
Single Serve, 1 pkt	10	0	3
One-Carb *(Heinz)*, 1 Tbsp, ½ oz	5	0	1
Tomato Paste, 2 Tbsp, 1 oz	25	0	6
Regular, ¾ cup, 6 oz	140	1	32
Tomato Puree, ½ cup, 4½ oz	50	0	10
Tomato Sauce:			
Regular, ½ cup, 4.4 oz	50	0	11
Spanish Style, ½ cup, 4.3 oz	40	0	9
w. Mushrooms, ½ cup, 4.3 oz	45	0	10
w. Onions, ½ cup, 4.3 oz	50	0	12
Tomato Seasoning, 3 tsp	20	0	4
Sundried Tomatoes:			
Natural, 5-6 pces, 0.4 oz	22	0	5
In Oil, drained, 6 pces, ½ oz	40	2.5	4

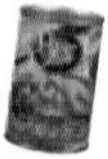

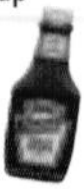

Sauces ~ Brands

	C	F	Cb
A-1			
Steak & Marinades Sauce: *Per Tablespoon (½ oz)*			
Bold & Spicy; Teriyaki; New York	20	0	5
Carb Well Steak Sauce	5	0	1
Chicago	20	1	3
Jamaican Jerk	25	0.5	5
New Orleans Cajun	25	0	5
Steak Sauce	15	0	3
Barilla: *Per ½ Cup*			
Olives; Garden Veggie	90	4	12
Roasted Garlic & Onion	60	1.5	11
Other varieties, average	70	2.5	12
Bertolli: *Per ½ Cup*			
Creamy Alfredo	200	18	6
Italian Sausage	100	3	15
Olive Oil & Garlic	90	3	14
Olive w. Sundried Tomato	100	4	13
Marinara; Rst Red Pepper, average	80	2	13
Traditional Basil Pesto	270	27	4
Best Foods/Hellmann's: *Per 2 Tbsp*			
Tartar Sauce	80	7	5
Buitoni			
Pasta Sauces: *Per ½ Cup Serving, 4½ oz*			
Garden Vegetable; Marinara	70	1.5	11
Green & Black Olive	80	3	10
Italian Baking	60	1	12
Mushroom & Garlic; Three Cheese	80	2.5	12
Roasted Garlic	70	1	12
Spicy Pepper	70	1.5	11
Sweet Peppers	60	2	10
Tomato & Basil	70	1.5	12
Bull's Eye: *Per 2 Tbsp*			
Barbecue Sauce	60	0	13
No Corn Syrup	50	0	13
Catelli			
Garden Select Pizza Sauce, 1 fl.oz	15	0.5	2.5
Meat Sauce, ½ cup, 4 oz	85	2.5	11
Garden Select 6 Vege Recipe Sauce: *Per ½ Cup*			
Parmesan & Romano	80	2.5	12
Thick & Chunky, Tomato Basil Blast	70	1	12
Other varieties, avg.	80	1.5	13
Cento: *Per ½ Cup*			
Sauces: Passata Tomatoes	40	0	8
Pasta, all natural	50	3	3
Pizza, fully prepared	25	0	5
Tomato: Arrabbiata; Vodka	70	3	6
Marinara; Puttanesca	115	9	6
White Clam	160	15	4

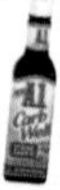

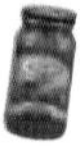

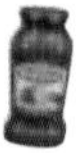

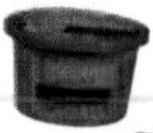

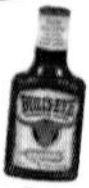

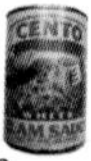

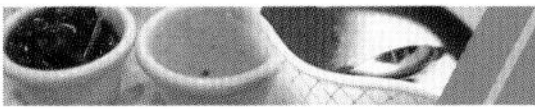

Sauces (Cont)

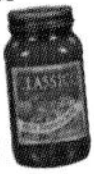

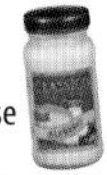

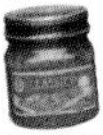

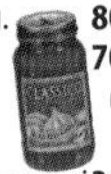

	C	F	Cb
Classico: *Per ½ Cup Unless Indicated*			
Caramelized Onion & Rstd Garlic	30	3.5	13
Homestyle Meat Selections Sce	125	5	14
Organic Spinach & Garlic	60	1	10
Roasted Red Pepper Alfredo	60	5	3
Spicy Tomato & Basil	90	3.5	12
Signature Recipes Sauce:			
Alfredo, avg., ¼ cup	80	7	3
Cabernet Marinara	60	2	10
Fire Rstd Tom. & Garlic	50	0.5	10
Florentine Spinach & Cheese	80	5	6
Mushrooms & Ripe Olives	60	1	11
Pesto, Sun-Dried Tomato, ¼ cup	90	5	8
Pesto, Traditional Basil, ¼ cup	230	21	6
Rstd Chicken w. Parm. & Garlic	90	2	13
Spicy Red Pepper	60	1.5	7
Spicy Tomato & Pesto	90	4	11
Sun-Dried Tomato Pesto	80	3	11
Traditional Favorites Sauce: *Per ½ Cup*			
Four Cheese	90	5	10
Italian Sausage w. Peppers & Onions	90	2	13
Rstd Garlic; Triple Mushr., avg.	80	3	11
Other varieties, average	70	1	12
Colgin, Liquid Smoke	0	0	0
Contadina: *Per ¼ Cup*			
Pizza Sauce: Flavored w. Pepperoni	35	1	5
Original; Four Cheese, avg.	30	0.5	6
Cooking Sauce: Sweet & Sour, 1 T.	40	1	8
Tomato Sauce, avg., ¼ cup	20	0	4
Crosse & Blackwell: *Per 1 Tbsp*			
Ham Glaze & Meat Sauce	30	0	7
Mint Sauce	5	0	1
Del Monte			
Spaghetti Sauces: *Per ½ Cup*			
w. Four Cheeses	70	1.5	15
w. Meat/Mushrooms, avg.	60	1	14
Other varieties, avg.	75	1	16
Chunky Sce: Garlic & Herb	60	1.5	11
Italian Herb	60	1	12
Sloppy Joe Sauce, Original, ¼ cup	50	0	11
Enrico's			
Sicilian	80	2.5	13
Traditional Italian Style	60	1.5	12
Mushroom Onion, ½ cup	70	1.5	13
Pizza, ¼ cup	40	1.5	6
Other varieties, ½ cup	60	1	12

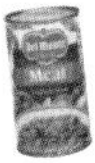

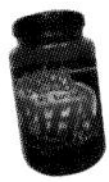

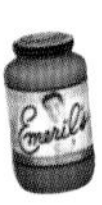

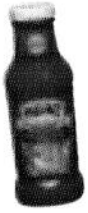

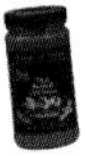

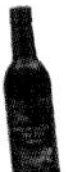

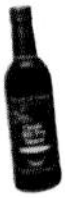

	C	F	Cb
Emiril's			
Pasta Sauces: *Per ½ Cup*			
Homestyle Marinara	90	4	11
Kicked Up Tomato	70	3	9
Puttanesca	80	5	9
Roasted Gaaahlic	70	3	9
Roasted Red Pepper	60	3	7
Vodka Sauce	130	8	13
French's			
Worcestershire Sauce, 1 tsp	5	0	1
Heinz: *Per 1 Tbsp (Approx. ½ oz)*			
Barbecue Sauces, all flavors	35	0	9
Chili Sauce	20	0	5
Horseradish Sauce	75	6	2
Steak Sauce 57	30	0	4
Tomato Ketchup: Regular	15	0	4
Reduced Sugar	5	0	1
Worcestershire Sauce, 1 Tbsp	10	0	1
Original Cocktail Sauce			
¼ cup, 2.2 oz	60	0	15
House of Tsang: *Per 1 Tbsp (Approx. ½ oz)*			
Bangkok Padang Peanut	45	2.5	4
Classic Stir Fry	25	1	4
General Tsao	45	0.5	10
Ginger Soy	20	0	4
Hibachi Grill: Kobe Steak Grill	50	4	2
Spicy Hunan Smokehut	40	0.5	8
Sweet Ginger Sesame	40	1	8
Thai Peanut	50	3	4
Tokyo Teriyaki	40	0	10
Hoisin, 1 tsp	15	0	4
Imperial Citrus Soy	25	0	5
Korean Teriyaki Stir Fry	35	1.5	5
Mandarin Marinade	25	0	6
Oyster	30	0	7
Saigon Sizzle Stir Fry	45	2	7
Spicy Brown Bean	15	0	3
Sweet & Sour	35	0	8
Szechuan Spicy Stir Fry	25	1	4
Hunt's			
BBQ Sauce: Original, 2 Tbsp	60	0	15
Hickory & Brown Sugar, 2 T.	60	0	15
Manwich Sloppy Joe Sce, ¼ cup	30	0	7
Family Favorites, avg., 2 oz	30	0	6
Spaghetti Sauce: *Per ¼ of 26 oz Can*			
Traditional, 6.5 oz	75	0	15
Meat Sauce, 6.5 oz	90	0	16
Light Sauce, 6.5 oz	70	0	13

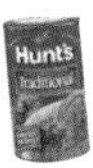

Brands (Cont)

	C	F	Cb
Jack Daniel's			
Original No. 7 BBQ Sce, 2 Tbsp	50	0	12
Steak Sauce,			
Original/Smokey, 1 Tbsp	15	0	5
Jim Beam			
Hot Wing Sauce, 2 Tbsp	20	2	0
KC Masterpiece: *Per Tbsp.*			
Marinades: Garlic & Herb	30	1	5
Honey & Teriyaki	40	0.5	9
Original BBQ	60	0	15
Kikkoman Marinades			
Black Bean Sce, 2 Tbsp	80	1.5	17
Hoisin Sce, 2 Tbsp	50	1	6
Honey Mustard, 1Tbsp	30	0	6
Rosted Garlic & Herbs, 1 Tbsp	20	0	4
Toasted Sesame, 1 Tbsp	40	0.5	6
Knorr			
Classic Sauce: *Per 2 Tbsp (Prepared)*			
Bernaise	20	0	4
Hollandaise	20	0	4
Classic Gravy, avg., ¼ cup	25	0	4
Kraft			
CarbWell Sauce, 2 Tbsp	15	0	3
Sauce: Cocktail, 1 Tbsp	30	0.3	6
Horseradish, 1 tsp	15	1.5	1
Sandwich & Burger Spread, 1 T.	45	3.5	3
Sweet 'n Sour, 1 Tbsp	30	0	7
Tartar: 1 Tbsp	70	6	4
Lemon & Herb, 1 Tbsp	75	8	0.5
Fat-Free Tartar, 1 Tbsp	12	0	3
Barbecue Sauces: Average, 2 T.	50	0.5	12
Las Palmas			
Red Chile Sauce, ¼ cup, 2 oz	20	0.5	2
Enchilada Sauces: Green Chile	25	1.5	3
Hot/Original, ¼ cup, 2 oz	15	0.5	2
Lawry's 30 Minute Marinade: *Per Tbsp*			
Caribbean Jerk; Teriyaki	20	0	5
Lemon Pepper	10	0	2
Mesquite	5	0	1
Mexican Chile & Lime	15	0	3
Thai Ginger; Herb & Garlic	10	0	2
Other varieties, average	15	0	2
Packet Seasonings: *Per 2 teaspoons (Dry)*			
Fajitas; Taco, average	10	0	3
Average other flavors	20	0	4

	C	F	Cb
Lea & Perrins			
Worcestgershire Sauce,			
1 tsp	5	0	1
Monterey			
Pesto Sauce, ¼ cup, 2 oz	280	28	4
Mr Yoshida's			
Original Gourmet, 2 Tbsp, 30ml	90	0	20
Hawaiian Sweet & Sour, 2 Tbsp	70	0	18
Mrs Dash Marinade (Salt-Free)			
Lemon Herb Peppercorn, 1 Tbsp	25	2	2
Spicy Teriyaki, 1 Tbsp	25	0.5	4
Muir Glen: *Per ½ Cup*			
Organic Pasta Sauce:			
Mushr. Marinara; Portobello Mushr.	50	0	11
Other varieties, average	50	1	11
Newman's Own: *Per ½ Cup*			
Bombolina (Tomato & Basil)	90	4.5	13
Five Cheese	80	3	10
Fra Diavolo	70	3	10
Marinara; Sockarooni	70	2	12
Roasted Garlic & Peppers	70	2.5	11
Vodka	110	5	11
Old El Paso			
Enchilada Sauce:			
Green Chile, ¼ cup	20	1	3
Other varieties, ¼ cup	25	1	4
Sauce Mixes, 2 Tbsp	10	0	2
Picante Sauce, 2 Tbsp	10	0	2
Taco Sauce, 1 Tbsp	5	0	1
Salsas: Make Mine Medium, 2 Tbsp	10	0	2
Wild for Mild, 2 Tbsp	10	0	2
Thick N' Chunky varieties, 2 Tbsp	10	0	3
Pace: *Per 2 Tbsp*			
Picante Sauce	10	0	2
Chunky Salsa	10	0	2
Salsa Con Queso	90	6	6
Prego: *Per ½ Cup*			
Pasta Sauce: Marinara	100	3	12
Diced Onion & Garlic	120	4.5	18
Flavored w. Meat	130	5	19
Fresh Mushroom	90	3	14
Italian Sausage & Garlic	100	3.5	13
Mini Meatball	150	6	20
Mushroom & Garlic	80	2.5	13
Ricotta Parmesan	90	3	13
Roasted Garlic Parmesan	100	1	20
Three Chse; Tom. Basil & Garlic, avg.	90	1.5	17
Other varieties, average	120	3.5	19

Updated Nutrition Data ~ www.CalorieKing.com
Persons with Diabetes ~ See Disclaimer (Page 24)

Brands (Cont)	C	F	Cb
Prego (Cont): *Per ½ Cup*			
Chunky Garden: Combination	90	1.5	17
Mushroom Supreme	120	4	19
Other varieties, average	110	3.5	17
Heart Smart: Traditional Italian	90	3	13
Mushroom Italian	100	3	15
Premier Japan (Organic)			
Garlic/Ginger/Wasabi Tamari, 1 T.	10	0	2
Ragu: *Per ½ Cup (Unless Indicated)*			
Pizza Quick Sauce: *Per ¼ Cup*			
Traditional	40	2	4
Homemade Style	30	1	4
Thick & Zesty	40	1.5	5
Cheese Creations: *Per ¼ Cup*			
Classic Alfredo	110	10	3
Double Cheddar	100	9	3
Light Parmesan Alfredo	70	5	3
Chunky Gardenstyle: *Per ½ Cup*			
Mushroom & Green Pepper	100	3	16
Other varieties, average	110	3	18
Light varieties, average	50	0	10
Old World Style: Marinara	80	4.5	11
Meat Sauce	80	4	7
Mushroom; Traditional	70	3	8
Organic: Garden Veggie	80	2.5	12
Cheese; Traditional	80	3	11
Rich & Meaty: Classic Italian Style	150	10	9
Mama's Meat Sauce	130	8	8
Sausage, Peppers & Onions	155	10	8.5
Robusto!: 7-Herb Tomato	80	3.5	9
Chopped Tom., Olive Oil & Garlic	95	5	10
Parmesan & Romano	90	3.5	10
Sauteed Beef, Onion & Garlic	90	5	9
Sauteed Onion & Garlic	80	4	9
Rainforest Organic			
Ginger Curry, 1 Tbsp	15	1	2
Papaya Pepper, 1 Tbsp	0	0	0
Rinaldi: *Per ½ Cup*			
3-Cheese	80	2	15
Original	80	3	12
Meat/Mushroom	80	3	12
Other varieties, average	70	2.5	12
S & W: *Per Tablespoon*			
Teriyaki, Light/Marinade	20	0	4

	C	F	Cb
Safeway Select			
Salsa: *Per 2 Tbsp*			
Chipotle; Southwest	15	0	3
Garlic Lovers	10	0	3
Peach P'apple; Salsa Verde	20	0	4
Sauce: *Per 2 Tablespoons*			
Fiesta Fajita	15	0	2
Mild Enchilada	20	0	4
Mild Taco	10	0	2
Roasted Tomato	15	0	2
Select Sauces: *Per ½ Cup*			
Arrabbiata	70	8	10
Four Cheese	70	3	10
Garlic & Basil	70	4	6
Marinara	60	2	10
Mushroom & Onion	60	3	6
Spicy Red Bell Pepper	50	1	9
Sundried Tomato & Olive	60	3	6
Vodka	130	10	9
Seeds of Change: *Per ½ Cup*	50	0.5	9
Tomato Basil Genovese	60	3.5	9
Marinara di Venezia	60	3.5	6
The Wizard's (Organic)			
Hot Stuff, 1 Teaspoon	0	0	0
Vegetarian Worcestershire, 1 tsp	2	0	0.5
Troy's Sauces (Organic)			
Ginger Sauce, 1 Tbsp	10	0	1
Peanut Sauce, 1 Tbsp	25	1.5	2
Timpone's: *Per ½ Cup*			
Spaghetti Sauce: Classic	50	2.5	8
Family Recipe	80	3	7
Mom's	70	3	7
Tony Roma's			
Wing Sauce, 1 Tbsp	15	1	1
Trader Joe's BBQ Sauce,			
Kansas City Style, 2 Tbsp	60	0	15
Tree of Life: *Per ¼ Cup*			
Tomato	50	2	9
Fat-Free Classic Tomato	40	0	9
Fat-Free Sweet Pepper	35	0	8
Walnut Acres: *Per ½ Cup (125g)*			
Organic Pasta Sauce, average	50	1	10

Home-Popped Popcorn

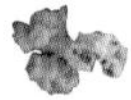

	C	F	Cb
Popping Corn Kernels:			
2 Tbsp, 1 oz	110	1	26
(makes approx. 5 cups)			
Air-popped (no oil), plain, 1 oz	110	1	22
1 cup (6g)	20	0	5
Oil-popped, plain, 1 oz	145	8	16
1 cup (11g)	55	3	6
Popcorn Oil, 1 Tbsp	120	14	0

Microwave Popcorn

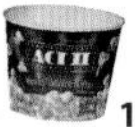

	C	F	Cb
Average All Brands (Popped)			
Butter: Regular, 1 cup	35	2	4
Light, 1 cup	25	1	4
Act II Popcorn:			
Butter, 1 cup, 0.3 oz	30	2	4
5 cups, popped, 1 oz	160	10	18
Light Butter, 1 cup, 0.2 oz	25	1	4
5 cups, popped, 1 oz	110	4.5	19
Butter Lovers,1 cup, 0.3 oz	35	2.5	4
4½ cups, 1 oz	170	12	16
94% Fat-Free Butter, 1 cup	30	1.5	4.5
4½ cups, 1 oz	130	2.5	28
American Fare (K-Mart):			
Butter, 0.3 oz	40	2	5
3 cups, 1 oz	120	2	23
Theater Butter, 1 cup	40	2	5
3.5 cups	140	8	15
Curves: 94% Fat-free, 6 cups	120	1.5	26
90% Calorie, 1 mini bag	90	3	19
Jolly Time: America's Best, 1 cup	20	0	5
Blast O Butter: Regular, 1 cup	45	3	4
Light, 1 cup	30	1.5	4
Caramel Apple Healthy Pop, 5 c.	110	2	23
Healthy Pop, 1 cup	20	0	4
Kettle Mania, 1 cup	45	3	4
Mallow Magic, 1 cup	60	5	6
Newman's Own: Butter, 1 oz	130	5	18
Light Butter Flavor, 3½ oz	120	4	19
Orville Redenbacher's: *Popped*			
Movie Theater Butter, 1 cup	30	2.5	4
4½ cups, popped, 1 oz	170	12	16
Smart Pop!: Butter, 7 cups	120	2	25
100 Calorie Mini Bags (1)	100	2	24
Tender White, 6½ cups	130	2.5	28
Pop Secret Popcorn: *Popped*			
100 Calorie Pop, 1 snack bag	100	3	20
94% Fat Free, 6 cups	120	2.5	26
Jumbo Pop Butter, all types, 3½ cups	180	11	18
Light Butter (1)	120	4.5	20
Movie Theater Butter, 4 cups	180	13	17
Other varieties, avg., 4 cups	170	12	17
Smart Balance, 1 cup	20	0	6

Bagged Popcorn

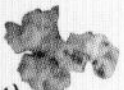

	C	F	Cb
Average All Brands (Ready-to-Eat)			
Regular/Plain: ½ oz pkg	80	5	8
1 oz pkg	160	10	16
4 oz pkg	640	40	64
2 oz Box (store/airport)	320	16	32
3 oz Bag (9" high x 5" wide)	480	24	48
Caramel Popcorn,			
without nuts, 1 cup, 2 oz	240	4	46

Brands ~ Bagged Popcorn

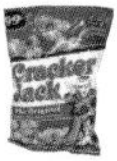

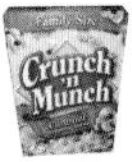

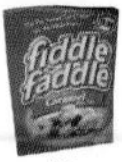

	C	F	Cb
Boston's: Fat Free, ⅔ cup, 1 oz	100	0	23
Lite, 2 cups, 1 oz	140	6	19
Gourmet Super Prem., 2 c., 1 oz	160	11	13
40% Less Fat, 2¾ cups, 1 oz	140	6	17
Cracker Jack: Original,			
½ cup, 1 oz	120	2	23
1 cup, 2 oz	240	4	46
99-Cents Pkg, 3⅜ oz	410	7	78
Crunch 'N Munch			
Caramel/Toffee, avg.:			
1 oz quantity	135	5	21
1 cup, 2 oz	270	19	42
4 oz box	540	20	84
7.5 oz box	1010	38	158
Fiddle Faddle:			
Butter Toffee/Caramel			
1 oz qty	120	3.5	22
1 cup, 2 oz	240	7	44
8 oz box	960	28	176
Jay's: Fat Free Caramel Corn, ¾ cup	110	0	26
Korn Krunch: *(Kornfections Treasures):*			
Almond Pecan (Sugar Free), 1 oz	150	8	19
Orville Redenbacher's:			
Popcorn Cakes, Minis, avg. (8)	60	1	11
Drizzles, avg., ⅔ cup, 1 oz	150	7	22
Poppycock: Pecan Delight, ½ cup	150	7	20
Original Clusters, ½ cup, 1 oz	160	8	20

Movie Theater Popcorn

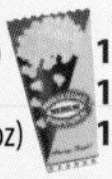

	C	F	Cb
Small (7 cups): Plain	385	21	44
with Butter (3 pumps, ¾ oz)	570	42	44
Medium (15 cups): Plain	825	45	94
with Butter (4 pumps, 1 oz)	1075	73	94
Large (20 cups): Plain	1100	60	124
with Butter (6 pumps, 1½ oz)	1485	102	124
Butter: 1 Pump, ¼ oz	65	7	0
4 Pumps (2 Tbsp), 1 oz	250	28	0

Updated Nutrition Data ~ www.CalorieKing.com
Persons with Diabetes ~ See Disclaimer (Page 24)

Corn & Tortilla Chips

Average All Brands

Corn Chips:

	C	F	Cb
Avg. all types, 1 oz	150	8	18
8 oz bag	1200	64	144
Doritos: 13 chips, avg., 1 oz	140	7	18
White Nacho Cheese, 1 oz	150	8	17
Fritos, 32 chips, 1 oz	160	10	15

Tortilla Chips: Average, 1 oz | 140 | 7 | 18

(1 oz = approx. 12 chips or 13 strips)

	C	F	Cb
Baked! Tostitos (15) 1 oz	120	3	22
Doritos: 13 chips, 1 oz	140	7	18
Light, 13 chips, 1 oz	100	2	19
Baked! Nacho Cheesier, 15 chips, 1 oz	120	3.5	21
Garden of Eatin', 1½ oz bag	210	11	27
Munchies Mix, ¾ cup, 1 oz	140	7	18
Snyder's, Multigrain, 1 oz	130	5	20
Stacy's, Baked, Pita Chips (14), 1 oz	130	4	18
Utz Low-Fat Baked, 10 chips, 1 oz	120	2	23

Tostitos: Regular, 1 oz | 140 | 7 | 18

	C	F	Cb
Light, 1 oz	90	1	20
6.75 oz bag	610	6	135

Potato Chips/Crisps

Average All Brands

Regular:

	C	F	Cb
Plain or flavored, 2 chips	15	1	1.5
1 oz pkg (20 chips)	150	10	15
4 oz quantity	600	40	60
14 oz pkg	2100	140	210

Brands:

	C	F	Cb
Lay's Classic, 1 oz	150	10	15
Lay's Stax, avg. all, 1 oz	150	10	15
Pringles: 14 Chips, 1 oz	160	11	14
Large, 6 oz can	920	63	86
Minis, 1 bag, 0.8 oz	120	7	13
Selects, 28 chips, 1 oz	145	9	16
Snack Stack, 23g tub	140	10	12
Ruffles, 12 chips, 1 oz	160	10	14

Reduced Fat: *Pringles,* 16 Chips, 1 oz | 140 | 7 | 17

Sun Chips; Terra, avg.,

	C	F	Cb
16 chips, 1 oz	140	6	18

Low-Fat/Baked:

	C	F	Cb
Lay's Baked!, 15 chips, 1 oz	110	1.5	23
Ruffles Baked!: 9 chips, 1 oz	120	3	21
Cheddar Sour Crm, 10 chips, 1 oz	120	3	22

Fat Free: *Lay's Light,* 1 oz | 75 | 0 | 17

	C	F	Cb
Pringles (Fat-Free), 15 chips, 1 oz	70	0	15

Pretzels

Average All Brands

Hard-Baked Pretzels:

	C	F	Cb
1 oz quantity	100	0	22
Sticks, thin, 2¼" (9/oz), 1	12	0	3
Twists, thin, ¼" thick, (5/oz),1	25	0	5
Dutch (2¾"x 2⅝") ½ oz, 1	55	1	11
Sourdough *(Snyder's),* ¾ oz, each	100	0	22

Soft Pretzels (Twists) average:

	C	F	Cb
Plain: Regular, 2.2 oz	210	2	43
King Size, 5.1 oz	485	4.5	99
New York Street Vendors, 7 oz	660	6	135
Big Cheese, 1.76 oz	130	3	22

Peanut Butter filled *(Tr. Joe's)* 1 oz | 150 | 8 | 14

Choc-coated *(Snyders),* 1 oz | 130 | 6 | 18

	C	F	Cb
White Choc covered, 7 pces, 1 oz	140	6	19

Brands

	C	F	Cb
American Fare, Mini Twists, 1oz	110	1	23

Auntie Anne's: *See Fast-Foods Section*

Rold Gold *(Frito-Lay)*

	C	F	Cb
Braided Twists (8), 1 oz	110	1	23
Classic Pretzel Sticks, 1 oz	100	0	23
Cheddar Cheese Tiny Twists, 1 oz	110	1	23
Hard sourdough pretzel, 1 pce	100	0.5	21
Tiny Twists, avg. all, 1 oz	110	1	23
Tiny Sticks (18), 1 oz	100	0	23
Thins (9), 1 oz	110	1	23

Snyder's of Hanover Pretzels

	C	F	Cb
100 Calorie Pretzel Pack, 0.9 oz	100	0	22

Multigrain:

	C	F	Cb
Pretzel Sticks/Twists, 1 oz	120	2	22
Pretzel Nibblers,			
Honey Mustard, 1 oz	140	5	20
Rods (3), 1 oz	120	1	24
Homestyle (15), 1 oz	120	1	25
Mini (20), 1 oz	110	0	25
Nibblers (16), 1 oz	120	0	25
Thins, 1 oz	110	1	23

SuperPretzel: Soft Pretzels (1) | 160 | 1 | 34

	C	F	Cb
Softstix (2)	130	3	22
Soft Pretzel Bites (5)	150	0.5	32

Pretzelfils: Pizza (2) | 130 | 2 | 22

	C	F	Cb
Pepperjack; Mozzarella, (2), avg.	130	3.5	21
Utz: Pretzels, avg., 1 oz	110	1	23
Real Choc-covered Pretzels (2)	120	5	17

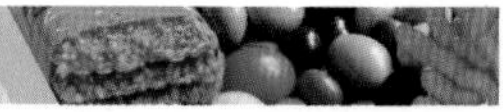

Snacks   C F Cb

Note: Actual weight of packaged snacks is usually 5-10% more than label Net Wt. For accuracy, weigh snack and allow extra calories for any extra weight.

	C	F	Cb
Bagel Crisps (N.Y. Style) 6 crisps, 1 oz	130	5	17
Banana Chips, ¼ cup, 13 chips, 1 oz	150	7	21
Beef Jerky (Lance), average, 1 oz	70	1	4
Beef Sticks (Lance), 1 oz	130	10	4
Bugles, Original, 1⅓ cup, 1 oz	160	9	18
Cheese Balls (Utz), 1 oz pkg	150	9	16
Cheese Crackers:			
Cheese Filled (Lance) (6), 1.4 oz	190	11	22
Cheese Curls: 1 cup, 1 oz	150	9	16
Cheese Nips (Nabisco) 1 oz	140	6	19
Cheese Puffs: Avg., 1 oz	160	10	15
American Fare, 1½ cup, 1 oz	160	11	13
Snyder's Multigrain, 1 oz	130	6	19
Cheese Twists, (27), 1 oz	160	12	13
Cheerios, Snack Mix:			
Cheddar, ⅔ cup, 1 oz	120	3	21
Original: ⅔ cup, 1 oz	110	3	20
Baked, Not Fried, ⅔ cup, 1 oz	120	3.5	21
Cheetos: Regular all flavors, 1 oz	160	10	15
Baked!, cheese flavored, 1 oz	130	5	19
Cheez Balls, 27 balls, 1 oz	150	9	11
Cheez-It Crackers:			
Avg. all flavors, 1 oz	150	8	18
1.25 oz pkg	165	7	23
3 oz pkg	450	24	54
Reduced Fat, 1 oz	130	4	20
Twisters, 1.25 oz pkg	165	7	23
Chex Mix (General Mills):			
100 Calorie Pouch, avg.	100	3	18
Bold Blend; Peanut, ½ cup, 1 oz	140	6	20
Traditional, ⅔ cup, 1 oz	130	4	22
Choc., avg., all varieties, 1.2 oz	150	5	23
Other varieties, avg., ½ cup, 1 oz	130	4	22
Churros (Mex. Pastry) 10", 1 oz	100	5	12
Combos (Oven Baked):			
Crackers, ⅓ cup, 1 oz	140	6	18
1 cup, 3 oz	420	18	54
Pretzels, ⅓ cup, 1 oz	130	4.5	19
1 cup, 3 oz	390	14	57
Cookies: See Pages 83–89			
Cool Cuts, Carrot & Ranch, 2.3 oz	70	5	5
Corn Chips: See Page 153			
Corn Crunchies/Spirals, 1 oz	95	0	22
Corn Nuts: ⅓ cup, 1 oz	130	4.5	20
1.7 oz bag	220	7.5	34
Corn Puffs: (Pirate's Booty), 1 oz	130	5	18
Wotsits (Walker), 21g, (¾ oz) pkg	105	6.5	11
Dunkin Stixs (Hostess), 3, 4oz	490	25	63

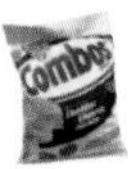

Snacks (Cont)   C F Cb

	C	F	Cb
Flavor Twists (Fritos), 1 oz	160	10	16
French's Potato Sticks ¾ c., 1 oz	180	12	16
Funyuns, Onion flavor (13), 1 oz	140	7	18
Genisoy Soy Crisps, avg., 1 oz	120	3	17
Goldfish (Pepperidge Farm) 1 oz	140	5	20
Gold-N-Chees (Lance), 1 oz	150	8	17
Handi-Snacks (Kraft), avg., 1 oz	110	5	16
Honey Mustard Onion Pieces			
(Snyder's) 1 pkg, 2 oz	280	14	36
Hot Peanuts (Lays), 3½ oz	310	25	10
Jerky (Beef) 1 oz stick	70	1	4
Lance Sandwich:			
Grilled Cheese, 1.4 oz	200	10	22
Other varieties, average, 1.4 oz	200	10	22
Munchies (Frito-Lay):			
Chse Fix; Flaming Hot, ¾ c.	140	7	18
Totally Ranch, ¾ cup	140	6	19
Munchos, 16 pieces, 1 oz	160	10	16
Nabisco: Chips Ahoy, 1.4 oz	160	8	21
Cheese Nips (13), 1 oz	140	5	20
Nutter Butter Bites, 1.2 oz	170	7	24
Oreo, 1.3 oz	160	7	24
Garden Harvest:			
Apple Cinnamon/Banana, 1 oz	120	3	22
Tom. Basil/Vege Medely, 1 oz	120	4	20
Ritz Bits Go-Pak Chse, 1 oz	150	9	18
Ritz Bits S'Mores, 1 oz	150	6	20
Nibblers (Snyder's): Reg. (13), 1 oz	130	3	24
Fat Free (16), 1 oz	120	0	25
Onion Rings (T.G.I. Friday), 1 oz	130	6	19
Oriental Mix (Rice Snacks), 1 oz	130	3.5	24
Rice Snacks (Trader Joe's), 1 oz	110	0	22
Oyster Crackers (Sunshine), 1 oz	60	1.5	11
Party Mix (Cheez-It) ½ c., 1 oz	130	4.5	21
Peanut Butter Nuggets (10), 1 oz	140	6	15
Pirate's Booty, 1 oz bag	130	5	18
4 oz bag	520	20	72
w. Caramel, 2.75 oz bag	330	5.5	63
Pirate's Cannon Balls, 1 oz	130	5	18
5 oz bag	715	27	99
Pita Chips, avg., (9) 1 oz	130	4	18
Popcorn: See Page 152			
Pork Cracklins, 1 oz	180	14	0
Pork Rinds, 1 oz	160	10	0
Potato Chips: See Page 153			
Potato Skins (TGI Friday) (16)	130	9	24
Potato Sticks (Ralphs), ⅔ c., 1.1oz	170	11	15

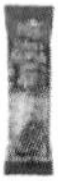

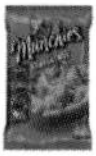

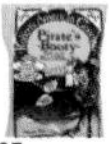

Updated Nutrition Data ~ www.CalorieKing.com
Persons with Diabetes ~ See Disclaimer (Page 24)

Snacks (Cont)

	C	F	Cb
Quakes Rice Snacks,			
Average, 7-10 mini cakes, ½ oz	65	2	13
Quaker Mini Delights, 1 bag	90	3.5	16
Rice Chips, Bar-B-Q/Onion, 1 oz	140	7	18
Sandwich Crackers (Austin): Per Pkg			
Chse Cracker w. Pnut Butter, 1.37 oz	140	7	15
Reduced Fat, 1.26 oz	170	7	25
Chse Cracker w. Cheddar, 1.37 oz	210	10	26
PB & J Cracker Sandwich, 1.37 oz	200	10	24
Santitas (Frito-Lay), 1 oz	130	6	19
Sesame Sticks (Cityfarm), 1 oz	160	9	13
Smart Puffs (Robert's), 1.37 oz bag	180	8	23
Soy Crisps, avg. 1 oz	120	3	17
Soy Nuts: Dry Roasted, ¼ cup, 1 oz	130	6	9
Choc-coated, 1 oz	140	7	13
Dr Soy Soy Nuts BBQ, 1 oz	150	8	8
Sun Chips (Frito-Lay), 1 oz	140	6	18
Sunflower Chips (Snyders), 1 oz	140	6	20
100 Calorie Snack Pack (1)	100	4	14
Sweet Snack Mix (Quaker):			
Cinnamon Crunch, 1 oz	130	5	20
Honey Graham, 1 oz	130	5	19
TastyKake: Koffee Kake Jr, 71g	280	10	44
Chocolate Jr, 94g	340	12	55
Creme Filled Koffee Kakes (2)	360	17	51
Tings (Robert's), 2 oz bag	300	14	36
Toasted Cheese Crackers, 1 pkg	220	11	23
Tortilla Chips: Page 153			
Tostitos:			
Regular, avg., 1 oz	140	7	19
Light, 1 oz	90	1	20
Trader Joe's, Baked Cheese Crunchies,			
33 pieces, 1 oz	130	6	19
7 oz pkg	910	42	133
Trail Mix (Nuts/Seeds/Dried Fruit):			
Regular, 3 Tbsp, 1 oz	140	9	13
Tropical, 3 Tbsp, 1 oz	130	7	16
w. Chocolate Chips, 1 oz	180	12	16
Dr Soy Trail Mix, 1 oz	110	4	12
Turkey Jerky Teriyaki (Oberto), 1 oz	80	1	8
Vegetable Snacks (Snyder's), 1 oz	140	7	19
Veggie Chips, (365/Wholefoods),1 oz	130	7	13
Veggie Straws, (365/Wholefoods),1 oz	130	7	16
Wasabi Peas, ¼ c., 1 oz	120	3	19
Wheatables (Keebler):			
Original, (17), 1 oz	140	6	20
Orig., Red.-Fat (19), 1 oz	140	4	22
Honey Wheat (17), 1 oz	140	6	20
Seven Grain (17), 1 oz	140	6	20
Yogurt Pretzels (7), 40g	190	7	30
Yogurt Raisins,			
(Sun-Maid), 1 oz	120	4.5	20

Fruit Snacks

	C	F	Cb
Betty Crocker: Fruit Gushers, 25g	90	1	20
Fruit by the Foot, 1 roll, 21g	80	1	17
Fruit Roll Ups, 1 roll, 14g	50	1	12
Scooby Doo; G-Force, 25g pkg	80	0	20
General Mills:			
Blues Clues; Dora the Explora (1)	60	0	14
Other varieties	80	0	21
Kellogg's: Disney Fruit Snacks, 25g	80	0	19
Fruit Streamers, 1 Roll	80	1	17
Twistables, 23g	70	0.5	17
Yogos, 23g	90	2	18
Sunkist: Fruit Snacks, 1 pouch	90	1	20
Fruit Smoothie Blitz, 1.3 oz	140	1	32

Vending Machines

	C	F	Cb
Brownie, frosted (Lance), 3 oz	400	18	56
Cheese Balls (Utz), 1 oz	150	9	11
Choc Chip Cookies (Nabisco), 40g	190	9	27
Choc Milk, 8 fl.oz	260	9	36
Coca-Cola Classic, 12 fl.oz	140	0	39
Diet Coke, 12 fl.oz	0	0	0
Corn Chips, 1 oz	160	10	16
Hostess Sweet Roll, 4¼ oz	420	13	68
Donut, plain, 1.4 oz	160	9	18
Fruit Pie (Hostess), 4½ oz	480	20	68
Granola/Cereal Bars	140	3	26
Hershey's, 1.55 oz bar	210	13	25
Hot Fries (Con Agra), 1 oz	150	7	17
Kellogg's Rice Krispies Treat	150	3.5	28
Lance Captain's Wafers, 1 pkg	190	8	23
M & M's: Plain, 1.7 oz	240	10	34
Peanuts, 1.7 oz	250	13	30
Milk: Whole, 8 fl.oz	160	9	13
Reduced Fat, 2%, 8 fl.oz	140	5	14
Milky Way, 2 oz	260	10	41
Orange Juice, 8 fl.oz	120	0	29
Peanuts, roasted (Lance), 1 oz	200	15	6
Popcorn, plain, 1 oz	160	10	16
Pork Skins, 1 oz	160	10	0
Potato Chips: 1 oz	150	10	15
Reduced Fat, 1 oz	120	3	21
Pretzels, 1 oz	110	1	23
Raisins, ½ oz pkg	45	0	11
Reese's Peanut Butter Cups, 1½ oz	230	13	23
Snickers, 2.1 oz bar	280	14	35
Tortilla Chips, 1 oz	140	7	18

Homemade & Restaurant

Restaurant & Take-Out
Average All Preparations, Per 8 fl.oz

	C	F	Cb
Bean Medley	200	3	34
Beef Consomme	30	0	2
Borscht (w. Sour Cream)	130	8	14
Bouillabaisse	400	15	10
Chicken & Corn	290	14	20
Chicken & Wild Rice	80	4	9
Chicken Consomme	50	0	2
Chicken Curry	180	8	18
Chicken Jambalaya	160	7	8
Chicken Noodle	80	2	12
w. Chicken	160	4	12
Chicken Soup	80	2	6
Chili with Beans	250	12	25
Clam Chowder	240	15	11
Corn & Crab	120	3	18
Corn Chowder	150	8	16
Cream of Broccoli	200	12	20
Cream of Potato	150	6.5	17
Cream of Mushroom	200	13	15
Fish Chowder	220	15	6
French Onion	420	15	25
Gazpacho	50	0	5
Lentil Soup	250	9	28
Lobster Bisque	320	15	10
Matzo Ball (w. 1 large ball)	180	7	24
Minestrone	125	2.5	20
Mulligatawny	300	15	8
Pea & Ham	240	10	25
Potato & Bacon	170	7	19
Pumpkin, Creamy	210	10	26
Shark Fin Soup	100	4	8
Spicy Shrimp Soup, 1 bowl	160	7	10
Split Pea Soup	180	2.5	30
Vegetable (Fat Free)	75	0	18
Vegetable Beef	80	2	10
Vichyssoise	200	9	15
Watercress	90	4	13

Other Soups: *See International & Fast-Foods Sections (Arby's, Au Bon Pain, Boston Market, Dunkin' Donuts, Denny's, Schlotzsky's, Sizzler, Souplantation, Sweet Tomatoes, Zoup!)*

Homemade Soups: *Calculate calories, fat and carbohydrates from recipe ingredients.*

Bouillon Cubes & Powders

	C	F	Cb
Bouillon Cubes: *Average all Types*			
Regular, 1 cube	5	0	1
Low Sodium (LiteLine)	12	0	1
Powders: *Average, 1 tsp*	10	0	1
Herb-Ox: *Instant Broth & Seasoning,*			
Beef, 1 envelope	5	0	1
Chicken; Vegetarian	5	0	1
Herbs, Spices: 1 tsp	5	0	1
Soup Oyster Crackers			
40 small/3 large, ½ oz	60	2	8

Amy's (Organic)
Per Cup (½ Can)

	C	F	Cb
Alphabet (Fat-Free)	80	0	16
Black Bean Vegetable	130	1.5	25
Butternut Squash	100	2.5	20
Chunky Tomato Bisque	120	3.5	21
Chunky Vegetable	60	0	13
Corn Chowder	190	10	25
Cream of Mushroom, ¾ cup, (½ can)	140	9	13
Cream of Tomato	100	2	17
Lentil	150	4.5	19
Minestrone	90	1.5	17
No Chicken Noodle	90	3	12
Pasta & 3 Bean	130	5	19
Potato Leek	180	10	21
Split Pea (Fat-Free)	100	0	21
Vegetable Barley	70	1	13
Other varieties, average	150	4	23

'Light in Sodium' Range *(50% less sodium),*
(Calories/Fat/Carb ~ Same as Regular Range)

Andersen's ~ *Per Cup*

	C	F	Cb
Lentil	110	2	19
Split Pea	130	0	24
Split Pea w. Bacon	140	1	23
Tomato	130	3.5	22

Baxters
Per Cup (Prepared as Directed)

	C	F	Cb
Cream of Asparagus	160	10	15
Cream of Scottish Smoked Salmon	150	8	16
French Onion	70	0	15
Stilton Cheese & White Port	210	15	14
Vichyssoise	210	15	16

Updated Nutrition Data ~ www.CalorieKing.com
Persons with Diabetes ~ See Disclaimer (Page 24)

Bean Cuisine

Per Cup (Prepared as Directed)

	C	F	Cb
13 Bean Boullabaisse; Lentil, avg.	220	0	17
Island Black Bean	210	0	17
Santa Fe Corn Chowder	160	0	18
White Bean Provencal	250	1	32

Bear Creek ~ *Per Cup*

	C	F	Cb
Cheddar Potato	190	7	30
Chicken Noodle	120	1.5	22
Hot & Sour	90	0.5	18
Minestrone	110	0	23
Split Pea	110	1.5	20
Vegetable Beef	110	0.5	22
Other varieties, average	145	5	28

Campbell's

Classic Red & White: *Per ½ Cup*

	C	F	Cb
Bean w. Bacon; Fiesta Chili Beef, avg.	170	4	25
Beef Noodle	70	2	8
Beef w. Vegs/Barley; Minestrone, avg.	90	1.5	16
Cheddar Cheese	100	5	11
Chicken & Dumplings	70	2.5	10
Chicken Won Ton	60	1	8
Cream of Asparagus	110	7	9
Cream of Broccoli	90	3.5	12
Cream of Chicken & Mushroom	80	6	7
Cream of Mushroom	100	6	9
Cream of Onion	100	6	10
Cream of Potato	90	2	15
Cream of Shrimp	90	5	8
Creamy Chicken Noodle	120	7	11
French Onion	45	1.5	6
Green Pea	180	3	28
Manhattan Clam Chowder	70	0.5	12
New England Clam Chowder	90	2.5	13
Old Fashioned Vegetable	80	1.5	14
Split Pea w. Ham & Bacon	180	3.5	27
Tomato	90	2	20
Tomato Bisque	130	3.5	23
Vegetable	100	0.5	20

Healthy Request Condensed: *Per ½ Cup*

	C	F	Cb
Chicken Rice	70	1.5	13
Vegetable Beef	90	1	15
Other varieties, average	80	2	15

Kids Condensed Soup: *Per ½ Cup*

	C	F	Cb
Batman; Dora; Jimmy Neutron	70	2	11
Chicken Alphabet/& Stars	70	1.5	11
Chkn Noodle O's; Curly Ndle	80	2	12
Chicken Noodle Soup	60	2	8
Goldfish Pasta w. Meatballs	80	3	11
Tomato Goldfish Pasta	130	0.5	28
Tomato Soup	90	0	20

Campbell's (Cont)

Chunky: *Per 8 fl.oz Cup*

	C	F	Cb
Baked Potatoes w. Bacon Bits	160	6	23
Clam Chowder Manhattan	120	3.5	19
Classic Chicken Noodle	110	2.5	15
Gr. Chkn & Sausage Gumbo	140	2.5	21
Hearty Vegs.w. Pasta	120	2	23

Select Gold Label: *Per 8 fl.oz Cup*

	C	F	Cb
Golden Butternut Squash	90	1.5	18
Iralian Tomato with Basil/Garlic	90	0	19

Select Harvest: *Per 8 fl.oz Cup*

	C	F	Cb
Beef w. Roasted Barley	130	1	22
Chicken & Dumpling	180	7	19
Chicken Vegetable Medley	110	0.5	19
Chicken w. Egg Noodles	120	4	12
Creamy Chicken Alfredo	220	13	15
Creamy Potato w. Roasted Garlic	180	10	20
Harvest Tomato w. Basil	100	0	20
Italian Saus. w. Pasta & Pepperoni	160	7	18
Italian Style Wedding	160	7	16
Mexican Style Chicken Tortilla	130	2.5	20
Minestrone; Tom. Garden; Vege	110	1	20
New England Clam Chowder	170	10	15
Potato Broccoli Cheese	150	9	15
Savory Chicken & Rice	110	0.5	20
Savory White Bean w. Roasted Ham	170	1	30
Slow Roasted Beef & Vegetable	100	0.5	16
Split Pea w. Roasted Ham	150	1	29
Other varieties, average	140	3	20

Select Bowls: *Per Microwave Bowl*

	C	F	Cb
Chicken w. Egg Noodles	240	8	24
Italian Style Wedding	260	8	32
Mexican Style Chicken Tortilla	260	5	38
Minestrone	200	1	38
New Eng. Clam Chowder	220	4	34
Savory Chicken & Rice	220	2	36

Heat & Serve Bowls: *Per Bowl*

	C	F	Cb
Chicken Noodle Soup	140	4	20
Creamy Tomato Soup	320	10	50
Tomato Soup	220	0	48
Vegetable Soup	220	1	44
Vegetable Beef Soup	160	1	30

Soup at Hand: *Per Container*

	C	F	Cb
Chicken w. Mini Noodles	80	2	11
Cream of Broccoli	150	7	17
Creamy Tomato	190	4	34
New England Clam Chowder	120	6	13
Vegetable Beef	60	1	10

Dr McDougall's

	C	F	Cb
Big Cups: *Per Full Serving*			
Hot & Sour w. Noodles	320	1	45
Miso Soup w. Noodles	180	1	34
Pad Thai/Ramen, average	200	1	42
Black Bean & Lime	340	2	60
Minestrone & Pasta	200	1	40
Split Pea w. Barley	240	2	42
Tamale/Tortilla w. Baked Chips, avg.	200	2	34
Light Sodium: *Per Container*			
Chicken Noodle, Vegan	140	0.5	28
Chinese Chicken Noodle	140	1	28
Lentil Couscous	190	1	37
Split Pea	200	1	35
Tomato, Basil Pasta	100	0.5	21
White Bean & Pasta	170	1	34

Dixie Diners' Club

Per Cup (Prepared as Directed)

Carb Counters, Dine 'n Dash:			
Broccoli & Cheese	70	5	3
Chicken Cheese Enchilada	95	6	4
Chicken Noodle	40	1	3
Cream of Mushroom	50	4	2

Fantastic Cup Soups

Vegetarian Soup Cups: *Per Container*			
Baja Black Bean Chipotle	130	0.5	31
Buckaroo Bean Chili	160	2	33
Classic French Onion	90	2.5	15
Creamy Potato Leek	120	2.5	22
Great Lakes Cheddar Broccoli	100	3	15
Green Onion Miso w. Tofu	140	1.5	26
Hot & Sour	170	2	33
Mama's Minestrone	160	2.5	30
Sesame Miso	140	2	27
Southwest Tortilla Bean	170	3.5	34
Spicy Thai	150	0.5	32
Split Pea	140	0.5	28
Summer Vegetable Rice	110	0.5	25
Three Onion Noodle	180	2	36
Tuscan Tomato & Shells	140	1	31
Vegetarian Chicken Noodle	90	1	17

Health Valley

	C	F	Cb
Per Cup			
Broths: Beef Flavored, Fat-Free	10	0	0
Chicken: Fat-Free	25	0	0
Low-Fat	35	1.5	0
Vegetable, Fat-Free	20	0	5
Fat-Free Soup: Split Pea & Carrots	110	0	24
Chicken Flav. Noodles w. Veggie	110	0	24
Tomato Veggie	80	0	17
Vegetable Barley	90	0	19
Other varieties, average	80	0	17
Organic Soup: Black Bean	110	0	5
Chicken Noodle	80	2	11
Garden Vegetable	100	2	17
Lentil	100	1	21
Minestrone	70	1	17
Mushroom Barley	70	0	17
Potato & Leek	70	0	15
Split Pea	120	0	26
Tomato	80	0	18
Vegetable	80	0	18
Soup Cup: *Per ⅓ Cup*			
Fat Free: Lentils with couscous	130	0	28
Zesty Black Bean w. Rice	100	0	22

Healthy Choice

Per Cup			
Bean & Ham	180	2	29
Chicken & Dumplingsf	140	2.5	21
Chicken w. Rice Soup	110	1.5	17
Chicken Tortilla Style	160	2	25
Country Vegetable	110	1	19
Fiesta Chicken	120	2	20
Garden Vegetable	120	0.5	24
Hearty Chicken	130	2	19
New England Clam Chowder	110	1	19
Old Fashioned Chicken Noodle	100	1.5	13
Split Pea and Ham	170	2	22
Vegetable Beef	130	1	22
Zesty Gumbo	100	2	16

Kikkoman

Mixes			
Chinese Style Egg Flower: 1⅓ tsp	40	1	7
w. Corn, 1 Tbsp	50	6	11
Instant Miso:			
Shiro (White): 1 pkt	35	1	4
w. Tofu, 1 pkt	35	1	3

Updated Nutrition Data ~ www.CalorieKing.com
Persons with Diabetes ~ See Disclaimer (Page 24)

Imagine

	C	F	Cb
Per Cup			
Broths: Beef	20	1	1
No-Chicken	10	0	2
Vegetable	20	0	2
Organic, Creamy: Acorn Squash	70	1.5	14
Broccoli	60	1.5	10
Butternut Squash	90	2	18
Chicken	70	1.5	12
Portobello Mushroom	80	3	10
Potato Leek	110	3	18
Sweet Corn	120	3	20
Sweet Pea	80	1.5	14
Tomato	80	1	15
Tomato Basil	90	1.5	17

Knorr

Recipe Classics: *Dry Mix*			
Cream of Spinach, 2 T.	60	1.5	11
French Onion, 2 Tbsp	45	1	8
Leek Soup, 2 Tbsp	60	1	11
Spring Vegetable, 2 Tbsp, 0.3 oz	25	0	6
Tomato w. Basil, 3 Tbsp, 0.7 oz	70	1	15
Vegetable, 2 Tbsp, 0.6 oz	30	0	6
Bouillon Cubes: *Per ½ Cube (1 Cup, Prepared)*			
Beef; Chicken, average	20	1.5	0.5

Lipton

Cup-a-Soup: *Per Envelope*			
Cream of Chicken	60	1	15
Chicken Noodle	45	1	8
Recipe Secrets: *Per Serving (Dry Mix)*			
Beefy Onion, 1 Tbsp	25	0.5	5
Onion, 1 Tbsp	20	0	4
Onion Mushroom, 1⅓ Tbsp	35	0	6
Soup Secrets: *Per Cup (Prepared)*			
Noodle Soup	60	1	10
Chicken Noodle	60	1	10

Manischewitz

Condensed: *Per ½ Cup*			
Chicken Broth, Clear	15	0	2
Chicken w. Kreplach	40	1	6
Chicken w. Matzo Balls	80	3.5	9
Quart Jars: *Per 8 fl.oz (Prepared)*			
Borscht w. Beets	90	0	21
Borscht Low Calorie	25	0	6
Ready To Serve: Matzo Balls in Broth	220	9	27
Dry Mixes: *Per Cup*			
Matzo Ball & Soup Mix	40	0.5	9
Split Pea Cello	140	0	25
Vegetable Soup Cello	120	0	22

Maruchan

	C	F	Cb
Instant Lunch,			
Avg. all flavors, 1 pkg	290	12	38
Ramen, all flavors, ½ pkt, 1½ oz	190	7	26

Miso Cup (Edward & Sons)

Per Cup (Prepared as Directed)			
Golden Vegetable; Savory Seaweed	30	1	3
Traditional with Tofu	35	1	4
Reduced Sodium	25	1	3

Nile Spice ~ *Per Cup*

	C	F	Cb
Black Bean; Lentil	170	1.5	35
Chicken Flavored Vegetable	110	1.5	21
Country Mushroom	140	2.5	26
Minestrone	140	1	30
Split Pea, low-fat	200	1	35
Minestrone Couscous	180	1.5	34
Other varieties, average	190	2	36

Nissin ~ *Per Whole Package*

	C	F	Cb
Choice Ramen (Low-Fat),			
Slow Stewed Beef	280	2	56
Top Ramen: Beef Flavor	380	14	54
Chicken Flavor	380	14	52
Cup Noodle: Beef Flavor Minestrone	540	22	74
Shrimp w. Tomato & Garlic	570	24	74

Pacific Foods ~ *Per Cup*

	C	F	Cb
Chicken Broth	10	0	1
Natural, Beef Broth	20	0	1
Organic: French Onion	35	0	6
Creamy Butternut Squash	90	2	17
Creamy Tomato	100	2	16
Roasted Red Pepper & Tomato	110	2	16
Vegetable Broth	15	0	3
Hearty Soups: Chicken Fajita	150	2.5	24
Other varieties, average	170	5	22

Pritikin ~ *Per Cup*

	C	F	Cb
Fat Free Chicken Broth	5	0	1
Hearty Vegetable	80	0	15
Split Pea	130	0.5	23
Vegetarian Vegetable	80	0	15

Progresso

	C	**F**	**Cb**
Vegetable Classic: *Per Cup*			
French Onion	50	1.5	8
Green Split Pea	170	1	28
Garden Vegetable	90	0	20
Hearty Tomato	110	1	23
Lentil; Tomato Basil, avg.	155	2.5	29
Minestrone	110	2	19
Tomato Rotini	140	1	29
Vegetable	80	0.5	16
Traditional: *Per Cup*			
Beef Barley	140	3.5	18
Chkn Herb Dumpling; Minestrone	100	2.5	14
Italian-Style Wedding; Chickarina, avg.	130	5	15
Manhattan Clam Chowder	100	2	17
New England Clam Chowder	190	10	20
Potato Broccoli & Cheese Chowder	180	10	18
Southwestern Style Chicken	120	2.5	19
Split Pea w/ Ham	150	1	25
Other varieties, average	100	2.5	14
Rich & Hearty: *Per Cup*			
Chicken & Homestyle Noodles	110	2	14
Chicken Pot Pie Style	170	6	21
Crmy Chicken Wild Rice	150	8	13
New England Clam Chowder	190	9	22
Savory Beef Barley Veg.	130	1	22
Slow Cooked Veg. Beef	120	1	20
Steak & Homestyle Noodles	110	2	16
Steak & Sauteed Mushrooms	110	2	18
Other varieties, average	125	2	21
Microwaveable Bowls: *Per Bowl*			
Chicken & Wild Rice/Noodle, avg.	100	1.5	17
Minestrone Soup	90	1.5	17
Vegetable Soup	80	0.5	17
Light, Low-Fat/Low-Carb:			
Vegetable & Noodle, 8.75 oz	60	0.5	13
Southwestern-Style Veg., 8.5 oz	60	0	12
All other varieties, 8.5 oz	60	0	14

Signature (Safeway)

	C	**F**	**Cb**
Signature Soups: *Per Cup (8.6 oz)*			
Baked Potato; Craving Crab, avg.	420	33	20
Broccoli & Cheesy Cheddar	280	21	14
Chkn Noodle; Harvest Veg. Beef, avg.	130	4	14
Clam Chowder, all varieties	330	24	19
Fajita Chicken & Corn Chowder	350	23	25
Golden Split Pea	200	3	31
Savory Chicken & Wild Rice	170	6	20
Stompin' Steakhouse Chili	260	8	17
Tuscan Tomato & Basil Bisque	310	26	17

Shelton's

	C	**F**	**Cb**
All Natural: *Per Cup*			
Black Bean & Chicken	190	4	22
Chicken Noodle	80	2	9
Chicken Rice	90	1	14
Chicken Tortilla	120	1.5	18
Broths: Chicken	35	2.5	0
Organic Turkey	0	0	0

Simply Asia

	C	**F**	**Cb**
Noodle Bowls: *Per Bowl*			
Miso Tofu	420	3.5	82
Sesame Chicken	430	4.5	82
Soy Ginger	330	5	61
Spring Vegetable	270	3	56
Szechwan Garlic	650	12	121
Szechwan Hot & Sour	480	7	88

Spice Hunter

	C	**F**	**Cb**
Mixes ~ Per Bowl			
Chicken Noodle	140	1.5	25
Chicken Vegetable	160	1	31
Creamy Thai Noodle	200	5	31
Split Pea	250	1.5	43

Swanson

	C	**F**	**Cb**
Per Cup			
99% Fat Free Chicken Broth	15	0.5	1
Beef Broth	15	0	1
Chicken Broth	15	0	1
Vegetable Broth	15	0	3

Tabatchnick

	C	**F**	**Cb**
Per Single Pouch			
Balsamic, Tomato & Rice	110	3.5	18
Barley Mushroom; Wild Rice, avg.	80	1	17
Black Bean	230	2.5	39
Broccoli & Cheese	200	12	15
Cabbage	90	1	21
Chicken w. Dumplings	150	6	19
Corn Chowder	130	4.5	21
Cream of Broccoli	130	5	18
Cream of Mushroom/Spinach, avg.	95	5	11
Creamed Spinach	40	1	7
Lentil	160	0	29
Macaroni & Cheese	250	8	34
Minestrone; Vegetable, avg.	100	1.5	18
New England Potato	110	5	17

Updated Nutrition Data ~ www.CalorieKing.com
Persons with Diabetes ~ See Disclaimer (Page 24)

Tabatchnick (Cont)

	C	F	Cb
New York Chicken	70	1	13
Old Fashioned Potato	100	1.5	21
Onion	60	1.5	11
Pea	140	1	34
Salmon Chowder	80	1.5	15
Seafood Chowder	130	6	15
Southwest Bean	220	5	35
Tomato Rice	110	3.5	18
Yankee Bean	180	1.5	33
Vegetarian Chili	180	3.5	28
Low Sodium: Mushroom	80	1	17
Pea	140	0	34
Vegetable	90	1.5	17

Thai Kitchen

	C	F	Cb
Instant Rice Noodle: Per Package (Prep. as Directed)			
Bangkok Curry; Thai Ginger	190	3.5	37
Garlic & Veggie; Spring Onion	190	3	37
Lemongrass & Chili	190	3.5	37
Rice Noodle Soup Bowls: Per ½ Bowl			
Hot & Sour	120	2.5	23
Lemongrass & Chili	110	1.5	23
Thai Ginger	120	2	23

Trader Joe's

Per Cup

	C	F	Cb
Barley w. Vegetables	110	3	19
Black Bean	130	1.5	25
Chicken Broth	15	0	1
Chicken Noodle	90	1	14
Chunky Minestrone	110	2.5	19
Creamy Corn Chowder	170	6	28
Lentil w. Vegetables	140	3	21
Organic Lentil Vegetable	130	1.5	25
Rich Onion	90	3.5	12
Split Pea, Low Fat	100	0	19
Condensed: Clam Chowder	160	4	22

Vermont Country Soup

Per Cup

	C	F	Cb
Chicken Noodle	180	8	16
Chicken Pomodoro	150	6	17
Country Vegetable	90	1	20
Cream of Potato	290	16	31
New England Clam Chowder	320	23	23
Tuscan Minestrone	120	1.5	22

Walnut Acres

Per Cup

	C	F	Cb
Autumn Harvest	100	2	19
Chicken & Wild Rice	60	2	11
Chicken Noodle	100	3	13
Classic Minestrone	100	0	22
Country Corn Chowder	150	3	28
Creamy Portobello Mushroom	80	4	9
Creamy Tomato	100	2.5	17
Four Bean Chili	140	1.5	28
Roasted Garlic Potato	110	2.5	21
Savory Meatball w. Orzo	140	4	18
Savory Tomato	120	2	23

Westbrae Natural

	C	F	Cb
Instant Miso, all flavors	35	1.5	3
Ready-to-Eat: Per Cup, 8 fl.oz			
Fat-Free: Split Pea	150	0	28
Alabama Black Bean Gumbo	140	0	26
Hearty Milano Minestrone	120	0	24
Louisiana Bean Stew	130	0	25
Mediterranean Lentil	140	0	24
Santa Fe Vegetable	160	0	31
Spicy Southwest Vegetable	130	0	25
Low-Fat, New York UnChicken Ndle	60	1	10
Semi-Condensed: Per ¾ Cup, 6 fl.oz			
Monte Carlo Creamy Mushroom	70	3	10
Low-Fat, California UnChicken Broth	15	0.5	2
Fat-Free, Tuscany Tomato	70	0	16

Wolfgang Puck

Per Cup

	C	F	Cb
Original: Chicken and Egg Noodles	130	6	11
Chicken and Dumpling	220	13	17
Creamy Roast Chicken with Rice	200	10	16
New England Clam Chowder	210	12	19
Old Fashioned Beef Barley	120	3.5	17
Organic: Chicken with Rice	130	4	18
Classic Minestrone	110	3.5	17
Country Tom. & Basil	130	6	18
Spicy Bean	160	0.5	30
Thick Hearty Vegge	130	5	19

Wylers

	C	F	Cb
Dry Mix: Mrs Grass Onion, 10g	35	0.5	6
Homestyle Vegetable, 12g	35	0	7
Mrs Grass Soup Mix:			
Chicken Noodle, 1 cup	70	1.5	11
Beef Vegetable, 1 cup	90	0.5	18

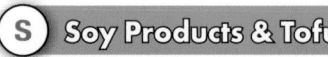

Soybean Products — C F Cb

Cheeses (Soy): See Page 80
Miso Soy Bean Paste

	C	F	Cb
Cold Mountain: Light Yellow, 1 tsp	10	0	1
Mellow Red, 1 tsp	15	0	3
Red, 1 tsp	10	0	1
Miso (dry mix), average			
1 Tbsp., dry mix	35	1	5
1 cup, prepared	35	1	5
Natto, ½ cup, 3 oz	160	7	14
Okara (Tofu fiber residue), ½ c., 2 oz	47	1	8
Tempeh: 1 piece, 3 oz	180	8	12
Fried, 3 oz	250	14	14
Seitan *(White Wave),* Trad., 3 oz	90	1	3
Soybean Protein *(TVP),* 1 oz	95	0	8
Soy Bean Paste, 1 tsp	10	0	2
Soy Beans: See Page 167			
Soy Drinks: See Page 48			

Tofu ~ Packaged — C F Cb

	C	F	Cb
Tofu Stir-Fried, average all, 4 oz	120	8	3
Azumaya Tofu: Soft (Silken), 3.2 oz	40	2	1
Soft, Light (Silken), 3.2 oz	40	1	3
Firm; Extra Firm, 2.8 oz	70	4	2
Light Extra Firm, 2.8 oz	60	2	3
Seasoned Tofu, avg., 3 oz	90	5	3
House Foods			
Premium Tofu: Soft (Silken), 3 oz	50	2.5	2
Medium Firm (Regular), 3 oz	60	3	1
Firm, 3 oz	70	3.5	2
Extra Firm, 3 oz	80	4	1

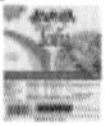

Tofu ~ Packaged (Cont) — C F Cb

	C	F	Cb
House Foods (Cont)			
Organic Tofu: Firm, 3 oz	60	3	0
Extra Firm, 3 oz	90	4.5	0
House Tofu: Tokusen Kinugoshi, 3 oz	90	4	3
Sukui/Soon (Extra Soft), 3 oz	45	2	2
Yaki Tofu: Yaki (Broiled), 3 oz	90	5	2
Tofu Steak: Grilled, 3 oz	90	5	2
Garlic & Pepper, 4.8 oz	80	9	1
Mori-Nu Tofu *(Silken)*			
Soft, 3 oz, 1" slice	45	2.5	2
Firm, 3 oz, 1" slice	50	2.5	2
Extra Firm, 3 oz, 1" slice	45	1.5	2
Organic, 3 oz, 1" slice	60	2.5	2
Lite, Firm, 3 oz, 1" slice	30	0.5	1
Seasoned Tofu: *Per 3 oz*			
Japanese Miso	60	2.5	3
Chinese Spice	50	2	3
Nasoya Tofu: Soft, ⅕ pkg, 2.8 oz	60	3	1
Silken, 3.2 oz	45	2	1
Firm, ⅕ pkg, 3.2 oz	70	3	2
Extra Firm, ⅕ pkg, 2.8 oz	80	4	2
Super Firm, cubed, ⅕ pkg, 2.8 oz	100	5	3
Chinese 5 Spice, ¼ pkg, 3 oz	90	5	3
White Wave: Baked Tofu, 1 square	90	5	2
Soft/Firm Tofu, ⅕ block, 3.2 oz	110	6	3
Reduced Fat, ⅕ block, 3.2 oz	90	4	4
Firm, 3 oz	100	6	3

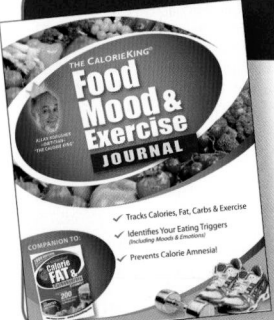

Spices & Herbs

	C	F	Cb
Per Teaspoon: Average all types	5	0	1
All Purpose, 1 tsp	0	0	0
Allspice, ground	5	0	1
Chili Powder	8	0	1
Cinnamon, ground	6	0	2
Curry Powder	6	0	1
Garlic Powder	9	0	2
Nutmeg, ground	12	0	1
Onion Powder	7	0	2
Parsley, dried	4	0	1
Pepper, black/red/white, avg.	6	0	1
Saffron	2	0	0
Salt-Free Blends, 1 tsp	0	0	0
Tumeric, ground	8	0	1
Seeds: Fenugreek	12	1	2
Mustard, Poppyseed	15	1	1
Other types, average	7	0	1

Seasonings & Flavorings

	C	F	Cb
Accent Flavor Enhancer, 1 tsp	0	0	0
Angostura Bitters, 1 tsp	15	0	4
Bacon Bits, average, 1 Tbsp	35	2	2
Bacon Chips (Durkee), 1 Tbsp, 7 g	30	1	2
Bac-Os (Betty Crocker), 1½ Tbsp, 7g	20	1	1.5
Bragg Liquid Aminos, 1 tsp	5	0	0
Butter Buds, 1 tsp	5	0	2
Garlic Bread Sprinkle, 1 tsp	8	0.5	1
Garlic Salt, 1 tsp	2	0	0
Italian Seasoning, 1 tsp	4	0	1
Lemon Pepper Seasoning, 1 tsp	7	0	1
Meat Tenderizer, avg., 1 tsp	7	0	1
Molly McButter, 1 tsp	5	1	1
Mrs Dash Blends, 1 tsp	0	0	0
Salad Crunchies (*McCormick*), 1 tsp	10	0.5	2
Salt: Regular, Sea Salt, Lite Salt	0	0	0
Seasoning Mixes, avg., ¼ pkg	70	1	9
Taco Seasoning, avg., ¼ pkg	30	0.5	4
Old El Paso: Chili Season. Mix, 1 T.	8	0.5	1.5
Cheesy Taco Season. Mix, 1 Tbsp	10	0.5	2
Taco/Burrito Seasoning Mix, 2 tsp	15	0	4
Fajita Seasoning Mix, 1 tsp	5	0	1.5
Vegit Seasoning Mix, ¼ tsp	10	0	2

Supplements

	C	F	Cb
Aloe Vera Juice, undiluted, 2 fl.oz	5	0	1
Brewer's Yeast: Tablets, 2 tabs	4	0	0.5
Flakes, 1 heaping Tbsp, ⅓ oz	30	0.5	4
Powder, 1 heaping Tbsp, ½ oz	50	0.5	6
Cod Liver Oil, 1 Tbsp	125	13	0
Evening Primrose Oil, capsules, 1	5	0.5	0
Fiber Supplements: Tabs, 1	1	0	0
Metamucil Powder:			
Orange, 1 rounded Tbsp, 11g	45	0	12
Sugar-Free, 1 rounded tsp, 6g	20	0	5
Fish Oil Capsules, average, 1	10	1	0
Flax Oil: Capsules, 2	10	1	0
Barlean's, 3 softgels	110	11	0
Garlic Tablets/Capsules, each	3	0	0
Glowelle: Beauty Drink, 8 fl.oz	100	0	24
Powder Stick (1)	50	0	12
Lecithin Granules, 1 Tbsp, 10g	55	4	0.5
Protein: Powders, average, 1 oz	100	0.5	0
Powder Stick pack (1)	50	0.5	12
Seaweed: Dried, 1 oz	85	0.5	22
Soaked, drained, 1 oz	15	0.5	3
Spirulina, 1 tablet	2	0	0.5
Vitamins/Minerals: Tabs/Caps, 1	2	0	0
Vitamin E Capsules, each	5	0	0
Viactiv Chews (1)	20	0.5	4

Cough & Pharmaceutical

	C	F	Cb
Cough/Cold Syrups: *Per Tablespoon*			
Regular: w. sugar, 1 Tbsp	35	0	9
w. alcohol, 1 Tbsp	46	0	9
Sugar-Free (*Diabetic Tussin*), 1 T.	0	0	0
Cough Drops/Lozenges: *See Page 77*			
Antacids: Average, 1 tablet	4	0	1
Liquid, 1 Tbsp	6	0	1
Sudafed Syrup, 1 tsp	14	0	3
Tylenol Liquid: Child, 1 tsp	17	0	4
Extra Strength, 1 tsp	11	0	3
(Antacid Sodium Counts ~ See Page 293)			

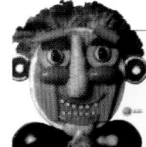

Eat at least 5 servings of fruit and vegetables every day . . . and Enjoy Better Health!

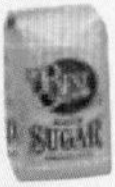

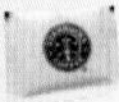

Sugar

	C	F	Cb
White Sugar, granulated:			
1 level teaspoon, 4g	15	0	4
1 heaping teaspoon, 6g	25	0	6
Single portion, 1 pkg	10	0	3
1 Tablespoon, 12g	50	0	12
1 ounce, 1 oz	110	0	20
1 cup, 7 oz	770	0	200
1 pound	1760	0	464
Single Portion Packages:			
1 Stick, 4g	15	0	4
Square Pkg, 6g	25	0	6
Starbucks, 8g	30	0	8
1 cube, ½", 6g	25	0	6
Brown Sugar: 1 Tbsp, 13g	50	0	13
1 ounce, 1 oz	110	0	28
1 cup, not packed, 5 oz	540	0	140
1 cup, packed, 7¾ oz	845	0	218
Powdered/Confectioners:			
Sifted, 1 cup, 3½ oz	385	0	98
Unsifted, 1 cup, 4¼ oz	460	0	117
Cinnamon Sugar, 1 tsp, 4g	15	0	4
Dextrose, 1¼ tsp	15	0	4
Fructose: Dry, 1 tsp, 4g	15	0	4
Liquid, 1 oz	80	0	21
Glucose, 1 oz	110	0	27
Glucose Tablets (1), 5g	20	0	5
Palm Sugar, 3 Tbsp, 12g	45	0	11
Piloncillo (Brown Sugar), 3oz cone	325	0	81
Turbinado Sugar, 2 Tbsp, 1 oz	110	0	27
Unrefined Cane Sugar, 1 oz	110	0	27

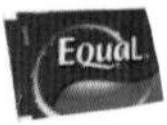

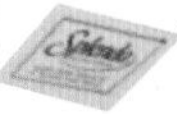

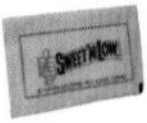

Sugar Substitutes

	C	F	Cb
DiabetiSweet, 1 teaspoon	9	0	4
(Carbohydrate as Sugar Alcohol)			
Equal: Tablet/Liquid	0	0	0
Granulated, 1 pkg	4	0	1
Powdered, packet	0	0	0
Sugar Lite, 1 tsp	8	0	2
NutraSweet Spoonful, 1 tsp	2	0	0
Nutra Taste; Sweet One, 1 pkt	0	0	0
PerfectSweet, 1 tsp	15	0.5	4
Splenda: Powder, 1 c.	95	0	24
Packet	0	0	0
Granular, 1 tsp	5	0	1
Sugar Blend, for Baking, ½ cup	385	0	96
Stevia, Single Serving	0	0	0
Sugar Twin: 1 pkt	3	0	0
Sugar Substitute, 1 tsp	2	0	1
Sweet 'N Low, 1 pkt	0	0	0
Walgreens Wal-Sweet, 1 pkt	0	0	0
Weight Watchers; Whey Low, 1 tsp	4	0	1

Syrups, Molasses

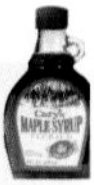

Syrups: *Average All Brands*
(Corn/Rice/Maple/Pancake/Sundae/Waffle)
Includes Aunt Jemima, Cary's, Karo, Hershey's,
Hungry Jack, Log Cabin, Mrs Butterworth's

Regular/Dark/Light Color:	C	F	Cb
1 Tbsp, ½ fl.oz	55	0	14
¼ cup (4 Tbsp)	220	0	55
Single Portion: 1½ oz pkg	170	0	42
Lite: 1Tbsp	25	0	6
¼ cup (4 Tbsp)	100	0	25
Sugar-Free: *Cary's,* 2 Tbsp, 1 oz	18	0	5
Cozy Cottage, 2 Tbsp, 1 oz	10	0	3
Da Vinci, 2 Tbsp, 1 oz	5	0	1
Honey Cream Syrup, ¼ c., 2 oz	220	0	55
Molasses: Dark/Light: 1 T., ¾ oz	55	0	14
1 cup, 11½ oz	880	0	224
Blackstrap: 1 Tbsp, ¾ oz	47	0	13
1 cup, 11½ oz	750	0	208

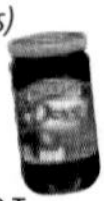

Ice Cream Toppings

	C	F	Cb
Average All Types & Brands			
(Hershey's, Kraft, Smuckers)			
Butterscotch, Caramel, 2 T.	140	1	30
Chocolate: Hot Fudge, 2 T.	140	4	22
Fat Free Chocolate, 2 T.	100	0	23
Pineapple, Strawberry, 2 T.	110	0	28
Smuckers: Guilt-Free/Lite, 2 T.	100	0	24
Magic Shell, 2 Tbsp	210	15	18
Milky Way, 2 Tbsp	130	3.5	24

Honey, Jam, Preserves

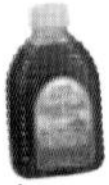

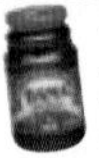

Average All Brands	C	F	Cb
Honey: 1 tsp, ¼ oz	22	0	5.5
1 Tbsp, ¾ oz	65	0	17
1 ounce, 1 oz	85	0	23
1 cup, 12 oz	1030	0	269
Single Portion, ½ oz pkg	45	0	11
Jams/Jellies/Marmalade/Preserves:			
Regular, 1 tsp, ¼ oz	20	0	5
1 Tbsp, ¾ oz	55	0	14
1 ounce, 1 oz	80	0	20
Single Portion, ½ oz pkg	40	0	11
Apple/Fruit Butters, 1 T., 0.6 oz	20	0	6
Fruit Spreads: Regular, 1 tsp	15	0	4
Low Sugar, 1 tsp	8	0	2
Low Cal. *(Featherweight),* 1 tsp	8	0	2
Jelly: Regular, average, 1 tsp	18	0	4.5
Imitation, Low Calorie, 1 tsp	4	0	1

Updated Nutrition Data ~ www.CalorieKing.com
Persons with Diabetes ~ See Disclaimer (Page 24)

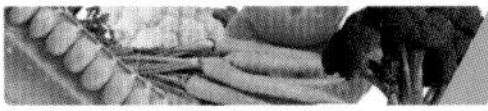

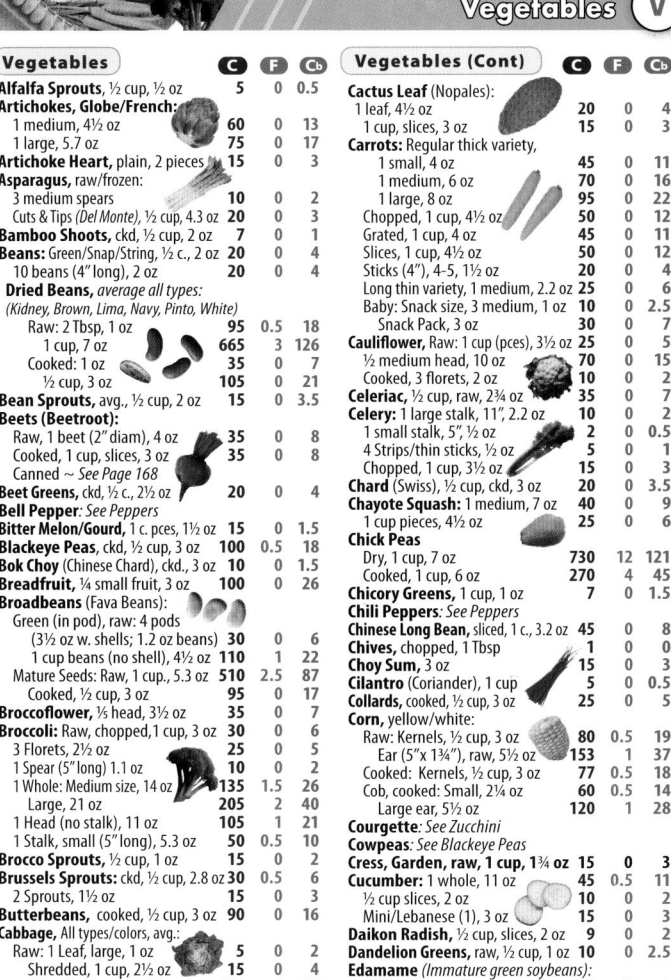

Vegetables	C	F	Cb
Alfalfa Sprouts, ½ cup, ½ oz	5	0	0.5
Artichokes, Globe/French:			
1 medium, 4½ oz	60	0	13
1 large, 5.7 oz	75	0	17
Artichoke Heart, plain, 2 pieces	15	0	3
Asparagus, raw/frozen:			
3 medium spears	10	0	2
Cuts & Tips *(Del Monte)*, ½ cup, 4.3 oz	20	0	3
Bamboo Shoots, ckd, ½ cup, 2 oz	7	0	1
Beans: Green/Snap/String, ½ c., 2 oz	20	0	4
10 beans (4" long), 2 oz	20	0	4
Dried Beans, *average all types:*			
(Kidney, Brown, Lima, Navy, Pinto, White)			
Raw: 2 Tbsp, 1 oz	95	0.5	18
1 cup, 7 oz	665	3	126
Cooked: 1 oz	35	0	7
½ cup, 3 oz	105	0	21
Bean Sprouts, avg., ½ cup, 2 oz	15	0	3.5
Beets (Beetroot):			
Raw, 1 beet (2" diam), 4 oz	35	0	8
Cooked, 1 cup, slices, 3 oz	35	0	8
Canned ~ *See Page 168*			
Beet Greens, ckd, ½ c., 2½ oz	20	0	4
Bell Pepper: *See Peppers*			
Bitter Melon/Gourd, 1 c. pces, 1½ oz	15	0	1.5
Blackeye Peas, ckd, ½ cup, 3 oz	100	0.5	18
Bok Choy (Chinese Chard), ckd., 3 oz	10	0	1.5
Breadfruit, ¼ small fruit, 3 oz	100	0	26
Broadbeans (Fava Beans):			
Green (in pod), raw: 4 pods			
(3½ oz w. shells; 1.2 oz beans)	30	0	6
1 cup beans (no shell), 4½ oz	110	1	22
Mature Seeds: Raw, 1 cup., 5.3 oz	510	2.5	87
Cooked, ½ cup, 3 oz	95	0	17
Broccoflower, ⅕ head, 3½ oz	35	0	7
Broccoli: Raw, chopped,1 cup, 3 oz	30	0	6
3 Florets, 2½ oz	25	0	5
1 Spear (5" long) 1.1 oz	10	0	2
1 Whole: Medium size, 14 oz	135	1.5	26
Large, 21 oz	205	2	40
1 Head (no stalk), 11 oz	105	1	21
1 Stalk, small (5" long), 5.3 oz	50	0.5	10
Brocco Sprouts, ½ cup, 1 oz	15	0	2
Brussels Sprouts: ckd, ½ cup, 2.8 oz	30	0.5	6
2 Sprouts, 1½ oz	15	0	3
Butterbeans, cooked, ½ cup, 3 oz	90	0	16
Cabbage, All types/colors, avg.:			
Raw: 1 Leaf, large, 1 oz	5	0	2
Shredded, 1 cup, 2½ oz	15	0	4
½ Lge Head (7" diam), 22 oz	150	1	35
Cooked, shredded, ½ cup, 2½ oz	15	0.5	3.5

Vegetables (Cont)	C	F	Cb
Cactus Leaf (Nopales):			
1 leaf, 4½ oz	20	0	4
1 cup, slices, 3 oz	15	0	3
Carrots: Regular thick variety,			
1 small, 4 oz	45	0	11
1 medium, 6 oz	70	0	16
1 large, 8 oz	95	0	22
Chopped, 1 cup, 4½ oz	50	0	12
Grated, 1 cup, 4 oz	45	0	11
Slices, 1 cup, 4½ oz	50	0	12
Sticks (4"), 4-5, 1½ oz	20	0	4
Long thin variety, 1 medium, 2.2 oz	25	0	6
Baby: Snack size, 3 medium, 1 oz	10	0	2.5
Snack Pack, 3 oz	30	0	7
Cauliflower, Raw: 1 cup (pces), 3½ oz	25	0	5
½ medium head, 10 oz	70	0	15
Cooked, 3 florets, 2 oz	10	0	2
Celeriac, ½ cup, raw, 2¾ oz	35	0	7
Celery: 1 large stalk, 11", 2.2 oz	10	0	2
1 small stalk, 5", ½ oz	2	0	0.5
4 Strips/thin sticks, ½ oz	5	0	1
Chopped, 1 cup, 3½ oz	15	0	3
Chard (Swiss), ½ cup, ckd, 3 oz	20	0	3.5
Chayote Squash: 1 medium, 7 oz	40	0	9
1 cup pieces, 4½ oz	25	0	6
Chick Peas			
Dry, 1 cup, 7 oz	730	12	121
Cooked, 1 cup, 6 oz	270	4	45
Chicory Greens, 1 cup, 1 oz	7	0	1.5
Chili Peppers: *See Peppers*			
Chinese Long Bean, sliced, 1 c., 3.2 oz	45	0	8
Chives, chopped, 1 Tbsp	1	0	0
Choy Sum, 3 oz	15	0	3
Cilantro (Coriander), 1 cup	5	0	0.5
Collards, cooked, ½ cup, 3 oz	25	0	5
Corn, yellow/white:			
Raw: Kernels, ½ cup, 3 oz	80	0.5	19
Ear (5"x 1¾"), raw, 5½ oz	153	1	37
Cooked: Kernels, ½ cup, 3 oz	77	0.5	18
Cob, cooked: Small, 2¼ oz	60	0.5	14
Large ear, 5½ oz	120	1	28
Courgette: *See Zucchini*			
Cowpeas: *See Blackeye Peas*			
Cress, Garden, raw, 1 cup, 1¾ oz	15	0	3
Cucumber: 1 whole, 11 oz	45	0.5	11
½ cup slices, 2 oz	10	0	2
Mini/Lebanese (1), 3 oz	15	0	3
Daikon Radish, ½ cup, slices, 2 oz	9	0	2
Dandelion Greens, raw, ½ cup, 1 oz	10	0	2.5
Edamame *(Immature green soybeans):*			
Shelled, ½ cup, 2.6 oz	110	5	8
With shells, 10 pods, 1¼ oz	30	1	3

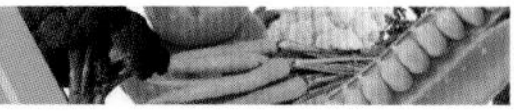

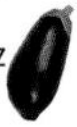

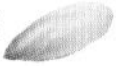

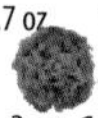

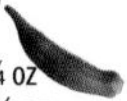

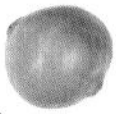

Vegetables (Cont)

	C	F	Cb
Eggplant: Raw, ¼ med, 4 oz	30	0	7
Raw, ½ cup, 1" pieces, 1½ oz	10	0	2.5
1 slice, fried, 1 oz	75	4	10
Endive, Belgian/French: Raw, 1 med. head (6"), 2½ oz	12	0	2.5
Fennel, 1 cup, sliced, 3 oz	25	0	6.5
Gai Choy Cabbage, ckd, 1 cup, 6 oz	20	0	3
Gai Lan (Chinese Kale), ckd, 1 cup	35	0.5	7
Garlic, 1 clove	4	0	1
Ginger: ¼ cup slices, 1 oz	20	0	4.5
Crystallized (sugared), 7 pce, 1½ oz	130	0	35
Horseradish, 1 Tbsp, ½ oz	5	0	1
Jerusalem Artichoke, raw, ½ cup	55	0	13
Jicama, raw, sliced, ½ cup, 2¼ oz	25	0	5.5
Kale, 1 cup, chopped, 2½ oz	35	0.5	7
Kohlrabi, ½ cup, cooked, 1¾ oz	17	0	4
Leek, cooked, 1 whole, 4½ oz	40	0	9
Lentils, green/brown: Dry, 1 oz	100	0.5	17
Dry, 1 cup, 6¾ oz	680	2	115
Cooked, ½ cup, 3½ oz	115	0.5	20
Lettuce, 1 cup, chop./shred., 2 oz	7	0	1.5
Butterhead, 2 leaves, ½ oz	2	0	0.5
Cos/Romaine, shred'd, 1 c., 1.7 oz	10	0	1.5
Iceberg: 1 outer leaf, ½ oz	2	0	0.5
1 medium head, 16 oz	75	1	16
Lima Beans, baby, ckd,½ c., 3 oz	105	0	20
Lotus Root, 10 slices, ckd, 3 oz	60	0	14
Mung Bean Sprouts, ½ cup, 2 oz	15	0	3
Mushrooms: Raw, 1 medium, 0.6 oz	4	0	0.5
Raw, 1 large, sliced, ¾ oz	5	0	1
Raw, ½ cup pieces, 1¼ oz	8	0	1
Cooked, ½ cup pieces, 2½ oz	20	0.5	4
Mustard Greens, Raw, ½ cup, 1 oz	7	0	1.5
Nopales: *See Cactus Leaf.*			
Okra, 8 pods, 4 oz	30	0	7
Cooked, ½ cup, slices, 2¾ oz	20	0	3.5
Onions, Raw: 1 small, 2½ oz	30	0	7
1 medium, 4 oz	50	0	11
1 large, 5½ oz	65	0	15
1 jumbo, 16 oz	190	0.5	46
Chopped, Raw, ½ cup, 3 oz	35	0	8
1 Tbsp, 0.4 oz	4	0	1
Slices: 1 cup, 4 oz	50	0	12
1 medium slice (⅛"), ½ oz	5	0	1
1 large slice (¼"), 1⅓ oz	15	0	4
Dehydrated flakes, ¼ c, ½ oz	50	0	12
Rings, breaded/fried, 2 rings	80	5	9
Scallions, ½ cup, 2 oz	15	0	3.5
Spring, ½ cup, chopped, 2 oz	15	0	3.5
(*French's* Fried Onions: *See Page 72*)			
Blossom/Blooming: See Fast-Foods (Chili's/Outback)			

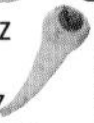

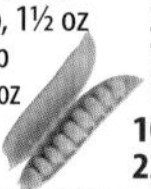

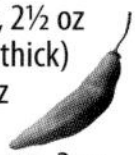

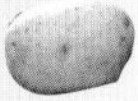

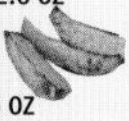

Vegetables (Cont)

	C	F	Cb
Parsley, chopped, ½ cup, 1 oz	10	0	2
Parsnip: 1 medium, 4 oz	85	0	20
Cooked, ½ cup slices, 2¾ oz	55	0	13
Peas: Raw, Green, ¼ cup, 1½ oz	30	0	5
Raw, with pods, ½ lb	70	0	13
Snow Peas, 10 pods, 1.2 oz	15	0	2.5
Split: Dry, hulled, 1 oz	100	0.5	17
Cooked, 1 cup, 7 oz	230	1	42
Peppers: Sweet, 1 medium, 4.2 oz	30	0	6.5
Bell: 1 medium, 4.2 oz	30	0	6.5
½ cup, chopped, raw, 2½ oz	20	0	4.5
1 ring (3" diam. x ¼" thick)	3	0	0.5
Chili: Green/Red, 1½ oz	20	0	4.5
Habanero, 1 only, 8g	10	0	2
Pigeon Peas, cooked, ½ cup, 3 oz	95	1	17
Pimientos, 3 medium, 3½ oz	25	0	5
Poi, ½ cup, 4.2 oz	135	0	33
Potatoes: Raw (with skin)			
1 Baby, Gourmet, 2 oz	45	0	10
1 Small, 6 oz	130	0	30
1 Medium, 7.5 oz	165	0	37
1 Peeled, 4 oz	90	0	20
1 Large, 8 oz	175	0	40
1 Extra large (Russet), 13 oz	285	0.5	65
1 Jumbo (Russet), 16 oz	350	0.5	80
Baked (no fat); large, 10 oz raw:			
Plain, with skin, 7 oz	185	0.3	42
without skin, 5½ oz	145	0	34
Garlic Potatoes, mashed, 4 oz	130	5	19
w. Skin/Toppings: + 2 tsp fat	270	8	58
+ Sour Cr./Chives, 2 Tbsp	320	6	60
+ Plain Yogurt, 2 Tbsp	260	1	60
+ Grated Cheese, 1 oz	370	9	58
+ Cottage Cheese, 2 oz	315	2	60
Mashed w. milk and fat, ½ c.	120	4.5	18
Potato Skins: (w. Cheese topping):			
½ whole (8 oz baking), 4 oz	240	13	22
French Fries: Small svg, 2.6 oz	250	13	30
Medium svg., 4 oz	380	20	47
Froz., uncooked, 18 fries, 4 oz	165	5.5	28
Oven-heated, 18 fries, 4 oz	165	5.5	28
Take-Out, 1 cup, 5 oz	440	25	60
McDonald's: Small, 2.6 oz	250	13	30
Medium, 4 oz	380	20	47
Fried, 18 pieces, 4 oz	167	5.5	24
Au Gratin, ½ cup, 4.3 oz	162	9	14
Pancakes, 2 small, 2 oz	120	6.5	12
Kugel, 5 oz	300	20	26
Puffs, fried, 4 puffs, 1 oz	53	2.5	8
Scalloped, ½ cup, 4¼ oz	114	5.5	15
Ore-Ida Frozen Potatoes: See Page 168			

Updated Nutrition Data ~ www.CalorieKing.com
Persons with Diabetes ~ See Disclaimer (Page 24)

Vegetables (Cont)

	C	F	Cb
Potato Salad, ½ cup, 4½ oz	180	10	14
Pumpkin:			
Mashed, ½ cup, 4⅓ oz	25	0	6
Raw, 1" cubes, 1 cup, 4 oz	30	0	7.5
Pumpkin Flowers, 1 cup, 1.2 oz	5	0	1
Purslane: Cooked, ½ c., 2 oz	10	0	2
Raw, 1" cubes, 1 cup, 1.5 oz	7	0	1.5
Radicchio, 2 leaves, ½ oz	4	0	1
Shredded, 1 cup, 1½ oz	18	0	3.5
Radish: Avg., 10 only, 1½ oz	7	0	1.5
Oriental, ½ c. slices, 1½ oz	8	0	2
Rhubarb, raw, ½ cup, 2 oz	15	0	3
Rutabaga, ckd., ½ c. cubes, 3 oz	33	0	7.5
Salsify, ckd, ½ c. slices, 2½ oz	48	0	11
Sauerkraut, ½ cup, 2½ oz	13	0	3
Seaweed: Average, dried, 1 oz	7	0	2
Soaked, drained, 1 oz	15	0	4
Nori/Laver, dried, 6 sheets, ½ oz	35	0	5
Shallots, chopped, 1 T,, ½ oz	7	0	1.5
Sorrel, raw, ½ cup, 4 oz	23	0.5	4
Soybeans: Mature, dry, 1 oz	118	5.5	9
Dry, ½ cup, 3⅓ oz	387	18	28
Cooked, ½ cup, 3 oz	150	7.5	8.5
(Soy Products/Tofu/Tempeh: See Page 77)			
Spinach: Cooked, ½ cup, 3 oz	20	0	3.5
Raw: 3 leaves/1 cup, 1 oz	7	0	1
1 Bunch, 12 oz	78	1.5	12
Creamed, avg., ½ cup, 4½ oz	187	15	8
Squash: Summer, raw, ½ c., 2½ oz	10	0	2
Cooked, ½ cup slices, 3 oz	14	0	3.5
Winter, cooked,			
Acorn, ½ cup cubes, 3½ oz	34	0	9
½ medium (10 oz raw wt.)	114	0	30
Butternut, ½ c. cubes, 3½ oz	40	0	10
¼ medium (9 oz raw wt.)	115	0	30
Spaghetti, ½ cup, 1¾ oz	16	0	3.5
Succotash, ckd, ½ cup, 3⅓ oz	110	1	23
Sweetcorn: *See Corn*			
Sweet Potatoes:			
Cooked with skin (no fat)			
1 medium, 4 oz	103	0	24
No skin, mashed, ½ c., 5½ oz	125	0	29
Swiss Chard, ckd, chopped, 1 c., 6 oz	35	0	7
Taro, cooked, ½ cup, 2⅓ oz	94	0	23

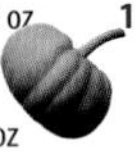
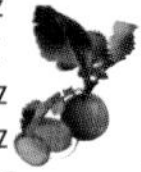
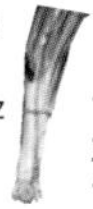
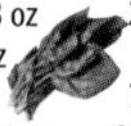
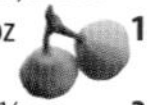
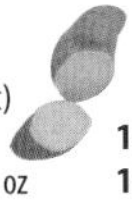

Vegetables (Cont)

	C	F	Cb
Tomatoes: 1 small (2¼" diam.), 3 oz	15	0	3
1 medium (2¾" diam.), 5 oz	25	0	5
1 large (3½" diam.), 8 oz	40	0.5	9
1 extra lge (3" diam.), 12 oz	60	0.5	14
Chopped, 1 cup, 6½ oz	35	0.5	7
Extra Listings: *Page 145*			
Tomatillo, 1 medium, 1.2 oz	10	0	2
Turnip: ckd, ½ cup, 2¾ oz	17	0	4
Greens, cooked, ½ cup, 2½ oz	14	0	3
Water Chestnuts: 5-6 nuts, 1 oz	56	0.5	13
½ cup slices, 2¼ oz, raw	60	0	15
Canned, 1 oz	14	0	3.5
Watercress, 10 sprigs, 1 oz	3	0	0.5
Yams: Cooked, ½ cup, 2½ oz	80	0	19
Baked, 1 medium (6") 8 oz	264	0.5	63
1 large (9") 12 oz	395	0.5	94
Yardlong Bean, 1 pod, ½ oz	6	0	1
Yucca Root, ½ cup, 3½ oz	165	0.5	39
Zucchini: 1 medium, 7 oz, raw	30	0.5	6.5
½ cup slices, cooked, 3 oz	14	0	3.5

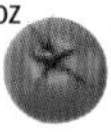
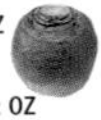
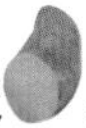
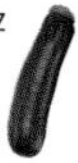

Frozen Vegetables

	C	F	Cb
Birds Eye			
Broccoli/Corn/Vegetables, ⅔ cup	50	1	9
Chopped Spinach, ⅓ cup, 3 oz	30	0	3
Other varieties, average, 1 cup	30	0	6
Baby: Corn & Veg. Blend, ⅔ cup	50	1	9
Broccoli Florets, 1 cup, 3 oz	30	0	4
Corn, Pea & Bean Blend, ¾ cup	70	0.5	13
Sweet Peas, ⅔ cup, 3 oz	70	0	12
Whole Green Beans, 1 cup, 3 oz	35	0	5
Deluxe Vegetables: *Per Cup*			
Sugar Snap Stir Fry, 3½ oz	40	0	7
Broccoli, Cauliflower & Peppers	25	0	3
Broccoli, Carrots & Water Chestnuts	35	0	6
Seasoned: *Per ⅔ Cup, 3 oz*			
Southwestern Corn	90	2	16
Asparagus, Corn & Carrots	70	0.5	13
Singles: *Per 3.25 oz Packet*			
Super Sweet Corn	80	1	14
Sweet Peas	70	0	13
Baby Brussel Sprouts	50	0	9
Steam Fresh: *Per Serving*			
Broccoli Cuts, 1 cup	30	0	4
Mixed Veggies, ⅔ cup	60	0	12
Super Sweet Corn, ⅔ cup	70	1	14
Vegetables & Sauce: *Prepared (Includes Pasta)*			
Asian, 1 cup	60	1	12
Green Bean & Almonds, ¾ cup	80	4	8

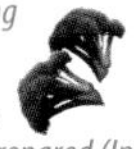

Frozen Vegetables (Cont)

	C	F	Cb
Green Giant			
Just for One,			
Broccoli & Cheese Sauce, 4.25 oz	60	3	7
Vegetables: Asparagus Cuts, ⅔ c.	20	0	3
Corn: Nibblers, ½ ear, 2.2 oz	70	0.5	14
Extra Sweet Niblets, ⅔ cup	70	1	13
Shoepeg, no sauce, ½ cup	70	1	15
Honey-Glazed Carrots, 1 cup	90	3	15
Le Sueur Baby Sweet Peas, ¾ cup	60	0.5	11
Spinach, no sauce, ½ cup, 3½ oz	25	0	3
Veggies In Cheese & Cream Sauce: *Prepared*			
Alfredo Vegetables, ¾ cup	70	2.5	9
Broccoli, Cauliflower, Carrots, 1 c.	50	1.5	7
Cauliflower & Cheese Sce, ½ cup	60	2.5	6
Creamed Spinach, ½ cup	70	2.5	9
Rice & Vegetables: *Per ½ Pkg (Prepared)*			
Cheesy Rice & Broccoli	135	2.5	25
Rice Medley	140	2	26
Rice Pilaf	115	1.5	22
White & Wild Rice	140	3	25
Ore-Ida (As Purchased):			
French Fries: Country, 18 fries, 3 oz	120	4	19
Crispers 20 pces, 3 oz	210	12	23
Crispy Crunchies, 13 fries, 3 oz	160	8	20
Fast-Food Fries, 27 fries, 3 oz	180	7	21
Waffle Fries, 8 fries, 3 oz	160	6	22
Golden Crinkles, 12 pces, 3 oz	130	4	17
Golden Fries, 14 pces, 3 oz	120	2.5	20
Oven Chips, 7 pces, 3 oz	160	7	22
Shoestrings, 32 pces, 3 oz	150	6	19
Steak Fries, 7 fries, 3 oz	120	3	17
Zesties, 12 pces, 3 oz	140	5	22
Hash Browns: Toaster, 2 patties	220	12	25
Potatoes O'Brien, ¾ c., 2 oz	60	0	13
Onion Rings: Gourmet, 3 pces, 3 oz	190	9	24
Onion Ringers, 6 pces, 3.2 oz	220	12	25
Sweet Potatoes: 4 oz	80	0	18
Steam n' Mash			
Cut Russet, ¾ Cup, 3.3 oz	80	0	1
Cut Sweet Potatoes, 1 cup, 4.4 oz	90	0	20
Garlic Seasoned Potatoes, ¾ cup	110	4	17
Three Chse Potatoes, ¾ c.	80	0.5	16
Tater Tots: 9 pces, 3 oz	150	7	22
Mini, 19 pces, 3 oz	190	10	19
Onion, 9 pces, 3 oz	160	7	22
Extra Crispy, 12 pces, 3 oz	145	7	19
Twiced Baked: Potatoes, 1, 5 oz	190	7	26

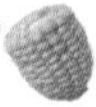

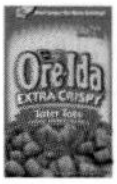

Canned/Bottled

	C	F	Cb
Solids & Liquid			
Artichoke Hearts *(Fanci Foods):*			
Plain, 1 oz (1)	8	0	1
Marinated, ¼ bottle, 1 oz	25	1.5	2
Asparagus, Drained: 3 spears, 2 oz	10	0	1.5
Pieces, ½ cup, 4.3 oz	25	0.5	3
Bamboo Shoots, 1 cup, 4½ oz	25	0	4
Bean Salad, ½ cup, 4⅓ oz, no oil	90	0	20
Beans: Green, ½ cup, 2½ oz	15	0	3
Baked Beans, ½ cup, 4½ oz	120	0.5	27
Butter Beans, ½ cup, 4½ oz	90	0	16
Italian, cut, ½ cup, 4½ oz	30	0	6
Kidney Beans, ½ cup, 3½ oz	105	0.5	19
Lima Beans, ½ cup, 4½ oz	80	0	15
Pinto Beans, ½ cup, 4½ oz	105	1	18
Beets: Sliced, ½ cup, 3 oz	26	0	6
Crinkle/Pickled *(Del Monte)* ½ cup	80	0	20
Carrots: Sliced, ½ cup, 2½ oz	20	0	4
Honey Glazed *(Del Monte)* ½ cup	75	0	18
Corn: Kernels, ½ cup, 4½ oz	80	0.5	18
Creamed style, ½ cup, 4½ oz	92	0.5	23
Garbanzo/Chick Peas, ½ c., 4.2 oz	143	1.5	27
Green Chilies, diced, 2 Tbsp, 1 oz	6	0	1.5
Hearts of Palm (1), 1.2 oz	7	0	1
Mushrooms: ½ cup, 2½ oz	20	0	4
in Butter Sauce, 2 oz	20	1	2
Onions: Pickled, 1 med., ½ oz	10	0	2
Cocktail, 1 onion	0	0	0
French's Fried Onions: *See Page 72*			
Peas, ½ cup, 3 oz	60	0.5	10
Peppers: Hot Chili, Jalapeno, (1), 1 oz	6	0	2
Sweet, undrained, 2½ oz	13	0	3
Jalapeno, w. liq., ½ c. chopped	18	0.5	3
Fried, drained, 2 Tbsp, 1 oz	60	5	3
Salsa, average all types, 2 Tbsp	10	0	2
Sauerkraut, undrained, ½ c., 4 oz	22	0	5
Spinach, ½ cup, 3½ oz	25	0.5	3.5
Succotash: w. Cr. Style Corn, ½ c.	100	0.5	23
w. whole kernels, undrained, ½ c.	80	0.5	18
Sweetcorn: *See Corn*			
Sweet Potato: ½ cup, 3½ oz	90	0	24
Tomatoes, Sundr.: Natural, 5-6 pce	22	0	5
In Oil, drained, 6 pces, ½ oz	38	2.5	4
Tomato Products: *See Page 85*			
Vegetables, mixed, ½ cup, 4 oz	45	0	8
Yams: in Light Syrup, ½ cup, 4 oz	105	0	25
Candied, ½ cup, 5 oz	170	0	46
Zucchini in Tom. Sce., ½ c., 4 oz	30	0	8

Updated Nutrition Data ~ www.CalorieKing.com
Persons with Diabetes ~ See Disclaimer (Page 24)

Quick Guide | C | F | Cb

Yogurt
Average All Brands: Per 8 oz Cup

	C	F	Cb
Plain Yogurt: Whole	140	8	10
Low-Fat	145	3.5	16
Fat-Free	125	0.5	17
Fruit Flavored: Whole, 8 oz	225	8	32
Low-Fat	230	4	43
Fat-Free, regular	215	0.5	43
Fat-Free, no sugar added	80	0	15

Yogurt Parfait/Deli Cups | C | F | Cb

	C	F	Cb
With Fruit Pieces:			
(⅔ Yogurt + ⅓ Fruit)			
Small, 8 oz cup	140	3	20
Large, 12 oz cup	210	4.5	30
With Fruit + Granola:			
Small, 8 oz cup (+ ¾ oz Granola)	235	7	30
Large, 12 oz cup (+ 1½ oz Granola)	400	13	58

Yogurt ~ Brands | C | F | Cb

	C	F	Cb
Albertson's (Low-Fat): Plain, 8 oz	140	2	19
Swiss, avg. all flavors, 8 oz	240	2	49
Fruit on the Bottom (low-fat):			
Average all flavors, 8 oz	230	2	45
Alta Dena: Low-Fat: Plain, 8 oz	170	4.5	20
Average other flavors	220	2	41
Non-Fat: Fruit Flavors	190	0	38
Plain, 8 oz	110	0	16
Vanilla, 8 oz	160	0	30
America's Choice: Swiss Style	210	2.5	41
Non-Fat, all flavors, 8 oz	100	0	15
Blue Bunny			
Light, avg. fruit flavors, 6 oz	100	0	14
No Sugar Added, 6 oz	80	0	14
Superfruit, avg., 6 oz	100	0	14
Omega 3, avg., 4 oz cup	80	1	15
Breyers			
YoCrunch: *Per 6 oz*			
Fun: Cookies n' Crm w. Oreo	190	3.5	34
Strawb. w. Nestle Crunch	210	4.5	37
Vanilla w. Butterfinger	200	4	36
Vanilla w. M&M's Minis	210	4.5	35
Light: Cookies n' Cream w. Oreo	120	2.5	19
Peach/Strawberry w. Granola	120	1	22
Disney Swirled, Low-Fat, avg., 4 oz	110	1	22
Brown Cow			
Cream Top: Plain, 6 oz	130	7	9
Fruit Flavors, average, 6 oz	170	6	27
Low-Fat: Plain, 8 oz	130	3	15
Flavors, average, 8 oz	150	2	27
Non-Fat: Plain, 8 oz	110	0	16
Fruit Flavors, avg., 8 oz	130	0	26
Raspb. Pear & Grains, 6 oz	150	2.5	26

Cabot	C	F	Cb
Non-Fat: Plain, 8 oz	100	0	19
Fruit flavors, 8 oz	130	0	24
Greek Style: Reg., 6 oz	210	17	9
Low-Fat (2%), 6 oz	160	3	25
Cascade Fresh:			
Low-Fat, 6 oz	140	2	23
Fat-Free, all flavors, 6 oz ctn	110	0	20
Whole Milk: Plain, 8 oz	170	8	12
Flavors, average, 8 oz	200	7	24
Colombo			
Light, all flavors, 8 oz	120	0	21
Classic, avg., 8 oz	220	2	42
Fat-Free, Plain, 8 oz	100	0	16
Dannon:			
Plain (Natural), 8 oz	160	8	12
Activia: Avg. all flav.	110	2	19
Light, avg. all flav.	70	0	13
All Natural:			
Flavors, average, 6 oz	160	2.5	26
Non-Fat, Plain, 6 oz	80	0	12
Danimals:			
Drinkables, Strawberry, 4 oz	90	1.5	16
Extreme, 3.1 fl.oz	70	0.5	15
Fruit Blends, avg., 6 oz	170	1.5	33
Fruit on the Bottom, avg.,6 oz	150	1.5	28
Frusion Smoothie, 10 fl.oz bottle	260	3.5	50
La Creme, Regular, avg., 4 oz	140	5	19
Light & Fit (0% Fat): Avg., 6 oz	60	0	11
Carb + Sugar Control Smoothie, 4 oz	60	3	3
Non-Fat Carb, 4 oz	40	0	7
Light & Fit 0% Plus: Vanilla, 4 oz	50	0	10
Avg. other flavors	60	0	11
Emmi Swiss (Low-Fat):			
Fruit flavors, 6 oz	160	2.5	26
Bircher Muesli, 6 oz	180	3	30
Fage			
Peach/Cherry/Strawb., 5.3 oz	210	12	18
Honey, 5.3 oz	250	12	28
0%, 8 oz	120	0	9
2%: Plain 8 oz	150	4.5	9
Fruit, 5.3 oz	140	5	19
Honey, 5.3 oz	180	2.5	29
Horizon Organic			
Whole Milk, Plain Vanilla, 8 oz	220	6	32
Low-Fat: Blended, 6 oz	150	1.5	27
Yogurt Tubes (1)	70	1	12
Fat-Free, all varieties, 6 oz	140	0	27
32 oz Carton, Plain, 8 oz	110	0	15

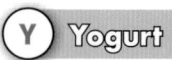

Brands (Cont)   C   F   Cb

	C	F	Cb
Jewel: *8 oz Ctn (Low-Fat)*			
Fruit On The Bottom, avg.	240	2.5	46
Swiss, average	200	2	38
Vanilla	210	2	40
32 oz Tubs: Plain, 1 cup, 8 oz	170	3	20
Plain, Non-Fat, 1 cup, 8 oz	130	0	19
Kemps: '100 Calories' (Non-Fat), 5 oz	100	0	22
Light '80 Calories', 6 oz ctn	80	2	16
Yo Stix, average, 2.25 oz tube	80	2	13
Yo-J Drink, average, 8 fl.oz	150	0	35
Kirkland			
Low-Fat: Blueb./Peach/Strawb. 8 oz	240	2	48
Knudsen: 70 Calories, 6 oz	70	0	11
Free, average, 6 oz	170	0	33
Kroger:			
Blended: Plain, 8 oz	150	54	17
Flavors, 8 oz	250	2.5	47
Active Lifestyle, Vanilla, 6 oz	80	0	12
Carb Master, avg. all flavors, 6 oz	80	1.5	4
Fruit On The Bottom, avg all flav.	220	3	41
Lite, avg. all flavors, 8 oz	100	0	17
Fat-Free, Vanilla, 8 oz	200	0	39
Low-Fat, Plain, 8 oz	150	4	17
La Yogurt:			
Original, average, 6 oz	150	2	30
Light, average, 6 oz	90	0	15
Rich & Creamy, 6 oz	160	2	30
Enriched, average, 6 oz	160	2	30
Fruit on the Bottom, average, 8 oz	220	2.5	43
Sabor Latino: Dulche De Leche, 6 oz	190	1.5	36
Fruit Flavors, average, 6 oz	170	2	34
LALA, Reduced-Fat:			
Fruit Flavors, avg., 8 oz	200	4	36
Smoothies, avg., 9 oz bottle	200	4	34
Light n' Lively			
Fruit Flavors, average, 4.4 oz	135	1	27
Lucerne			
Low-Fat: Plain, 8 oz	150	3.5	18
Fruit Flavors, avg., 8 oz	240	2.5	45
Vanilla	240	2.5	44
Fat-Free: Plain, 8 oz	120	0	20
Light Fat-Free, fruit, 8 oz	130	0	27
Meadow Gold, avg., 6 oz ctn	90	2.5	10
Mountain High			
Original Style, Plain, 8 oz	180	8	17
Strawb./Vanilla, 8 oz	210	7	27
Low-Fat: Classic, all flav., 8 oz pkg	140	1.5	25
Large Containers: Plain, 8 oz	140	2.5	18
Fruit Flavors, avg., 8 oz	180	2.5	30
Fat-Free: Plain, 8 oz	120	0	18
Strawberry/Vanilla, avg., 8 oz	160	0	28

	C	F	Cb
Nancy's			
Whole Milk: Honey, plain, 8 oz	180	8	16
w. Fruit Cup, avg, 9.5 oz	230	5	41
Low Fat: Plain/Lemon/Vanilla, avg	150	3	16
Other flavors, average, 8 oz	180	3	27
Non-Fat: Plain, 8 oz	120	0	17
Vanilla (32 oz ctn), swtn'd, 8 oz	220	0	40
Soy Cultured: (6 oz ctn): Plain	150	3	25
Berry flavors, average	140	3.5	24
O Organics (Safeway), avg., 6 oz	150	2.5	25
Publix: Fat-Free, Plain, 8 oz	140	0	23
Swiss Style, Low-Fat, 8 oz	240	2.5	41
Ralphs: *Same as Kroger*			
Roberts:			
Plain, 8 oz	130	2.5	15
Lemon, 8 oz	200	2	34
Fat-Free, all flavors, 8 oz	90	0	14
with splenda, 6 oz	70	0	11
Silk (Soy): Plain, 1 cup, 8 oz	150	4	22
Vanilla, 6 oz ctn	180	4	31
Other flavors, average, 6 oz	150	2	30
Stater Bros: Plain, 8 oz	140	2	19
Fruit on the Bottom, avg., 8 oz	220	2	44
Blended Low-Fat, avg., 8 oz	240	2	48
Stonyfield Farm (Organic)			
All Natural Fat-Free: Plain, 8 oz	80	0	14
Fruit Flavors, avg., 6 oz	120	0	24
Choc. Underground, 6 oz	170	0	37
Low-Fat: Caramel	180	1.5	35
Plain	90	1	11
Other flavors, avg.	200	2.5	35
Whole Milk Yogurt: Vanilla Truffle	220	5	38
French Vanilla, 6 oz	170	6	23
Other flavors, average, 6 oz	160	6	21
Oikos: Plain, 5.3 oz ctn	90	0	6
Blueberry/Honey, avg., 5.3 oz	120	0	17
O'Soy: Choc.; Vanilla, avg., 6 oz	160	3	26
Fruit on Bottom, average, 6 oz	170	2.5	30
YoKids: Cups, 4 oz	120	2	22
Stop & Shop			
8 oz Ctn: Light (0% Fat), avg.	110	0	20
Fruit on the Bottom, avg.	220	2.5	42
32 oz Tub: Low-Fat, Plain, 8 oz	140	3	16
Non-Fat: Plain, 8 oz	130	0	18
Vanilla, 8 oz	190	0	34
Trader Joe's: Low-Fat, avg., 8 oz	220	3	40
Non-Fat: Regular 8 oz	170	0	34
French Village, Vanilla, 6 oz	130	0	26
Organic Vanilla, 8 oz	160	0	27
Organic Low-Fat, average, 6 oz	150	2.5	25
Cultured Soy, average all, 6 oz	150	3	28
Fruit on the Bottom, Crm Top, 6 oz	170	6	23

Updated Nutrition Data ~ www.CalorieKing.com
Persons with Diabetes ~ See Disclaimer (Page 24)

Brands (Cont)

	C	F	Cb
Trader Joe's (Cont):			
Greek Style; 8 oz Tubs: Fig	310	17	26
Honey	375	22	34
Strawberry	365	18	34
16 oz Tubs: Plain	295	22	9
Non-Fat Plain	120	0	7
Weight Watchers, all flav., 6 oz ctn	100	0.5	17
Wildwood: Soyogurt Plain, 6 oz	90	3.5	11
Other flavors, avg., 6 oz	130	3	23
Smoothie, average, 10 oz	210	4	40
Whole Foods (365)			
365: Non-Fat, Plain, 6 oz	90	0	13
Fruit flavors, avg., 6 oz	150	0	30
Vanilla, 6 oz	130	0	23
365 Organic:			
Fruit flavors, avg., 6 oz	150	0	29
Whole Soy: Plain, 6 oz	150	3	27
Berry, Strawb. Ban., avg.	180	3	35
Other flavors, avg., 6 oz ctn	160	3	30
YoCrunch: *Low-Fat (6oz Cup)*			
With Oreo Cookies	190	3.5	34
With Granola	190	2	38
Vanilla w. Candy pces	200	4.5	35
Yoplait			
Original, average all flavors, 6 oz	170	1.5	33
99% Fat-Free Orig. Flavors, 4 oz	110	0	20
Fiber One, 4 oz	80	0	19
Fizzix, 2 oz	80	2	18
Light: Fruit Flavors, 6 oz	100	0	19
Indulgent Flavors, 6 oz	110	0	20
Thick & Creamy, Light, 6 oz	100	0	20
Thick & Creamy Custard Style, 6 oz	190	3.5	32
Go-Gurt!, Fruit Flavors, 2.2 oz tube	80	2	13
Grande!: Fat-Free Plain, 8 oz cup	130	0	19
99% Fat-Free Flavors, 8 oz cup	250	2.5	48
Trix, Fruit Flavors, 4 oz	120	1.5	23
Whips!: Choc. Flavors, 4 oz	160	4	26
Fruit Flavors, 4 oz	140	2.5	25
Yo-Plus, avg., all flav., 4 oz	110	1.5	20
Yoplait Kids, 4 oz	100	2	17

Yogurt Drinks & Probiotics

	C	F	Cb
Dairy Delite:			
Blueberry; Peach, 16 oz	420	7	82
Strawberry/Banana, 16 fl.oz	380	7	74
Dannon: Danimals, 3.4 fl.oz	90	1.5	15
Danup, 7 fl.oz	150	3.5	27
DanActive, 3.4 fl.oz	95	1.5	17
Frusion, 10 fl.oz	260	3.5	50
Light 'n Fit Smoothies, all flav., 7 fl.oz	70	0	13
Glen Oaks, all flavors, avg., 1 cup	240	3.5	45
Kemps, Yo-J Drink,			
Average all flavors, 8 fl.oz	150	0	35
Lightful, Satiety Smoothies: *Per 8.25 oz*			
(Contain 5g Protein)			
Caffe Latte	90	0.5	37
Mango Oasis	90	0	38
Peachy Cream	90	0	37
Strawberry Bliss	90	0	37
(Note: Carbs include Erythritol natural sweetener)			
Nouriche, Regular, 11 fl.oz	260	0	55
Promise, Activ, 3.3 fl.oz	70	3.5	8
Ralphs: Smoothies			
Peach, 7 fl.oz	200	2.5	37
Raspberry, 7 fl.oz	210	2.5	40
Strawberry, 7 fl.oz	190	2.5	35
Silk Live! 10 oz	230	4	33
Stonyfield Farm			
Smoothies, avg., 10 oz	230	3	39
Light, all flavors, 10 oz	130	0	41
WholeSoy, 12 fl.oz bottle	230	4.5	36
Yonique: Pina Colada, 6 fl.oz	190	4	30
Peach; Banana; Guava, 6 fl.oz	170	2	30
Yoplait Go Gurt, 5 fl.oz	120	0.5	23
Yoplait: Smoothie, 8 fl.oz	220	2.5	44
Light Smoothie, 8 fl.oz	90	0	16

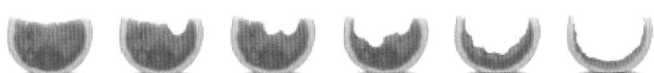

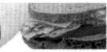
Cafeteria-Style Foods C F Cb

Average All Preperations

	C	F	Cb
Beef Stroganoff, 5 oz	195	13	7
Beef Stroganoff w. 4 oz noodles	350	14	36
Chicken Lasagna, 1 piece	300	11	32
Chicken Chop Suey w. 4 oz rice	245	4	37
Deep Dish Burrito, 7 oz	265	13	20
Grnd Beef Casserole, 2 scoops, 6 oz	245	13	17
Italian Meat Sce for Spagh., 5 oz	150	9	9
w. 5 oz Spaghetti	350	10	49
Lasagna, 1 piece	275	11	25
Meatloaf, 3 oz	205	13	4
Ranch Beans, 2 scoops, 6 oz	350	11	45
Red Beans & Rice, 7 oz	280	9	37
Scalloped Potato/Ham, 2 scp, 6 oz	160	6	20
Stuffed Shells in Sauce (1)	105	3	17
Swedish Meatballs (3)	205	12	9
Sweet & Sour Pork/Rice, 9 oz	240	3	40
Swiss Steak w/Mushr. Gravy, 6 oz	280	11	4
Tator Tot Casserole, 2 scoops, 6 oz	260	15	20
Tenderloin Tips/Mushr. Gravy, 5 oz	210	13	3
w. 5 oz noodles	395	15	38
Tuna Noodle Casserole, 2 scp, 6 oz	180	6	17
Turkey Tetrazzini, 2 scoops, 6 oz	195	7	17
Vegetable Lasagna, 1 piece	250	13	21

Croissants

	C	F	Cb
Unfilled: Medium 1½ oz	180	10	21
Filled: w. Ham (2 oz), garnish	280	14	24
w. Ham (2 oz), Cheese (2 oz)	470	30	20
w. Chick (2 oz) Cheese (2 oz)	470	30	20
w. Turkey/Ham/Chse (2 oz ea.)	580	36	20
Au Bon Pain: Ham & Cheese	340	10	46
Spinach & Cheese	250	9	32

7-Eleven: *Page 244*

Bagels

	C	F	Cb
Plain: Large, 4 oz (no filling)	320	2	65
with 2 oz Cream Cheese	500	27	54
with 2 oz Lox (Smoked Salmon)	400	4	65
Also see Bagels Section: *Page 104*			
Fast-Foods Restaurants: *Page 183*			

Au Bon Pain: *Page 185*

Bruegger's: *Page 192*

Einstein Bros Bagels: *Page 206*

Sandwiches C F Cb

No Spreads Unless Indicated
(Includes 2 Slices Bread ~ 3 oz)

	C	F	Cb
BLT (5 strips Bacon, 2 Tbsp Mayo)	600	40	46
Breaded Chicken & garnish	540	28	46
Chicken Salad w. Mayo., 5 oz	580	30	49
Chopped Liver, Egg, Mayo.	630	25	44
Corned Beef w. Mustard., 5 oz	560	28	44
Egg Salad w. Mayonnaise	570	29	49
Egg Salad Club w. Bacon, Mayo.	780	53	49
Grilled Cheese (3 oz)	540	30	44
Ham (4 oz); Cheese (4 oz), Mayo.	910	56	44
Lobster Salad (4 oz) w. Mayo.	530	25	45
Overstuffed Tuna Salad (7 oz)	870	39	75
Philadelphia Cheese Steak S'wich	550	23	42
Reuben (6 oz Beef/Pastrami, 2 oz Cheese, 2 Tbsp Dressing)	920	60	28
Roast Beef (4 oz) w. Mustard	460	12	45
Roast Pork (4 oz) w. Apple Sauce	500	16	55
Shrimp Salad Club w. Bacon, Mayo.	800	57	48
Sloppy Joe w. Sauce (7 oz)	600	30	45
Steak Sandwich (5 oz cooked)	680	32	41
Triple Cheese (4 oz) Melt	720	45	46
Tuna Salad w. Mayo., 5 oz	610	30	49
Turkey Breast (5 oz) w. Mayo.	460	18	44
Turkey Breast (5 oz) w. Mustard	360	7	44
Turkey Club w. Bacon, Mayo.	830	38	31
Vegetarian w. Avocado, Cheese	820	49	72

7-Eleven: *Page 244*

Schlotzsky's: *Page 246*

Subway: *Page 257*

Wraps & Roll-Ups C F Cb

Average All Types
(Meat/Chicken/Fish/Veggie)

	C	F	Cb
Small size, approx. 9 oz	500	25	48
Regular, approx. 15 oz	830	40	80
Large, approx. 22 oz	1400	70	134
Fast-Foods Restaurants: *Page 182*			

Au Bon Pain: *Page 185*

Sonic Drive-In: *Page 251*

Subway: *Page 257*

WAWA: *Page 266*

Updated Nutrition Data ~ www.CalorieKing.com
Persons with Diabetes ~ See Disclaimer (Page 24)

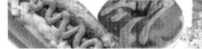

Fair & Carnival Foods

Mexican	C	F	Cb
Burritos w. Bean/Beef, 17 oz	1100	41	104
Carne Asada, 14.5 oz	820	44	58
Fish Tacos, 1 taco, 5 oz	270	13	31
Nachos w. Cheese, 9" plate	860	59	70
Taco Chicken, 3.3 oz	210	12	16
Tamale (1), 3.5 oz	180	8	21
Taquitos, 5 oz	370	17	43

Greek			
Baklava, 2" square	245	13	32
Falafel, 11.6 oz	660	27	85
Greek Salad, 14 oz	520	48	17
Gyros, 7.5", 12 oz	680	40	55
Spanakopita, 8 oz	200	7.5	23

Italian			
Garlic Bread, ½ loaf, 10 oz	1135	40	147
Pizza Bread, Pepperoni, ½ loaf, 12 oz	1115	32	151
Pizza on a Stick, 1 piece	535	28	55
Personal Pizza: 7": Cheese (1)	670	24	80
Pepperoni (1)	795	35	80
Ham & Pineapple (1)	800	31	87

Low Carb			
Beef Patty, wrapped in lettuce, 4 oz	480	33	0

Sandwiches: Per 7½" Roll			
Ham, 11 oz	645	39	47
Hot Pastrami, 9 oz	760	17	62
Roast Beef, 11 oz	620	36	46
Philadelphia Cheese Steak, 13 oz	680	36	49
Tuna, 12 oz	830	60	46
Turkey, 11 oz	665	24	65
Veggie, 11 oz	490	23	49
Oriental: Fried Egg Roll, 6 oz	400	19	44
Rice Bowl: Beef, 6" Bowl	880	13	136
Chicken, 6" Bowl	870	15	135

Hamburgers			
⅓ Pound Burger, 7.5 oz	670	41	26
Cheeseburger, 6 oz	550	36	25

Hot Dogs/Franks: With Bun			
Hot Dog: Regular, (1)	215	14	28
with Chili, 6 oz	450	32	32
with Chili & Cheese, 7.3 oz	500	36	31
⅓ Pound Hot Dog	550	41	31
Foot Long Hot Dog	470	26	41
Corn Dog: Regular, 4 oz	250	14	23
Jumbo, 6 oz	375	21	36
Jumbo Franks w. Bun:			
Bratwurst; Sausage; Kielbasa, avg.	800	60	28

Fair & Carnival Foods (Cont)

Barbeque Items (Weights with Bone)	C	F	Cb
Chicken, 15 oz	740	24	34
Corn on the Cob, 8" (1), 16 oz	200	1	42
Pork Ribs, 18 oz	1360	68	21
Smoked Turkey Legs (w/ skin), 19 oz	1135	54	0
Beef Stew over Rice, 2 cups	440	14	61

Potatoes & Fries			
Australian Battered Potato, 12 oz	1290	66	155
Baked Potato, 14 oz	435	0.5	100
Fries: French, 7 oz	560	24	70
Cheese Fries, 10 oz	645	38	62
Chili Fries, 10 oz	700	36	83
Chili/Cheese Fries, 13 oz	745	45	57
Curly Fries, 7 oz	620	30	78
Tasti Chips, 40 chips, 6.5 oz	780	33	117
Sweet Potato, 14 oz	405	0.5	97
Ranch Dip, 3 oz	165	14	9

Finger Foods			
Artichoke: Steamed, 6 pieces	65	0	16
Fried, 9 pieces	250	14	24
Chicken Nuggets (6)	340	17	26
Chicken Strips (4), 4.5 oz	445	21	33
Finger Steaks (2), 4 oz	400	20	26
Mushrooms, Fried, 10-12 pieces	395	26	34
Onion Rings, 3 rings	310	13	40
Onion Flower	1320	72	140
Shrimp, Fried, 10-12 pieces, 5 oz	555	30	36
Sweet Potato Strips, Fried, 4 pces	750	30	106
Zucchini, Fried, 4 slices	620	40	42

Salads/Sides			
Baked Beans, 4 oz	140	2	38
Chili, 1 cup	280	11	24
Cole Slaw, 5 oz	350	21	37
Pickle, whole (6")	30	0	8
Potato Salad, 5 oz	290	15	35
Popcorn: Plain, small, 3 oz	450	24	48
Large, 6 oz	900	48	96
Kettle Corn: Small, 5 oz	600	15	110
Large, 10 oz	1200	30	220

Cakes, Donuts, Cookies			
Funnel Cake: Plain	760	44	80
Toppings: Cinn. & Sugar, 2 tsp	30	0	8.5
Apple Cinnamon, 2 oz	85	3	36
Strawberries & Cream, 2 oz	70	0	16
Cinnamon Roll, large	730	24	114
Churro, 1½ oz	165	8	21
Donuts, Jumbo Twist, 7.5 oz	905	49	109

Fair & Carnival Foods (Cont)

	C	F	Cb
Cakes, Donuts, Cookies (Cont)			
Fried Snicker Bar, 5 oz	445	29	42
Fried Oreos, 3 cookies	300	10	33
Fried Twinkie, 1	420	34	45
Cotton Candy, 5½ oz bag	625	0	156
Red Rope Licorice, (24"), 2 oz	200	0	46
Cream Puff, 4.3 oz	500	43	22
Puff-on-a-Stick (4), 8.6 oz	995	86	44
Strawberry Crepe, 4.3 oz	280	14	36
Choc. Dipped Strawberry, 1 pce	125	7	15
Fudge, 1.5 oz	200	11	25
Twinkie Dog (Sundae)	500	14	89
Key Lime Pie Bar, 6 oz	635	40	59
Cheesecake on a Stick, 6 oz	655	47	56
Cobbler, 5 oz	350	10	62
Soft Pretzel, 4.5 oz	340	2	70
Candied Apple, 7 oz	330	0.5	80
Ice Cream & Frozen Treats			
Dippin' Dots Ice Cream: Small, 4 oz	150	7	17
Medium, 8 oz	305	14	35
Large, 16 oz	600	28	70
Snow Cone (includes 3 oz syrup)	270	0	68
Frozen Yogurt in sugar cone, 14 oz	475	2	94
Ice Cream: Small, sugar cone, 10 oz	775	42	83
Large, sugar cone, 14 oz	935	54	96
Sherbet, 8 oz	270	4	59
Frozen Banana, choc cover, 5 oz	240	4	53
Drinks			
Lemonade, 18 fl.oz	210	0	52
Orange Julius, 20 fl.oz	490	10	96
Strawberry Julius, 20 fl.oz	430	0	98
Icee, 16 fl.oz	235	0	59
Malt, 16 fl.oz	690	33	85
Slushies, 16 fl.oz	260	0	65
Soft Frozen Lemonade, 12 fl.oz	300	0	78
Smoothies: Berry Flavors, 16 fl.oz	350	1	80

Stadium Foods

	C	F	Cb
Sandwiches			
Bacon Burger, 8.3 oz	470	25	34
Cheeseburger, 8.3 oz	450	23	33
Chicken Sandwich: w. Cheese, 8.3 oz	510	29	40
no Cheese, 7.7 oz	460	25	40
w. Bacon, 8.3 oz	530	31	41
Hamburger, 7.8 oz	400	19	33
Polish Sausage Sandwich, 7 oz	565	33	46
French Fries, 6.4 oz	470	34	39
Fruit Cup, 6 oz	80	0	20
Hot Dogs			
Chili Dog, 7.7 oz	520	29	45
Hot Dog, 6.4 oz	465	21	50
Jumbo Dog, 8 oz	490	25	38
Kraut Dog w. Sauerkraut, 7.8 oz	490	27	41
Nachos, 40 chips w. 4 oz cheese	1100	59	132
Individual Pan Pizza (6"): *Per 10 oz Pizza*			
BBQ Chicken	630	24	71
Cheese	630	27	71
Pepperoni	660	30	70
Snacks			
Brownie, 2.5" x 4.5"	360	18	44
Cheese Sauce, 1.25 oz	100	8	4
Cheetos, 2.75 oz pkg	440	28	42
Chocolate Chip Cookie, 2.3 oz	280	12	40
Churros, 8", 3 oz	325	15	42
Doritos, Nacho, 2.75 oz pkg	390	20	48
King Size Candy:			
Butterfinger, 3.75 oz	485	18	75
Nestle Crunch, 2.75 oz	390	21	85
Lays Chips, 2.75 oz pkg	440	28	42
Peanuts in shell, 8 oz	930	80	24
Popcorn: Small (9 cup size)	575	35	56
Large (15 cup size)	950	58	93
Red Vines, 5.5 oz box	560	0	136
Soft Pretzel: Regular, 5.5 oz	490	3.5	101
Giant, 8 oz	710	5	147
Beverages: Orange Juice, 12 fl.oz	180	0	2
Beer: Heineken, 16 fl.oz	200	0	16
Light Miller, 16 fl.oz	165	0	10
Miller Draft, 16 fl.oz	205	0	18
Jack Daniels Punch, 12 fl.oz	235	0	34
Wine, White, 9 fl.oz	190	0	6
Soda (with ½ ice), average: 20 fl.oz	160	0	40
32 fl.oz	260	0	65
Snow Cone, 18 oz (incl. 3 oz syrup)	270	0	68
Starbuck's Frappuccino, 12 fl.oz	195	2.5	39

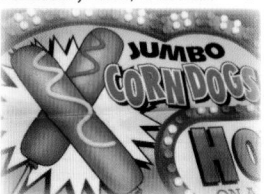

Updated Nutrition Data ~ www.CalorieKing.com
Persons with Diabetes ~ See Disclaimer (Page 24)

Chinese & Asian Dishes

	C	F	Cb
Appetizers			
Crab Cake, 63g	105	5	0.5
Curried Meat Triangles, 1 pce	150	5	12
Dumplings: Pork, steamed, 1	40	3	4
Pork, fried, 1 dumpling	75	7	4
Vegetable, steamed, 1	25	0.5	4
Egg Rolls, mini, 3 rolls	100	3	11
Rice Paper Roll, 1	80	2	10
Spring Roll: Small, 1½ oz	100	7	10
Medium, 3 oz	200	12	20
Large, 5 oz	350	15	33
Wonton, 1 only	55	3	4
Soup: Egg Flower, bowl	90	2	16
Hot & Sour Soup, bowl	110	4	14
Rice: Plain, 1 cup (½ Pint), 6½ oz	240	0.5	54
2 cups (1 Pint), 13 oz	480	1	108
Fried: 1 cup, 5 oz	320	13	42
Large dish, 16 oz	1010	40	134
Noodles: Chinese Egg, ckd, 1 cup	200	3	42
Entrees & Mains: *Per Whole Dish*			
Almond Chicken, 18 oz	685	50	18
Beef Satay, 17 oz	760	50	15
Beef in Black Bean Sce, 17 oz	530	33	17
Broccoli Beef, 16 oz	650	30	31
Chicken (sliced) & Broccoli	280	12	13
Chop Suey: Chicken, 20 oz	560	37	7
Pork, 20 oz	680	50	12
Chow Mein, Beef/Chicken, 24 oz	940	60	50
Crab Puff/Rangoon, 1 dumpling	80	4.5	7.5
Crispy Fried Chicken, 8 oz	485	33	12
Egg Drop Soup: w. Noodles, 1 cup	120	3	15
w/out Noodles, 1 cup	70	3	3
Egg Foo Yung w. Sauce, 1 cup	225	12	11
Kung Pao Chicken, 6 oz	240	15	12
Lemon Chicken, 10 oz	580	32	25
Lo Mein (stir-fried)	620	29	61
Moo Shu Chicken, 2 wrapped crepes	430	16	43
Omelet, Chicken/Shrimp, 16 oz	990	82	10
Orange Chicken, 6 oz	500	27	42
Steamed Whole Fish: ½ Red Snapper	500	11	1
Sweet & Sour: Fish, 20 oz	1160	58	106
Pork, 18 oz	950	50	92
Vegetable Combination, w. oil, 6 oz	250	17	19
Vegetables, Steamed (no oil), 6 oz	120	1	25
Bubble Tea, average, 12 fl oz	240	0	55
Fortune Cookie: each	25	0.5	5

Cajun & Creole

	C	F	Cb
Alligator, 4 oz cooked	160	2	0
Baked Herb Chicken, 1 serving	850	53	2
Bouillabaisse	400	15	10
Cajun Fried Turkey, 1 serving	630	25	0
Cocktail Sauce, 2 Tbsp	30	0	6
Couche-couche, ½ cup	80	0	17
Crawfish Bisque, 1 serving	500	10	10
Crawfish, cooked, 2 oz	45	0.5	0
Creole Jambalaya, 1 serving	550	30	15
Frog Legs, steamed (2)	45	0	0
Guinea Fowl, flesh, 4 oz, ckd	160	4	0
Hogshead Cheese, ¼ cup	80	5.5	0
Jambalaya, Shrimp & Crabmeat	520	14	12
Red Beans & Rice, 1 serving	400	17	52
Roasted Quail, w. Bacon on Toast	550	25	15
Remoulade Sauce, 2 Tbsp, 1 oz	110	11	2
Shrimp Creole, 1 serving	450	20	10
Stuffed Smothered Steak, w. 1 cup Rice	890	50	50
Turtle, cooked, 3 oz	120	3	0

Cuban

	C	F	Cb
Bl. Beans w. Rice (Moros con Cristianos)	510	22	76
Blk.-eyed Pea Fritters (Bollitos de Carita)	80	5	6
Casserole Corn Tamale	445	20	55
Chkn w. Yellow Rice (Arroz con Pollo)	925	49	87
Cuban Bread (Pan Cubano)	80	1.5	15
Donuts in Syrup (Bunuelos)	170	5	10
with Melado	100	5	10
Grilled Plantains	145	0	40
Gypsy's Arm Cake (Brazo Gitano)	260	18	42
Roast Pork S'wich (Pan con Lechon)	640	30	62
Seasoned Beef w. Olives & Raisins (Picadillo)	435	36	10
Shredded Beef (Ropa Vieja)	550	35	10
Taro Root Mash (Pure de Malanga)	315	3	69
Yuca with Citrus Garlic Dressing (Yuca con Mojo)	190	9	25

French Foods

	C	F	Cb
Blanquette d'Agneau (Lamb Stew)	800	30	17
Brioche, 1 cake	280	14	34
Bouillabaisse (Fish Stew)	400	15	10
Coq au Vin (Chicken in Wine)	800	30	16
Coquilles St. Jacques	320	13	36
Crème Brulée, 1 serving	460	40	21

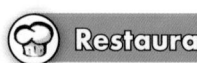

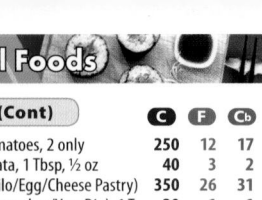

French Foods (Cont) | C | F | Cb

Item	C	F	Cb
Baguette, 3 slices, 2.2 oz	150	1	35
Creme Caramel (Caramel Custard)	260	10	38
Crepe Suzette, 1x6" crepe w. sauce	220	10	13
Duck a l'Orange	780	35	47
Escargot (Snails), garlic butter (6)	200	10	4
Frog Legs, fried, 4 med. pairs	400	20	10
Lamb Noisettes, fried, 2 chops	500	40	1
Mousse au Chocolat	380	15	33
Potage Creme Crecy (Carrot Soup)	360	18	14
Salade Nicoise (Tuna/Oliv./Veg.)	450	13	14
Veal Cordon Bleu (Veal/Ham/Ch)	650	25	18
Vichyssoise (Pot./Leek Soup), 1 c.	200	9	15

Baguette & French Stick: *Page 102, 103*
Croissants: *Pages 113, 173*

German

Item	C	F	Cb
Bavarian Bread Dumpling, 3 small	330	10	28
Beef Goulash with Veggies	520	20	46
Black Forest Cake, 1 slice	380	16	30
Bratwurst, grilled, 1 medium, 6 oz	450	37	2
Chicken: Fried, Viennese-style	530	20	28
Livers w. Apple/On., 6 oz	460	28	10
Herring, Pickled: Rollmops, 4 oz	260	16	3
with Sour Cream, 4 oz	310	20	3
Hot Sausage Curry	300	7	6
Kugelhupf Cake, 1 lge slice, 4 oz	400	23	40
Sauerbraten Pork (Pot Roast)	650	35	15
Torte: Linzer (Alm./Raspb. Jam)	430	18	58
Sacher (Choc./Apricot Jam)	260	12	23
Weiner Schnitzel, 1 medium	750	35	38

Greek

Item	C	F	Cb
Baklava Pastry: Small	240	13	32
Large, 3¾ oz	400	21	45
Calamari, deep fried, 1 cup	300	13	17
Chicken Kebob Plate	345	13	8
Galactobureko, 1 only			
(Filo, Custard, Pastry in Syrup)	360	15	48
Greek Chicken Salad	400	18	9
Gyros, 4 oz	380	33	6
Hummus & Pita, 4 oz	260	12	30
Kataifi, (Filo, Nut, Pastry in Syrup)	350	11	56
Moussaka, 1 serve, 8 oz	350	22	22
Soup: Argolemono (Egg Lemon Soup			
with Chicken & Rice)	85	6	5
Souvlaki (Lamb), each, 2 oz	120	6	1

Greek (Cont) | C | F | Cb

Item	C	F	Cb
Stuffed Tomatoes, 2 only	250	12	17
Taramosalata, 1 Tbsp, ½ oz	40	3	2
Tyropita (Filo/Egg/Cheese Pastry)	350	26	31
Tzatziki (Cucumber/Yog. Dip), 1 T.	20	1	1
Vine Leaves (Dolma), stuffed, 3 rolls, 6 oz	200	5	13

Daphne's Greek Cafe: *See Fast-Foods Section*

Hawaiian

Item	C	F	Cb
Ahi Tuna, grilled (6 oz fillet), no fat	220	2	0
Chicken Long Rice, 1 cup, 7 oz	240	14	12
Gyoza, 1 only	55	2	6
Haupia (Coconut Pudd.), 1 pce (4"x 2½")	120	6	17
Hawaiian Sweet Bread, ½ sl., 2 oz	180	4.5	29
Kalua Chicken, 4 oz	280	16	0
Pork, 4 oz	350	24	0
Kim Chee (pickled cabbage), ½ c., 4 oz	20	0	5
Kulolo (Taro Pudding), 1 slice	125	5	19
Lau Lau: Chicken (1) 7 oz	280	21	3
Pork (1) 7 oz	320	26	5
Loco Moco (rice/burger/egg/gravy)	650	27	63
Lomi Salmon, ¼ cup, 4 oz	20	1	2
Malasadas (Donut), 2 oz	240	13	26
Manapua (Char Siu Pork Bun), 2.3 oz	180	8	25
Poi (mashed ckd taro), 1 c., 8½ oz	270	0.5	65
Poke, avg all types, 3 oz	90	1	9
Portuguese Sausage, 2 oz	180	15	2
Potato Salad, ½ cup, 5 oz	170	10	17
Shave Ice *(Matsumoto)*, all flavors:			
w. Icecream, 1 large	300	4	64
w. Beans, 1 large	290	0	72
Spam Musubi: w. Regular Spam	265	11	34
(4 oz rice+1.3 oz Spam/7-Eleven Hawaii)			
Homemade: w. Lite Spam (50% less fat)	220	5	34
Taro Pancake Mix, ⅓ cup (makes 2)	140	2	26
Plate Lunches:			
Chicken Katsu (9 oz) w. 2 scp Rice	1110	48	108
+ Macaroni Salad, ¾ cup	1360	68	123
or Tossed Salad + Fr. Dress. (2 T.)	1240	61	111
Hamburger (5 oz) w. 2 scoops Rice	710	24	81
Gravy + Macaroni Salad	1135	49	112
MahiMahi (7 oz) w. 2 scoops Rice	650	12	90
+ Macaroni Salad + Tartar Sce	1150	58	109
or Macaroni Salad, no Tartar Sce	935	34	108
or Tossed Salad + Fr. Dress. (3 T.)	815	27	96
or Tossed Salad, no dressing	670	12	93
Teri Beef (5 oz) w. 2 scoops Rice	790	23	94
+ Macaroni Salad, ¾ cup	1095	47	113
or Tossed Salad, no dressing	800	23	95

Updated Nutrition Data ~ www.CalorieKing.com
Persons with Diabetes ~ See Disclaimer (Page 24)

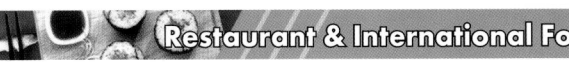

Indian & Pakistani | C | F | Cb |

Per Serving
(Meat dishes allow 4 oz meat/serving)

	C	F	Cb
Aloo Samosa, each	155	12	12
Alu Gosht Kari (Meat/Pot. Curry)	600	40	23
Chicken Korma	500	35	6
Chicken Pilaf (Murgh Biriyani)	700	53	50
Chicken Tikka	260	16	2
Chicken Vindaloo	400	20	8
Chapati/Roti, 7″ diam. piece	60	0.5	11
Dal (Lentil Puree): 1 cup, no oil	230	1	37
1 Tbsp Tadka (oil topping)	120	13	0
Dhakla (Lentil Dish), 1″ sq., 1 oz	105	5	13
Dhansak, ½ cup	105	3.5	11
Gosht Kari (Meat Curry/Tom./Pot.)	460	25	17
Lamb Pilaf	520	35	40
Lassi (Sweet or Mango), 1 cup, 8 oz	160	4	24
Masala Gosht (Beef/Tom./Gravy)	400	25	18
Mulligatawney Soup, average	300	15	8
Murgh Tikka, 1 cup	300	4	7
Naan Bread, ¼ (8″ x 2″), 1 oz	75	2	11
Pappadum, 1 large/2 small	50	3	5
Pesrattu (Lentil Crepe), 9″, 2.6 oz	130	5	15
Pork Vindaloo Curry	620	47	3
Rajmah (Kidney Bean Curry), 1 cup	225	5	35
Rogan Josh (Lamb/Yogurt Sce)	500	30	3
Shahi Chicken (Braised Lamb)	430	28	3
Tandoori Chicken: Breast	260	13	5
Leg/Thigh portion	300	17	6

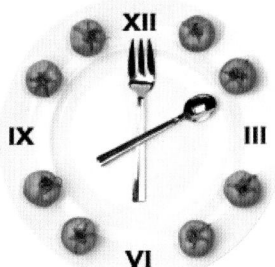

Italian Dishes | C | F | Cb |

	C	F	Cb
Baked Ziti: Small	370	27	32
Regular	575	42	49
Breadstick (1), 2 oz	120	2.5	25
Broccoli Fettucine Alfredo, reg.	815	23	125
Bruschetta, 2 slices	380	17	53
Calzones, average, all types	840	34	101
Cannelloni, 1 tube, 6 oz	280	15	18
Cheese Breadstick (1), 2.4 oz	180	8	20
Cheese Ravioli w. Sauce	495	17	65
Chicken Alfredo	775	29	82
Chicken Parmigiana, 11 oz	520	22	16
Chicken Scallopine, dinner	1110	71	68
Eggplant Parmigiana	900	39	78
Fettucine Alfredo: Small	525	15	80
Lunch	775	22	119
Dinner	1130	81	68
Linquine & Seafood, dinner	1130	71	79
Manicotti Formaggio	800	38	57
Meat Lasagne: Small, 10 oz	440	23	39
Large, 16 oz	700	36	60
Meat Ravioli	725	22	102
Minestrone Soup, 1 bowl	110	2	18
Penne Rustica: Lunch	1300	71	76
Dinner	1540	80	101
Ravioli, over-stuffed, average	990	67	57
Spaghetti & Meatballs			
With Tomato Sauce: Kids	500	20	58
Medium/Lunch	1080	63	89
Large/Dinner	1430	81	119
With Meat Sauce: Kids	550	25	56
Medium/Lunch	1300	79	84
Large/Dinner	1700	103	110
Veal Marsala, dinner	1320	66	132
Veal Parmigiana, dinner	1270	65	116
Vegetable Primavera	610	8	116
Macaroni & Cheese ~ *Page 135*			
Panini S'wich (Restaurant):			
Chicken, 16 oz	900	38	81
Meats, avg., 18 oz	940	39	81
Vegetarian, 15 oz	750	31	83
Pizza: Ready-To-Eat ~ *Page 137*			
Gourmet Deep Dish (*Gino's East*) ~ *Page 209*			
Desserts: Lemon Ice	180	0	45
Gelato: Vanilla (Milk Base), ½ cup	200	15	18
Choc. Hazelnut (Milk), ½ cup	370	29	26
Water Base, ½ cup	100	0	25
Tiramisu, 1 piece, 5 oz	400	29	30

For more listings see Fast-Foods Section

Japanese

	C	F	Cb
Sushi Rice: cooked, 1 Tbsp	25	0	5
1 cup, 5¼ oz	380	3	82
Sushi (Maki) Rolls: *Per Piece*			
Average all types (California Rolls; Crm Cheese w. Crab; Eel; Salmon; Shrimp; Tuna; Yellowtail; Vegetable)			
Small (1⅛" diam. x 1⅛" high), 0.8 oz	25	0.5	3.5
Med. (1¾" diam. x 1¾" high), 1.6 oz	50	1	7
Large (2¼" diam. x ⅞" high), 2 oz	60	1.5	9
Sushi Packs: *Per Pack*			
Average all types: 6 large pces	370	5	55
9 medium pieces	360	6	60
12 small pieces	265	3	45
Futomaki (thick roll), 6 pieces	380	5	72
Hand Roll (Cone) 4 oz	120	2	18
Inari (rice filled soybean pocket), 4 pce	420	9	73
Sushi-Nigiri (fish on rice):			
average all types, 1 piece	70	0.5	12
Sushi Plate: Assorted, 6 pieces	420	3	36
Combination (Sushi & Sushi Rolls)			
2 Sushi + 6 sm. & 3 med. rolls	400	7	72
Sashimi (Sliced Raw Seafood/Beef)			
Ika (Squid), 4 oz	105	2	0
Hamachi (Yellowtail), 4 oz	165	6	0
Maguro (Yellowfin Tuna), 4 oz	120	1	0
Niku (Beef), 5 oz	200	10	0
Saba (Mackerel), 4 oz	160	7	0
Suzuki (Sea Bass), 4 oz	110	0.5	0
Tako (Octopus), 4 oz	95	1	0
Dipping Sauces: Average, 2 Tbsp	30	0	7
Ginger Vinegar Dressing, 2 Tbsp	20	0	5
Edamame (young green soybeans):			
Steamed (in pods), 4 oz	60	3	5
Boiled beans (no pods), 4 oz	160	7	12
Katsu-don Pork w. Rice	1100	39	141
Miso Soup w. Tofu pieces, 1 cup	85	3	11
Seaweed Salad, 1.5 oz	20	2	0
Sukiyaki (Beef/Tofu/Veg.), 8 oz	400	24	32
Tempura (Batter-fried Shrimp & Veggies)			
3 large shrimp & veggies	320	18	25
1 shrimp only	60	4	3
Teppan Yaki (Steak, Seafood & Veggies)			
10 oz serving	470	30	15
Teriyaki: Beef, 4 oz serving	350	25	4
Chicken, 4 oz serving	260	9	7
Salmon, 6 oz serving	270	8	3
Sake Wine (16% alc.), 3 fl.oz	115	0	7
Yakatori, 1 skewer, 2½ oz	140	5	1

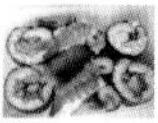

Kosher/Deli Foods

	C	F	Cb
Bagel/Bialy, 1 small, 2 oz	160	2	32
Beiglach (Cheese Knish)	350	17	35
Blintzes: Average, 1 only	120	1	25
w. Sour Cream. & Preserves	370	10	30
Borscht: (no sour cream), 1 cup	85	3	14
Diet/Reduced Cal., 1 cup	30	1	7
Cabbage Roll (meat/rice), 5 oz	170	6	21
Chicken Broth: 1 cup	80	8	0
with vegetables	100	8	5
with noodles	150	9	16
Lowfat, plain, 1 cup	25	1	0
Cholent, 1 med. serving, 1 cup	350	16	48
Chopped Liver: 1 serving, 3 oz	110	6	5
with Egg Salad, ¼ cup	100	7	3
Farfel, dry, ½ cup	90	0.5	21
Hallah (Yeast Bread), 1 sl., 1 oz	85	2	14
Gefilte Fish Balls: Reg., medium, 2 oz	55	2	4
with jelled broth	80	2	6
Cocktail size, 1 oz	30	1	2
Sweet, medium, 2 oz	55	2	4
with jelled broth	95	2	9
Herring: Smoked, 2 oz	120	8	0
in Sour Cream, 2 oz	150	10	0
Kasha, cooked, ½ cup	100	0.5	20
Kipfel (Vanilla/Almd. Cookie), 1 pce	60	2	7
Knaidlach ~ See Matzo Balls			
Knish: Kasha/Potato, 1 only	130	4	22
Cheese, 1 only	350	17	35
Kreplach, beef, 1 piece	40	1	6
Kugel, potato/noodle, 1 serving	300	20	25
Latkes (Potato Pancake), 2 oz	200	11	22
3 Latkes w. Sour Cr./Apple Sce	750	25	95
Lochshen: Plain, 1 cup	130	2	26
Pudding, 1 cup	380	13	48
Lox (Smoked Salmon), 2 oz	65	2	0
Mandelbrot (Almond Bread), 1 slice, ¼" thick	45	2	5
Matzo *(See Page 105)*, 1 oz board	110	0.5	21
Matzo Balls: 2 small, or 1 large, 2"	90	3	12
Extra large ball, 3"	180	6	24
Matzo Ball Soup:			
Cup w. 2 small or 1 large ball	150	5	27
Bowl with Chicken & Noodles	325	13	34
Jerry's Deli, large bowl	560	17	56
New York Cheesecake, 4 oz	350	24	26
Pierogi, potato/cheese, 1 pce	90	4	11
Reuben S'wich w. ½ lb corned beef	920	60	28
Schmaltz (Rend'd chick. fat), 1 T.	90	10	0

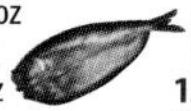

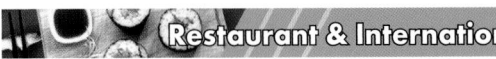

Korean Food

	C	F	Cb
Bibimbab (Veggies & Beef on Rice), 1 cup	565	15	89
Bulgogi (Barbeque Beef), 3.5 oz	325	12	15
Galbi (Short Ribs), 16 oz	975	61	16
Gujeolpan (Pancake w. Meat & Vegetables), cup w. 1 pancake	340	11	39
Japchae (Noodle w. Veggies & Meat), 1¼ cup	365	19	34
Sides:			
Kimchee (Cabbage Relish), ½ cup	30	0	6
Namool (Assorted Veggies) 1 cup	125	6.5	9
Soups: *Per Serving*			
Muguk (Radish & Chive Soup), 6 oz	105	7	6
Samgyetang (Ginseng Chicken Soup)			
no Chicken Skin, 1 cup	520	11	60
w. Chicken Skin, 1 cup	725	35	60
Yuk Gae Jang (Spicy Beef Soup), 1¼ cup	180	13	5

Lebanese/Middle East

	C	F	Cb
Baba Ghannouj, 2 Tbsp, 1 oz (Eggplant/Sesame Dip)	70	6	2
Baklava, 1 pastry, 1¾ oz (Pastry, Nuts, Syrup)	245	18	18
Cabbage Rolls, 1 roll, 3 oz (Cabbage Leaf, Meat, Rice)	100	3	12
Cous Cous, 1 serving (Semolina, Milk, Fruit, Nuts)	400	21	43
Felafel (Chick Pea Fritter): Fried, 1 medium, 1 oz	60	4	4
Hummus, ¼ cup, 2.2 oz	105	3	5
Fried Kibbi, 1 piece, 3 oz (Wheat, Meat, Pinenuts)	180	8	15
Kafta, 1 skewer, 1½ oz (Ground Lamb Ssg. on Skewer)	85	5	2
Kibbeh Naye, 1 cup, 9 oz (Raw Lamb, Bulgur & Spices)	450	18	28
Lebanese Omelet, 1 serving, 4 oz (Egg, Spinach, Pinenuts, Onion)	200	12	13
Pilaf, 1 cup (Rice, Onion, Rais., Apr. Spice)	400	11	60
Shawourma, 1 serving, 4 oz (Spit-Roast Beef)	280	15	2
Shish Kabob, 1 stick, 2½ oz	130	7	2
Spinach Pie, 1 piece, 3½ oz	290	21	20
Sweet Almond Sanbusak, 1 pce (Pastry, Almonds, Spices)	200	15	11
Tabouli, 1 serving, 4 oz	125	7	13
Tahini Sauce, avg., 1 Tbsp	90	8	2

Mexican

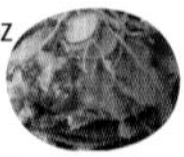

	C	F	Cb
Black Bean Soup, 1 bowl	200	3	34
Burritos *(Taco Bell):* Bean	370	10	55
Supreme® Beef	440	18	50
Chili, plain, ¼ cup	90	6	8
Chili con Carne: w. Beans, 1 cup	310	17	15
w/o Beans, 1 cup	370	28	10
Chimichangas, Beef, 5 oz	400	19	43
Chorizo Sausage, 2 oz	265	23	0
Churros, 1½ oz	150	8	18
Corn Chips, ½ c., 1 oz	160	10	17
Costillas Ribs, 6 oz	675	52	0
Enchilada, average	330	10	18
Fajitas, Chicken	200	7	20
Guacamole, avg., 2 Tbsp, 1 oz	45	4	2
Horchata: *Don Jose,* 1 cup, 8 fl. oz	140	4	25
Cacique, 1 pint bottle, 16 fl. oz	320	7	62
Margarita (w. 1½ oz Tequila)	160	0	6
Masa (Pre-mixed for Tamales), 1 oz	80	5	9
Menudo, ½ cup	55	1.5	10
Nachos: *Del Taco,* Regular	395	24	40
Macho Nachos	1145	63	113
Taco Bell: BellGrande®	760	43	80
Supreme®	470	26	42
Nachos: with cheese, peppers, 1 portion (6-8 nachos), 7 oz	600	33	60
with cheese, beans, ground beef, peppers, 1 portion (6-8 nachos), 9 oz	570	31	56
Nopal Cactus Salad, 1 serving	130	9	11
Papas Fritas (Fried Potatoes) (1), 6 oz	325	18	40
Piloncillo (Brown Sugar): 1 Tbsp, 13g	50	0	13
Cone, small, 3", 3 oz	325	0	81
Quesadilla, Cheese *(Taco Bell)*	490	28	39
Queso Fresco, ¼ cup	80	4.5	8
Refried Beans, ¾ cup, 6 oz	160	3	26
Rice Pudding (Arroz Con Leche), 4 oz	140	3	24
Sopes (Gorditas), 2 oz	120	0	27
Taco *(Taco Bell):* Regular, Crispy	170	10	13
Ranchero Chicken	270	15	21
Taco Supreme®	220	14	14
Double Decker® Taco	340	14	39
Taco Salad w. Salsa	840	52	85
Taco Sauce, average, ¼ cup	15	0	3
Taco Shell, regular	50	2	8
Tamales, Beef/Chicken, avg, 4.5 oz	250	11	27
Taquitos, Beef & Cheese, 4.5 oz	330	15	36
Tostada *(Taco Bell)*	250	10	29
Tortilla, Corn, 6" diam.	70	1	14
Tortilla Chips, 1 oz	150	8	18

Extra Listings of Mexican Dishes:
• **Fast-Foods Section** *(Taco Bell, Del Taco)*
• **Canned Bean/Chili Products:** See Pages 113-118

Mexican (Cont)

	C	F	Cb
Breads: Bolillos, 1 roll, 3½ oz	240	4	42
Telera, 2 oz	150	1.5	19
Mexican Cornbread, 4" square	210	11	19
Cakes, Cookies, Pastries			
Banderilla (Pastry Puff), 1 shell	140	10	8
Bigotes, 7"	570	22	44
Calvos, 2½ oz	320	18	38
Capirotada (Bread Pudding), 10 oz	810	38	107
Cinnamon Cookies, 2	125	8	13
Cocadas, 1 oz	120	6	15
Cortadillo, 1 cookie, 1.9 oz	300	11	48
Concha (All Colors):			
Small (3" diam), 2½ oz	250	8	38
Medium (4" diam), 3½ oz	350	11	53
Large (5" diam), 5½ oz	550	18	84
Cream Puff with Custard, 4¼ oz	255	14	25
Cuerno, 2 oz	200	4.5	34
Cuerno Fine, 2¾ oz	330	17	40
Donut, large, 4", 3½ oz	440	21	58
Elotes, 3½ oz	450	24	51
Empanadas (Average all types):			
Small, 2 oz	230	10	28
Regular, 3 oz	300	14	42
Fiesta Cookie, 2¼ oz	280	8	47
Galletas Mixtas (1), 1 oz	100	2.5	16
Guayaba, 3¼ oz	360	14	53
Jelly Rolls, 3¼ oz	240	4	46
Mantecadites (Almond Shortbread), 4½ oz	670	42	64
Mini Pound Cake, 3 oz	260	12	33
Mini Cupcakes, 1¾ oz	180	8	25
Muffins/Nino Enbuelto, large, 6 oz	465	11	49
Nuez, 3¼ oz	380	17	52
Ojo De Buey, 4 oz	360	15	55
Oreja (Elephant Ear), 3 oz	310	15	38
Pan Dulce (Mexican Sweet Bread), 1 bun	330	10	45
Panquecitos, 2½ oz	260	11	36
Piedras, 4 oz	470	15	76
Polvorones, 3 oz	370	18	48
Puerquitos, 5 oz	600	24	88
Rebanadas, 3½ oz	390	18	51
Roles De Canela (Cin. Roll), 4½ oz	490	15	81
Roscas, 2¾ oz	360	18	44
Semitas, 3 oz	300	10	46
Sopapillas (flaky pastry puffs), 1 pce	100	7	10
w. Honey & Cream	200	14	18
Strawberry Crema Roll (⅙), 2½ oz	240	5	45
Extra Food Listings ~ See CalorieKing.com			

Polish

	C	F	Cb
Cabbage Rolls w. Sour Cr., 2 sm.	220	10	30
Chicken Casserole w. Mush., 1 cup	520	27	5
Kielbasa (Sausages, Onions, fried), 2 large	350	28	2
Meatballs in Sour Cream, 3 x 1½" balls	300	16	11
Pierogi, Fruit/Veg, 3" ball	80	2	15
Pork Goulash (Pork/Veg. Stew)	550	21	38
Pot Roast with Vegetables	630	21	28

Soul Foods

	C	F	Cb
Breakfast Sausage, fried, 2 patties	250	17	0
Brunswick Stew, 1 cup, 8.5 oz	320	14	19
Cornbread, homemade, 3 oz	200	7.5	28
Fatback, raw, ¼ oz	60	6.5	0
Ham Hock	90	6.5	2
Hog Maw	45	2.5	0
Hominy, cooked, ¾ cup	110	0.5	25
Hush Puppies, 5 pieces	260	12	35
Kale, cooked, ½ cup	20	0.5	4
Oxtail	70	3.5	0
Pig's Ear, ¼ ear	50	3	0
Pig's Foot, ½ foot	70	4.5	0
Pig's Tail, ⅓ tail	115	10	0
Poke Salad, cooked, ½ cup	16	0.5	3
Pork Brains	40	2.5	0
Pork Chitterlings, simmered, 3 oz	260	25	0
Pork Cracklings, ½ oz	80	6	0
Pork Neck Bones	65	4	0
Pork Skin, 1 cup	70	4.5	0
Pork Tongue, ⅓ tongue	75	5.5	0
Possum	65	3	0
Sousemeat	60	4.5	0
Succotash, ½ cup	80	1	17
Sweet Potato Pie, ⅛ of 9" pie	250	12	34
Tripe, 2 oz	55	2	0
Vienna Sausage, 2 small	90	8	1
small	45	4	0.5

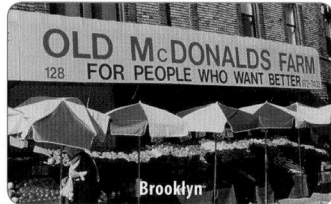

Brooklyn

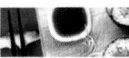
Spanish | C | F | Cb
Arroz Abanda (Fish with Rice)	340	8	31
Arroz Con Pollo (Rice/Chick. Sal)	500	23	50
Clams Marinara, 8 clams	330	16	22
Cochifrito (Lamb w. Lemon/Garlic)	650	25	5
Cochinillo Asado, 2 sl. (Rst Suckling Pig)	300	15	3
Cocido Madrileno			
(Madrid-Style Boiled Dinner)	450	27	18
Flan de Leche (Caramel Custard)	325	9	52
Fritadera de Ternera (Sauteed Veal)	450	27	2
Gazpacho, 1 bowl	60	0	15
Paella a la Valenciana			
(Chicken & Shellfish Rice)	900	42	70
Pollo a la Espanola (Chicken)	475	30	4
Ternera al Jerez (Veal w. Sherry)	660	29	6
Zarzuela (Fish & Shellfish Medley)	530	27	40

Thai Foods | C | F | Cb
Appetizers: Satay Pork, 1 oz	100	4	2
Spring Roll, 1¼ oz	110	6	13
Soups: Tom Yam (Hot & Sour):			
Spicy Shrimp/Seafood, 1 cup	100	4	6
1 bowl	160	7	10
Vegetarian, 1 cup	50	0	11
Curries: Chicken w. Ginger, 1 cup	390	34	4
Thick Red Curry w. Beef, 1 cup	600	50	7
Thai Chicken Curry, 1 cup	340	23	4
Massaman Curry, 1 cup	680	57	8
Green Curry w. Pork, 1 cup	480	44	5
Pad Thai, Large serving, 18 oz	990	38	125
Fish: Steamed w. Spicy Thai Sce	450	8	46
Crispy Fried, 5 oz	290	15	9
Spicy Chicken (w. veggies), stir-fry	450	22	14
Spicy Garlic Tofu w. veggies, stir-fry	340	18	8
Sticky Thai Rice: Plain 1 cup, 6 oz	170	0.5	36
w. Coconut & Sugar, 1 cup	880	28	120
Stir-fried Rice Noodles, 1 c., 5½ oz	270	9	40
Stir-fried Vegetables, 1 cup	100	3	14
Salads: Green Papaya Salad	160	0	40
Spicy Prawn, 9 shrimp	170	3	15
Thai Chicken, 1 serving	330	9	17
Thai Beef Salad, 1 serving	260	9	15
Thai Noodle, 1 serving	410	13	45
Satay Chicken & Peanut Sauce:			
1 satay stick	390	24	20
Sauces: Peanut Satay, ½ cup, 4 oz	160	10	13

Vietnamese | C | F | Cb
Banh Cuon (Steam Rice w. Pork), 1 roll	105	7	8
Bo Nuong (Beef Satay), 2 sticks	265	9	4
Bo Xao Dau Phong			
(Ginger Beef w.Onion, Fish Sce.)	750	30	10
Ca Chien Gung (Whole Snapper/Ging.)	600	16	6
Canh Chay (Veg./Tofu Soup)	80	3	13
Cari (Curry) Chicken, 1 cup	475	29	16
Cari (Curry) Chicken, w. Rice Noodle,			
cup curry & cup cooked noodles	660	29	60
Cari (Curry) Chicken, w. Steam Rice,			
cup curry & cup rice	650	29	55
Cuu Xao Lan (Curried Lamb,			
Veggies in Coconut)	900	40	80
Ga Chien (Crisp Chick + Plum Sce)	900	40	105
Ga Nuong (Chicken Satay + Sce)	240	10	4
Ga Xao Rau (Marinated Chicken			
Braised w. Veg.)	800	26	100
Gio Lua (Lean Pork Pie), ⅛ of pie	245	12	0
Goi Cuon (Cold Spring Rolls), each	60	1	7
Rau Cai Xao Chay (Stir Fried Vege.)	400	15	65
Thit Bo Vien (Beef Balls), 6 balls	225	14	2
Thit Heo Goi Baup Cai, each			
(Spicy Cabbage Rolls w. Pork)	200	7	11
Soup: Per Bowl (1½ Cup)			
Bun Bo Hue (Hot & Spicy Soup			
no Pork Feet	340	9	35
w. Pork Feet	830	45	35
Chicken & Rice Noodle Soup	400	3	55
Pho Bo (Beef Noodle Soup)	410	7	59
Pho Ga (Chicken Noodle Soup)	460	6	58
Pho Tai (Rare Beef & Noodle Soup)	440	7	73
Salad: Per ½ Cup			
Goi Du Du (Green Papaya Salad)	155	3	29
Sauce: Nuoc Cham (Hot Sauce)	5	0	1

Gourmet & Miscellaneous
	C	F	Cb
Ants Eggs/Larvae, 1 Tbsp	20	0	0
Ants, Choc. coated, 3 Tbsp	140	7	2
Bee Maggots, canned, 3 Tbsp	65	2	0
Caviar, black/red, 1 Tbsp	40	3	0
Caterpillars, canned, 2 oz	60	2	0
Frog Legs, fried, 1 pair (large)	125	7	0
Haggis, boiled, 4 oz	350	24	22
Locusts, roasted, 1 oz	35	1	0
Silkworms, raw, 1 oz	60	2	0
Snails in garlic butter, 6 large	200	10	4
Snake, roasted, 4 oz	160	6	0

Fast - Foods & *Restaurants*

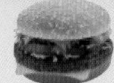

***For Complete Menu Listings
& Extended Nutritional Data
~ See CalorieKing.com***

A&W® (Oct '08)

Sandwiches & Burgers	C	F	Cb
Bacon Cheeseburger	570	33	41
Bacon Double Cheeseburger	800	48	47
Double Cheeseburger	720	42	46
Papa Burger	720	42	46
Kids Cheeseburger	460	24	39
Kids Hamburger	430	22	37
Sandwiches: Crispy Chicken	550	23	55
Grilled Chicken	400	13	35
Chicken			
Strips, 3 pieces	500	29	32
Hog Dogs: Cheese	320	20	25
Coney Chili	310	18	24
Coney Chili Cheese	350	21	27
Plain	280	17	22
Fries & Sides			
Fries: 4 oz	310	13	45
Cheese Fries, 4 oz	310	12	45
Chili Fries, 6 oz	370	15	49
Chili Cheese Fries, 7 oz	410	17	52
Cheese Curds, 5 oz	570	40	27
Chili Bowl, 8 oz	190	6	22
Dipping Sauces: Per 1 oz Serving			
BBQ	40	0	10
Honey Mustard	100	6	12
Ranch	160	17	2
Sweet & Sour	45	0	12
Desserts: Per Small Serving			
Polar Swirl: M&M	720	25	107
Oreo	720	25	107
Reese's	750	31	97
Sundae: Caramel	340	9	57
Chocolate	320	8	53
Hot Fudge	350	11	54
Strawberry	300	8	47
Vanilla	310	8	52
Milkshakes & Floats: Per 16 fl.oz			
Chocolate	700	29	100
Strawberry	670	29	90
Vanilla	720	31	97
Floats: *Medium*			
A&W Root Beer Float	330	4.5	70
A&W Root Beer Float, Diet	150	4.5	23
Drinks			
A&W Root Beer: Regular, 20 fl.oz	270	0	72
Diet, 20 fl.oz	0	0	0
Coca Cola: 15 fl.oz	200	0	51
Diet, 15 fl.oz	0	0	0

Applebee's® (Oct '08)

(Author Estimates)	C	F	Cb
Appetizing Starters			
Buffalo Chicken Wings:			
With Ranch Dressing	1100	81	48
Without Ranch Dressing	735	42	44
Boneless Buffalo Wings: With Dress.	1105	81	48
Without Dressing	670	50	10
Mozzarella Sticks (9) plus dip	1005	57	7
Veggie Patch Pizza (10") ⅙ Pizza	150	9	12
Entree Meals: Includes Sides/Sauces			
Applebee's Riblets	2025	130	106
Chicken Broccoli Alfredo	1255	57	87
Crispy Buttermilk Shrimp	845	34	83
Crispy Orange Chicken Skillet	1710	69	209
Fiesta Lime Chicken	1285	47	136
Burger & Sandwiches			
Angus Bacon Cheeseburger	940	53	58
Cheeseburger: No Fries	720	37	50
With Fries	1000	51	89
Clubhouse Grill S'wich: No Fries	880	51	57
With Fries	1340	72	119
Cowboy Burger: No Fries	1100	64	64
With Fries	1450	80	111
Bruschetta Burger	1280	90	53
Turkey & Bacon Ciabatta: No Fries	715	35	57
With Fries	1140	55	114
Salads: Full Serving with Dressing			
Apple Walnut Chicken Salad	1160	92	26
Bourbon Street Steak Salad	1255	81	68
Oriental Chicken Salad	1015	50	111
Pecan Crusted Chicken Salad	1180	65	63
Shrimp and Spinach Salad	570	41	14
Sizzling Fajitas: Includes 4 Tortillas			
Average all types	1900	76	174
Flour Tortilla (8"), each, 1.6 oz	145	3	25
Weight Watchers: Complete Meal			
Cajun Lime Tilapia	360	4	31
Confetti Chicken	370	7	34
Grilled Shrimp Skewer Salad	210	2	22
Italian Chicken & Portobello S'wich	360	6	50
Steak & Portobellos	330	10	24
Onion Soup au Gratin	150	8	10
Southwest Cobb Salad	440	8	59
Teriyaki Steak 'N Shrimp Skewers	370	7	33
Tortilla Chicken Melt	480	13	50
Soup, Onion Soup au Gratin	150	8	10
Cakes/Desserts: Per Serving			
Chocolate Raspberry Layer Cake	230	3	46
Sizzling Apple Pie w. Ice Cream	1085	56	146
Triple Chocolate Meltdown Cake	725	31	107

Arby's® (Oct '08)

Breakfast: Per Serving	C	F	Cb
Blueberry Muffin, 3 oz	320	12	49
Biscuits: Plain	275	15	28
Bacon Egg & Cheese	460	28	30
Ham, Egg & Cheese	445	23	31
Sausage, Egg & Cheese	555	38	30
Croissants: Plain	190	10	21
Bacon & Egg	335	22	23
Ham & Cheese	275	12	22
Sausage & Egg	435	32	23
French Toastix, 4.4 oz	310	13	44
Sourdoughs			
Bacon, Egg & Cheese	435	16	41
Egg & Cheese	390	12	41
Ham, Egg & Cheese	440	13	42
Sausage Egg & Cheese	555	28	41
Wraps: Bacon, Egg & Cheese	515	29	50
Sausage, Egg & Cheese	690	45	51
Sandwiches & Burgers			
Arby's Melts, w/o sauce	305	12	36
Bacon Beef 'n Cheddar	520	26	45
BBQ Bacon 'n Jack 2for	360	15	42
Corned Beef Reuben	590	32	55
French Dip & Swiss	475	18	38
Roast Beef: Regular	320	13	34
Medium	415	20	34
Large	545	28	42
Super	400	18	40
Roast Beef & Swiss	775	41	71
Roast Ham & Swiss	690	30	73
Roast Turkey & Swiss	710	29	73
Roast Turkey Ranch & Bacon	815	37	73
Roast Turkey Reuben	595	30	55
Spicy Cajun Fish	595	32	58
Ultimate BLT	780	45	76
Chicken Naturals Sandwich			
Chicken Bacon & Swiss: Crispy	625	29	52
Grilled	460	16	38
Chicken Cordon Bleu: Crispy	660	31	49
Grilled	495	18	35
Chicken Fillet: Crispy	580	29	50
Grilled	416	16	36
Sandwich Melts: Ham & Swiss	270	5	35
Sourdough Ham	380	14	39
Sourdough Roast Beef	355	14	40
Swiss	305	12	37
Subs, Toasted: Classic Italian	785	38	68
French Dip & Swiss	620	19	68
Philly Beef	740	35	64
Turkey Bacon Club	620	17	66

Sandwiches & Burgers (Cont)	C	F	Cb
Wraps: Chicken Salad with Pecans	640	38	48
Corned Beef Reuben	560	29	42
Roast Turkey Ranch & Bacon	680	36	42
Roast Turkey Reuben	565	27	42
Southwest Chicken	570	30	40
Ultimate BLT	650	44	46
Regular Combos: Includes Medium Fries & 22 fl.oz Pepsi			
Bacon Beef 'n Cheddar S'wich	1130	50	149
Beef 'n Cheddar Sandwich	1050	44	148
Chicken Bacon & Swiss	1050	40	144
Chicken Fillet Sandwich	1005	40	142
Corned Beef Reuben Sandwich	1195	56	159
Pecan Chicken Salad Wrap	1245	62	152
Popcorn Chicken Shakers	1135	48	143
Roast Beef	925	37	138
Roast Turkey & Swiss S'wich	1315	53	177
Rst Turkey Ranch & Bacon Wrap	1290	60	146
Roast Turkey Reuben Sandwich	1200	54	159
Salads: *Without Dressing*			
Market Fresh: Chicken Club	425	22	26
Martha's Vineyard	275	8	24
Santa Fe	415	18	37
Santa Fe with Grilled Chicken	285	9	20
Sides			
Fries: Curly, 1 small, 3.7 oz	340	20	39
Homestyle, 1 small, 4 oz	300	20	44
Jalapeno Bites, 5 bites	305	22	29
Loaded Potato Bites, 5 bites	345	22	27
Mozzarella Sticks, 4 sticks	425	28	38
Onion Petals, 4 oz	330	23	35
Potato Cakes, 2 cakes	245	19	26
Southwest Eggrolls, 4 pieces	225	7	29
Sauces			
Arby's, 1 packet, 0.5 oz	15	0	4
Cheddar Cheese, 0.7 oz	30	2	2
Horsey, 0.5 oz	60	5	3
Marinara, 1.5 oz	30	2	4
Spicy Three Pepper, 0.5 oz	20	1	3
Tangy Southwest, 2 oz	335	35	5
Dipping: BBQ, 1 oz	45	1	11
Bronco Berry, 2 oz	120	0	30
Buffalo, 1 oz	10	1	2
Chile Lime Ranch, 1.5 oz	190	19	2
Desserts			
Cheesecake Poppers with sauce	330	15	44
T.J. Cinnamon: Cinnamon Roll	505	10	73
Chocolate Twist	250	12	34
Pecan Sticky Bun	690	22	91
Turnovers, Apple with Icing	375	16	64
Shakes: Per Regular, 14 fl.oz			
Chocolate	515	13	85
Strawberry	500	13	82
Strawberry Banana Swirl	565	16	87
Vanilla	440	13	65

Arthur Treachers® (Oct '08)

Meals: Per Serving	C	F	Cb
Fish & Chips Platter, 22.10 oz	1535	95	153
Shrimp and Chips Platter, 24 oz	1850	120	185
Seafood Sampler, 20 oz	1560	94	166
Fish Sandwich, 7 oz	435	18	50
Breaded Clam Order, 5.6 oz	470	27	40
Sides: Coleslaw, 5 oz	180	12	15
Hush Puppies (2) 4.5 oz	120	16	84

Atlanta Bread Co® (Oct '08)

Sandwiches	C	F	Cb
Chicken Salad on Sourdough	440	9	42
Chicken Waldorf	450	29	65
Honey Maple Ham	410	5	64
Kid's Peanut Butter & Jelly	550	15	89
Kid's Grilled Cheese	390	15	46
Turkey Bacon Rustica	960	56	62
Tuna Salad on French	630	33	57
Turkey on Nine Grain	370	6	50
Veggie on Nine Grain	500	25	52
Signature Sandwiches On Focacia			
Bella Chicken, Tomato	610	38	34
California Avocado, Tom. On.	930	50	98
Chicken Waldorf on Asiago	450	29	26
ABC Special On French Baguette	750	30	57
NY Hot Pastrami on Rye	660	29	59
Paninis: Chicken Pesto	800	35	83
Cordon Bleu	670	19	80
Cubano	650	19	80
Italian Vegetarian	570	16	84
Turkey Club	710	24	81
Salads: Caesar	150	9	7
Balsamic Bleu Salad	330	18	35
Chopstix Chicken	240	10	22
Fruit Salad,	130	0	34
Greek Salad	240	16	15
House Salad, without dressing	90	2	13
Salsa Fresca Salmon Salad	560	29	40
Muffin Tops: Banana Nut	420	26	39
Blueberry	250	12	31
Chocolate Chip	390	19	51
Mocha Chip	410	20	53
Pumpkin	200	2	43

For Extra Menu Items ~ see CalorieKing.com

Au Bon Pain® (Oct '08)

Bagels: Per Bagel	C	F	Cb
Asiago Cheese	340	6	55
Cinnamon Raisin	310	1	66
Honey 9 Grain	360	4	71
Plain	280	1	57
Spreads: Plain Cream Cheese, 2 oz	170	16	4
Honey Pecan	120	10	5
Veggie, 2 oz	170	16	3
Breakfast Sandwiches			
Egg on a Bagel	360	4	59
with Bacon	420	8	60
with Bacon & Cheese	500	15	59
with Cheese	430	10	58
Croissants: Ham & Cheese	400	20	38
Spinach & Cheese	290	16	28
Filled: Plain	300	17	31
Almond	600	38	55
Apple	270	11	44
Chocolate	430	22	58
Raspberry Cheese	320	15	41
Sweet Cheese	380	19	48
Café Sandwiches			
Arizona Chicken	750	29	61
Baja Turkey	640	24	63
Mozzarella Chicken	750	25	67
Chicken Tarragon w. Romaine	740	31	61
Prosciutto Mozzarella	770	41	64
Chicken Pesto	720	26	62
Spicy Tuna on Multigrain	500	18	59
Hot Sandwiches and Melts			
Steakhouse on Ciabatta	720	31	71
Tuna Melt	670	30	62
Turkey Melt	780	34	73
Wraps: Chicken Caesar Asiago	660	28	62
Fields & Feta	480	18	67
Mediterranean Wrap	610	31	73
Southwest Tuna	760	42	65
Soups: Per Medium 12 oz Bowl			
Broccoli Cheddar	310	21	20
Corn Chowder	350	18	40
Low Fat: Chicken Noodle	130	3	20
Garden Vegetable	80	2	14
Vegetarian Chili	230	3	40

Au Bon Pain® cont... (Oct '08)

Breads	**C**	**F**	**Cb**
Artisan Multigrain Bread, 1 slice	190	1.5	26
Bread Bowl (1)	620	3	121
Foccacia (1)	350	7	61
Rosemary Garlic Breadstick	180	5	30
Bread Rolls, Soft (1)	410	11	65
Salads: Per Container			
Asiago Salad, 6 oz	210	12	18
Chef's Salad, 8 oz	250	15	8
Chickpea, Tomato & Cucumber	230	12	23
Garden Salad, Side, 3.5 oz	50	2	8
Green Bean and Beet	210	8	27
Mandarin Sesame Chicken	350	18	30
Mediterranean Chicken, 9.8 oz	330	16	12
Riviera 9.5 oz	260	7	46
Thai Peanut Chicken, 11 oz	240	8	19
Tuna Garden, 10.5 oz	250	13	14
Turkey Medallion Cobb, 11 oz	340	19	15
Cookies: Per Cookie			
Chocolate Chip	260	12	37
English Toffee	210	11	26
Oatmeal Raisin	230	8	36
Shortbread	310	18	34
Blonde	330	19	61
Choc Chip Brownie	380	17	62
Desserts: Apple Strudel	430	24	48
Cherry Strudel	460	26	49
Pecan Roll	630	32	80
Fruit Cup: Small, 6 oz	70	0	16
Large, 12 oz	140	1	32
Muffins: Blueberry	450	17	66
Carrot Walnut	520	25	66
Corn	460	16	69
Cranberry Walnut	500	23	61
Raisin Bran	410	9	74
Cakes: Per Slice			
Banana Nut Pound Cake, 4.7 oz	520	28	60
Cappuccino Pound Cake, 5.2 oz	530	26	68
Chocolate Pound Cake, 5 oz	500	29	58
Beverages:			
Caffe Latte, 16 fl.oz	260	14	21
Frozen Mocha Blast, 16 fl.oz	440	17	80
Peach Iced Tea, 22 fl.oz	120	0	30

For Complete Nutritional Data ~ see CalorieKing.com

Auntie Anne's® (Oct '08)

Pretzels: With Butter	**C**	**F**	**Cb**
Almond	400	8	72
Cinnamon Sugar	450	9	83
Garlic	350	4.5	68
Glazin' Raisin	510	4	107
Jalapeno	310	4.5	59
Original	370	4	72
Sesame	410	12	64
Sour Cream & Onion	340	5	66
Whole Wheat	370	4.5	72
Stix, 6 sticks	370	4	72
Pretzels: Without Butter			
Almond Pretzel; Whole Wheat	350	1.5	72
Cinnamon Sugar	350	2	74
Garlic Pretzel; Sour Crm & Onion	320	1	66
Glazin' Raisin	470	0.5	104
Jalapeno	270	1	58
Original	340	1	72
Sesame	350	6	63
Stix, 6 sticks	340	1	72
Dipping Sauces			
Caramel Dip, 1.5 oz	135	3	27
Cheese Sce; Hot Salsa Chse, avg.	100	8	4
Light Cream Cheese, 1¼ oz	70	6	1
Marinara Sauce, 1¼ oz	30	0.5	5
Sweet Dip, 1¼ oz	40	0	10
Sweet Mustard, 1¼ oz	60	1.5	8
Beverages: Per Serving			
Auntie Anne's Lemonade, 22 fl.oz	180	0	43
Dutch Ice (20 fl.oz): Kiwi-Banana	270	0	63
Blue Raspberry	230	0	55
Lemonade	450	0	110
Mocha	570	15	105
Orange Crème	400	0	92
Pina Colada; Strawberry	535	0	125
Wild Cherry	300	0	69
Dutch Smoothie: *Per 20 fl.oz*			
Blue Raspberry	400	14	61
Kiwi-Banana	430	14	68
Lemonade	540	14	95
Mocha	590	23	90
Orange Crème	500	14	83
Pina Colada	470	14	79
Strawberry; Wild Cherry, avg.	450	14	74

Back Yard Burgers® (Oct '08)

Burgers	C	F	Cb
Back Yard Burger ⅓ lb	470	29	38
Cheeseburger ⅓ lb	520	34	38
Bacon Cheddar	620	42	38
Barbecue Bacon	630	39	47
Black Jack	580	39	36
Chili Cheese	560	36	41
Garden Veggie Sandwich	240	6	47
Jr Burger	310	17	38
Hawaiian	550	33	44
Miz Grazi	530	34	39
Mushroom Swiss	540	36	37
Low-Carb Burger	350	27	3

Chicken Sandwiches			
Bacon Swiss	390	20	37
Barbecue	280	8	44
Blackened	290	11	39
Buffalo Ranch	540	30	51
Hawaiian Chicken	280	8	45
Honey Mustard	320	11	46
Lemon Butter Chicken	260	9	37
Savory Chicken	230	6	36
Specialities: BLT	270	16	36
Chicken Tenderloins, 3 piece	400	28	22
Chili Dog	340	20	29
Chili Cheese Dog	400	25	29
Hot Dog	310	18	27

Baked Potatoes			
Chili & Cheddar, 9 oz	330	11	48
Ranch, 7.7 oz	410	22	45
Salsa, 7.7 oz	250	5	47
Traditional/Plain, 6 oz	190	0	43

Fries			
Chili Cheese Fries, 6.7 oz	350	22	28
Seasoned Fries, regular, 3 oz	260	16	26
Waffle Fries, regular, 3 oz	240	16	23

Salads (No Dressing)			
Blackened Chicken	160	4	11
Charbroiled Chicken	140	3	11
Garden Fresh	25	0	5

Cobblers: Apple, 6 oz	430	20	61
Blackberry; Peach, 6 oz	420	20	60
Cherry, 6 oz	460	20	68

Shakes: Per 12 fl.oz			
Chocolate; Strawberry	560	26	79
Vanilla	540	26	71

For Complete Nutritional Data ~ see CalorieKing.com

Baja Fresh® (Oct '08)

Burritos: No Tortilla Chips	C	F	Cb
Baja Burrito: with Chicken	790	38	65
with Steak	850	46	67
Bare Burrito: with Charbroiled Chkn	640	7	97
Veggie and Cheese	580	10	101
Bean & Cheese Burrito: with Chkn	970	35	96
with Steak	1030	43	97
Vegetarian	840	33	96
Burrito Dos Manos: with Chicken	760	26	94
with Steak	795	30	95
Burrito Mexicano: with Chicken	790	13	117
with Steak	860	21	118
Burrito Ultimo: with Chicken	860	36	84
with Steak	950	44	85
Grilled Vegetarian	800	33	94

Fajitas			
Chicken with Corn Tortillas	860	24	105
Chicken with Flour Tortillas	1140	33	147
Nachos: with Charbroiled Steak	2120	118	163
with Cheese	1890	108	163
with Chicken	2020	110	164
Quesadilla: with Charboiled Chkn	1330	80	84
with Charbroiled Steak	1430	87	84
with Cheese	1200	78	84
Vegetarian	1260	78	96

Tacos: No Tortilla Chips			
Baja Fish Taco, Fried	250	13	27
Fried Mahi Mahi Taco	230	9	26
Baja Style Taco with Chicken	210	5	28
with Steak	230	5	28
with Gulf Shrimp	200	5	28

Salads: No Dressing or Tortilla Chips			
Baja Ensalada:			
with Charbroiled Chicken	310	7	18
with Charbroiled Shrimp	230	6	18
with Charbroiled Steak	450	18	18
Tostadas: Charbroiled Chicken	1140	55	98
Charbroiled Fish	1130	55	99
Charbroiled Shrimp	1120	55	99
Charbroiled Steak	1230	63	98
Savory Pork Carnitas	1180	62	100

For Complete Nutritional Data ~ see CalorieKing.com

Baskin Robbins® (Oct 08)

Ice Creams: Per 4 oz Scoop

	C	F	Cb
Classic Flavors: Cherries Jubilee	240	12	30
Chocolate	260	14	33
French Vanilla	280	18	26
Gold Medal Ribbon	260	13	34
Jamoca	240	13	24
Old Fashioned Butter Pecan	280	18	24
Oreo Cookies 'n Cream	280	15	32
Peanut Butter 'n Chocolate	320	20	31
Reese's P'nut Butter Cup	300	18	31
Vanilla	260	16	26
Very Berry Strawberry	220	11	28
World Class Chocolate	280	16	31
Frozen Yogurt, avg., 4 oz scoop	200	4	38
Fruit Blast Bars, all flavors	50	0	13
Ice, all flavors, 4 oz scoop	130	0	33

Sherbets: Per 4 oz Scoop

	C	F	Cb
Blue/Red Raspberry; Orange	160	2	34
Rock 'n Pop Swirl	190	4	37

Sundaes:

	C	F	Cb
Classic Sundaes: Banana Royale	630	31	87
Brownie Sundae	890	42	123
Classic Banana Split	980	31	172
Premium Sundaes:			
Chocolate Oreo	1100	55	151
Jamoca Oreo	830	32	130
Oreo,	1330	61	189
Reese's Peanut Butter Cup	1250	81	108

Soft Serve Sundaes: Per 10 oz Regular

	C	F	Cb
Caramel; Hot Fudge, avg.	600	25	87
Strawberry	450	18	59
Sundae Cups: Oreo	330	15	45
Peanut Butter Cup	390	24	36
Pralines 'n Cream	330	16	43

Soft Serve, '31 Below' Blends: Per 16 oz Cup

	C	F	Cb
Chocolate Oreo	1280	55	185
Fudge Brownie	1390	62	194
Heath	1150	54	149
Oreo	980	41	141
Reese's P'nut Butter Cup	1230	67	132
Strawberry Banana	690	23	110
York Peppermint Pattie Brownie	1610	80	222

Soft Serve, Cups/Cones:

	C	F	Cb
Chocolate Dipped: Reg., 6 oz	505	31	50
Large, 9 oz	760	47	75
Kid's, 3 oz	255	16	25
Vanilla: Regular, 6 oz	280	11	37
Large, 9 oz	420	17	56
Kid's, 3 oz	140	5.5	19
Fruit Cream: avg, Medium, 16 oz	670	19	112
Large, 24 oz	1000	27	168

Baskin Robbins cont... (Oct 08)

Beverages

	C	F	Cb
Freezes w. Orange Sherbet:			
Small	370	4	82
Medium	510	5	112
Large	740	8	164
Cappuccino Blast: *Per Medium, 24 fl.oz*			
Original	460	19	66
Original with Whipped Cream	480	21	67
Original, Non-Fat	340	0	78
Caramel	720	24	121
Jamoca Oreo	910	31	156
Mocha	540	18	87
Oreo 'n Cookies	800	31	118
Fruit Blast: *Per Medium, 24 fl.oz*			
Berry Pomegranate/Peach, avg.	510	0	128
Strawberry Citrus/Wild Mango	480	1	120
Fruit Blast Smoothie: *Per Medium, 24 fl.oz*			
Berry Pomegranate Banana	710	1	172
Mango	620	2	148
Strawberry Banana	730	2	178
Ice Cream Soda: *Per Medium*			
with Vanilla Ice Cream	720	30	103
Ice Cream Float: *Per Medium*			
w. Vanilla Ice Cream & Root Beer	680	30	99
Milk Shakes: *Per Medium, 24 fl.oz*			
Choc Chip	750	28	106
Vanilla	980	45	125
Choc with Vanilla Ice Cream	1000	45	133
Strawberry w. Strawb. Ice Cream	650	19	104
Cones: Cake	25	0	5
Sugar	45	0.5	9
Waffle	90	2	20

For Complete Nutritional Data ~ see CalorieKing.com

Ben & Jerry's®

Ice Cream & Frozen Yogurt ~ See Page 106
Novelty Bars ~ See Page 110

Big Apple Bagels®

	C	F	Cb
Bagels: All types, avg., 5 oz	340	2	68
½ bagel, 2.5 oz	170	1	34
Choice Bagels: *Per Bagel*			
Blueberry Cobbler	392	8	70
Cheddar Nacho	352	6	60
Cinnamon Apple Pie	386	8	68
Cinnamon Bun	400	8	70
Cinnamon Danish	396	8	72
French Toast	372	4	74
Quiche Lorraine	354	8	54
Strawberry White Chocolate	364	4	72
Swiss Melt	368	8	58
White Chocolate Swirl	396	8	70

Updated Nutrition Data ~ www.CalorieKing.com
Persons with Diabetes ~ See Disclaimer (Page 24)

Big Apple cont... (Oct '08)

Cream Cheese: Per 2 Tbsp , 1 oz	C	F	Cb
Plain	90	9	2
Plain Lite	60	4.5	3
Whipped: Classic Plain	70	7	1
Brown Sugar Cinnamon	70	5	5
Reduced-Fat Spring Veggie	60	5	2
Other varieties, avg	90	8	2
My Favorite Muffin: Per Jumbo, 5.8 oz			
Regular: Blueberry	505	24	66
Chocolate Chip	635	33	81
Cinnamon Swirl Cheesecake	640	33	84
Pumpkin Spice	545	24	78
Fat Free: Blueberry	325	0	78
Chocolate Marble	375	0	87
Cinnamon Bun	505	0	126
Soups: Per Cup (8 oz)			
Boston Clam/Potato Chowder	210	13	20
Chicken Noodle; Beef Pot Roast	110	4	12
Garden Vegetable	110	1	22
Minestrone	150	3	26
Split Pea w. Ham; Hearty Veggie	95	2	16

For Complete Nutritional Data ~ see CalorieKing.com

Big Boy

~ Same Menu and Data as Frisch's Big Boy ~ Page 209

Biggby Coffee (Oct '08)

Hot Drinks	C	F	Cb
Caffe Latte: with 2% Milk	175	7	16
with Non-fat Milk	115	0	16
with Soy	145	5	15
Cappuccino: with 2% Milk	105	4.5	9.5
with Non-Fat Milk	70	0	9.5
with Soy	90	3	9
Chai Latte: with 2% Milk	350	7	58
with Non-Fat Milk	295	0	58
Cocoa Caramella: with 2% Milk	300	9	48
with Whipped Cream	380	15	52
Hot Caramel Cider: with 2% Milk	300	8	57
Mocha Mocha: with 2% Milk	235	6	31
with Whipped Cream	315	12	36
Nutty Buddy, with 2% Milk, no sugar	165	7	18
Cold Drinks: *Per Tall, 16 fl.oz*			
Banana/Berry Creme Freeze, avg.	350	10	67
Berry Fruizen-T	335	0	84
Chai Big Chill	415	11	74
Chocolate Magic Milk	385	18	44
Mocha Big Chill	405	20	56
Original Big Chill	190	9	27

Extra Menu Listings ~ See CalorieKing.com

Blimpie® (Oct '08)

	C	F	Cb
Cold Deli Subs: Per 6" Sub on White with Cheese			
Blimpie Best	420	14	49
Club	385	10	49
Cuban	415	11	43
Ham & Swiss Cheese	390	10	50
Roast Beef & Provolone	410	11	47
Seafood	335	7	56
Tuna	485	21	46
Turkey & Provolone	395	10	49
Wraps: Chicken Caesar	605	29	56
Zesty	570	26	59
Steak & Onion	775	16	49
Hot Deli Subs: Per 6" Sub on White			
BLT	345	11	46
Meatball	605	32	51
Pastrami	455	17	48
VegiMax	520	20	56
Salads: Chef Salad	175	7	10
Macaroni Salad Side	330	22	28
Seafood Salad	120	4	17
Tuna Salad	270	18	7
Dressings & Sauces:			
Creamy Caesar	210	21	2
Creamy Italian	180	18	4
Soups: Per Serving			
Cream of Broccoli & Cheese	190	8	15
Harvest Vegetable	100	1	19
Chicken Noodle	130	4	18
Vegetable Beef	80	1.5	13
New England Clam Chowder	170	3	28
Desserts			
Cookies: Oatmeal Raisin Walnut	170	7	26
Sugar	325	17	41
Other varieties, average	195	11	22

For Complete Nutritional Data ~ see CalorieKing.com

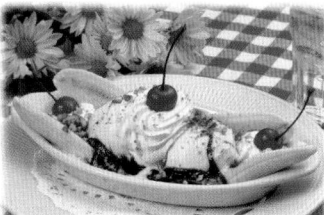

Bob Evans® (Oct '08)

Breakfast	C	F	Cb
Combinations: Country Biscuit	660	45	40
Pot Roast Hash Breakfast	650	39	34
Sausage Benedict	935	66	40
Farm Fresh Eggs: Hardboiled (1)	60	4	1
Over Easy (1)	100	8	1
Scrambled	255	17	2
Hotcake: Blueberry (1)	330	9	55
Buttermilk (1)	320	9	53
Omelets: Three Cheese	645	52	4
Border Scramble Omelet	725	56	14
Lite (with No Cholesterol Eggs)	500	31	14
Farmer's Market	780	60	13
Ham & Cheddar	635	48	3
Western	655	48	8
Crepes: Plain (1)	460	36	27
Sandwiches & Burgers			
Burgers: Bacon Cheeseburger	715	48	32
Cheeseburger	645	41	32
Hamburger	540	32	31
Ranch Steak Burger	940	68	35
Sandwiches: Fried Chicken Club	660	35	44
Bob-B-Q Pulled Pork	660	30	68
Grilled Chicken Club	605	35	31
Grilled Chicken, plain	400	15	30
Pot Roast	610	28	58
Turkey Bacon Melt	615	29	53
Meat/Steak			
Country Fried Steak: with Gravy	550	38	37
w/o Gravy, 5 oz	500	33	31
Cranberry Apple Pork Loin (1)	500	28	43
Meatloaf with Gravy, 4.5 oz	285	20	9
Open Faced Roast Beef, 10 oz	510	25	24
Pot Roast Beef Stew Deep-Dish	765	39	65
Steak Tips & Noodles, 28 oz	1025	46	81
Steak Tips Stir-Fry	1020	47	84
Dinners: *Side Dishes not Included*			
Chicken:			
Chicken-N-Noodles Deep-Dish	845	43	67
Slow-Roasted, 11 oz	295	16	23
Chicken Parmesan, 23 oz	800	29	85
Chicken Stir-Fry	640	20	77
Fried Chicken Breast (1), 5 oz	285	13	13
Grilled Chicken Breast, 4½ oz	230	13	0
Garlic Butter Grilled Chkn Breast	270	16	3
Turkey: Slow-Roasted Turkey, 3 oz	115	4	1

Dinners (Cont)	C	F	Cb
Fish: Fried Haddock, 6½ oz	365	18	27
Potato-Crusted Flunder, 5 oz	255	17	8
Salmon Stir-Fry, 29 oz	750	27	77
Wildfire Salmon, 9 oz	380	13	22
Pasta: Garden Vegetable Alfredo	900	45	99
Garden Veg. & Chicken Alfredo	950	44	85
Garden Veg. & Salmon Alfredo	1075	52	86
Italian Sausage & Pepper, 22 oz	820	40	76
Vegetarian: Vegetable Stir-Fry	505	15	86
Side Dishes: Baked Potato, 11 oz	205	0	54
Bread & Celery Dressing, 6 oz	30	0	6
Caramelized Onions, 2 oz	40	2	6
Coleslaw, 4 oz	205	14	19
Corn, 5 oz	170	8	25
Garden Vegetables, 6 oz	120	7	14
Glazed Carrots, 4 oz	85	3	14
Grilled Mushrooms, 8 oz	150	12	10
Loaded Baked Potato, 12½ oz	375	13	56
Mashed Potatoes, 6 oz	205	7	17
Rice Pilaf, 6 oz	130	4	20
Sweet Corn Griddle Cakes, 5½ oz	400	18	54
Fries: French Fries, 5 oz	355	15	51
Home Fries, 5 oz	185	7	27
Sauces/Condiments: Apple Sce, 4 oz	85	0	21
Beef Gravy, 2 oz	22	1	3
Chicken/Country Gravy, 2 oz	55	4	3
Cranberry Relish, 1 oz	55	9	13
Hollandaise Sauce, 2 oz	50	3	5
Marinara Sauce, 3 oz	35	1	5
Mayonnaise, ½ oz	90	10	0
Pork-Roasted Gravy, 2 oz	65	5	3
Sour Cream, 1 oz	55	5	2
Tarter Sauce, 1 oz	165	18	1
Wildfire BBQ Sauce, 1½ oz	95	0	22
Kid's Menu: Mac & Cheese	320	1	45
Mini Cheeseburgers (2)	305	19	21
Pasta	205	5	35
Plenty-O-Pancakes	500	17	79
Smiley Face Potatoes, 6 oz	525	31	57
Salads: Cobb	700	46	14
Country Spinach	605	41	13
Fruit & Yogurt Plate	405	2	93
Desserts, Pies, Sundaes			
Pie: Apple Pie, N.S.A., 1 slice	490	30	55
Coconut Cream Pie, 1 slice	535	27	65
Kids Sundae: Fudge Blast, 4.4 oz	250	11	34

Bojangles® (Oct '08)

Cajun & Southern Style Chicken	C	F	Cb
Breast, average	280	17	12
Leg, average	265	16	11
Thigh, average	310	23	11
Wing, average	355	25	11
Sandwiches			
Cajun Filet: no Mayo	340	11	41
w. Mayonnaise	440	22	41
Grilled Filet: no Mayo	235	5	25
w. Mayonnaise	335	16	25
Snacks: Buffalo Bites	180	5	5
Chicken Supremes	335	16	26
Biscuit Sandwiches: Biscuit, plain	245	12	29
Bacon	290	17	26
Bacon, Egg & Cheese	550	42	27
Cajun Filet	455	21	46
Country Ham	270	15	26
Egg	400	30	26
Sausage	350	23	26
Smoked Sausage	380	26	27
Steak	650	49	37
Fixins': Botato Rounds	235	11	31
Broccoli Florets	30	0	6
Cajun Pintos	110	0	18
Corn on the Cob	140	2	34
Dirty Rice	165	6	24
Green Beans	25	0	5
Macaroni & Cheese	200	14	12
Marinated Cole Slaw	135	3	26
Potatoes, no Gravy	80	1	16
Seasoned Fries	345	19	39
Sweet Biscuits: Bo Berry	220	10	29
Cinnamon	320	18	37

For Complete Nutritional Data ~ see CalorieKing.com

Boston Market® (Oct '08)

Sandwiches & Burgers	C	F	Cb
Roasted Sirloin Open Faced	410	15	32
Meatloaf Open Faced	670	38	48
Boston Chicken Carver	700	29	68
Boston Turkey Carver	770	27	68
Half Boston: Chicken Carver	340	15	29
Sirloin Dip Carver	500	25	35
Turkey Carver	390	14	34
Half Turkey Dip Carver	380	14	33
Salads			
Caesar Entree: with dressing	500	45	12
without dressing	140	8	8
Roasted Sirloin	160	6	0
Roasted Turkey	140	6	1
Rotisserie Chicken	160	1	3
Market Chopped: w. Dressing	580	48	30
no Dressing	210	9	28
w. Roasted Sirloin & Dressing	740	54	31
w. Roasted Turkey & Dressing	720	54	32
Sides			
Broccoli w. Garlic Butter	80	6	6
Butternut Squash	140	4.5	25
Caesar Salad	40	2	3
Creamed Spinach	280	23	12
Fresh Steamed Vegetables	60	2	8
Garden Fresh Coleslaw	170	9	21
Garlic Dill New Potatoes	140	3	24
Green Beans	60	3.5	7
Green Been Casserole	60	2	9
Macaroni & Cheese	300	11	35
Mashed Potatoes	270	11	36
Seasonal Fresh Fruit Salad	60	0	15
Squash Casserole	320	24	21
Sweet Corn	170	4	37
Sweet Potato Casserole	460	17	77
Soups			
Chicken Noodle	170	5	17
Chicken Tortilla: with toppings	340	22	24
without toppings	90	5	7
Desserts			
Chocolate Cake	580	34	67
Chocolate Chip Fudge Brownie	580	23	81
Cornbread	180	5	31
Nestle Toll House, Choc. Chip Cookie	370	19	49
Individual Meals			
Pastry Top Chicken Pot Pie	780	47	60
Meatloaf	530	26	31

For Complete Nutritional Data ~ see CalorieKing.com

Be sure to balance 'eating out' with adequate fruit and veggies.

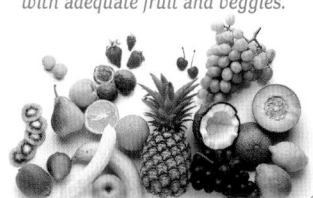

Fast - Foods & *Restaurants*

Boston Pizza® (Oct '08)

	C	F	Cb
Starters: Cactus Cut Potatoes/Dip	1150	89	72
Boston's Pizza Bread, no dip	500	12	84
Oven Rstd Boston's BBQ Wings	740	46	25
Soup: Baked French Onion	310	14	35
Salads: Caesar, reg., w. dressing	250	20	17
Spinach	250	22	6
Citrus Chicken Grilled	800	19	24
Sandwiches: Boston Brute & Fries	920	29	111
Boston Cheesesteak & Fries	1520	71	131
Chkn Santa Fe Stromboli & Caesar	770	24	106
New York Steak & Tossed Greens	850	62	28
Pizzas (Medium): *Per 2 Slices*			
BBQ Chicken	380	12	50
Boston Royal	420	12	54
Cheeseburger	560	24	50
Hawaiian	420	10	56
Meateor	520	22	50
Spicy Perogy	560	26	54
Ultimate Pepperoni	460	18	48
Vegetarian	340	8	52
Pastas (Full Order):			
Homestyle Lasagna	640	33	46
Chicken & Mushroom Fettucini	1430	79	139
Spicy Italian Penne	1410	78	134
Desserts: Chocolate Explosion	870	49	98
New York Cheesecake	600	32	76

For Complete Nutritional Data ~ see CalorieKing.com

Braum's® (Oct '08)

	C	F	Cb
Cinnamon Rolls, with Icing	500	12	88
Frozen Yogurt: Per ½ Cup			
Vanilla; Peach; Strawb./Banana	120	4	18
Other flavors, average	140	5	20
Ice Cream: Per ½ Cup			
Light: Average all varieties	115	4	19
Premium: Peanut Buttercup	190	12	18
Other flavors, average	150	7	18
Pies (Baked): Average, 1 slice	400	20	50

For Complete Nutritional Data ~ see CalorieKing.com

Buck's Pizza® (Oct '08)

	C	F	Cb
Buck's Deluxe: Med. (12"), 1 sl, ⅙	265	13	28
Large (14"), 1 slice, ⅛	270	13	29
X-Large (16"), 1 slice, ¹⁄₁₂	240	11	38
Small (9"), Whole Pizza	900	44	96
Personal (6"), Whole Pizza	400	17	69

Bruegger's Bagels® (Oct '08)

	C	F	Cb
Bagels			
Average all flavors, 4.3 oz	330	2	65
Softwiches (Square): Asiago	360	4.5	66
BLT	600	25	73
Chicken Breast	630	11	81
Everything	320	2	64
Garden Veggie	380	3	76
Hummus	540	13	85
Plain	350	2.5	70
Roast Beef	750	40	72
Breakfast S'wiches: Egg & Cheese	420	18	71
Egg, Cheese & Ham	460	18	73
Egg, Cheese & Sausage	640	38	72
Bagel Sandwiches: Chicken Fajita	530	11	81
Herby Turkey	560	14	78
Santa Fe Turkey	490	9	75
Smoked Salmon	490	10	74
Deli Softwich: Chicken Breast	630	11	81
Chicken Salad w. Mayo	670	27	76
Ham	510	6	85
Tuna Salad w. Mayo	720	34	76
Turkey w. Mayo	550	15	74
Salads: Caesar	270	17	22
Chicken Caesar	370	20	23
Sesame Chicken	480	28	30
Muffins: Blueberry	450	19	64
Chocolate	460	24	57
Cake: Lemon Pound, 3.3 oz slice	320	13	48
Cookies: Chocolate Chunk	500	22	71
Oatmeal Raisin	460	19	71
Slices: Luscious Lemon	300	16	36
Seven Layer	650	43	58
Chocolate Chunk Brownie	330	18	40
Raspberry Sammies	340	16	44

For Complete Menu & Data ~ see CalorieKing.com

Burgerville® (Oct '08)

	C	F	Cb
Hamburger	300	15	29
Cheeseburger	350	19	29
Double Beef Cheeseburger	430	25	29
Half Pound Colossal	730	45	31
Colossal	520	30	31
Tillamook Cheeseburger	630	40	31
Turkey Club Sandwich	550	32	38
Crispy Chicken	490	19	59
Grilled Chicken	320	4.5	44
Chicken Strips, 5 pieces	320	14	26
French Fries: Regular, 5 oz	360	17	48

For Complete Menu & Data ~ see CalorieKing.com

Updated Nutrition Data ~ www.CalorieKing.com
Persons with Diabetes ~ See Disclaimer (Page 24)

Burger King® (Oct '08)

Breakfast	**C**	**F**	**Cb**
Biscuits			
Bacon Egg & Cheese	410	25	31
Ham Egg & Cheese	390	22	31
Sausage, 1 biscuit, 4.2 oz	390	26	28
Cheesy Tots: Small, 6 pces, 2.7 oz	215	12	20
Medium, 9 pieces, 4.1 oz	325	18	30
Croissan'wich: Bacon Egg & Chse	340	20	26
Ham Egg & Cheese	340	18	26
Sausage & Cheese	370	25	23
Double Croissan'wich			
with Bacon, Egg & Cheese	430	27	27
with Double Bacon	430	27	27
with Double Ham	420	22	28
with Double Sausage	680	51	26
with Ham, Bacon, Egg & Cheese	420	24	27
with Sausage, Egg & Cheese	550	37	27
Hash Browns: Small, 3 oz	260	17	25
Medium, 4.9 oz	430	28	42
Sandwiches & Burgers			
Burgers: Bacon Cheeseburger	355	17	31
BK Stackers: Double	620	39	32
Quad	1010	70	34
Triple	820	55	33
BK Veggie: Burger	420	16	46
with Cheese	470	20	47
Cheeseburger	340	16	31
Double Cheeseburger	510	29	31
Hamburger	290	12	30
Steakhouse	950	59	55
Steakhouse Loaded	970	55	63
Sandwiches			
Original Chicken, with Mayo	650	38	48
BK Big Fish with Tartar Sauce	640	31	67
Chick'N Crisp w/o mayo	320	13	36
Spicy Chick'N Crisp	480	30	30
TenderCrisp Chicken	780	43	67
TenderGrill Chicken	510	19	49
Whopper Sandwiches			
Original	680	40	51
Double	920	58	51
Triple	1160	76	51
Whopper JR.:	370	21	31
with Cheese	420	25	32

Salads: Without Dressing or Croutons	**C**	**F**	**Cb**
Garden: with TenderCrisp Chicken	400	21	27
with TenderGrill Chicken	240	9	8
Kids Menu			
BK Fresh Apple Fries w. Dipping Sce	60	0	15
French Toast,w. Apple Sce, 5 pces	680	24	100
Kraft Macaroni & Cheese, 4 oz	180	7	22
Sides			
BK Chicken Fries			
w/o Buffalo Sauce, 6 pces, 4 oz	270	16	17
9 pieces, 5.5 oz	400	24	25
Chicken Tenders: Box, 5 pces, 2.7 oz	230	14	11
Big kids meal, 6 pces, 3.2 oz	275	17	13
Box, 8 pieces, 4.3 oz	370	23	18
French Fries: Small, 2.6 oz	230	13	26
Medium, 4.1 oz	360	20	41
Large, 5.6 oz	495	27	57
King, 6.8 oz	600	33	69
Onion Rings: Small, 1.5 oz	140	7	18
Medium, 3.2 oz	310	15	37
Large, 4.6 oz	440	22	53
King, 5.3 oz	500	25	62
Sauces & Condiments: Per 1 oz Container			
Dipping Sauces: Barbecue	40	0	11
Buffalo	80	8	2
Honey Mustard	90	6	8
Ranch	140	15	1
Sweet & Sour	45	0	10
Desserts			
Oreo Sundae Shakes: *Per Medium, 22 fl.oz*			
Chocolate	960	32	154
Strawberry	940	31	151
Vanilla	830	33	119
Beverages			
BK Joe Coffee, 16 fl.oz	10	0	1
Mocha Iced Coffee, 16 fl.oz	380	10	66
Icee, Coca-Cola: Small, 16 fl.oz	100	0	29
Medium, 22 fl.oz	140	0	40
Shakes:			
Chocolate: Small, 16 fl.oz	470	14	75
Medium, 22 fl.oz	690	20	114
Large, 32 fl.oz	950	29	151
Strawberry: Small, 16 fl.oz	460	14	73
Medium, 22 fl.oz	660	19	111
Large, 32 fl.oz	930	28	148
Vanilla: Small, 16 fl.oz	470	14	75
Medium, 22 fl.oz	560	21	79
Large, 32 fl.oz	820	30	117

For Complete Nutritional Data ~ see CalorieKing.com

California Pizza Kitchen
~ See CalorieKing.com

Captain D's Seafood® (Oct '08)
Platters: Per Platter, Includes Fries and Cole Slaw

	C	F	Cb
Fish, Shrimp & Chicken	1700	107	138
Jumbo Fish, average	1610	102	130
Super Shrimp	1380	83	122

Dinner: Per Order

	C	F	Cb
Chicken	1200	72	102
Crab	1050	60	106
Fish & Chicken	1460	93	121
Fish & Shrimp	1510	96	126

Sandwiches:

	C	F	Cb
Deluxe Classic Fish	890	59	62
Double Bacon Ranch Grilled Chicken	870	60	45
Desserts: Carrot Cake	390	19	50
Cheesecake	425	26	45
Chocolate Cake	300	10	49

Caribou Coffee® (Oct '08)
Classic: *Per Medium, 16 fl.oz*

	C	F	Cb
Coffee, with Steamed 2% Milk	120	5	11
Coffee Of The Day with 2% Milk	15	0.5	1

Cold: *Per Medium, 21 fl.oz*

	C	F	Cb
Iced Americano	15	0	2.5
Iced Coffee	235	12	30
Iced Latte with 2% Milk	150	6	14
Iced Mocha with 2% Milk	225	3.5	45

Coolers: *Per Medium, 16 fl.oz*

	C	F	Cb
Chocolate	295	4	61
Coffee	645	36	75
Espresso	125	2	24
Mint Oreo	515	20	82

Espresso: *Per Medium*

	C	F	Cb
1 medium, 4.4 fl.oz	5	0	0.5
Breve	425	36	15
Cappuccino with 2% Milk	75	3	7
Macchiato with 2% Milk, 4.5 oz	40	1	0

Hot Coffee: *Per Medium, 16 fl.oz*

	C	F	Cb
Pumpkin Pie Latte	375	15	48
Wild Cherry Mocha	535	15	88

Smoothies: *Per Medium, 21 fl.oz*

	C	F	Cb
Creampop	600	28	83
Passion Green Tea	250	0.5	61
Pom-a-Mango	310	0.5	74

Snowdrift: *Per Medium*

	C	F	Cb
Cookies 'n' Cream, 18.5 fl.oz	570	16	98
Mint with 2% Milk, 17 oz	420	11	71

Wild: *Per Medium*

	C	F	Cb
Hot Apple Blast	345	0.5	84
Mint Condition with 2% Milk	430	8.5	77

For Complete Menu & Data ~ see CalorieKing.com

Carl's Jr.® (Oct '08)
Charbroiled Burgers:

	C	F	Cb
Big Hamburger	470	17	53
Chili Cheeseburger	790	41	59
Famous Star	600	34	53
with Cheese	660	39	53
Kids Hamburger	460	17	53
Prime Rib Burger	730	43	45
Super Star with Cheese	660	39	53
Western Bacon Cheeseburger	710	33	70
Double	970	52	71
The Six Dollar Burger: Original	1010	68	60
Bacon Cheese	1070	76	50
Chili Cheese	1110	70	60
Guacamole Bacon	1140	85	54
Low-Carb	490	37	6
Prime Rib	1060	70	45

Chicken Sandwiches:

	C	F	Cb
Charbroiled: BBQ Chicken	360	4.5	48
Bacon Swiss Crispy Chicken	720	35	64
Chicken Club	550	25	43
Santa Fe Chicken	610	32	43
Spicy Chicken Sandwich	560	30	59
Chicken Breast Strips, 5-piece	710	41	46
Chicken Stars, 6-piece	260	16	14
Fish: Fish & Chips	630	28	68
Carl's Catch Fish Sandwich	660	31	75
Breakfast: Breakfast Burger	830	47	65
Bacon & Egg Burrito	570	33	37
Steak & Egg	660	36	44
Loaded Breakfast Burrito	820	51	52
Hash Brown Nuggets	330	21	32
Monster Breakfast Sandwich	730	47	39
Sourdough Ham Sandwich	460	21	39
Sunrise Croissant Sandwich	560	41	27
Fries: Chili Cheese, 12 oz	1410	76	100
CrissCut Fries, 14½ oz	410	24	43
Natural Cut: Small, 4 oz	540	25	47
Medium, 5½ oz	710	33	62
Onion Rings, 4½ oz	430	24	53

Salads: Without Dressing

	C	F	Cb
Taco	940	57	74
Charbroiled Chicken Salad	260	7	16
Side Salad	50	2.5	5

Dressings: Per 2 oz Pkg

	C	F	Cb
Blue Cheese	320	34	1
Thousand Island	240	23	7
Low-Fat Balsamic	35	1.5	5
Shakes: Van./Choc./Strawb. avg.	710	33	85
Malts, average all flavors	780	35	98

Updated Nutrition Data ~ www.CalorieKing.com
Persons with Diabetes ~ See Disclaimer (Page 24)

Carvel® (Oct '08)

Ice Creams: Per Regular 7.5 oz

	C	F	Cb
Cups: Chocolate	415	21	49
Vanilla	450	26	46
No Sugar Added, Vanilla	300	7	57
No-Fat, Chocolate/Vanilla	265	0	62
Dashers: Banana Barge	970	46	128
Mint Choc. Chip	800	42	96
Peanut Butter Cup	1060	60	95
Novelties: Brown Bonnet	390	23	43
Deluxe Flying Saucer w. Sprinkles	350	17	49
Flying Saucer, Chocolate	230	10	33

Desserts: Per Regular Sundae

	C	F	Cb
Classic Sundae: Caramel	670	34	81
Bittersweet Fudge	690	38	77
Strawberry	580	33	63

Thinny-Thin Classic Sundae

	C	F	Cb
No-Fat: Fudge	380	0	81
Strawberry	320	0	69

Fountain: Per Small, 16 fl.oz

	C	F	Cb
Carvelanche: Butterfinger	730	38	92
M&M; Reece's	760	39	88
Fried Ice Cream: Arctic Blender	850	29	132
Light Arctic Blender	630	5	132
Thick Shake: Float-Chocolate	790	34	109
Float-Strawberry	750	39	85
Float-Vanilla	810	39	102
Strawberry	600	31	70

Checkers®

Same Menu & Data as Rally's ~ See Page 239

Cheesecake Factory® (Oct '08)

(Author Estimates)

10" Cheesecake: Per Slice

	C	F	Cb
Adam's P'nut B'cup Fudge Ripple	930	59	93
Banana Cream	860	63	70
Brownie Sundae	970	63	96
Choc Chip Cookie Dough	1910	72	102
Dulce de Leche Caramel	1010	74	83
Kahlua Cocoa Coffee	840	55	80
Key Lime Cheesecake	710	49	64
Original Cheesecake	630	45	53
Vanilla Bean Cheesecake	870	64	69
White Choc. Raspberry Truffle	900	62	80
Appetizer: Avocado Eggrolls, 1 roll	435	27	48

Dinners: Complete Meal

	C	F	Cb
Cajun Jambalaya Pasta	1960	43	290
Chicken Madeira	1430	76	82
Famous Factory Meatloaf	1955	96	162
Fresh Fish Tacos	1130	23	160
Herb Crusted Filet of Salmon	1040	60	68
Lemon-Herb Roasted Chicken	1790	108	94
Salad: BBQ Ranch Chkn, no bread	1415	113	65

Charley's Grilled Subs® (Oct '08)

	C	F	Cb
Subs: Regular 7½" without Dressings/Mayo/Toppings			
BBQ Cheddar	585	20	70
Bacon 3 Cheese Steak	645	30	55
Buffalo Chicken	530	16	61
Chicken Bacon Club	580	23	54
Cordon Bleu	530	17	55
Chicken Teriyaki	530	16	60
Italian Deli	560	26	55
Mushroom Swiss Steak	520	19	57
Philly Cheesesteak	525	19	58
Philly Chicken	525	16	60
Philly Ham & Swiss	450	13	60
Philly Steak Deluxe	530	19	60
Philly Veggie	460	15	66
Sicilian Steak	620	28	55
Turkey Cheddar	460	12	55
Ultimate Club	515	20	55

Salads: Cheese/Dressings not included

	C	F	Cb
Chicken, Grilled/Teriyaki/Buffalo, avg.	290	13	16
Fresh Garden Salad	140	8	13
Grilled Steak Salad	290	16	14
Dressings: Italian/Ranch, avg., 1 oz	170	19	1
Mayo, 1 Tbsp., ½ oz	100	11	0
Fries: Regular	610	45	41
Ultimate, Chse, Ranch & Bacon	1250	103	57
Original Lemonade, 16 fl.oz	160	0	40

Extra Menu Items & Data = www.CalorieKing.com

Chevys Fresh Mex® (Oct '08)

	C	F	Cb
Sizzling Fajitas: Without Tortillas			
Original Famous Chicken	910	31	92
Sizzling Steak	1000	45	90
Portobello Mushroom & Asparagus	920	44	108
Grilled Tacos: Chicken	1020	34	121
Fish (Sea Bass)	970	33	121
Steak	1090	43	120
Grande Salads: Santa Fe	670	39	30
Santa Fe w/o Cheese or Bacon	320	11	28
Tostada Salad with Chicken	1550	94	102
w/o Tortilla Strips/Chse/Sour Cream	920	45	80
Tortilla Soup	400	17	36
Sides: Black Beans	190	2	33
Refried Beans	290	15	28
Guacamole, 2 oz	105	10	3
Mexican Rice	210	3	39
Salsa for Chips, 5 oz	40	0	8
Sour Cream	120	12	2
Tamalito (Sweetcorn), 2	180	7	29
Tortilla (El Machino), 2	140	4	22

Chick-fil-A® (Oct '08)

	C	F	Cb
Chick-fil-A Sandwiches			
Chargrilled Chicken w/o Sauce	270	3	37
Chargrilled Chicken Club w/o Sce	380	11	37
Chicken	410	16	39
Chicken Salad	500	20	53
Cool Wraps: Without Dressing			
Chargrilled Chicken	410	12	47
Chicken Caesar	480	16	44
Spicy Chicken	410	12	45
Breakfast			
Biscuits:			
Plain: w. Bacon Egg & Cheese	470	27	39
w. Gravy	330	15	43
Chicken	420	19	44
Sausage	490	32	38
Burritos: Chicken	420	18	40
Sausage	420	24	37
Chick-n-Minis, 1 box, 3 pces, 3.3 oz	275	11	28
Chicken, Egg & Cheese Bagel	500	20	49
Cinnamon Cluster	400	15	61
Hash Browns, 3 oz	260	17	25
Salads: Without Dressing & Condiments			
Chargrilled Chicken & Fruit	220	6	20
Chargrilled Chicken Garden	180	6	10
Chick-n-Strips	450	22	25
Southwest Chargrilled Chicken	240	9	17
Salad Dressings & Condiments			
Garlic & Butter Croutons, 0.5 oz	60	2	9
Tortilla Strips, 0.5 oz	80	4	8
Dressings: Blue Cheese, 1 oz	150	16	1
Buttermilk Ranch, 1.1 oz	160	17	1
Caesar, 1 oz	160	17	1
Light Italian, 1.1 oz	15	0.5	2
Thousand Island, 1.1 oz	150	14	5
Sauces: Barbecue, 1 oz	45	0	11
Buffalo, 0.7 oz	10	1	1
Buttermilk Ranch, 0.7 oz	110	12	1
Chick-fil-A, 1 oz	140	13	6
Honey Mustard, 1 oz	45	0	10
Honey Roasted BBQ, 0.4 oz	60	6	2
Polynesian, 1 oz	110	6	13
Sides			
Carrot & Raisin Salad, 6 oz	260	12	39
Chicken Salad Cup, 6 oz	350	24	7
Cole Slaw, 6.5 oz	370	32	20
Fruit Cup, 3.3 oz	50	0	12
Side Salad w/o Dressing, 3.8 oz	50	3	4
Waffle Potato Fries, 1 small, 3 oz	280	15	33
Soup: Hearty Breast of Chicken, 9.8 oz	150	4.5	19
Desserts			
Cheesecake	320	23	23
Fudge Nut Brownie	370	19	45
Icedream Cone w/o Toppings	170	4	31
Icedream Cup	260	7	44
Lemon Pie	350	11	59

Chili's® (Oct '08)

	C	F	Cb
Starters: Per Order			
Big Mouth Bites	850	75	29
Boneless Wings: Buffalo with Dress.	1170	85	50
Shanghai w. Dressing	1140	60	109
Bottomless Tostada Chips w. Sauce	480	36	26
Classic Nachos: w. Fajita Beef	1740	127	55
with Fajita Chicken	1630	112	55
with Pico de Gallo & Sour Cream	1450	108	53
Hot Spinach and Artichoke Dip	905	36	74
Skillet Queso w. Tostada Chips	1070	89	30
Southwestern Eggrolls	810	51	59
Wings Over Buffalo w. Dressing	1340	117	4
Meals: Cajun Chicken Pasta	1500	78	123
Chicken Club Tacos	1140	45	126
Chicken Crispers w. Side	1880	130	133
Chicken Tacos w. Rice & Beans	1200	41	137
Country Fried Chicken Steak	1660	101	141
Crispy Honey Chipotle Crisper	1890	99	203
Fajitas: Buffalo Chicken	1090	76	56
Citrus Fire Chicken & Shrimp	720	42	34
Classic Chicken	330	11	23
Classic Combo Steak & Chicken	560	30	21
Classic Steak	790	49	20
Mushroom Jack	750	45	31
Steak & Portobello	1130	84	26
Fire-Grilled Steaks: No sides or Toast			
Cajun Ribeye	870	76	3
Classic Sirloin	540	42	1
Ribeye	960	87	1
Country Fried Steak	1890	107	148
Salads: No Dressing Unless Indicated			
Boneless Buffalo Chicken	910	58	44
Caesar: with Chicken & Dressing	1010	76	39
with Grilled Shrimp & Dressing	980	77	39
Side Salad House	140	7	12
Mesquite Chicken	800	43	53
Quesadilla Explosion w. Dressing	980	53	78
Southwestern Cobb, no dressing	970	60	56
Guiltless Grill: Black Bean Burger	650	12	96
Chicken Sandwich	490	8	63
Desserts: Cheesecake, 1 slice	720	44	68
Chocolate Chip Paradise Pie	1600	78	215
Frosty Chocolate Shake	850	36	123
Molten Chocolate Cake	1270	62	172
For Complete Nutritional Data ~ see CalorieKing.com			

Chipotle® (Oct '08)

Breads	C	F	Cb
Flour Tortillas (13"), 1 tortilla	290	9	44
Flour Tortillas (6"), 3 tortillas	255	8	38
Taco Shells, Crispy, 4 shells	180	7	26
Meal Components			
Barbacoa, 4 oz	170	7	2
Black Beans, 4 oz	130	1	22
Carnitas, 4 oz	210	11	2
Cheese, 1 oz	110	9	0.5
Chicken, 4 oz	200	7	2
Lettuce, 1 oz	5	0	0.5
Pinto Beans, 4 oz	140	1	23
Rice, 3½ oz	160	4	30
Steak, 4 oz	190	7	2
Condiments			
Salsa: Corn, 4 oz	100	1	22
Green Tomatillo, 2 oz	15	0.5	3
Red Tomatillo, 2 oz	30	1	4
Tomato, 4 oz	25	0	6
Sour Cream, 2 oz	120	10	2
Vinaigrette, 2 oz	330	31	12
Extras: Chips, serving, 4 oz	570	27	73
Guacamole, 4 oz	140	10	10

Chuck E. Cheese® (Oct '08)

Appetizers: Per Serving	C	F	Cb
Buffalo Wings (12)	660	45	3
Italian Bread Sticks (1)	195	8	27
Mozzarella Sticks, 1 stick	105	6	7
Pizzas: Per Slice (Medium)			
BBQ Chicken	270	8	43
Cheese	235	7	33
Pepperoni	265	10	33
Vegetarian	235	7	36
Individual Pizza, Whole: Cheese	930	30	198
Pepperoni	1030	36	198
Sandwiches, No Fries: Ham & Chse	620	27	70
Grilled Chicken Sub	650	31	70
Italian Sub	730	40	69
Hot Dog	170	17	27
Hot Dog w. Cheese	335	30	28
French Fries: S'wich/Hotdog, 5 oz	240	9	37
Large Serving (a la carte), 10 oz	480	17	74
Desserts: Apple Pie Pizza, 1 slice	195	2	40
Birthday Cake (8"), 1 slice, 1/10	310	13	45
Cinnamon Sticks, 1 stick	200	5	33

Church's Chicken® (Oct '08)

Chicken: Per Serving	C	F	Cb
Crunchy Tenders: 1 piece	120	6	6
Spicy, 1 piece	135	7	7
Original: Breast, piece	200	11	3
Leg, piece	110	6	3
Thigh, piece	330	23	8
Wing, piece	300	19	7
Spicy: Breast, piece	320	20	12
Leg, 1 piece	180	11	8
Thigh, 1 piece	480	35	20
Wing, 1 piece	430	27	17
Sides: Per Regular Serving			
Cajun Rice, 3 oz	130	7	16
Cole Slaw, 4 oz	150	10	15
Collard Greens, 3½ oz	25	0	5
Corn on the Cob (1)	140	3	24
French Fries, 3½ oz	290	14	38
Honey Butter Biscuits (1), 1.7 oz	240	12	28
Jalapeno Bombers, 4 pieces, 4 oz	240	10	29
Macaroni & Cheese, 5.2 oz	210	11	23
Mashed Potatoes & Gravy, 3.6 oz	70	2	12
Okra, 4 oz	350	22	36
Sweet Corn Nuggets, 7.4 oz	600	29	72
Whole Jalapeno Peppers (2), 1.3 oz	10	0	2
Sauces: Per Packet			
BBQ; Sweet & Sour	30	0	7
Creamy Jalapeno	100	11	1
Honey Mustard	110	11	4
Purple Pepper	45	0	12
Ranch	130	13	1

Cici's Pizza® (Oct '08)

Buffet: Per 1/10 of 12" Pizza	C	F	Cb
Alfredo	140	4.5	18
Bacon Cheddar	145	5.5	18
Bar-B-Que	170	6.5	21
Beef	170	6.5	18
Cheese	150	4.5	20
Ham & Pineapple	140	4.5	19
Pepperoni & Jalapeno	165	6	20
Sausage	195	6.5	19
Spinach Alfredo	150	5	20
Zesty Ham & Cheddar/Pepperoni	155	6	18
To-Go: Per 1/10 of 15" Pizza			
Alfredo	215	8.5	27
Bacon Cheddar	255	8	36
Bar-B-Que	290	10	36
Beef	260	10	28
Cheese; Ham & Pineapple	225	8	27
Pepperoni & Jalapeno	220	8.5	25
Sausage	290	10	28
Spinach Alfredo	245	8	32
Zesty Ham & Cheddar	230	11	24
Zesty Tomato Alfredo/Veggie	215	9	25

Fast - Foods & *Restaurants*

Cinnabon® (Oct '08)

Sweet Rolls:	C	F	Cb
Cinnabon Bites (6)	510	19	77
Classic Cinnamon Roll (1)	815	32	117
Cinnabon Stix, 5 pieces, 85g	380	21	41
Minibon (1) 92g	340	13	49
Caramel Pecanbon (1)	1100	56	141
CinnaPretzel (1)	755	6	156
Sweet Roll Icing: Frosting Cup, 1.4 oz	180	11	20
Drinks: Mochalatta Chill, 480ml	360	13	55

For Complete Nutritional Data ~ see CalorieKing.com

CinnaMonster® (Oct '08)

Cinnamon Roll: Per Roll	C	F	Cb
Caramel Pecan	840	32	120
Original	880	24	100

Cosi® (Oct '08)

Sandwiches	C	F	Cb
Chicken Caesar	745	36	54
Italiano	745	42	49
Roasted Turkey & Brie	690	32	62
Sesame Ginger Chicken	480	7	69
Turkey Rustica	620	27	60
TBM	565	34	50
Tuna Cheddar	955	57	46
Melts			
Bacon, Turkey Cheddar	570	24	48
Grilled Chicken Parmesan	620	25	54
Pesto Chicken	670	31	52
Tuna Melt	875	40	51
TBM Melt	705	39	58
Pizza: Individual Flatbread			
Margherita	700	31	96
Pepperoni	805	40	94
Traditional Cheese	665	28	95
Soup: Per Regular Cup			
Pollo & Pasta Soup	160	4	14
Tomato Basil Aurora	225	15	20
Moroccan Lentil	200	3	32
Three Bean Chili	150	1	36
Salads: No Dresssing			
Greek Salad	270	20	17
Grilled Chicken Caesar	355	16	16
Signature Salad	325	18	34
Dressings: Per 2 oz			
Cosi Vinaigrette	355	39	2
Caesar	265	28	4

For Complete Menu & Data ~ see CalorieKing.com

Costco Food Court (Oct '08)

Pizza: Per Slice	C	F	Cb
Combo, 10.7oz	680	29	72
Cheese, 9.8 oz	700	28	70
Pepperoni , 8.9 oz	620	24	68
Dogs: Sinai Hot Dog, 7.9 oz	540	30	48
Hebrew National Hot Dog, 7.9 oz	530	32	42
Sinai Polish Sausage, 7.9 oz	570	32	44
Hebrew Polish Sausage, 7.9 oz	540	32	44
Salad, Chicken Caesar, 19.8 oz	800	57	32
Meals: Chicken Bake 11.5 oz	810	30	77
Ital. Sausage Sandwich, 12.6 oz	700	42	46
Beverages: Hot Latte, 9.6 fl oz	190	5	24
Hot Mocha, 11.3 fl oz	310	9	45
Mocha Freeze, 16.3 fl .oz	320	7	49
Latte Freeze, 15.3 oz	240	7	32
Churro, 5.2 oz	430	18	62
Smoothies: Per 16 fl.oz			
Fruit Smoothie	290	0	72
Straw/Banana Smoothie	300	0	74
Tropical Smoothie	270	0	65
Desserts: Ice cream Bar, 8 oz	870	65	60
Berry Sundae, 12.3 oz	410	0	87
Frozen Yogurt, 12 oz	390	0	82

Cousins Subs® (Oct '08)

7½" Subs	C	F	Cb
BLT	590	38	47
Cheese Steak	505	19	49
Chicken Breast	570	27	50
Chicken Cheddar Deluxe	670	39	51
Club	655	35	51
Double Cheese Steak	745	36	49
Garden Veggie	390	12	51
Gyro	710	41	61
Ham & Provolone	610	34	50
Hot Veggie	470	17	55
Italian Special	820	51	50
Meatball & Provolone	725	38	54
Pepperoni Melt	730	45	50
Philly Cheese Steak	530	19	55
Pizza	710	39	55
Roast Beef	610	30	50
Seafood w. Crab	640	38	60
Spicy Chicken Sedona	530	18	54
Three Cheese	685	44	50
Tuna	665	40	49
Turkey Breast	535	28	50

Cousins Subs® cont... (Oct '08)

	C	F	Cb
5" Mini Subs: Without Mayo, Cheese			
Club	195	3	26
Garden Veggie	135	1	26
Ham	180	2	26
Hot Veggie	145	1	27
Turkey Breast	175	2	26
French Fries: Small, 2.8 oz	250	13	30
Medium, 4 oz	365	19	43
Large, 5.3 oz	485	25	57
Salads: Without Dressings			
Chef Salad	330	14	26
Chicken Sedona	230	5	16
Garden: Salad	240	11	24
with Chicken Breast	355	12	26
Italian	410	24	25
Seafood Salad	320	11	35
Side Salad	135	6	14
Tuna Salad	630	46	24

For Complete Menu & Data ~ see CalorieKing.com

Cold Stone Creamery® (Oct '08)

Ice Creams	C	F	Cb
Amaretto: Like it, average all flav.	330	20	33
Love it, average all flavors	525	31	53
Gotta have it, average all flavors	790	47	80
Sorbet			
Like it, average all flavors	160	0	41
Love it, average all flavors	255	0	65
Gotta have it, average all flavors	380	0	97

Culver's® (Oct '08)

Culver Burgers:	C	F	Cb
Bacon Deluxe Double	750	50	34
Deluxe Burger: Single	495	31	34
Double	670	43	34
Low-Carb Burger	445	32	1
Favorite Sandwiches:			
Angus Philly Steak	520	20	46
Beef Pot Roast	365	16	33
Blackened Chicken	370	8	48
Crispy Chicken Fillet	625	29	68
Grilled Chicken Breast	375	8	47
Grilled Ham 'n Swiss on Rye	500	25	33
North Atlantic Cod Filet	740	42	58
Pork Tenderloin	595	29	62
Turkey Sourdough BLT	560	31	36
Turkey Stacked	450	19	47

Culver's® cont... (Oct '08)

Favorite Sandwiches:	C	F	Cb
Garden Fresh Salads: Cobb Salad	530	31	19
Avocado Pecan Bleu w. Chicken	555	41	16
Chicken Cashew w. Grilled Chicken	440	25	17
Classic Caesar w. Gr. Chicken	360	14	15
Crispy Chicken	615	42	34
Garden Fresco	235	12	19
Side Salad	85	5	6
Sides			
Chili Cheddar Fries, 9.3 oz	660	34	73
French Fries, regular, 5 oz	385	17	53
Mashed Potatoes & Gravy, small	140	2	26
Onion Rings, breaded, 6.7 oz	630	36	70
Desserts: Classic Lemon Ice, 7 oz	140	0	35
Lemon Ice Smoothie, 11 oz	405	16	61
Root Beer Float, 15 oz	465	18	70
Custard Dishes, Vanilla:			
1 Scoop	305	18	30
2 Scoops	590	35	58
3 Scoops	745	44	73

For Complete Nutritional Data ~ see CalorieKing.com

D'Angelo's® (Oct '08)

	C	F	Cb
Sandwiches:			
Cheeseburger: Pokket	460	25	31
Sub	525	26	44
Wrap	610	33	48
Chicken Stir Fry: Pokket	380	9	39
Sub	450	11	53
Wrap	535	17	57
Classic Veggie: D'Lite	360	7	63
Wrap	485	13	68
Roast Beef: D'Lite	340	5	51
Sub	320	5	48
Turkey: D'Lite	345	4	51
Sub	315	4	45
Grilled Chicken Breast, D'Lite	390	7	52
Italian Sub	615	31	54
Number 9 Steak Sub	460	19	41
Salads: No Dressing Unless Indicated			
Caesar Salad w. Dressing	475	39	25
Chicken Stir Fry Salad	170	3	11
Greek Salad	300	23	17
Roast Beef Salad	130	3	10
Lobster Salad	375	26	12
Tossed Salad	50	1	10
Turkey Salad	155	2	10

Fast - Foods & *Restaurants*

Dairy Queen® (Oct '08)

Burgers/Sandwiches		C	F	Cb
DQ All Beef Hot Dogs: Hot Dog		250	14	21
Chili Cheese		430	23	39
GrillBurgers: Per Burger				
DQ Original Cheeseburgers		400	18	34
Double Burger		640	34	34
Bacon Double		730	41	35
Bacon Cheddar		710	42	41
Classic without Cheese		530	28	42
DQ Ultimate		780	48	33
Hamburgers		350	14	33
½ lb burger		780	47	42
Sandwiches: Crispy Chicken		530	29	47
Grilled Chicken		400	16	32
Chicken				
Chicken Strips Basket, 4 Pieces		1340	96	82
G&C Quesadilla Chicken		1140	68	81
Salads: Without Dressing				
Crispy Chicken Caesar w. Croutons		540	26	44
Grilled Chicken		320	11	14
Sides				
DQ French Fries, 4 oz		295	13	41
DQ Onion Rings, 4 oz		470	30	45
Desserts: Per Medium Serving				
Blizzard Treats: Banana Cream Pie		790	30	118
Caramel Waffle Crisp		800	31	119
Cherry Cheesecake		700	28	95
Choco Cherry Love		750	35	95
Chocolate Chip		920	53	95
Chocolate Chip Cookie Dough		1030	40	151
Oreo Cookies		690	26	103
Reese's P'nut Butter Cups		770	32	104
Tin Roof Brownie		860	36	119
DQ Blizzard Cakes (8"): Per ⅛ Cake				
Cotton Candy		570	17	104
Reese'sP'nut Butter Cup		610	28	78
Tin Roof Brownie		550	26	70
DQ Dipped Cones: Per 7 oz Cone				
Butterscotch		485	23	60
Chocolate		480	23	60
DQ Soft Serve: Per ½ Cup, 3.3 oz				
Chocolate		150	5	22
Vanilla		150	5	22
Beverages: Per Medium, 20 fl.oz				
Malts: Blueberry		855	21	145
Chocolate		880	21	151
Cocoa Fudge		1110	49	145
Hot Fudge		940	29	145
Maple Walnut		1035	41	144
Marshmallow		875	21	154
Peanut Butter		1180	62	127

For Complete Nutritional Data ~ see CalorieKing.com

Daphne's® Greek Cafe (Oct '08)

Meals: Without Dressing	C	F	Cb
Chicken Kabob	425	21	84
Chicken Salad & Soup	570	27	49
Falafel Zesta Lunch	570	36	100
Salad & Soup	470	25	47
Zesta Lunch	545	35	91
Plate: Calamari	565	32	97
Chicken Kabob	525	23	88
Shrimp	440	26	85
Salads: Without Dressing			
Greek: Regular	385	19	41
w. Shrimp	585	30	54
Side	330	16	36
Sandwiches			
Pita: Calamari	500	28	44
Chicken	515	22	36
Greek Veggie	485	33	36
Gyros Jr.	475	32	35
Shrimp	405	24	35
Steak	595	41	34
Soups			
Avgolemono, 1 cup, 8 fl.oz	320	17	33

Davanni's® (Oct '08)

Hoagies: Per Half Hoagie (6") w. Mayonnaise	C	F	Cb
Assorted	390	29	21
3 Cheese	385	28	21
Chicken Breast	510	31	22
Chicken Parmigiana	415	19	22
Club	385	25	22
Italian Sausage	520	37	28
Meatball	465	31	31
Pastrami	440	25	22
Pizza	315	18	22
Salami	485	38	21
Tuna	550	42	24
Turkey	355	22	22
Veggie	350	23	25
Without Cheese ~ Deduct	40	3	0
Without Mayo ~ Deduct	100	11	1
Calzones, average all varieties	695	33	66
Pizzas			
5 Meat: Thin, 1 slice	240	12	18
Traditional: 1 slice	300	12	30
Solo Thin	1010	62	45
The Works: Thin, 1 slice	250	13	18
Traditional: 1 slice	310	14	30
Solo Thin	595	32	42
Veggie: Thin, 1 slice	210	9	18
Traditional: 1 slice	265	9	30
Solo Thin	495	22	42

Del Taco® (Oct '08)

	C	F	Cb
Breakfast			
Breakfast Burrito	250	11	24
Bacon & Egg Quesadilla	450	23	40
Egg & Cheese Burrito	450	24	39
Macho Bacon & Egg Burrito	1030	60	82
Steak & Egg Burrito	580	34	41
Hash Brown Sticks (5)	250	19	20
Tacos: Big Fat Chicken Taco	340	13	38
Big Fat Steak Taco	390	19	38
Big Fat Taco	320	11	39
Chicken Del Carbon	170	5	19
Crispy Fish Taco	290	16	30
Macho Taco	310	17	16
Spicy Mole Chicken Soft Taco	190	17	18
Steak Taco Del Carbon	220	11	19
Taco; Soft Taco, average	160	10	13
Burritos: Del Combo Burrito	530	22	61
Bean & Cheese Red/Green Burrito	270	8	38
Chicken Works Burrito	520	23	57
Del Beef Burrito	550	30	42
Del Classic Chicken Burrito	560	36	41
Deluxe Combo Burrito	570	25	64
Deluxe Del Beef Burrito	590	33	45
Half Pound Red/Green Burrito, avg.	430	12	46
Macho Beef Burrito	1170	62	89
Macho Combo Burrito	1050	44	113
Spicy Chicken/Veggie Works, avg.	500	17	68
Steak Works Burrito	590	31	58
Quesadillas: Cheddar; Spicy Jack	495	27	39
Chicken Cheddar; Spicy Jack Chkn	600	32	43
Salads: Deluxe Chicken Salad	740	34	77
Deluxe Taco Salad	780	40	76
Taco Salad	350	30	10
Burgers: Cheeseburger	330	13	37
Double Del Cheeseburger	560	35	35
Del Cheeseburger	430	25	35
Nachos: Regular, 4 oz	380	24	40
Macho Nachos, 16 oz	1100	63	113
Sides: Rice Cup, 4 oz	140	2	27
Beans 'n Cheese Cup, 7.8 oz	415	9	47
Chips & Salsa, small	155	7	22
Fries: Chili Cheese, 10.5 oz	670	46	51
Deluxe Chili Cheese, 12 oz	710	49	53
Small, 5 oz	350	23	34
Macho, 10 oz	690	46	68
Shakes: Chocolate, 15 fl.oz	685	14	119
Vanilla; Strawb. avg., 15 fl.oz	590	11	103

Denny's® (Oct '08)

	C	F	Cb
Breakfast			
Center Cut Sirloin & Eggs	370	15	1
Meat Lover's	1230	66	109
Moons Over My Hammy	760	40	52
Ultimate Omelette with Hash Browns	830	62	26
Platters: *Without Sides*			
Buttermilk Pancake	660	25	83
Scrambles, Heartland	1080	63	93
Sides, Two Eggs & More Breakfast	630	47	21
Slams: All-American	950	75	21
French Toast	1180	75	74
Grand Slam: Original	740	43	56
Slugger w. Hash Browns	1040	55	97
Lumberjack with Hash Browns	1040	53	84
Soups: Per 12 oz Bowl			
Chicken Noodle; Clam Chowder	170	11	13
Tomato Basil	240	15	21
Vegetable Beef	140	5	11
Sandwiches & Burgers: Without Fries or Condiments			
Burgers: Boca	510	16	64
Classic	780	45	56
Mushroom Swiss	900	55	62
Slam	1080	57	115
Sandwiches: Bacon, Lettuce & Tom.	570	37	36
Club	660	34	55
Fish	590	30	30
Grilled Chicken	490	13	57
Melts: Chicken Ranch	920	42	79
Philly	740	43	51
The Super Bird	570	27	43
Appetizers: Without Condiments			
Buffalo Chicken Strips, 5 strips	735	42	43
Buffalo Wings, 9 wings	975	72	11
Chicken Strips, 5 strips	720	33	56
Mini Burgers w. On. Rings, 6 burgers	2220	136	179
Mozzarella Sticks, 8 sticks, 8 oz	710	41	49
Sampler	1405	80	124
Smothered Cheese Fries	765	48	69
Meals: Without Sides, Bread or Condiments			
Country Fried Steak	645	46	30
Dinners: Fried Shrimp	260	12	18
Steakhouse Strip	390	14	0
Fish & Chips	960	54	83
Grilled Chicken	280	5	4
Gr. Shirmp Skewer w. Pilaf & Garlic Bread	570	24	58
Grilled Tilapia	530	18	33
Roast Turkey & Stuffing w. Gravy	510	14	66
Sirloin Steak	220	6	1
Sirloin Steak & Breaded Shrimp	440	15	23
T-Bone Steak	580	27	0

Denny's® cont... (Oct '08)

Sides	C	F	Cb
Butter Roll, 2 pieces	260	9	38
Corn, 4 oz	110	2	23
Fit Fare, Baked Potato	220	0	51
Fries, 5 oz	460	28	46
Garlic Dinner Bread, 2 pieces	170	11	15
Mashed Potatoes, Plain, 5 oz	170	7	23
Onion Rings, 1 serving, 4 oz	380	23	38
Salads: Without Dressing or Bread			
Chicken Caesar	660	41	27
Fried Chicken Strips	440	26	26
Grilled Chicken Breast	260	11	10
Side Caesar with Dressing	360	26	20
Side Garden	115	7	6
Salad Dressings: Per 1 oz Serving			
Blue Cheese	165	18	1
Caesar	135	14	1
French	105	10	3
Honey Mustard	160	15	20
Ranch	130	14	1
Thousand Island	120	11	5
Fat-Free Italian	15	0.5	3
Condiments			
Sour Cream, 1 serving, 1.5 oz	90	9	2
Desserts			
Banana Split	895	43	121
Carrot Cake	800	45	99
Cheesecake	580	38	51
Floats, Root Beer or Cola	280	10	47
Hershey's Chocolate Cake, 5 oz	630	33	79
Hot Fudge Brownie A La Mode, 10 oz	995	42	147
Pies: Apple, 7 oz	470	21	68
ChocolateP'nut Butter, 6 oz	655	39	64
French Silk, 7 oz	735	56	58
Sundaes: Double Scoop, w/o Topping	375	27	29
Single Scoop, w/o Topping	290	16	35
Beverages			
Cappuccino, French Van., 8 fl.oz	100	3	28
Fruit Medley, 4 oz	80	0	20
Iced Tea, Raspberry, w. Ice, 16 fl.oz	80	0	21
Juice, Ruby Red Grapefruit, 10 fl.oz	160	0	41

For Complete Nutritional Data ~ see CalorieKing.com

Dippin' Dots® (Oct '08)

Flavored Ices	C	F	Cb
All flavors, ½ cup, 3 oz	90	0	23
Frozen Yogurt: All flavors, ½ cup	100	0	21
Ice Cream: Per Serving (½ Cup)			
Average all flavors	180	9	20
Fat-Free, Fudge, No Sugar Added	90	1	18
Low-Fat, Vanilla, No Sugar Added	125	6	13
Sherbet, ½ Cup	100	1	21

Donato's® Pizza (Oct '08)

Thin Crust Pizza: ¼ Large Pizza	C	F	Cb
Chicken Vegy Medley	500	20	51
Classic Trio	675	37	52
Founder's Favorite	700	38	52
Hawaiian	590	27	56
Thicker Crust Pizza: ¼ Large Pizza			
Founder's Favorite	860	42	78
Mariachi Beef	795	36	81
Mariachi Chicken	805	35	81
Pepperoni	800	39	76
Serious Cheese	800	38	77
Vegy	715	29	83
Works	845	41	81
No Dough Pizza - Individual			
Chicken Vegy Medley	495	29	20
Classic Trio	530	37	18
Founder's Favorite	560	38	18
Hawaiian	435	26	22
Margherita	590	46	16
Mariachi Beef	530	34	23
Mariachi Chicken	495	30	21
Pepperoni	500	35	17
Pepperoni Zinger	585	42	17
Serious Cheese	455	31	17
Serious Meat	655	46	19
Vegy	420	25	23
Works	545	37	21
Stromboli: 3 Meat	690	31	67
Cheese	695	31	66
Deluxe	615	25	68
Pepperoni	715	34	67
Vegy	605	24	69

For Complete Nutritional Data ~ see CalorieKing.com

Domino's® Pizza (Oct '08)

C F Cb

14" Crunchy Thin Crust: Per ⅛ Slice

	C	F	Cb
Beef	230	14	20
Cheese Only	180	9.5	20
Green Pepper, Onion & Mushroom	180	9.5	20
Ham	195	10	20
Ham & Pineapple	200	10	22
Pepperoni	230	14	20
Pepperoni & Sausage	275	18	21
Sausage	240	15	22

14" Feast Crunchy Thin Crust: Per ⅛ Slice

	C	F	Cb
America's Favorite	350	24	26
Bacon Cheeseburger	380	25	24
Barbecue	350	21	31
Deluxe	310	20	25
ExtravaganZZa	380	26	27
Hawaiian	310	18	27
MeatZZa	390	27	26
Pepperoni	360	25	25
Philly Cheese Steak	310	19	22
Vegi	300	18	26

14" Classic Hand-Tossed : Per ⅛ Slice

	C	F	Cb
Beef	280	12	34
Cheese Only	230	7.5	34
Green Pepper, Onion & Mushroom	290	9	42
Ham	245	8	34
Ham & Pineapple	310	9.5	44
Pepperoni	280	12	34
Pepperoni & Sausage	385	17	43
Sausage	290	13	36

14" Feast Classic Hand-Tossed: Per ⅛ Slice

	C	F	Cb
America's Favorite	460	23	48
Bacon Cheeseburger	490	24	46
Barbecue	460	20	53
Deluxe	420	19	47
ExtravaganZZa	490	25	49
Hawaiian	420	17	49
MeatZZa	500	26	48
Pepperoni	470	24	47
Philly Chse Steak	420	18	44
Vegi	410	17	48

14" Ultimate Deep Dish: Per ⅛ Slice

	C	F	Cb
Beef	370	19	40
Cheese Only	320	14	40
Green Pepper, Onion & Mushroom	320	14	40
Ham	335	15	40
Ham & Pineapple	340	15	42
Pepperoni	370	19	40
Pepperoni & Sausage	415	22	41
Sausage	380	20	42

Domino's® Pizza cont... (Oct '08)

C F Cb

14" Feast Ultimate Deep Dish: Per ⅛ Slice

	C	F	Cb
America's Favorite	490	28	46
Bacon Cheeseburger	520	29	44
Barbecue	490	25	51
Deluxe	450	24	45
ExtravaganZZa	520	30	47
Hawaiian	450	22	47
MeatZZa	530	31	46
Pepperoni	500	29	45
Philly Chse Steak	450	23	42
Vegi	440	22	46

Salads: Per ½ Container

	C	F	Cb
Garden Fresh, 4.2 oz	70	4	5
Grilled Chicken Caesar, 5.6 oz	100	4.5	6

Salad Dressings & Condiments: Per Package

	C	F	Cb
Blue Cheese, 1.5 oz	230	24	2
Buttermilk Ranch, 1.5 oz	220	24	2
Creamy Caesar, 1.5 oz	210	22	2
Golden Italian, 1.5 oz	220	23	2
Light Italian, 1.5 oz	20	1	2

Sauces: Per Container

	C	F	Cb
Dipping: Blue Cheese, 1.5 oz	210	22	2
Garlic, 1.8 oz	440	49	0
Hot, 1.5 oz	120	12	3
Marinara, 2 oz	25	0	5
Ranch, 1.5 oz	190	21	2

Sides

	C	F	Cb
Breadsticks: 8 sticks, 8.5 oz	880	48	88
w/o sauce, 1 stick, 1.1 oz	110	6	11
Buffalo Chicken Kickers: (2), 1.8 oz	90	3	6
w/o dipping sauce (1), 0.9 oz	45	1.5	3
Buffalo Wings			
Barbecue, 2 wings, 3.1 oz	230	14	6
Hot, 2 wings, 3 oz	210	14	5
Cheesy Bread: 8 sticks, 10.2 oz	960	48	88
w/o sce, 1 stick, 1.3 oz	120	6	11
Cinna Stix: 8 sticks, 9.3 oz	960	48	112
w/o sweet icing, 1 stick, 1.2 oz	120	6	14

Desserts

	C	F	Cb
Sweet Icing, Dipper Cup, 2.5 oz	250	3	57

For Complete Nutritional Data ~ see CalorieKing.com

Don Pablos® (Oct '08)

	C	F	Cb
Appetizers: Per Serving			
Beef Taquito (1), without garnish	65	3	5
Chicken Flauta (1), w/o garnish	65	4	6
Dips: *Without Chips*			
Queso Blanco, 6 oz cup	340	27	13
Prairie Fire Bean w. Cheese, 6 oz	380	25	23
Guacamole Dip Sampler, 2 oz	85	8	4
Nachos (1 order): Taco Beef	1625	113	85
Cheese	1320	98	48
Quesadillas: *Incl. Sour Cream & Guacamole*			
Cheese Quesadilla, small, 4 slices	810	50	52
Mesquite Grilled Chicken, 4 slices	665	32	55
Mesquite Grilled Steak, 8 slices	1560	91	122
Burritos (No Sides): Chicken	880	48	70
Beef & Bean	1390	73	123
Carnitas: Trad'l Pork with Cold Set	1240	52	137
Chimichangas: *Includes Rice & Refritos*			
Spicy Beef Chimi De Oro	1350	68	131
Chicken Chimi	1100	42	114
Relienos: *With Sauce/Cheese Topping*			
Cheese (1)	400	26	19
Chicken (1)	235	11	21
Tamales: Chicken with Sauce (1)	220	10	25
Lunch, 1 Order: Don Pablo's	755	39	54
Dos Beef Tacos (Soft)	850	37	92
Dos Chicken Enchiladas	730	35	63
El Favorito	980	52	81
Fajitas: Chicken	600	20	74
Steak	770	39	83
Mamma's Skinny Enchiladas	475	14	51
Quesadillas: Cheese	900	55	61
Mesquite-Grilled Chicken	770	39	63
Salads:			
Chicken Caesar, with Dressing	1560	118	85
Steak Caesar, with Dressing	1790	144	97
Tortilla Salad, without Dressing	550	29	59
Flour Tortilla Taco Shell	485	27	50
Salad Dressing, 3 oz: Ranch	320	34	3
Blue Cheese	450	48	3
Honey Mustard	315	27	17
Low Fat French	150	4	30
Sides: Chips & Salsa, 1 order	340	17	43
Guacamole, 1¼ oz	50	5	2
Mexican Rice, 3 oz	105	1	21
Refritos, 5 oz	260	10	31
Sour Cream, 1¼ oz	75	7	2
Flour Tortilla , 7"	125	4	20
Soup: Tortilla, 6 oz cup	130	6	13
White Chicken Chili, 6 oz cup	235	13	23

Extra Menu Items ~ see CalorieKing.com

Dunkin Donuts® (Oct '08)

	C	F	Cb
Donuts: Apple N' Spice	260	11	35
Bavarian Kreme	250	11	35
Boston Kreme	270	12	38
Chocolate Frosted; Glazed	230	11	29
Chocolate Kreme Filled	300	14	39
French Cruller	150	8	17
Gingerbread	280	4	56
Jelly Filled	270	10	38
Mini M&M	270	12	39
Old Fashioned Cake	280	18	26
Powdered Cake	310	18	34
Pumpkin Glazed	280	6	52
Strawberry Frosted	240	10	32
Sugar Raised	210	10	27
Vanilla Kreme Filled	320	16	39
Fancies: Bow Tie Donut	300	17	34
Coffee Roll, avg, all varieties	340	20	36
Eclair,	300	15	39
Fritter: Apple	290	13	35
Glazed	250	13	31
Munchkins: Plain Cake, 4	230	15	21
Glazed, avg all varieties, 4	300	15	38
Jelly Filled, 5	240	8	37
Powdered Cake, 4	260	15	29
Sugar Raised, 5	190	8	26
Bagels: Plain	320	2.5	62
Cinnamon Raisin	330	3	65
Everything; Poppyseed	370	6	67
Multigrain	410	8	67
Onion; Wheat	320	3.5	61
Reduced Carb w. Cheese	380	12	45
Salt	320	2.5	62
Sesame	380	8	64
Croissant, Plain	270	14	30
Danish: Apple	330	20	32
Cheese	340	22	30
Muffins: Banana Walnut	540	25	69
Blueberry	470	17	73
Reduced-Fat	400	5	78
Chocolate Chip	630	26	89
Coffee Cake	580	19	78
Corn	510	18	77
Cranberry Orange	440	17	66
English	160	1.5	31
Honey Bran Raisin	480	15	79
Pumpkin	560	24	82

Continued Next Page ...

Updated Nutrition Data ~ www.CalorieKing.com
Persons with Diabetes ~ See Disclaimer (Page 24)

Dunkin Donuts® cont... (Oct '08)

Breakfast	C	F	Cb
Bagel Sandwiches			
Bacon Egg & Cheese	540	18	69
Ham Egg & Cheese	510	16	65
Sausage Egg & Cheese	660	35	63
Biscuit Sandwiches			
Sausage Egg & Cheese	800	52	54
Croissant Sandwiches			
Bacon Egg & Cheese	440	25	33
Ham Egg & Cheese	460	27	31
Sausage Egg & Cheese	630	45	34
Supreme Omelet	530	33	35
English Muffin Sandwiches			
Bacon Egg & Cheese	360	16	36
Ham Egg & Cheese	310	10	34
Sausage Egg & Cheese	530	32	37
Hash Browns: 3 pieces	60	3	7
9 pieces	180	9	22
Sandwiches, Bacon Lover's Supreme	640	43	36
Oven Toasted Breakfast Sandwiches:			
Supreme Omelet & Cheese:			
on Bagel	540	18	67
on Croissant	490	30	35
on Biscuit	660	38	56
Salads: With Dressing			
Dunkin' Deli: Caesar	390	33	14
Chicken Caesar	520	36	16
Garden	240	12	24
Sandwiches & Burgers			
Dunkin' Deli Sandwiches			
Cravings: Chicken Bruschetta	580	25	48
Chipotle Chicken	620	26	49
Pastrami Supreme	760	42	47
Pressed Cuban Sandwich	730	31	64
Deli Classics: Ham & Swiss	360	11	44
Tuna (Albacore)	550	26	49
Turkey & Cheese	510	22	45
Favorites: Avocado & Turkey	500	22	49
Steak & Cheese	510	23	45
Toasted Italian	630	34	49
Smarts: Egg White, Turkey Saus.	280	6	37
Egg White, Veggie	290	9	39
Beverages			
Cappuccino, 10 fl.oz	80	4.5	7
Coolatta: Cherry Lime SoBe, 16 fl.oz	250	0	62
Coffee: w. 2% Milk, 16 fl.oz	190	2	41
w. Cream, 16 fl.oz	350	22	40
w. Milk, 16 fl.oz	210	4	42
Lemonade, 16 fl.oz	240	0	59
Vanilla Bean, 16 fl.oz	500	17	85
Hot Chocolate: Milky Way, 14 fl.oz	280	9	52
White, 1 medium, 14 fl.oz	335	13	54
Iced Coffee: 16 fl.oz	15	0	3
Pumpkin Spice, 24 fl.oz	255	8.5	41
Smoothie: Red. Calorie Berry, 16 fl.oz	250	2	49

Eat 'N Park® (Oct '08)

Breakfast	C	F	Cb
Apple Waffles	960	44	126
Strawberry Waffle	725	29	100
Cornbeef Hash, 7.5 oz	340	23	16
Egg Beaters Breakfast	75	0	5.5
Fruit Cup	60	0.5	15
Hash Browns, 6 oz	235	12	28
Homefries, 6 oz	210	12	24
Omelette: Cheese	390	30	2.5
Ham & Cheese	465	32	3
Supreme	420	30	9
Oatmeal & Fruit	425	10	68
Pancake, Plain (1)	225	3	43
Burgers: American Grill	615	37	32
Bacon Cheeseburger	590	31	33
BBQ Bacon Cheeseburger	885	55	53
Classic Gardenburger	250	6	41
Cheeseburger	520	26	33
Mushroom & Onion	705	40	46
Hamburger	475	22	32
Black Angus Superburger	1085	73	28
Original Superburger	705	50	38
Sandwiches:			
BLT	290	14	27
Buffalo Chicken	785	41	71
Chicken Chargrill/Spicy, 4 oz	350	7	39
Chicken Portabella Hoagie	845	56	47
Croissant Tuna	580	39	35
Grilled Cheese	505	36	26
Hot Turkey	260	5	27
Pot Roast Melt	970	53	66
Reuben	720	49	31
Shedded Pot Roast	530	30	28
Steak & Cheese	1010	71	38
Turkey Club	770	44	49
Turkey Pastrami	715	46	40
Appetizers: Cheese Sticks	410	25	17
Buffalo Chicken Tenders	435	21	24
Cheese Sticks	410	25	17
Chicken Quesadillas	905	55	51
Onion Rings	210	13	19

Fast - Foods & *Restaurants*

Eat 'N Park® cont... (Oct '08)

	C	F	Cb
Dinners: Baked Lemon Sole	280	17	11
Chicken Fillets (5)	530	26	28
Chicken Parmigiana: Marinara	840	33	90
Meat Sauce	900	38	86
Chicken Stir-Fry	505	22	43
Chicken Broccoli Alfredo	630	19	66
Ground Sirloin	420	26	0
Scrod Floridian, 4 oz	120	1.5	4
Spaghetti Marinara	620	8	120
Spaghetti with Meat Sauce	820	19	140
T Bone	570	39	1
Turkey	435	18	31
Salads			
Buffalo Chicken Salad	605	42	42
Chicken Portabella Salad	320	11	23
Chicken & Strawberry	215	6	13
Fajita	730	43	41
Garden Salad	95	3	16
Spinach & Chicken	375	17	9
Dressings: Bleu Cheese, 2 Tbsp	90	7	7
French Fat Free	70	0	17
Italian Fat Free	10	0	3
House, 2 Tbsp	115	11	2
Thousand Island , 2 Tbsp	95	9	3
Desserts: Cheesecake, Plain	505	36	40
Cheesecake with strawberries	750	36	105
Grilled Stickies a la Mode	730	39	81
Ice Cream, 2 scoops	285	16	33
Pies: 1 Slice, Apple (NAS)	340	10	61
Peach (NAS)	300	10	50
Cherry	455	24	58
Pecan	680	40	79

Edo Japan® (Oct '08)

Meals: Per Regular Serving	C	F	Cb
Beef Yakisoba	575	26	54
Chicken & Beef	560	17	68
Chicken Yakisoba	430	6	52
Curry Chicken	395	5	87
Ginger Pork	520	10	71
Grilled Vegetables	325	1	71
Hawaiian Chicken	500	7.5	71
Seafood Grill	495	8	73
Sukiyaki Beef	635	26	68
Teriyaki Chicken	490	7.5	68
Teriyaki Shrimp	465	6	72

Einstein Bros®/Noahs® (Oct '08)

Bagels:	C	F	Cb
Asiago Cheese	320	5	58
Blueberry Bagel	290	1.5	64
Chocolate Chip	290	3	60
Garlic Dip'd	290	2.5	60
Onion Dip'd	290	1	63
Cinnamon Sugar	310	2.5	66
Egg Bagel	300	6	52
Everything	290	2	60
Honey Whole Wheat; Onion; Plain	270	1	61
Poppy Dip'd Bagel	290	3	60
Potato Bagel	260	1	58
Power Bagel, Fruit & Nut	380	6	72
Sesame Dip'd Bagel	310	3	62
Sundried Tomato Bagel	270	1.5	58
Gourmet Bagels: Green Chile Bagel	360	8	60
Dutch Apple Bagel	350	4	71
Spinach Florentine Bagel	350	8	59
Six-Cheese Bagel	340	6	58
Breakfast Sandwiches			
Egg Way: Original	540	20	62
with Bacon ; with Sausage	610	25	63
with Black Forest Ham	580	22	62
Spinach Mushr. & Omelette	540	21	65
Bacon & Spinach Panini	860	50	67
Sausage Ranchero Panini	690	30	64
Vegetable Breakfast Panini	740	36	68
Wraps: California Chicken	630	28	63
Chipotle Turkey	730	37	70
Bagel Dogs: Without Cheese			
Original	570	25	64
Original Asiago	590	26	64
Pizza Bagels: Cheese	440	11	66
Cream Cheese: Per 2 Tablespoons			
Blueberry	70	5	6
Garlic Herb/Garden Veggie/Jalapeno	60	5	3
Honey Almond; Strawberry	70	5	6
Onion and Chive	70	6	3
Plain	70	7	1
Salmon; Sun Dried Tomato Basil	60	6	2
Salads: Bros Bistro	820	68	38
Bros Bistro with Chicken	940	71	39
Chipotle	590	38	53
Chicken Chipotle	710	41	54
Caesar Salad with Chicken	700	54	23
Coffee, Specialty: Per Regular, 12 fl.oz			
Café Latte, Regular	140	5	13
Cafe Latte, Non-Fat	100	1	14
Cappuccino, Whole Milk	150	8	13
Mocha Whole Milk	270	9	38
Espresso, Regular 2 fl.oz	1	0	0
Americano Regular 8 fl.oz	1	0	0

Updated Nutrition Data ~ www.CalorieKing.com
Persons with Diabetes ~ See Disclaimer (Page 24)

El Pollo Loco® (Oct '08)

	C	F	Cb
Burritos:			
Classic Chicken	500	14	63
Pollo Asado	600	23	58
Twice Grilled	825	37	58
Ultimate Grilled	650	20	80
Flame-Grilled Chicken: Breast	220	9	0
Leg	80	4	0
Thigh	215	15	0
Wing	90	5	0
Bowls: Caesar	520	25	46
BBQ Black Bean Pollo	535	6	86
The Original Pollo	525	4	84
Ultimate Pollo	875	26	90
Loco Favorites: Chicken Taquito	220	11	20
Nachos: Grilled Chicken	1095	56	96
Loco	310	18	31
Cheese Quesadilla	420	23	35
Chicken Verde Quesadilla	590	27	53
Taco: Al Carbon	155	5	17
Crunchy Chicken	190	8	16
Soft Chicken	270	13	19
Salads: Caesar Pollo	530	40	18
Chicken Tostada	780	37	73
Garden Salad Small	125	7	10
Loco with Creamy Cilantro Dressing	170	14	8
Salad Dressings: Per Packet			
Creamy Cilantro	220	23	2
Light Creamy Cilantro	70	5	6
Light Italian	20	1	2
Ranch	230	24	2
Thousand Island	220	21	6
Condiments			
Guacamole, 1 oz	45	3	4
Jack & Poblano Queso, 1.8 oz	100	8	4
Salsa: Avocado, Hot, 1 oz	30	2	2
Chipotle, Hot, 1 oz	7	0	1
House, Mild, 1 oz	7	0	1
Pico de Gallo. 1 oz	11	0	2
Sides			
Corn Cobbette, 5 oz	90	1	19
French Fries, 5½ oz	440	21	55
Fresh Vegetables, 4 oz	35	0	8
Macaroni & Cheese, 5½ oz	275	17	28
Mashed Potatoes with Gravy, 6 oz	105	1	22
Pinto Beans, 6 oz	140	0	24
Refried Beans with Cheese, 6.3 oz	265	7	36
Spanish Rice, 4½ oz	160	1	35
Desserts: Caramel Flan, 5½ oz	305	12	46
Churros (2)	415	25	43

For Complete Nutritional Data ~ see CalorieKing.com

Fatburger® (Oct '08)

	C	F	Cb
Burgers: Baby Fat	300	15	24
Sausage & Egg Sandwich	620	44	33
Chicken Sandwich	360	13	32
Hot Dog	380	22	31
Fatburger	520	29	32
Fatburger with American Cheese	590	35	32
Kingburger	820	41	64
Kingburger w. Cheese	890	47	64
Turkey Burger	550	31	38
Shakes (17 fl.oz): Chocolate	880	38	103
Strawberry	700	32	91
Vanilla	730	30	103
Fries & Sides: Chili Cup, 7.6 oz	270	15	13
Fat Fries, 8 oz	550	26	72
Skinny Fries, 5.5 oz	490	20	71
Onion Rings, 5.5 oz	520	29	57

For Complete Nutritional Data ~ see CalorieKing.com

Fazoli's® Italian Food (Oct '08)

	C	F	Cb
Pasta Bowl: Per Serving			
Classic Ziti w. Meat Sauce, regular	700	23	91
Classic Ziti w. Meat Sauce, small	480	16	63
Ravioli with Marinara Sauce	500	15	71
Ravioli with Meat Sauce	570	21	70
Spaghetti with Marinara Sauce	670	4	132
Sampler Platter: Per Serving			
Classic Sampler Platter	810	25	108
Ultimate Sampler Platter	990	31	132
Oven-Baked Pasta: Per Serving			
Baked Chicken Parmesan	1110	56	100
Baked Spaghetti	680	22	90
Baked Spaghetti with Meatballs	940	40	100
Meat Lasagne	520	26	42
Rigatoni Romano	1090	54	101
Paninis: Four Cheese & Tomato	510	22	53
Grilled Chicken	480	14	55
Smoked Turkey	550	24	55
Pizzas: Per Slice			
Cheese, 4 oz	270	11	31
Pepperoni, 4.3 oz	310	14	31

Continued next page...

Fast - Foods & Restaurants

Fazoli's® cont... (Oct '08)

Submarinos (7")	C	F	Cb
Club	730	34	65
Ham n' Swiss	680	30	65
Original	940	58	68
Salads: Dressing Not Included			
Caesar Side Salad	40	2	4
Chicken & Fruit Salad	220	15	28
Chicken & Pasta Caesar Salad	440	15	41
Chicken BLT Ranch	270	10	13
Garden Side Salad	25	0	4
Parmesan Chicken	360	15	31
Pasta Side Salad	320	12	41
Salad Dressing: Italian Dressing	160	14	7
Fat Free Honey Mustard	60	0	15
Caesar Dressing	230	25	1
Honey French	220	18	14
Ranch Dressing	220	24	2
Lite Ranch Dressing	120	12	2

For Complete Nutritional Data ~ see CalorieKing.com

Fox's Pizza Den® (Oct '08)

12" Pizzas: Per Slice (⅛ Pizza)	C	F	Cb
Cheese	155	5	21
Pepperoni	180	7	21
16" Pizzas: Per Slice (¹⁄₁₀ pizza)			
Cheese	220	7	30
Pepperoni	250	9	30

Firehouse Subs® (Oct '08)

Subs: Per Medium	C	F	Cb
Chicken Salad	760	46	63
Engine Company	390	6	52
Engineer	380	5	55
Ham	410	7	58
Hero	430	7	54
Hook & Ladder	410	7	68
Italian	560	25	55
NY Steamer	410	12	48
Roast Beef	410	6	48
Tuna Salad	610	28	62
Turkey	370	4	58
Veggie	300	5	56

Five Guys (Oct '08)

Burgers	C	F	Cb
Cheeseburger	1110	70	52
Hamburger	970	58	51
Little Cheeseburger	760	45	52
Little Hamburger	690	39	51
Bacon Cheeseburger	1190	77	52
Bacon Burger	1050	65	51
Little Bacon Cheeseburger	680	51	51
Little Bacon Burger	770	46	51
Dogs			
Hot Dog	585	35	51
Cheese Dog	655	41	52
Bacon Dog	665	42	51
Bacon Cheese Dog	735	48	52
Five Guys Fries: Regular 8½ oz	620	30	78
½ Regular Order	310	15	39

Freshens® (Oct '08)

Frozen Yogurt: Per Serving	C	F	Cb
Soft Serve Yogurt, 1 oz	35	0.5	7
Smoothies: 100% Juice (21 fl.oz)			
Acai Energy Smoothie	320	3	72
All That Razz	360	0	79
Berry Breeze	305	0	77
Caribbean Craze	290	0	73
High Test Energizer	300	0	74
Jamaican Jammer	355	0	78
Mango Beach	90	0	48
Maui Mango	290	0	74
Mystic Mango	355	3	82
Orange: Shooter	335	3	77
Sunrise	355	3	81
Orange Passion	135	3	35
Peach: Passion	150	0	32
Sunset	270	0	67
Peachy Pineapple	335	0	73
Peanut Butter Energizer	475	10	83
Pineapple Paradise	330	4	77
Raspberry Royale	270	0	67
Strawberry: Oasis	90	0	49
Shooter	245	0	64
Squeeze	315	0	68
Sunrise	155	0	35
Invigorate: Per 4 oz Muffin			
Banana Nut Muffin	440	22	53
Blueberry Cranberry Muffin	460	22	68
Fudge Brownie, 3½ oz	380	17	48

Updated Nutrition Data ~ www.CalorieKing.com
Persons with Diabetes ~ See Disclaimer (Page 24)

Frisch's Big Boy® (Oct '08)

	C	F	Cb
***Breakfast,* HealthSmart, Egg Beaters:**			
Plain Omelette	310	8.5	38
Scrambled	310	8.5	38
Vegetarian Omelette	340	8.5	45
Health Smart Meals: Tossed Salad	45	0.5	6
Grilled Chicken Breast	325	10	22
Lemon Baked Cod	490	4.5	72
Spaghetti Marinara	420	6.5	76
Vegetable Stir-Fry	610	3.5	134
Sandwiches: Big Boy	600	26	35
Brawny Lad	420	21	30
Buddie Boy	760	34	80
Fish Sandwich	690	48	41
Small Hamburger	445	30	30
Super Big Boy	830	66	35
Swiss Miss	635	44	28
Sides: Chili	315	18	19
French Fries	360	19	45
Onion Rings	580	41	45
Tartar Sauce	370	40	1
Trio Salad	620	46	18
Soups: HealthSmart Cabbage Soup	50	0.5	9
Beverages: HealthSmart Shake	160	0	33

Gold Star Chili® (Oct '08)

	C	F	Cb
Meals			
Bowls: Low Carb Coney, 10.4 oz	570	47	7
Veggie Chili, 9 oz	160	2	29
Coney	285	14	30
Cheese Coney, 5.6 oz	345	18	31
Chili, 8 oz	215	12	8
Chili Cheese Nachos, 8½ oz	410	25	30
Chili Cheese Sandwich	290	12	30
Chili Sandwich	210	5	32
Regular 2-Way	420	11	58
Bean	490	12	71
Onion	435	11	62
Onion Bean	505	12	75
Regular 3-Way	650	30	59
Regular 4-Way	665	30	63
Regular 5-Way	735	30	76
Super 5-Way	1140	51	109
Tex Mex, 8 oz	210	9	17
Sides: Fries, 5 oz	365	19	44
Garlic Bread: Without Cheese, 2 oz	215	13	19
w. Cheese, 2½ oz	270	18	19

Gino's East® (Oct '08)

	C	F	Cb
***Deep Dish Pizza:** Medium 11" ~ Per Slice (⅙ Pizza)*			
Cheese	410	11	58
Crumbled Sausage	420	21	38
Pepperoni	450	15	57
Spinach	410	11	59
***Deep Dish Pizza:** Small 6" ~ Per Whole Pizza*			
Cheese	720	16	116
Crumbled Sausage	800	22	116
Pepperoni	780	20	116

Golden Corral® (Oct '08)

	C	F	Cb
Meals			
Bourbon Street Chicken, 3.5 oz	210	11	5
Cajun Whitefish, 3 oz	110	7	0
Fish Fillet Cajun Style, 2 pces	210	10	18
Fresh Fried Chkn, Leg or Thigh (1)	250	19	2
Meatloaf, 3.5 oz	190	10	10
Sirloin Steak, Buffet, 3 oz	220	13	0
Steakburgers, Lunch, 6 oz	860	55	0
Turkey Breast w. Wing, 2 oz	70	3	1
Sides: Baked Potato, plain (1)	110	0	25
Glazed Sesame Carrots	260	16	27
Macaroni Salad, ½ cup	190	8	26

Godfather's™ Pizza (Oct '08)

	C	F	Cb
***Golden Pizza:** Per Slice*			
Cheese: Medium, ⅛ pizza	220	8	25
Large, ⅒ pizza	250	9	28
Combo: Medium, 1/8 pizza	290	13	27
Large, slice, ⅒ pizza	330	15	30
Original Pizza			
Cheese: Mini, ¼ pizza	150	4	20
Medium, ⅛ pizza	260	7	34
Jumbo, 1/12 pizza	350	10	44
Combo: Mini, ¼ pizza	200	8	21
Medium, ⅛ pizza	350	14	36
Jumbo, 1/12 pizza	480	20	47
Thin Pizza			
Cheese: Medium, ⅛ pizza	170	8	15
Large, ⅒ pizza	210	10	17
Combo: Medium, ⅛ pizza	240	13	17
Large, ⅒ pizza	280	16	20
Sides			
Breadstick (1)	80	2	14
Cheesestick, 1 piece, ⅙ whole	130	3.5	18
Choc. Chip Cookie, slice , ⅙ whole	195	8	30
Potato Wedges, 4 oz	190	9	24

(The) Great American Bagel Co® (Oct '08)

Bagels:	C	F	Cb
4-Grain Honey	390	4	80
Apple Cinnamon Oat Bran	370	4	73
Apple Cinnamon Sugar	390	4	78
Apple Crumb	620	11	118
Asiago	520	16	72
Banana Nut	410	9	69
Blueberry	370	3.5	75
Cheddar Bacon	600	23	71
Chocolate Chip	420	8	78
Cinnamon Delight	640	18	108
French Toast	430	8	77
Jalapeno Cheddar	370	7	63
Onion	380	4	74
Plain; Pumpernickel; Salt	360	4	71
Strawberry	380	3.5	76
Stuffed Pepperoni	570	17	78
Stuffed Spinach	640	20	86
Sun-Dried Tomato Basil	390	4	74
Tomazzo	520	13	77
Veggie	310	3.5	61

Green Burrito (Oct '08)

Burritos:	C	F	Cb
Bean & Cheese	830	38	99
Grilled Chicken	1080	54	91
Meat Bean & Cheese: Chicken	660	28	67
Ground Beef	760	39	69
Steak	690	30	70
The Green Burrito w. Steak	950	35	122
Specialties:			
Enchiladas w. Cheese (2)	430	28	30
Super Nachos: Chicken; Steak	945	48	99
Ground Beef	1070	60	100
Taco Salad: Chicken	820	44	73
Ground Beef	940	57	75
Steak	850	47	76
Taquitos: Chicken, 2 taquitos	150	7	16
Chicken, 5 taquitos	350	15	39
Tacos: Fish, 6 oz	300	12	36
Hard: Chicken; Steak	210	11	15
Ground Beef	250	15	15
Soft: Chicken	210	7	18
Ground Beef	260	13	19
Sides: Chips, 2 oz	300	15	37
Chips & Cheese, 5 oz	690	40	65
Guacamole, 1.4 oz	45	4	3
Make Any Entree a Plate			
Pinto Beans & Cheese	320	16	43
Rice, 5 oz	340	10	58
Sour Cream, 1.4 oz	50	3.5	3

(The) Great Steak & Potato Company® (Oct '08)

Breakfast Sandwiches	C	F	Cb
Bacon, Egg & Cheese	605	36	39
Potatoes, Deluxe Home	285	17	33
Potatoes, Fresh Cut Home	275	17	31
Egg and Cheese	510	29	39
Ham and Cheese	570	31	42
Ham, Egg and Cheese	570	31	42
Sausage, Egg and Cheese	705	48	39
Steak, Egg & Cheese	600	33	41
Sandwiches			
Chicken Philly	940	53	63
Chicken Teriyaki	960	53	66
Ham Delight	930	55	72
Ham Explosion	930	55	71
Reuben	850	48	64
Super Steak	970	58	65
Turkey Philly	890	52	65
Veggie Delight	830	53	67
Sides			
Fried Onion Petals, 3 oz	190	11	22
Chicken Nuggets, Kids, 2.8 oz	165	9	10
Fries: Kids, 6.5 oz	290	14	38
Small, 12 oz	545	28	69
Regular, 14 oz	670	37	80
Large, 28.5 oz	1250	60	165
Potato Skins, 7 oz	440	30	26
Baked Potato, Plain, 6 oz	160	0	36
Meat: Per 4 oz Serving, No Sides			
Chicken	140	3	0
Gyro	205	12	5
Ham	120	4	6
Salami	145	11	1
Steak	160	7	0
Turkey	91	1	2
Salads: Without Dressing			
Chef Salad	245	11	13
Garden	37	0	8
Grilled Steak	395	25	13
Sauces: Cheese, 2 oz	80	5	0
Buffalo 1 oz	10	0	2
Teriyaki , 1 oz	25	0	3
Tzatziki, 1 oz	46	4	2
Breads/Pita			
Bread, 12"White, 7 oz	420	4	82
Bread, 7"Wheat, 4 oz	310	4	56
Pita, 3 oz	165	1	33

Haagen-Dazs® (Oct '08)

Ice Cream: Per ½ Cup

	C	F	Cb
Baileys Irish Cream	260	17	21
Banana Split	280	16	31
Black Walnut	300	22	21
Butter Pecan	310	23	21
Caramelized Pear & Toasted Pecan	270	15	30
Cherry Vanilla	240	15	23
Chocolate	270	18	22
Chocolate Chip Cookie Dough	310	20	29
Chocolate Chocolate Chip	300	20	26
Coffee	270	18	21
Cookies & Cream	270	17	23
Dulce de Leche	290	17	28
Green Tea	250	17	20
Mango	250	14	28
Pineapple Coconut	230	13	25
Pistachio	290	20	22

Extra Flavors ~ See CalorieKing.com

	C	F	Cb
Light Ice Cream: Dutch Chocolate	190	5	29
Light: Caramel Cone	250	8	39
Coffee	210	7	32
Dulce de Leche	220	7	33
Dutch Chocolate	190	5	33
Mint Chip	230	8	34
Vanilla Bean	200	7	29
Sorbet: Chocolate, Low-Fat	130	0.5	28
Coconut	170	7	26
Fat-Free: Orchard Peach	130	0	31
Raspberry/Strawberry	120	0	31
Zesty Lemon	110	0	28
Tropical	150	0	38

Frozen Yogurt: Per ½ Cup

	C	F	Cb
Chocolate Fudge Brownie	200	2.5	35
Vanilla Honey & Granola	200	4	32
Wildberry	180	2	34
Low-Fat: Coffee/Vanilla	200	4.5	31
Dulce de Leche	190	2.5	35
Vanilla Raspberry Swirl	170	2.5	32

Ice Cream Bars ~ See Page 111

Hardee's® (Oct '08)

Breakfast

	C	F	Cb
Big Country Platter: Bacon	980	56	90
Chicken	1140	61	105
Country Steak	1150	68	98
Biscuit: Egg	450	29	35
Bacon, Egg & Cheese	560	38	37
Country Ham	440	26	36
Breakfast Sandwiches: Frisco	420	20	37
Smoked Sausage	710	54	30
Loaded Breakfast Burrito	780	51	38
Loaded Omelet	640	44	37
Low Carb Breakfast Bowl	620	50	6
Sunrise Croissants with Ham	430	26	28

Hardee's® cont... (Oct '08)

Burgers:

	C	F	Cb
Cheeseburger ⅓ lb	680	39	52
Double Cheeseburger ¼ lb	510	26	38
Hamburger	310	12	36
Double Hamburger ¼ lb	420	19	37
Six Dollar Burger ½ lb	1060	73	58
Thickburger: Original, ⅓ lb	910	64	53
Double Thickburger ⅔ lb	1250	90	54
Grilled Sourdough ½ lb	1030	77	42
Double Bacon Cheese	1300	97	50
Monster ⅔ lb	1420	108	46
Double Bacon Cheese ⅔ lb	910	64	50
Low-Carb ⅓ lb	420	32	5
Mushroom 'N' Swiss ⅓ lb	720	42	48
Hot Dog	420	30	22

Sandwiches:

	C	F	Cb
Chicken: Spicy Chicken	470	21	46
Buffalo Chicken	780	36	74
Charbroiled BBQ Chicken	415	5	58
Charbroiled Chicken Club	550	30	35
Big Chicken Fillet	800	37	76
Fish Supreme	540	36	33
Hot Ham 'N' Cheese	420	18	39
Big Hot Ham 'N' Cheese	520	24	40
Big Roast Beef	470	23	38
Regular Roast Beef	330	16	29
Kids Meals: Cheeseburger w. Kids Fries	600	27	68
Hamburger w. Kids Fries	560	24	67
2 Chicken Strips w. Kids Fries	500	25	50
Fried Chicken: Breast portion	370	15	29
Leg portion	170	7	15
Thigh portion	330	15	30
Wing portion	200	8	23
Chicken Strips: 3 Strips, 5 oz	380	20	27
5 Strips, 8.5 oz	630	34	45
Sides: Chili Cheese Fries	850	48	76
Coleslaw, Small, 4 oz	170	10	20
Crispy Curls, 3.8 oz	340	16	43
medium, 4.7 oz	415	20	52
Mashed Potato & Gravy, small	90	2	17
French Fries: Kids 2.8 oz	205	9	28
Small, 4.2 oz	325	14	45
Medium, 5.7 oz	435	19	60
Large, 6.2 oz	470	21	65
Desserts: Apple Turnover	290	15	36
Chocolate Chip Cookie	290	11	44
Malts: Average all flavors, 16 fl.oz	780	35	97
Shakes: Average all flavors, 16 fl.oz	700	34	85

Harvey's® (Oct '08)

Sandwiches & Burgers	C	F	Cb
Angus Burger	390	17	34
Angus Burger w. Cheese	440	21	35
Angus Patty, 1 patty	215	15	3
Cheeseburger	440	23	35
Hamburger	380	18	35
Grilled Chicken Sandwich	340	6	32
VeggieBurger	315	9	39
Hot Dog	320	14	34
Patties: Original, 1 patty	210	16	4
Chicken, 1 patty	170	4	1
Veggie Burger, 1 patty	150	7	7
Sides			
Chicken Strips, 3 pieces	310	16	24
French Fries: Large, 5.3 oz	400	17	58
Regular, 4.2 oz	320	14	47
Value, 3.1 oz	240	10	35
Gravy, 3.2 oz	35	1	5
Onion Rings: Large, 4.3 oz	420	21	52
Regular, 2.8 oz	280	14	35
Poutine, 10 oz	640	33	67
Salads: Dressing Not Included			
Garden Salad	40	0	8
Entree: Chicken Salad	140	1.5	16
Garden Salad	70	0.5	16
Salad Dressings			
Creamy Caesar	140	14	2
Creamy Garlic Peppercorn Ranch	140	14	2
Fat-Free Honey Dijon	50	0	12
Light Italian	60	4	6
Sauces			
Barbecue Sauce	50	0	12
Ketchup	10	0	2
Light Mayonnaise, ½ oz	45	5	1
Spicy Buffalo, 1 oz	50	3.5	5
Dipping: Barbecue	90	0	21
Honey Mustard	160	12	13
Plum	125	0	31
Sweet n' Sour	80	0.5	17
Breakfast: Bacon, 3 Strips	40	2	0
Extra Egg (1)	90	6	0
Homefries	300	19	29
Sandwich: Breakfast Club	440	22	33
Breakfast Club Deluxe	480	24	33
Sausage (1)	130	9	3
Toast: White, 2 slices	180	2	35
Whole Wheat, 2 slices	170	2	32

Hogi Yogi® (Oct '08)

Frozen Yogurt: Per ½ Cup	C	F	Cb
Chocolate Base, 2.5 oz	80	0	17
Vanilla (No Sugar Added): Base, 2.6 oz	100	0	22
Regular Sandwiches: Club	340	5	47
BBQ Chicken	360	4.5	59
Roast Beef	300	4.5	46
Smokey Turkey	320	3	46
Turkey	290	3	57
Vegetarian	240	2.5	45
Smoothies: Per 24 oz			
Berry Blast	310	0	70
Fruit Safari	370	3.5	84
Jungle Mist	430	4	101
Peach Treat	430	0	105
Pina Collision	450	4.5	105
Pure Passion	430	4	99
Ragin Raspberry	370	3.5	84
Strawberry Kist	420	0.5	98

Hot Dog on a Stick® (Oct '08)

Menu Items	C	F	Cb
Hot Dog on a Bun	470	26	41
Hot Dog on a Stick	250	14	23
Veggie Dog	180	3	24
American Cheese on a Stick	240	13	22
Pepper Jack Cheese on a Stick	240	13	21
French Fries, 7 oz	700	37	83
Lemonade (12 fl.oz): Original	140	0	34
Cherry/Lime	165	0	40
Sugar Free Lemonade	10	0	2

Hot Stuff Pizza® (Oct '07)

	C	F	Cb
Pizza: Per Slice (⅛ Medium or ¹⁄₁₀ Large)			
Beef	320	12	34
Canadian Bacon	320	11	25
Cheese	350	12	25
Double Pepperoni	390	18	37
Garden Style	300	11	34
Italian Sausage	340	15	37
Masterpiece Supreme	330	14	34
Pepperoni	350	14	37
Pork Sausage	340	15	33
Western Omelet	320	15	30

Hungry Howie's Pizza® (Oct '08)

Pizzas: Per Slice	C	F	Cb
Cheese: Small, ⅙ pizza	160	3.5	20
Medium, ⅛ pizza	190	5.5	23
Large, ⅒ pizza	210	5	25
X-Large, ⅛ pizza	395	9.5	42
Oven Baked Subs : Pizza, ½ sub	690	34	67
Deluxe Italian, ½ sub	505	18	61
Sides: Chicken Tenders, 2 pieces	140	4.5	11
Howie Wings, 5 wings	180	13	0
Toppings:			
Anchovies	55	3	0
Bacon	30	0.5	0.4
Banana Peppers	6	0	1.1
Beef	30	2	0.5
Pepperoni; Sausage	25	1.5	0
Black Olives; Green Olives	5	0	0.5
Green Peppers; Mushroom	0	0	0.5
Ham	5	0.5	0
Onions	5	1	0.5
Pineapple	5	0.5	1.5

I Can't Believe It's Yogurt® (Oct '08)

	C	F	Cb
Original Frozen Yogurt: Per Serving (4 oz)			
Chocolate; Vanilla	140	8	17
Strawberry	150	7	19
Low-Fat Frozen Yogurt: Per Bar (5.5 oz)			
Chocolate	120	2.5	23
Smoothies: Per Serving (8.5 oz)			
Ana-Bana-Berry	80	0	21
Mighty Berry	130	0.5	30
Raspberry Rush	110	0.5	26
Strawbapple; Strawberry Skinny	60	0	16
Strawberry Banana	130	0.5	30

In-N-Out Burger® (Oct '08)

Burgers: Hamburger w. Onion	390	19	39
with Mustard/Ketchup	310	10	41
Protein Style, no Bun	240	17	11
Cheeseburger with Onion	480	27	39
with Mustard/Ketchup	400	18	41
Protein Style, no Bun	330	25	11
Double Double®	670	41	39
with Mustard/Ketchup	590	32	41
Protein Style, no Bun	520	39	11
French Fries, 4.4 oz	400	18	54
Drinks: Milk, 10 fl.oz	180	6	18
Coca-Cola®, 16 fl.oz			
Lemonade, 16 fl.oz	180	0	40
Root Beer, 16 fl.oz	220	0	54
Shakes, Strawb., Choc. 15 fl.oz	690	36	83

For Complete Nutritional Data ~ see CalorieKing.com

IHOP® (Oct '08) *(Author Estimates)*

Pancakes: (Syrup/Butter extra)	C	F	Cb
Buttermilk (1), 1.7 oz	110	3	17
Short Stack, 3	330	9	51
Full Stack, 5	550	15	85
Harvest Grain 'N Nut: (1) 2¼ oz	180	9	20
Combo	1035	65	80
Crepe-Style, 2 oz	120	6	14
IHOP For Me: Pancake Trio (3), 5.1 oz	330	9	51
w. Marg. & ¼ c. sugar-free syrup	470	20	63
Syrup: Regular, 1 Tbsp	50	0	12
Sugar-Free, 1 Tbsp	10	0	3
Whipped Butter/Margarine, 1 T.	80	9	0
Waffles (Plain): Regular (1), 3 oz	310	15	37
Belgian, Regular (1), 4 oz	390	19	48
Breakfast: Per Serving			
Classic Combos: Cntry Fried Steak/Eggs	1530	105	73
Signature: Rooty Tooty Fresh & Fruity, average all flavors	855	45	84
T-Bone Steak & Eggs	1310	86	63
Omelette Feast			
Colorado Omelette: No pancakes	790	68	5
with 3 buttermilk pancakes	1205	83	66
The Big Steak Omelette: No pancakes	910	72	14
with 3 buttermilk pancakes	1325	87	75
Burgers & Sandwiches			
BBQ Bacon Cheeseburger w. Fries	1510	87	131
Chicken Clubhouse Stacker w. Fries	1710	98	132
Ham & Egg Melt w. Onion Rings	1350	70	121
Patty Melt w. Fries	1480	72	145
Entrees: Old Fashioned Pot Roast	765	48	30
with Mashed Potatoes	965	53	65
Grilled Cod Hollandaise, w. sides	1335	97	66
Top Sirloin Steak, w. topping & sides	1775	121	95
Salad: Clubhouse Spinach w. Chkn	1450	115	53

Jack's® (Oct '08)

Sandwiches: Big Bacon Burger	700	42	45
Big Jack Burger	500	27	40
Cheeseburger	380	17	35
Chicken Fillet Sandwich	640	31	69
Double Big Jack Cheese Burger	930	60	43
Double Cheeseburger	590	33	37
Grilled Chicken Sandwich	410	15	44
Hamburger	270	8	35
Chicken Fingers, 3 pieces	470	24	33
Egg & Cheese Biscuit	550	34	35
Fries, regular	250	9	38

Additional Listings ~ see CalorieKing.com

Jack in the Box® (Oct '08)

Breakfast	C	F	Cb
Biscuit: Bacon, Egg & Cheese	430	25	34
Sausage	440	29	32
Sausage, Egg & Cheese	740	55	35
Spicy Chicken	460	22	44
Breakfast Jack: Regular	290	12	29
w. Sausage	450	28	29
Croissant: Sausage	580	39	37
Supreme	450	25	36
Sandwiches: Sourdough	420	24	21
Ultimate	570	27	49
Extreme Sausage Sandwich	670	48	31
Hash Brown Sticks (5)	230	16	20
Meaty Burrito	610	36	39
Sandwiches & Burgers			
Bacon Ultimate Cheeseburger	1090	77	53
Junior Bacon Cheeseburger	430	23	30
Ultimate Cheeseburger	1010	71	53
Hamburger	280	12	30
Hamburger w. Cheese	330	15	31
Deluxe Hamburger: No Cheese	370	21	31
w. Cheese	440	25	34
Jumbo Jack: Regular	600	35	51
w. Cheese	690	42	54
Sirloin Steak Melt	880	51	63
Sourdough Jack	710	51	36
Chicken & Fish			
Bacon Chicken Sandwich	440	24	39
Chicken Breast Strips (4)	500	25	36
Chicken Fajita Pita, no salsa	300	9	33
Chicken Sandwich	400	21	38
Ciabatta: Grilled Chicken Chipotle	690	28	65
Spicy Crispy Chicken	750	34	75
Fish & Chips, medium, 8.8 oz	660	34	70
Jack's Spicy Chicken Sandwich	620	31	61
w. Cheese	700	37	62
Sourdough Grilled Chicken Club	530	28	34
Tacos & Snacks			
Bacon Cheddar Potato Wedges	720	48	52
Beef Taco (1), regular	160	8	15
Egg Rolls (3)	400	19	44
Monster Beef Taco (1)	240	14	20
Stuffed Jalapenos (3)	225	13	22

Jack in the Box® cont... (Oct '08)

Fries & Rings	C	F	Cb
Natural Cut Fries: Medium, 5.9 oz	450	23	54
Kids portion, 2.8 oz	220	11	3
Seasoned Curly Fries, med., 4.4 oz	400	23	45
Onion Rings (8), 4.2 oz	500	30	51
Salads: No Dressing or Condiments			
Asian Chicken	160	1.5	18
Chicken Club	320	16	12
Side Salad	50	3	5
Southwest Chicken	310	12	28
Sauces & Dressings			
Dipping Sauce: Barbecue, 1 oz	45	0	11
Buttermilk House, 1 oz	130	13	3
Frank's Red Hot Buffalo, 1 oz	10	0	2
Sweet & Sour, 1 oz	45	0	11
Tartar, 1½ oz	210	22	2
Sauce: Mayo-Onion, ½ oz	90	10	1
Soy, 0.3 oz	5	0	1
Taco, 0.3 oz	0	0	0
Cheese: American, 1 slice	45	3.5	1
Swiss, 1 slice	40	3	1
Provolone, 1 slice	70	6	0
Condiments			
Ketchup	10	0	2
Mustard	5	0	1
Salsa	5	0	1
Sour Cream	60	5	2
Desserts			
Cheesecake, 3.6 oz	310	16	34
Chocolate Overload Cake, 3.3 oz	300	8	57
Ice Cream Shakes: Per Regular, 16 fl.oz			
Chocolate Ice Cream	750	36	95
Oreo Cookie Ice Cream	760	40	87
Strawberry Ice Cream	730	35	90
Vanilla Ice Cream	650	35	70

For Complete Nutritional Data ~ see CalorieKing.com

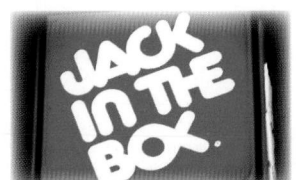

Jamba Juice® (Oct '08)

Juices: Per Original, 24 fl.oz	C	F	Cb
Carrot	200	1	45
Fit n' Fruitful	370	3.5	84
Pomegranate Heart Defender	440	1	103
Orange	330	1.5	77
Boosts:			
3G Charger Super Boost 3grams	5	0	2
Omega-3 Super Boost 10 grams	30	1.5	7
Green Caffeine Boost 2.7 grams	5	0	2
Shots:			
Matcha Green Tea: with Orange Jce	60	0	13
with Soymilk	80	0	16
Wheatgrass, 1 fl.oz	5	0	1
Yogurt Blend: Blueberry	350	1	70
Sunrise Strawberry	380	1	78
Smoothies: Per Original, 24 fl.oz			
Aloha Pineapple	470	1.5	111
Banana Berry	450	1.5	106
Caribbean Passion	420	2	97
Citrus Squeeze	440	2	104
Coldbuster	410	2.5	95
Mango A Go-Go	470	2	110
Mega Mango	340	1	85
Orange A Peel	400	1	93
Orange Dream Machine	490	2	107
Peach Perfection	320	0.5	78
Peach Pleasure	440	2	104
Peanut Butter Moo'd	840	21	139
Pomegranate Paradise	340	1	86
Strawberry Surf Rider	490	1.5	119
Protein Berry Workout w/whey	390	1	80
Razzmatazz	440	2	102
Strawberry Whirl	310	0.5	76
Strawberries Wild	400	0.5	94
Energy: Acai Super-Antioxidant	420	6	86
Matcha Green Tea Blast	440	0.5	97
Razz 'n Tea	320	0	74
Tahiti Green Tea	390	1.5	92
Light Smoothies:			
Berry Fulfilling	260	1	57
Mango Mantra	280	1	64
Strawberry Nirvana	250	0.5	55
Pretzels: Apple Cinnamon	380	4	76
Sourdough Parmesan	410	10	67
Cookies/Cake: Blueberry Oatcake	280	10	42
Omega 3 Oatmeal Cookie	150	6	26
Zucchini Walnut Loaf	270	9	43

Jimmy John's® (Oct '08)

Subs (8")	C	F	Cb
Figures Based on French Bread			
#1 Pepe	685	38	55
#2 Big John	565	27	54
#3 Totally Tuna	505	20	58
#4 Turkey Tom	555	26	54
#5 Vito	580	25	57
#6 Vegetarian	640	36	58
JJBLT	660	36	54
Giant Club Sandwiches			
Figures Based on French Bread			
#7 Gourmet Smoked Ham	850	40	76
#8 Billy	865	40	77
#9 Italian Night	975	53	77
#10 Hunter's	855	39	76
#11 Country	840	38	76
#12 Beach	795	37	78
#13 Gourmet Veggie	855	46	78
#14 Bootlegger	720	28	74
#15 Club Tuna	720	30	77
#16 Club Lulu	790	35	74
Plain Slims: Figures Based on French Bread			
Slim 1 Ham & Cheese	540	12	72
Slim 2 Roast Beef	420	1.5	71
Slim 3 Tuna Salad	575	19	72
Slim 4 Turkey Breast	405	0.5	70
Slim 5 Salami Capicola & Cheese	625	21	72
Slim 6 Double Provolone	590	20	72
The J.J. Gargantuan	1010	55	60
Low Carb Options:			
Hunter's Club Unwich	520	39	9
The JJ Gargantuan Unwich	770	55	11
Low-Fat Options:			
#4 Turkey Tom	555	26	54
Slim 4 Turkey Breast	405	1	70
Sides			
Jimmy Chips: BBQ, 1 oz	160	9	17
Jalapeno, 1 oz	150	7	18
Regular, 1 oz	160	8	18
Sea Salt & Vinegar, 1 oz	140	8	16
Pickle: Spear	5	0	1
Whole	15	0	3
Cookies, average	420	16	65

Johnny Rockets® (Oct '08)

Original Hamburgers	C	F	Cb
Hamburger #12	880	57	58
Original Burger	725	46	52
Chili Size	1255	84	67
Patty Melt	785	48	48
Rocket Double	1190	79	58
Rocket Single	830	52	57
Route 66	910	63	53
Smoke House	970	60	60
St Louis	1160	80	62
Streamliner	430	11	61
Turkey Single	730	42	56
Sandwiches: Chicken Club	1070	39	126
Grilled Breast of Chicken	630	33	52
Grilled Cheese	540	30	40
Grilled Ham & Cheese	515	24	40
Philly Cheese Steak	715	30	58
Tuna Melt	755	45	40
Tuna Salad	710	46	41
Other Favourites			
Chicken Club Salad:			
with Chicken Tenders	670	40	37
Chili Dog	815	55	46
Hot Dog	420	24	38
Extras: Bacon, 0.7 oz	100	7	0
Chili, 1 serving, 2.5 oz	170	15	3
Extra Patty, 3.1 oz	270	20	1
Grilled Mushrooms, or Onions	20	2	1
Starters			
Chili Bowl, 13 oz	870	69	24
American Fries, 8 oz	530	23	77
Cheese Fries, 10 oz	760	42	78
Chili Fries, 12 oz	710	40	76
Onion Rings, 6.8 oz	500	34	42
Rocket Wings, regular order	270	10	17
Desserts: Apple Pie	930	59	88
A la mode, scoop, 4 oz	260	16	26
Hot Fudge Sundae	830	47	93
Beverages: (Medium): Root Beer	170	0	49
Coke	170	0	28
Sprite	170	0	45
Lemonade	170	0	49
Float	420	26	42
Shakes: Chocolate, 20 oz	1100	60	120
Vanilla, 20 oz	1120	60	131
Extra for Malt	60	2	10

Kenny Rogers Roasters® (Oct '08)

Chicken	C	F	Cb
½ Chicken: w/o Skin or Wing	315	10	1
with Skin	515	28	2
¼ Dark Meat: w/o Skin	170	7	1
with Skin	270	17	1
¼ White Mea: w/o Skin or Wing	145	2	1
with Skin, serving	245	11	1
Grilled Breast Platter	990	52	100
Pies: Chicken Pot Pie	710	33	78
Pita, Roasted Chicken	690	35	42
Turkey: Sliced Breast	160	2	0
Salads: Without Dressing			
Chicken Caesar	285	9	18
Roasted Chicken	290	10	19
Sandwiches: Grilled Chicken	525	29	32
Turkey	385	12	30
Side Dishes: Corn Cob	70	0.5	14
Corn Muffin	165	6	25
Sweet Corn Niblets	115	0.5	28
Honey Baked Beans	150	1	32
Italian Green Beans	115	8	10
Macaroni & Cheese	200	6	24
Potatoes: Baked Sweet	265	0	62
Garlic Parsley	260	12	37
Real Mashed	295	14	39
Rice Pilaf	175	5	43
Steamed Vegetables	50	0	8
Soup: Chicken Noodle, 1 bowl	90	2	12

KFC® (Oct '08)

Original Recipe	C	F	Cb
Breast: 1 piece, 5.5 oz	350	20	7
w/o skin or breading	140	2	1
Drumstick, 1 piece, 1.85oz	110	7	2
Thigh, 1 piece, 3.75oz	280	20	7
Whole Wing, 1 piece	120	7	4
Chicken Strips			
Extra Crispy: Breast, 1 pce, 6 oz	460	28	16
Drumstick, 1 piece, 2 oz	150	9	6
Thigh, 1 piece, 3.9 oz	360	27	12
Whole Wing, 1 piece, 1.75 oz	160	10	6
Chicken Strips:			
Crispy, 2 Strips	250	13	13
3 Strips	370	19	19
Original, 3 Strips	280	14	10
Popcorn Chicken: Kids, 3 oz	290	19	16
Individual, 4 oz	400	25	22
Large, 5.6 oz	550	35	30

Updated Nutrition Data ~ www.CalorieKing.com
Persons with Diabetes ~ See Disclaimer (Page 24)

KFC® cont... (Oct '08)

Sandwiches	C	F	Cb
Double Crunch			
with Original Recipe Strip	440	22	35
with Crispy Strip	500	26	41
Crispy Twister:			
with Original Recipe Strip	520	25	48
with Crispy Strip	580	29	54
Filet Sandwich, Original Recipe	330	22	13
Oven Roasted Twister	440	18	42
Tender Roast Sandwich	390	15	30
Toasted Wraps:			
with Original Recipe Strip	330	17	27
with Crispy Strip	360	19	30
with Tender Roast Filet	310	14	24
KFC Snackers: With Crispy Strip			
Regular	300	13	30
Buffalo	260	9	32
Honey BBQ, no skin	210	3	31
Untimate Cheese	280	10	31
Twisters: Crispy	520	25	48
Oven Roasted with Sauce	440	18	42
Chicken Pot Pie	690	40	57
Wings: Fiery Buffalo (1)	80	5	4
Honey BBQ (1)	80	5	5
Teriyaki (1)	100	5	5
Hot Wings: Regular (1)	70	5	3
Fiery Buffalo (1)	80	5	5
Honey BBQ (1)	100	5	9
Sweet & Spicy (1)	80	5	6
Teriyaki (1)	100	5	9
Dipping Sauces: Fiery Buffalo, 1 oz	25	0	6
Creamy Ranch, 1 oz	140	15	1
Garlic Parmesan, 1 oz	130	13	2
Honey BBQ, 1 oz	40	0	9
Honey Mustard, 1 oz	120	10	6
Sweet & Sour, 1 oz	45	0	12
Sides: Per Single Portion			
Baked Beans, 4.6 oz	200	1.5	39
Biscuit, 2 oz	180	9	21
Cole Slaw, 4.6 oz	180	10	22
Corn on the Cob (3"), 3 oz	70	0.5	16
Macaroni & Cheese, 4.8 oz	180	8	18
Mashed Potatoes with Gravy, 5.4 oz	120	4	19
Potato Wedges, 3.6 oz	260	13	33

KFC® cont... (Oct '08)

KFC Famous Bowls	C	F	Cb
Mashed Potato with Gravy, 9 oz	680	32	74
Rice w. Gravy, 1 reg. bowl, 18 oz	800	28	108
Salads: Without Dressing or Croutons			
Crispy Chicken BLT	340	18	19
Crispy Chicken Caesar	320	17	17
House Side Salad	15	0	2
Roasted Chicken BLT	200	7	7
Roasted Chicken Caesar	190	6	5
Dressings:			
Original Ranch: 2 oz	200	20	3
Fat Free, 1½ oz	35	0	8
Creamy Parmesan Caesar, 2 oz	260	26	4
Golden Italian Light, 1½ oz	45	2.5	6
Original Ranch: 2 oz	200	20	3
Croutons, Parm. Garlic, Pouch (1)	70	3	8
Desserts:			
Apple Pie, Mini's, 3 pies	390	21	46
Double Chocolate Chip Cake, 1 pce	280	9	47
Lil' Buckets: Chocolate Cream, 4 oz	280	14	37
Lemon Creme, 4.5 oz	390	14	60

Koo♦Koo♦Roo® (Oct '08)

Rotisserie Chicken	C	F	Cb
Leg & Thigh, 4.8 oz	300	18	1
Breast & Wing, 6.5 oz	355	16	1
Half Rotisserie Chicken, 11.3 oz	655	34	2
Original Skinless Flame Broiled Chicken™			
3 Piece Original Dark, 5 oz	320	16	5
Original Breast, 4.1 oz	190	5.5	0
Roasted Turkey: Breast, sliced, 4 oz	180	8	0
Hand-Carved Turkey Sandwich	600	32	31
Traditional Turkey Dinner	690	29	67
Turkey Pot Pie	885	44	83
Salads: Per Regular (No Dressing)			
BBQ Chicken Salad	365	14	22
Chicken Caesar Salad	285	11	12
Chinese Chicken Salad	550	28	39
Koo Koo Roo House Salad	115	4	16

For Extra Menu Items ~ see CalorieKing.com

Kilwin's® ~ *see CalorieKing.com*

Kohr Bros® ~ *see CalorieKing.com*

Kolache® ~ *see CalorieKing.com*

Krispy Kreme® (Oct '08)

Doughnuts	C	F	Cb
Apple Fritter	380	20	47
Caramel Kreme Crunch	380	19	49
Chocolate Iced Glazed Cruller	290	15	37
Chocolate Iced Cake	280	14	36
Chocolate Iced Custard Filled	300	17	35
Chocolate Iced Glazed	250	12	33
Chocolate Iced Kreme Filled	350	20	39
Chocolate Iced with Sprinkles	270	12	38
Cinnamon Apple Filled	290	16	32
Cinnamon Bun	260	16	28
Cinnamon Twist	240	15	23
Dulce de Leche	300	18	30
Glazed: Chocolate Cake	300	15	42
Cinnamon	210	12	24
Cruller	240	14	26
Kreme Filled	340	20	39
Lemon Filled	290	16	35
Maple Iced	240	12	32
Original	200	12	22
Raspberry Filled	300	16	39
Sour Cream	300	13	43
New York Cheesecake	340	20	34
Powdered: Cake	290	14	37
Strawberry Filled	290	16	33
Sugar Doughnut	200	12	21
Traditional Cake Doughnut	230	13	25
Doughnut Holes: Orig. Glazed (5)	200	11	25
Glazed Cake, Regular/Choc. (4)	210	10	29
Chiller Beverages: No Cream Topping			
Fruity Chillers:			
Average all flavors,12 fl.oz	170	0	43
20 fl.oz	295	0	71
Kremic Chillers: Includes Whipped Cream Topping			
Orange & Kreme: 12 fl.oz	630	28	92
20 fl.oz	970	40	150
Lemon Sherbert: 12 fl.oz	630	28	95
20 fl.oz	980	40	155
Choc./Mocha: Avg. 12 fl.oz	670	29	104
Latte, 12 fl oz	670	28	49
Choc/Mocha: Avg., 20 fl.oz	1050	41	171
Latte, 20 fl.oz	1050	40	79

For Complete Nutritional Data ~ see CalorieKing.com

Krystal® (Oct '08)

Burgers/Sandwiches	C	F	Cb
B.A. Burger	470	27	39
w. Cheese	530	32	40
BA Double Bacon Burger	800	53	41
Krystal Burger	160	7	17
Krystal Chik	240	11	24
Bacon Cheese Krystal	190	10	16
Cheese Krystal	180	9	17
Double Krystal	260	13	24
Double Cheese Krystal	310	16	26
Chili Cheese Pup	210	12	17
Corn Pup	260	19	19
Plain Pup	170	9	15
Sampler Combo: Krystal, Chik, Pup, Fries + 16 fl.oz drink	1330	54	170
French Fries			
Regular, 4.2 oz	470	20	53
Chili Cheese Fries, 7.3 oz	540	28	59
Sides			
Krystal Chili	200	7	22
Chik'n Bites, Small, 4 oz	310	19	16
Chik'n Bites & Salad	290	20	12
Kryspers	190	13	17
Breakfast Items			
Krystal Sunriser Sandwich	240	14	14
Biscuit: Bacon, Egg & Cheese	390	23	33
Chik Biscuit	360	15	40
Plain Biscuit	270	13	33
Sausage Biscuit	480	33	33
Biscuit & Gravy	280	14	34
Country Breakfast	660	42	46
Scrambler, 11 oz	440	26	33
4-Carb Scrambler: Bacon	370	29	4
Sausage	600	51	3
Desserts: Apple Turnover, fried	220	10	31
Lemon Icebox Pie	260	9	41
Drinks: Per 16 fl.oz with ¼ ice			
Coca-Cola Classic	130	0	40
Diet Coke	0	0	0
Sprite	125	0	39

For Complete Nutritional Data ~ see CalorieKing.com

La Rosa's Pizzeria® (Oct '08)

	C	F	Cb
Focaccia Style: Per Slice, 1/10 of Medium Pizza			
Florentine	240	13	24
Roma	300	18	23
Hand Tossed: Per Slice			
Deluxe Topper	290	12	29
Buddy Topper	310	14	29
Cheese	230	8	29
Meat Topper	320	15	29
Pepperoni Topper	300	14	29
Veggie Topper	320	16	32
Pan Crust: Per Slice			
Buddy Topper	310	14	29
Cheese	300	16	30
Deluxe Topper	370	21	31
Pepperoni Topper	370	22	30
Stuffed Pizza: Per Slice			
Cheese	340	14	40
Meat	790	53	44
Traditional Crust: Per Slice			
Buddy Topper	275	15	20
Cheese	200	10	19
Deluxe Topper	270	16	20
Meat Topper	300	18	20
Pepperoni Topper	280	16	20
Calzones: Per Calzone, No Dipping Sauce			
3 Meat & 3 Cheese	1080	55	102
3 Veggie & 3 Cheese	860	34	105
Cheese & Pepperoni	960	45	101
Cheese	840	34	101
Philly Cheese Steak	870	39	90
Sausage Pelucci	1040	52	92
Pasta Dinner: No Sides			
Cheese Ravioli	660	26	80
Chicken Strips w. Traditional Sauce	285	10	21
Lasagna w. Meat Sauce	735	38	61
Link Sausage w. Traditional Sauce	415	26	21
Spaghetti: & Meatballs	870	28	119
with Alfredo Sauce	975	50	104
with Meat Sauce,	700	18	104
with Traditional Sauce	640	12	113
Appetizers			
Chicken Tender	540	31	30
Four Taste Sampler	1570	99	82
French Fry Basket w. Provolone	860	56	73
Mozzarella Cheese Sticks	635	43	36
Onion Twists, Regular, no Sauce	460	27	48
Wings: Special Recipe (12)	1260	87	21
Spicy Hot (12)	1245	85	26

For Complete Nutritional Data ~ see CalorieKing.com

La Salsa Fresh Mexican Grill® (Oct '08)

	C	F	Cb
Burritos: Black Beans w. Cheese	590	19	82
with Carnitas	695	22	82
with Chicken	730	23	89
Pinto Beans with Cheese	570	18	77
with Chicken	700	22	84
with Steak	675	24	77
Baja Fish Burrito	875	53	58
California Burrito	815	35	89
Overstuffed Grilled Burrito			
with Chicken	1260	59	110
with Carnitas	1200	59	108
with Steak	1290	66	109
Three Pepper Fajita: with Carnitas	780	35	79
with Chicken	780	34	81
with Steak	785	37	79
with Shrimp	940	34	80
Nachos: Includes Cheese, Salsa, Sauce & Sour Cream			
Black Beans with Carnitas	1570	83	141
with Chicken	1600	83	148
with Steak	1580	84	142
Pinto Beans with Carnitas	1560	83	139
with Chicken	1590	83	146
with Steak	1565	84	139
Guacamole, Salsa and Chips	970	55	103
Tacos: Baja Fish	395	22	29
Baja Shrimp	320	19	30
Carnitas Guadalajara	320	15	30
Quesadillas: With Chips unless indicated			
Classic: with Carnitas	1160	68	82
with Chicken	1155	67	83
with Steak	1165	69	82
Grande: with Carnitas	1335	71	116
with Chicken	1330	70	117
with Steak	1345	72	116
Stuffed Fajitas: *Without Chips*			
with Carnitas	855	51	53
with Chicken	865	52	56
with Steak	885	55	53
with Shrimp	800	49	54
Fire Roasted Bowl			
Black Beans: with Chicken	730	32	74
with Steak	735	34	73
w/o meat	630	29	71
Pinto Beans with Chicken	730	32	73
with Steak	720	34	70
w/o meat	620	29	69

Little Caesar® (Oct '08)

14" Pizza: Per Slice, 1/8 Pizza

	C	F	Cb
3 Meat Treat	350	18	20
Ultimate Supreme	310	14	31
Vegetarian	220	9	27
Deep Dish:			
Just Cheese	320	13	38
Pepperoni	360	16	38
Hot-N-Ready: Cheese Only	240	9	30
Pepperoni	280	11	39
Hula Hawaiian: with Ham	270	9	33
with Canadian Bacon	280	9	34
Baby Pan! Pan!, Single	360	18	33
Caesar Wings: Barbecue, 1 wing	70	4	3
Mild/Hot, 1 wing	60	4.5	1
Oven, Roastd, 1 wing	50	3.5	0
Caesar Dips: Per 1.5 oz Container			
Buffalo	140	14	4
Buffalo Ranch	230	24	3
Buttery Garlic	380	42	0
Cheezy	210	21	3
Chipotle	220	24	2
Ranch	250	26	3
Bread: Per Piece			
Crazy Bread, 1 stick	100	3	15
Crazy Sauce, 4 oz	45	0	10
Italian Cheese Bread	130	7	13
Pepperoni Cheese Bread	140	7	14
Churros, 1 stick, 1.5 oz	150	4	25
Churros Sauces, avg.	90	3	16

Lone Star Steakhouse® (Oct '08)

Starters

	C	F	Cb
Amarillo Chse Fries, 1/4 order, 8 oz	660	38	89
Chicken Tenders	1090	66	91
Lone Star Wings	950	62	15
Spinach Artichoke Dip	490	40	13
Texas Rose	1260	38	108
Texas Rose Sauce	155	17	1
Tostado Tortilla Chips	390	22	46
Steaks: Cajun Ribeye	820	52	6
Chopped Steak	710	52	0
Five Star Filet, 6 oz	335	18	2
Garlic Medallion & Shrimp	370	11	0
Lunch Steak, plain	390	27	1
NY Strip Steak	525	28	0
Sirloin Steak & Lobster	335	8	10
Texas Ribeye	700	40	6

Lone Star® cont... (Oct '08)

Seafood

	C	F	Cb
Fried Shrimp (5)	290	15	30
Grilled Shrimp (5)	190	7	17
Lobster Tail, grilled	85	0.5	8
Mesquite Grilled Shrimp: Dinner	230	8	17
Entree	310	18	0
Sweet Bourbon Salmon	240	11	0
Mesquite-Grilled Specialties: Sides not included			
Baby Back Ribs	400	26	5
Bubba (BBQ) Chicken Breast	165	1.5	5
Grilled Chicken	170	4	0
Grilled Pork Chop	320	16	0
Mesquite Grilled Shrimp Dinner	230	8	17
Superstar Combo	645	29	5
Burgers & Sandwiches			
Bubba Chicken Sandwich	170	2	5
Lone Star Cheeseburger	900	45	50
Steak Sandwich	640	22	55
Swiss & Mushroom Burger	845	38	52
Salads: Cobb	685	37	23
Chicken Caesar Salad	480	24	19
El Paso Salad	350	19	25
Steakhouse Salad	710	53	2
Dressings: Bleu Cheese	95	9	2
Catalina Dressing	90	5	9
Creamy Caesar Dressing	100	9	3
Honey Mustard Dressing	145	14	5
Lemon Butter	230	25	0
Ranch Dressing	110	11	2
Steakhouse Dressing	70	6.5	2
Texas Ranch Dressing	105	11	28
Thousand Island Dressing	65	4	5
Whipped Honey Butter	315	30	11
Sides & Partners:			
Baked Potato, plain	230	0.5	50
Chili: Cup, 4 oz	140	7	5
Bowl, 10 oz	345	18	14
Garlic Lovers Medallions & Shrimp	370	11	0
Sauteed Mushrooms	140	9	11
Sauteed Mushrooms & Onions	140	7	15
Sauteed Onions	85	2.5	14
Steak Fries, 8oz	610	26	86
Sweet Potato, plain	330	0.5	76
Soups: Steak Soup, Bowl, 10 oz	65	7	11
Chicken Pot Pie, Bowl, 10 oz	50	5	12

Long John Silver's® (Oct '08)

Sandwiches & Burgers	C	F	Cb
Chicken, 4.8 oz	360	15	40
Fish, 6.2 oz	470	23	48
Ultimate Fish, 7 oz	530	28	49
Seafood			
Alaskan Flounder, 1 piece, 3.7 oz	250	11	26
Baked Cod, 1 piece, 3.6 oz	120	4.5	1
Battered Fish, 1 piece, 3.2 oz	260	16	17
Battered Shrimp, 1 piece, 0.5 oz	45	3	3
Breaded Clams, 1 snack box, 3 oz	320	19	29
Buttered Lobster Bites, 1.8 oz	125	4.5	14
1 snack box, 3.5 oz	250	9	27
1 platter portion, 3.5 oz	250	9	27
Clam Strips, 3 oz	240	13	22
Lobster Stuffed Crab Cake, 2.2 oz	170	9	16
Popcorn Shrimp, 1 snack box, 2.9 oz	270	16	23
Chicken			
Chicken Plank, 1 piece, 1.8 oz	140	8	9
Salads: Without Dressing			
Crispy Chicken Club, 13.8 oz	510	30	35
Shrimp & Seafood, 12.6 oz	260	12	22
Salad Dressings & Condiments: Per 1.5 oz Pouch			
Garden Ranch	230	24	2
Lite Italian	20	1	3
Thousand Island	220	21	7
Fat-Free French	50	0	12
Sides			
Cheesesticks, 1 stick, 0.5 oz	45	2.5	4
Clam Chowder, 1 bowl, 8.6 oz	170	8	19
Cole Slaw, 4 oz	200	15	15
Corn Cobbette w/o butter, 3.4 oz	90	3	14
Crumblies, 1 oz	170	12	14
Fries: Regular, 3 oz	235	10	34
Large, 5 oz	390	17	56
Hushpuppies, 1 pup, 0.8 oz	60	2.5	9
Rice, 4 oz	180	3.5	34
Veggie Bites:			
Broccoli Cheese, 5 pieces, 3.1 oz	220	12	23
Jalapeno Cheddar, 5 pces, 3.1 oz	250	14	24
Dipping Sauces: Per 1 oz			
Cocktail	25	0	6
Tartar	100	9	4

For Complete Nutritional Data ~ see CalorieKing.com

Macaroni Grill (Oct '08)

Appetizers	C	F	Cb
Calamari Fritti	1210	78	66
Crab Stuffed Mushrooms	750	38	71
Parmesan Crusted Artichokes	820	62	40
Peasant Bread	520	11	89
Romano's Sampler, 3 Choices	1640	98	62
Tomato Bruschetta	1000	70	75
Meals			
Amore De Le Grill: *Includes Sides*			
Chianti Steak	1200	62	78
Chicken Sorrentino	1050	46	85
Grilled Salmon Teriyaki	1090	52	84
Honey Balsamic Chicken	1190	59	94
Classico Italian: *Dinner Size*			
Chicken Scaloppine	1110	71	68
Eggplant Parmesan	1240	64	118
Mama's Trio	1770	98	116
Parmesan Crusted Sole	2170	134	148
Primo Chicken Parmesan	2220	148	126
Veal Marsala	1320	66	132
Pastas			
Carmela's Chicken Rigatoni	1320	87	84
Classico Italian			
Fettuccine Alfredo with Shrimp	1320	95	70
Spaghetti & Meat Sauce	1110	63	87
Spaghetti & Meatballs w. Sauce	2430	128	207
Over Stuffed: Chicken Cannelloni	870	44	57
Lobster Ravioli	1090	78	55
Marsala Chicken Ravioli	1300	85	55
Pizzas: Per Pizza			
Brick Oven: Crowd Pleasers	840	24	114
Pesto Chicken	1940	101	163
Sicilian	1450	70	124
Salads: Without Dressing			
Chicken Florentine	540	20	56
Insalata Blu with Chicken	570	38	9
Parmesan Crusted Chicken	1060	49	59
Seared Sea Scallops	1050	68	22
Salad Dressings & Condiments: Per 1 fl.oz			
Parmesan Peppercorn Ranch	90	9	1
Roasted Garlic Lemon Vinaigrette	170	17	4
Low-Fat Caesar	30	2	4
Soups: Per 8 fl.oz Cup			
Chicken Toscana	260	16	18
Italian Sausage & Tomato	190	7	22
Dessert			
Dessert Ravioli	1630	74	223

For Complete Nutritional Data ~ see CalorieKing.co

McDonald's® (Oct '08)

Burgers/Sandwiches	C	F	Cb
Big Mac	540	29	45
Big N' Tasty	460	24	37
Big N' Tasty w. Cheese	510	28	38
Cheeseburger	300	12	33
Double Cheeseburger	440	23	34
Filet-O-Fish	380	18	38
Hamburger	250	9	31
McChicken	360	16	40
McRib	500	26	44
Quarter Pounder:	410	19	37
with Cheese	510	26	40
Double with Cheese	740	42	40
Premium Chicken Sandwiches:			
Crispy Chicken Classic	530	20	59
Crispy Chicken Club	630	28	60
Crispy Chicken Ranch BLT	580	23	61
Grilled Chicken Classic	420	10	51
Grilled Chicken Club	530	17	61
Grilled Chicken Ranch BLT	470	12	53
Snack Wraps:			
Chipotle BBQ: w. Grilled Chicken	260	9	28
with Crispy Chicken	330	15	35
Honey Mustard: w. Grilled Chicken	260	9	27
with Crispy Chicken	330	16	34
Ranch: with Grilled Chicken	270	10	26
with Crispy Chicken	340	17	33

Extra Value Meals	C	F	Cb
Large Fries & Large Soda, add	810	25	149

French Fries: (Fried in partially hydrogenated vegetable oil)

	C	F	Cb
Small, 2.5 oz	230	11	29
Medium, 4.1 oz	380	19	48
Large, 5.4 oz	500	25	63
Ketchup, 1 pkg	15	0	3

French Fries: (Fried in Canola Oil Blend ~ Zero Trans Fat)
(In New York City/Philadelphia ~ More locations during 2009)

	C	F	Cb
Small, 2.6 oz	230	11	29
Medium, 4 oz	360	18	45
Large, 6 oz	530	26	67

Chicken McNuggets®/Sauces	C	F	Cb
Chicken McNuggets: 4 pieces	190	12	11
6 pieces	280	17	25
10 pieces	460	29	27
Sauces: Barbecue, 1 oz pkg	50	0	12
Honey, ½ oz pkg	50	0	12
Hot Mustard, 1 oz pkg	60	2.5	9
Sweet 'N Sour, 1 oz pkg	50	0	12

McDonald's® cont... (Oct '08)

Chicken Selects® Breast Strips	C	F	Cb
Strips: 3 pieces	400	24	38
5 pieces	660	40	39
Sauces (1.5 oz pkg): Creamy Ranch	200	22	2
Spicy Buffalo	70	7	1
Tangy Honey Mustard	70	2.5	13
Chipotle Barbecue	70	0	18

Breakfast Menu	C	F	Cb
Biscuit: Regular	260	12	33
Large	320	16	39
Bacon Egg & Cheese, large	520	30	43
Bacon Egg & Cheese, regular	420	24	27
Sausage with Egg, large	570	37	42
Sausage with Egg, regular	510	33	36
Breakfast Steak	120	8	0
Big Breakfast, regular	740	48	51
Deluxe Breakfast, regular	1090	56	111
English Muffin	160	3	27
Grape/Strawberry Jam	35	0	9
Hash Browns (1)	150	9	15
Hotcakes: Plain (3)	350	9	60
w. Margarine (2 pats), no Syrup	430	18	60
w. Margarine (2 pats) & Syrup (1)	610	18	105
McGriddles: Bacon, Egg & Chse	420	19	48
Sausage	420	22	44
Sausage, Egg & Cheese	560	32	48
McMuffin: Egg	300	12	30
Sausage	370	22	29
Sausage with Egg	450	27	30
McSkillet: Burrito with Sausage	610	36	44
Burrito with Steak	570	270	44
Sausage, 1.4 oz patty	170	15	1
Sausage Breakfast Burrito	300	16	26
Scrambled Eggs (2)	170	11	1

Breakfast Value Meal (Extras)	C	F	Cb
Hash Browns & Coffee (black/no sugar,) add	150	9	15
Hash Browns & Orange Juice, add	290	9	48

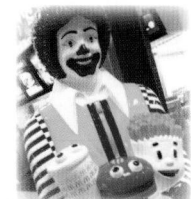

Updated Nutrition Data ~ www.CalorieKing.com
Persons with Diabetes ~ See Disclaimer (Page 24)

McDonald's® cont... (Oct '08)

Salads: Without Dressing

	C	F	Cb
Asian Salad: with Crispy Chicken	410	20	31
with Grilled Chicken	300	10	23
Bacon Ranch Salad: No Chicken	140	7	10
with Crispy Chicken	370	20	20
with Grilled Chicken	260	9	12
Caesar Salad: No Chicken	90	4	9
with Crispy Chicken	330	17	20
with Grilled Chicken	220	6	12
Southwest Salad: w. Crispy Chicken	430	20	38
with Grilled Chicken	320	9	30
Fruit & Walnut, Snack Size, 1 pkg	210	8	31
Side Salad	20	0	4
Butter Garlic Croutons, ½ oz	60	1.5	10

Salad Dressings: Per Package

Newman's Own: Ranch, 2 oz	170	15	9
Creamy Caesar, 2 oz	190	18	4
Creamy Southwest, 1.5 oz	100	6	11
Low-Fat: Balsamic Vinaigrette	40	3	4
Family Recipe Italian	60	2.5	8
Sesame Ginger Dressing	90	2.5	15

Desserts/Cookies

Apple Dippers with Caramel Dip	105	0.5	23
Apple Dippers, 1 pkg. 2.4 oz	35	0	8
Caramel Dip, 0.7 oz	70	0.5	15
Baked Apple Pie, 2.7oz	250	13	32
Cinnamon Melts, 4 oz	460	19	66
Cookies: Oatmeal Raisin (1), 1.1 oz	150	6	22
Sugar Cookie (1), 1.1 oz	150	6	21
McDonaldland® Cookies: 2 oz	250	8	42
Chocolate Chip Cookies, 2 oz	270	11	39
Fruit 'n Yogurt Parfait: Regular	160	2	31
without Granola	130	2	25
Ice Cream: Kiddie Cone, 1 oz	45	1	8
Vanilla Reduced Fat Cone, 3.2 oz	150	3.5	24
Van. Red'd-Fat Ice Cream only, 3 oz	130	3.5	20
McFlurry™: M&M®, 12 fl.oz cup	620	20	96
Oreo®, 12 fl.oz cup	550	17	88
Sundaes: Hot Caramel Sundae	340	8	60
Hot Fudge Sundae	330	10	54
Strawberry Sundae	280	6	49
Peanuts (for Sundaes)	45	3.5	2

Triple Thick Shakes: Average all Flavors:

12 fl.oz cup	430	10	75
16 fl.oz cup	565	13	100
21 fl.oz cup	720	18	132
32 fl.oz cup	1125	26	200

McDonald's® cont... (Oct '08)

Drinks:

	C	F	Cb
1% Low Fat Milk, 8 fl.oz	100	2.5	12
1% Chocolate Milk, 8 fl.oz ctn	170	3	26
Coffee (black), 16 fl.oz	0	0	0
Half & Half Creamer, 1 pkg	20	2	0
Sugar Packet (1), 4 g	15	0	4
Apple Juice, 6.8 fl.oz box	90	0	23

Cappuccino: *Per 12 fl.oz*

Caramel	240	6	41
French Vanilla	240	6	42
Hazelnut	240	6	42

Coca-Cola or Sprite (No Ice):

Child, 12 fl.oz cup	110	0	29
Small, 16 fl.oz cup	150	0	43
Medium, 21 fl.oz cup	210	0	58
Large, 32 fl.oz cup	310	0	86
Diet Coke	0	0	0

Hi-C Orange Lavaburst (No Ice):

Child, 12 fl.oz cup	120	0	32
Small, 16 fl.oz cup	160	0	44
Medium, 21 fl.oz cup	240	0	64
Large, 32 fl.oz cup	350	0	94

Iced Coffee, average all flavors:

Small, 16 fl.oz	130	5	21
Medium, 24 fl.oz	190	8	29
Large, 32 fl.oz	270	11	45
Iced Tea	0	0	0

Orange Juice: Small, 12 fl.oz

Small, 12 fl.oz	140	0	33
Medium, 16 fl.oz	180	0	42
Large, 21 fl.oz	250	0	57

Powerade Mountain Blast:

Child, 12 fl.oz	70	0	20
Small, 16 fl.oz	100	0	27
Medium, 21 fl.oz	150	0	39
Large, 32 fl.oz	220	0	58
Hot Chocolate, 12 fl.oz	380	15	53

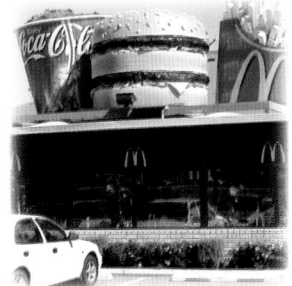

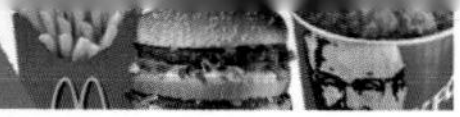

Manhattan Bagel® (Oct '08)

Bagel (East Coast): Per Bagel (4 oz)	C	F	Cb
Blueberry; Cheddar Cheese	320	1.5	68
Chocolate Chip	330	3	67
Cinnamon Raisin	330	1	70
Egg, 4 oz	320	2	67
Jalapeno Cheddar; Marble Rye	320	1.5	67
Plain, 4 oz	320	1	68
Pumpernickel; Rye	320	1.5	69
Spinach	320	1	67
Sundried Tomato; Whole Wheat	310	1	66
Cream Cheese: Reduced-Fat, 1.75 oz	150	12	5

For Complete Nutritional Data ~ see CalorieKing.com

Max & Erma's® (Jan '07)

Appetizers	C	F	Cb
Black Bean Roll-Ups	575	10	95
Entrees: Blue Cheese NY Strip	1340	107	9
Caribbean Chicken (lunch)	535	20	60
Salads: No Breadstick			
Hula Bowl with Dressing	575	7	79
Half Hula Bowl with Dressing	365	4	57
Baby Greens Salad, no dressing	120	11	6
Shrimp Stack Salad with dressing	320	12	33
Sandwiches & Hamburgers			
Burger Stack with Broccoli	1105	81	6.5
Chicken Stack with Broccoli	825	51	6.5
Sides			
Buttered Broccoli, 3.5 oz	105	9	4.5
Fruit Salad, 4.5 oz	55	0	16
Garlic Breadstick (1)	155	6	21
Hearty Beef Chili Soup	390	15	39
Fruit Smoothie	125	0.5	28
Dressings: Per 2 Tablespoons (1 fl.oz)			
Bleu Cheese	200	21	0.5
Italian	110	12	1
Ranch	120	12	0.5
Fat Free: French	125	0	31
Honey Mustard	60	0	14
Low-Fat Tex Mex Dressing	25	0	2.5

For Complete Nutritional Data ~ see CalorieKing.com

Mazzio's® (Oct '08)

Appetizers: Per Serving	C	F	Cb
Breadsticks, no sauce, ¼ order	150	3	26
Breadsticks, ¼ order	150	3	26
Cheese Dippers, ⅓ order	405	18	47
Cinnamon Sticks, ¼ order	625	36	70
BBQ Chicken Wings, ⅕ order	190	12	7
Nachos: Beef w. Jalapenos, ½ order	485	34	20
Cheddar with Jalapenos, ½ order	425	30	19
Calzones: Per 1/10 Whole			
Ham Bacon & Cheddar, no Sauce	245	7.5	32
Pepperoni	260	10	32
Pastas: Without Garlic Toast			
Fettuccine Alfredo	1060	56	106
Spaghetti with Marinara Sauce	640	8	120
Lasagna: with Meat Sauce	950	52	64
with Marinara Sauce	705	30	73
with Alfredo Sauce	1265	94	55
Sandwiches			
Focaccia: Chicken, Bacon & Swiss	1020	70	49
Ham & Cheddar	745	47	47
Mazzio's Sub	770	50	45
Turkey & Swiss	720	38	46
Tuscan Smash	645	34	45
Hoagie: Chicken, Bacon & Swiss	1360	73	120
Ham & Cheddar	1090	50	119
Mazzio's Sub	1110	52	117
Turkey & Swiss	1060	41	118
Tuscan Smash	985	36	117
Pizzas: Per ⅛ Medium, 12" Pizza			
Cheese: Original Crust	235	9	30
Thin Crust	180	9	18
Chicken Club: Original Crust	260	9	31
Thin Crust	205	9	19
Mazzio's Works: Original Crust	310	14	31
Thin Crust	255	14	20
Meatbuster: Original Crust	285	13	30
Thin Crust	235	13	19
Mexican: Original Crust	315	14	35
Thin Crust	260	14	23
Pepperoni: Original Crust	255	11	30
Thin Crust	200	11	18
Sausage: Original Crust	275	12	30
Thin Crust	225	12	19
Supremebuster: Original Crust	260	10	31
Thin Crust	205	11	19
Veggie: Original Crust	230	8	31
Thin Crust	180	8	19
Sides: Garlic Toast, 1 pce, 1.4 oz	160	10	15
Kosher Pickle Spear, 1 oz	5	0	1
Potato Chips, 1 oz	150	10	15

For Complete Nutritional Data ~ see CalorieKing.com

Updated Nutrition Data ~ www.CalorieKing.com
Persons with Diabetes ~ See Disclaimer (Page 24)

Mimi's Cafe® (Oct '08)

Breakfast	C	F	Cb
Hot off the Griddle, French Toast	305	13	40
Hot off the Griddle, Pancakes	955	35	139
Three Egg Omelette w. Sides, Low-Fat	480	5	69
Two Egg Breakfast w. Sides	385	25	26
Carb Conscious Specialties			
Mimi's Breakfast	680	22	21
Chicken & Vegetable Platter	765	42	24
Fresh Salmon w. Steamed Veggies	460	28	8
Half Pound Cheeseburger in Lettuce	730	41	13
Mediterranean Omelette w. Tomato	545	35	25
Petite Chopped Cobb Salad, no Dr.	605	51	13
Top Sirloin Steak w. Steamed Veg.	580	27	7
Two "AA" Large Eggs w. Tom./Saus.	415	32	5
Sandwiches			
Classic Beef Dip	520	15	43
Fresh Roasted Turkey Breast: Reg.	530	27	28
Low-Fat, ½ sandwich	335	9	42
Ham & Cheddar Grill	1210	77	74

For Complete Nutritional Data ~ see CalorieKing.com

Miami Subs® (Oct '07)

Burgers	C	F	Cb
Deluxe Burger	785	59	31
Deluxe Cheeseburger	860	65	32
Deluxe Bacon Cheeseburger	920	69	32
Platters: Chicken Breast	745	41	57
Gyros	1420	93	81
10 Wings w. Fries & Blue Cheese	1020	67	50
Salads: Caesar w. Dressing	460	34	26
Chicken Caesar w. Dressing	610	39	28
Chicken Club	490	25	23
Garden	310	18	21
Greek	285	15	24
Side Greek w. Dressing	80	5	4
Cheesesteaks (6"): Original	410	11	45
Classic	420	11	47
Chicken Philly Classic	550	27	46
Works	530	22	51
Pitas: Gyros	660	39	46
Chicken	390	13	33
Subs (6"): Ham & Cheese	450	18	79
Italian Deli	515	24	49
Meatball	490	22	49
Tuna	470	18	44
Turkey	485	18	51
Sides: Mozzarella Sticks	755	56	34
Onion Rings	870	68	55
Spicy Fries: Regular	530	39	39
Large	1040	72	85

Mr. Goodcents® (Oct '08)

Cold Sub: Per ½ Sub on Wheat Bread	C	F	Cb
Centsable	495	20	57
Cheese Mix	570	26	57
Italian Sub	620	34	57
Mr. Goodcents Original	510	23	56
Oven Roasted Chicken Breast	355	6	54
Penny Club	365	7	56
Pepperoni & Cheese	710	43	57
Roast Beef	370	7	54
Tuna Salad	500	21	62
Veggie Sub	295	4	57
Hot Sub: Per ½ Sun on Wheat Bread w. Cheese			
Chicken Bacon Ranch	670	31	55
Meatball	715	33	65
Pastrami & Swiss	530	18	56
Philly Jack 'n Cheese	520	17	59
Roast Beef 'n Cheddar	540	17	56
Pasta: Alfredo Sauce	1290	80	106
Chicken Alfredo	1425	85	106

Mr. Hero® (Oct '08)

7" Sandwiches & Burgers	C	F	Cb
Burgers: Cheeseburger	835	54	61
Romanburger	935	62	61
Grilled Chicken Philly	480	9.5	62
Deli Subs: Original Italian	715	40	61
Tuna & Cheese	790	54	58
Turkey	530	20	60
Ultimate Italian	770	43	61
Steak Subs: Tuscan	705	32	58
Hot Buttered Cheesesteak	750	43	59
Zesty Bacon & Swiss	675	31	57
4½" Taste Buddies: Per Sandwich			
Bacon Cheeseburger	430	30	33
Grilled Italiano	440	33	32
Tuna 'n Cheese	485	38	31
Zesty Chicken	495	25	48
Pasta: Spaghetti/Rigatoni Dinner	890	17	152
w. Meatballs	1115	36	153
Salads: Per Salad			
Chicken Caesar with Caesar dressing			
Grilled Chicken	165	3	13
Oriental Chicken w. sesame dress.	290	13	25
Tuna Salad	495	49	11
Sides			
Breadsticks (2), 6 oz	450	17	64
Cheddar Cheese Sauce, 1.5 oz	55	4	4
Potato Waffer, 5.6 oz	430	30	39
Jalapeno Poppers	430	28	37
Mozzarella Sticks, 8.7 oz	565	43	12
Onion Petals, 5.7 oz	600	37	58
Desserts: Oreo Cheesecake	340	19	38
Strawberry Swirl Cheesecake	290	16	32

Mrs Fields Cookies® (Oct '08)

	C	F	Cb
Brownies: Per 2.6 oz Brownie			
Butterscotch Blondie	350	14	52
Double Fudge	360	20	45
Pecan Fudge	360	20	46
Special Walnut Fudge & Blondie	330	16	43
Toffee Fudge, brownie	360	19	47
Walnut Fudge	360	20	45
Cake:			
Chocolate Chip, 3 oz piece	350	17	45
Cookies			
Bite Size Nibblers: Cinn. Sugar (3)	170	8	22
Debra's Special (3)	170	7	23
Peanut Butter (3)	180	10	20
Semi-Sweet Chocolate (3)	170	8	24
Triple Chocolate (3)	170	9	23
White Chunk Macadamia (3)	180	9	23
Butter Cookie (1)	200	8	29
Cut Out Cookie (1)	400	19	56
Debra's Special (1)	200	9	28
Peanut Butter (1)	210	12	24
Semi-Sweet Chocolate (1)	210	10	29
with Walnuts(1)	220	11	29
Triple Chocolate (1)	210	11	28
White Chunk Macadamia (1)	230	12	27
Muffins: Blueberry (1), ¾ oz	70	3	10
Chocolate Chip (1), ¾ oz	80	4	11
Mandarin Orange (1), ¾ oz	80	3	9
Raspberry (1), ¾ oz	70	3	10

For Complete Nutritional Data ~ see CalorieKing.com

Nathan's Famous® (Oct '08)

	C	F	Cb
Burgers:			
Burger with Cheese,10.2 oz	705	43	45
Double Burger w. Cheese, 15.6 oz	1180	84	45
Bacon Cheeseburger, 10.8 oz	780	50	45
Super Cheeseburger, 13.65 oz	295	18	24
Corn Dog with Stick, 3.2 oz	380	21	39
Nathan's Famous Hot Dogs			
All Beef (1), 3.5 oz	295	18	24
All Beef Cheese (1), 5.5 oz	390	25	30
All Beef Chili 5.5 oz	400	23	33
Chicken			
Chicken Tender, 6.2 oz	525	39	24
Chicken Tender Platter, 17.5 oz	1245	90	119
Chicken Wing w. Bleu Chse, 14.9 oz	1480	137	26
Gr. Chicken Breast Platter, 15 oz	840	56	58

Nathan's Famous® (Oct '08)

	C	F	Cb
Sides			
Cheese Fries: Med., 8 oz	560	39	46
Large, 11 oz	755	52	62
Super, 17 oz	1190	83	96
Corn on the Cob, 5.5 oz	140	1.5	34
Mozzarella Sticks with sauce, 5.5 oz	385	28	20
Onion Rings, regular, 5.6 oz	545	35	46
Soups			
Chicken Noodle, 12 oz	190	5	27
Manhattan Clam Chowder, 12 oz	270	4.5	48
New England Clam Chowder, 12 oz	250	4.5	42

For Complete Nutritional Data ~ see CalorieKing.com

Ninety Nine (Oct '08)

	C	F	Cb
Appetizers			
All Star Sampler, ¼ platter	450	29	23
Boneless Wings & Skins Sampler, ¼	360	21	18
Outrageous Potato Skins, ¼ platter	300	23	13
Toasted Ravioli	200	10	20
Sandwiches: No Sides			
Buffalo Chicken Sandwich	1120	60	87
Cajun Mushroom Steakburger	1210	81	64
Philly Steakburger	870	47	53
Tuscan Steakburger	1270	88	64
Veggie Burger	790	26	71
Meals			
Cape Cod Seafood Trio, no sides	650	38	20
Captain's Combo Platter	2020	131	134
Grilled Chicken Fajitas	1350	55	103
Grilled Double BBQ Turkey Tips	1650	72	148
Southwestern Quesadilla	340	19	18
Smothered Sirloin Tips, no sides	820	40	9
Salads			
Boneless Buffalo Wing	910	55	54
Calypso Coconut Shrimp	940	62	80
Wild Bleu Chicken & Spinach	1220	80	57
Sides			
Double Bleu Iceberg Wedge	450	41	9
Garlic Red-Skin Mashed Potatoes	290	13	48
Honey Butter Biscuit w. honey butter	300	14	38
Honey Butter, ¼ oz	35	2	3
Perfect: Baked Potato	330	6	65
Rice, 8.5 oz	310	7	57
French Fries, 8 oz. raw weight	550	36	51
Rustic Bread w. Garlic Sauce	150	4	27
Desserts			
Apple Fortune	870	39	123
Little Midnight Fudge Hero	440	24	54
Strawberry Mimosa Cake	700	35	89
Strawberry Shortcake	610	26	87
Towering Midnight Oreo Fudge Cake	880	48	108

Noodles & Company® (Oct '08)

Meals: Per Regular Order

	C	F	Cb
American: Buttered Noodles	620	16	84
House Marinara	650	12	107
Mushroom Stroganoff	780	31	100
Wisconsin Mac & Cheese	900	31	119
Asian Noodles: Bangkok Curry	490	13	85
Indonesian Peanut Saute	950	23	165
Japanese Pan	690	9	133
Pad Thai	700	20	117
Mediterranean: Pasta Fresca	780	22	111
Penne Rosa	810	26	119
Pesto Cavatappi	910	30	114
Whole Grain Tuscan Fettuccine	770	26	108
Proteins: Braised Beef	190	10	0
Organic Tofu	180	11	4
Parmesan Crusted Chicken	190	8	17
Sauteed Beef	210	12	0
Seasoned Chicken Breast	130	2.5	0
Salads: Caesar w. Dressing	320	28	11
Chinese Chop	310	15	23
The Med:	310	13	39
Side: Cucumber Tomato	80	0	18
Tossed Green	60	6	3
Sides: Potstickers, 3 Pieces	200	4.5	31
Ciabatta Roll (1)	160	1.5	31
Soups: Chicken Noodle	300	4	44
Thai Curry	480	19	70
Tomato Basil Bisque	420	23	45

Nothing But Noodles® (Oct '08)

Noodle Bowls

	C	F	Cb
American: Beef Stroganoff	510	31	33
Buttery Noodles	650	44	46
Santa Fe Pasta	705	54	40
Spicy Cajun Pasta	660	50	44
Southwest Chipotle	715	58	41
Asian: Sesame Lo Mein	410	11	64
Spicy Japanese Noodles	420	8	74
Thai Peanut	570	20	89
Pad Thai Noodles	600	10	118
Italian: Basil Pesto	575	42	36
Margherita Pasta	475	31	36
Fettuccini Alfredo	725	56	36
Marinara Pasta	490	11	77
Three-Cheese Macaroni	445	21	45
Cappellini Primavera	500	28	56
Rice Dishes: General Tso's Chicken	760	44	69
Kung Pao Chicken	935	51	89
Thai Peanut Stir Fry	595	27	59

For Extra Menu Items ~ see CalorieKing.com

O'Charley's® (Oct '08)

Appetizers: Per Serving

	C	F	Cb
Chicken Quesadilla Dip	990	59	53
Chicken O'Tenders w. Buffalo Sce (6)	810	53	31
Chips & Salsa	520	18	82
Fried Cheese Wedges (7)	880	60	55
Spinach & Artichoke Dip	940	51	107
Brunch: Per Order (w. Brunch Potatoes & Toast)			
Cajun Chicken Omelette	870	63	13
Spanish Omelette	1180	80	66
Ultimate Omelette	1180	79	68
Strawberry Waffle	1290	50	196
Chicken: Per Order			
Chicken Parmesan w. Vegetables	860	42	70
Chicken Tenders Dinner, w. Sauce	850	57	34
Chicken Teriyaki on Rice	500	6	57
Grilled Chicken Dinner	460	13	26
Salads: No Dressing			
Black & Bleu Caesar	920	65	21
O'Charley's Caesar Salad	490	30	13
Cajun Chicken	740	49	17
California Chicken	560	26	42
Southern Fried Chicken	720	41	34
Sandwiches: No Fries			
Bacon & Cheese Trio Chicken	800	40	53
Buffalo Kickin', no dressing	980	58	72
French Dip	650	23	70
Grilled Chicken Flatbread, no sides	770	28	83
Grilled Chicken Sandwich	610	27	52
Three Cheese Bacon Burger	1050	63	51
Seafood:			
Coconut Shrimp w. Sauce, no sides	650	26	88
Sides: Baked Potato, plain	420	24	52
Cole Slaw	250	19	19
French Fries, Adult Size	300	18	30
Rice Pilaf	200	5	31
Smashed Potatoes	370	12	47
Vegetable Medley	180	14	13
Steak & Ribs: Per Serving (No Sides or Fries)			
Steak Tips Monterey, 1 order	1000	64	47
Choice Sirloin, 5 oz	260	14	0
Filet Mignon, 9 oz	500	30	0
Flame Grilled Sirloin: 7 oz	430	28	0
10 oz	580	35	0
Prime Rib: 10 oz	1020	79	3
16 oz	1630	127	4
Full Rack of Ribs	1480	96	76
Ribeye Steak, 12 oz	810	55	0

Old Country Buffet® (Oct '08)

	C	F	Cb
Entrees: BBQ Beef Ribs, 5 oz	300	23	7
BBQ Smoked Sausage, 2.8 oz	140	10	9
Carved: Beef Brisket, 3 oz	210	11	2
Ham, 3 oz	140	9	0
Roast Beef, 3 oz	230	15	0
Roast Turkey, 3 oz	170	8	0
Salmon Filet, 3 oz	190	11	0
Chicken Hand Breaded Fried:			
Breast, 5.85 oz	280	12	3
Drumstick (1), 2.65 oz	130	8	1
Thigh (1), 4.3 oz	250	16	3
Chicken, Trad'l Baked: Breast	270	12	0.5
Drumstick (1), 2.65 oz	130	9	0.5
Thigh (1), 4.3 oz	240	16	0.5
Roasted Jerk-Wing 2 oz (1)	80	4	0
Chicken Wings: Hot, Drummies (1)	50	3.5	0
Hot, Wing (1)	70	4	0
Fish: Patties, 1 piece, 2.6 oz	180	9	17
Fried, 1 piece, 1.3 oz	90	4.5	10
Shrimp: Fried, 6 shrimp, 2oz	200	10	22
Butterfly Shrimp, fried, (1)	35	1.5	4
Sausage: 1 link	90	8	0
Smoked Saus. & Sauerkraut (1)	195	17	3
Salads:			
California Coleslaw, 3.5 oz	100	0	24
Macaroni Vegetable Salad, 3.5 oz	240	16	21
Marinated Vegetables, 3.5 oz	50	3.5	5
Seven Layer Salad, 2.6 oz	190	17	4
Spanish Rice, 1 Tbsp, 3 oz	140	7	9
Tossed Green Salad, 1 cup, 1.6 oz	5	0	1
Sides: Baked Potato (1), 6.3 oz	180	0	31
Hashed Browns, 3.5 oz	100	6	11
Soups: Chili Bean, 4 fl.oz ladle	80	3.5	9
Corn Chowder, 4 fl.oz ladle	130	8	14
Navy Bean Soup, 4 fl.oz ladle	50	0.5	9
Desserts			
Cheesecake, plain, 1 piece, 2.8 oz	230	12	28
Chocolate Decadence Cake, 1 piece	220	10	30
Cookie, Sugar Free Ranger (1)	90	5	10
Hot Fudge Sundae Cake, 3 oz	160	3	33
Lemon Cream Pie, 2.3 oz	170	4	32
Pudding: Chocolate, 1 Tbsp, 3 oz	120	4.5	19
Reduced Sugar/Calorie, 3 oz	70	1	12
Vanilla, 1 Tbsp, 3 oz	130	5	19
Red. Sugar Pie Cherry, 3.3 oz	170	10	18

Olive Garden® (Oct '08)

	C	F	Cb
Appetizers			
Bruschetta	440	21	57
Muscles Di Napoli	515	35	13
Sicilian Scampi	460	31	16
Stuffed Mushrooms	415	31	20
Entrees (Includes Vegetables):			
Lunch: Lasagna Classico	860	47	54
Eggplant Parmigiana	900	39	78
Fettuccine Alfredo	850	58	70
Five Cheese Ziti al Forno	880	44	83
Dinner: Pork Fillettino	1010	58	116
Chicken Scampi	1181	46	120
Manicotti Formaggio	800	38	57
Stuffed Chicken Marsala	1315	87	72
Garden Fare Selections (Lower Fat)			
Lunch: Capellini Pomodora, 13 oz	480	11	54
Linguine alla Marinara, 10.6 oz	310	4	47
Shrimp Primavera, 19 oz	485	12	65
Venetian Apricot Chicken	280	3	20
Dinner: Capellini Pomodora, 21 oz	840	17	87
Linguine alla Marinara, 17 oz	430	6	80
Shrimp Primavera, 26 oz	730	12	84
Venetian apricot Chicken	380	4	30
Soups: Minestrone Soup, 6 fl.oz	160	1	30
Zuppa Toscana	420	28	24
Dressing (Low Fat): Italian	35	2	4
Parmesan Peppercorn, 2 fl.oz	45	2	5

(The) Old Spaghetti Factory® (Oct '08)

	C	F	Cb
Lunch Entrees: Fettuccine Alfredo	1200	80	93
Chicken Parmigiana, 19 oz	830	32	80
Sicilian Garlic Cheese Bread	310	20	21
Hearty Sicilian Meatballs, 31 oz	1350	36	86
Lasagna Vegetariano 20¾ oz	830	48	68
Pot Pourri, 26 oz	1280	43	176
Spinach & Cheese Ravioli, 11 oz	480	16	63
Spinach Tortellini w. Alfredo, 12 oz	930	56	86
Spaghetti: w. Clam Sauce, 15 oz	660	14	104
w. Sicilian Meatballs, 21 oz	960	31	114
w. Marina Sauce, 15 oz	560	5	108
w. Meat Sauce, 15 oz	610	9	105
w. Clam Sauce, 15 oz	660	14	104
Chicken Penne, 18¾ oz	900	32	113
Crab Ravioli, 11 oz	810	46	73
Meatloaf, Italian Style, 18½ oz	1180	68	83

On the Border® (Oct '08)

C F Cb

Salads: *With Dressing Unless Indicated*

	C	F	Cb
Chicken Fiesta, Grilled	1140	74	52
Grande Taco Salad, Beef, no dress.	1450	102	78
Grand Taco Salad, Spicy Chicken	1280	89	74
House Salad, no dressing	170	10	15
Original Shrimp Fajitas	750	63	18
Sizzling Steak Fajita, no dressing	910	65	24
Sizzling Chicken Fajita, no dressing	760	48	23

Dressings: *Per 2 fl.oz Serving*

	C	F	Cb
Chipotle Honey Mustard	310	29	11
Jalapeno Ranch	180	19	2
Ranch Dressing	220	23	2
Smoked Jalapeno Vinaigrette	230	22	8
Salsa, 2 oz	25	1	3
Fat-Free, Balsamic Vinaigrette	50	0	10
Salsa Fresca, 2 oz	20	0	3
Soups: Chicken Tortilla, 1 bowl	350	22	24

For Complete Nutritional Data ~ see CalorieKing.com

Orange Julius® (Oct '08)

C F Cb

Orange Julius: *Small, 16 fl.oz*

	C	F	Cb
Small, 16 fl.oz	130	0.5	33
Medium, 20 fl.oz	160	0.5	41
Large, 32 fl.oz	260	1	65

Other Julius Originals: *Per 16 fl.oz*

	C	F	Cb
Bananarilla	320	7	65
Cool Cappuccino	300	10	45
Pina Colada	260	7	52
Pomegranate Julius	160	0	42
Strawberry Banana	300	7	60

20 fl.oz Size ~ Add 25% to above figures
  ~ Double the above figures

Premium Fruit Smoothies: *Per 20 fl.oz*

	C	F	Cb
Blackberry Storm	680	15	128
Blackberry Toner	410	0.5	94
Blueberrathon/Wild Blue Twist	440	1	110
Cocoa Latte Swirl	960	23	156
Mango Passion	370	0	86
Orange Swirl	640	15	114
Pomegranate & Berries	400	0	92
Raspberry Creme	650	15	118
Raspberry Crush	480	1.5	121
Strawberry Sensation/Tropical Tango	430	0	100
Strawberry Xtreme	390	0	89
Tart 'N' Berry	570	0.5	139
Tropi-Colada	620	15	112
Add Banana, 1, 4.45 oz	110	0	29
Nutrition Boosts: Fiber Plus, 6g	5	0	4
Heart Health, 4g	15	0	3
Joint Care, 6g	20	0	5
Protein (Soy), 19g	90	3	8

Outback Steakhouse® (Oct '08)

C F Cb

(Author Estimates)

Aussie-Tizers

	C	F	Cb
Aussie Chse Fries (28 oz), w. dress.	2900	182	240
Bloomin Onion (23 oz), w. dressing	2210	134	241
Gold Coast Coconut Shrimp, w. Sce	690	30	97
Grilled Shrimp on the Barbie w. Sce	660	42	32
Kookaburra Wings w. Sauce (10)	1160	75	65
Darling Point Crab Cakes w. Sce (2)	840	72	33

Steaks: *Meat Only ~ Add Extra for Sides*

	C	F	Cb
Ayers Rock Strip (New York Strip) 12 oz	850	66	0
Outback Special, 12 oz Sirloin	780	55	0

Prime Ribs:

	C	F	Cb
8 oz cut	450	38	0
12 oz cut	675	57	0
16 oz cut	905	77	0
Rib-Eye, 14 oz	730	40	0
The Melbourne, P/house, 20 oz	1365	110	0
Lean meat only	700	37	0

Victoria's "Center Cut Filet": *With ¼" Fat*

	C	F	Cb
Tenderloin, 7 oz	490	37	0
Tenderloin, 9 oz	630	48	0

Victoria's "Crowned Filet": *No Sides*

	C	F	Cb
Tenderloin (7 oz) w. Horseradish	840	64	21
Tenderloin (7 oz) w. Bleu Chse	1110	86	22
Tenderloin (9 oz), w. Horseradish	1005	79	22
Tenderloin (9 oz), w. Bleu Chse	1270	101	22

	C	F	Cb
Meals: Hearts of Gold Chicken	870	55	22
Hearts of Gold Tilapia	640	31	23
Alice Springs Chicken	1080	60	23
Salad: Queensland w. Dressing	1100	88	45
Queensland Salad, no Dressing	705	47	37
Sides: Aussie Chips, 7½ oz, w. Ketchup	725	32	100
Fresh Veggies	80	1	14
Grilled Onions, 7.5 oz	180	11	19
Jacket Potato, Plain, 9 oz	270	0	63
Jacket Potato, w. Butter/Cheese	400	14	63
Mushrooms, Sauteed, 8 oz	150	11	12
Desserts: Cheesecake Olivia	700	38	79
Choc. Thunder from Down Under	1220	78	134

Note: Most figures above are author estimates and not intended for clinical use.

Panda Express® (Oct '08)

Appetizers

	C	F	Cb
Chicken Egg Roll, (1), 3 oz	170	8	17
Chicken Potsticker, 3 pieces	220	12	25
Veggie Spring Roll, (1)	80	3.5	11

Meals

	C	F	Cb
Chicken: Black Pepper, 5½ oz	200	12	11
Chicken Kung Pao Cashew, 5½ oz	240	15	12
Orange Chicken, 5½ oz	500	27	42
Beef & Broccoli, 5½ oz	150	7	11
BBQ Pork, 5½ oz	400	23	15
Sweet & Sour Pork, 5½ oz	400	23	35
Mixed Vegetables, 5½ oz	90	7	8
Fried Tofu with mixed Vegies, 5½ oz	120	8	10

Rice & Noodles: Per Order (8 oz)

	C	F	Cb
Chow Mein	390	12	59
Fried Rice	450	14	67
Steamed Rice	380	2.5	81

Panera Bread® (Oct '08)

Bagels: Blueberry

	C	F	Cb
Blueberry	350	2	71
Dutch Apple & Raisin	340	2.5	73
Plain	310	1.5	62
Spreads: Plain Cream Cheese, 2 oz	180	18	2
Reduced-Fat, average, 2 oz	135	11	5

Salads: With Dressing

	C	F	Cb
Asian Sesame Chicken	410	19	31
Caesar	400	27	26
Classic Cafe	170	11	19
Greek	440	39	15
Grilled Chicken Caesar	510	28	27

Sandwiches: Asiago Roast Beef

	C	F	Cb
Asiago Roast Beef	710	32	56
Bacon Turkey Bravo	830	31	86
Chicken Salad on Whole Grain	590	25	71
Italian Combo	1070	50	93
Sierra Turkey	970	54	80
Smoked Ham & Swiss on Rye	700	35	55
Smokehouse Turkey Panini	800	30	80
Tuna Salad on Honey Wheat	720	45	59
Turkey Artichoke Panini	700	22	87

Soups: Per 8oz

	C	F	Cb
Broccoli Cheddar	230	16	14
Cream of Chicken & Wild Rice	200	12	19
French Onion, no Cheese/Croutons	90	3	12
Chicken Noodle	100	2	16
Vegetarian: Black Bean	150	1	29
Garden Vegetable	90	1	17
Muffins: Chocolate Chip Muffie	270	12	40
Pumpkin Muffie	250	10	39
Wild Blueberry Muffin	400	16	59

For Extra Listings ~ see CalorieKing.com

Papa Gino's® (Oct '08)

Appetizers: Per Serving

	C	F	Cb
BBQ Chicken Tenders, Small, 4.3 oz	290	13	27
Buffalo ChknTenders, Small, 4.2 oz	230	10	18
Cheese Breadsticks, Small, 5.8 oz	430	19	46
Cheese Garlic Bread, Large, 4.5 oz	275	10	37
Cinnamon Sticks, Small, 3.6 oz	310	10	50
French Fries, Small, 6.5 oz	360	22	38
Mozzarella Sticks, Small, 5 oz	345	15	35

Pastas: Entree Size

	C	F	Cb
Papa Platter, Penne, Spagh., plain	1065	41	137
Ravioli	445	20	49
Spaghetti & Meatballs	955	36	124
Spaghetti Chkn Parmigiana	1060	40	129

Pizzas: Per Slice

	C	F	Cb
Large Thin Crust: BBQ Chicken	240	9	28
Buffalo Chicken	220	9	23
Cheese	210	9	24
Chicken Pepper	245	11	24
Garlic Chicken	250	11	25
Meat Combo	275	14	25
PapaRoni	275	14	25
Pepperoni	240	11	24
Super Veggie	220	9	26
Works	260	12	25

Subs: Per Small Sub

	C	F	Cb
BLT	685	31	72
Italian	905	48	69
Meatball	820	42	78
Meatball Parmesan	920	50	78
Seafood Salad	680	34	69
Steak	600	23	65
Steak & Cheese	695	30	68
Super Steak	740	30	78
Tuna	735	38	67
Turkey Club	600	19	70

Salads

	C	F	Cb
Buffalo Chicken Tender	320	15	32
Caesar	190	8	20
Chicken Bacon Cheddar	480	22	25
Chicken Tender	325	14	29
Garden	175	6	27
Italian Chopped	575	50	12
Side: Caesar	70	3	7
Garden	65	2	10
Dressings: Bleu Cheese, 1.1 oz	150	15	3
Caesar, 3 oz	395	43	0
Ranch, 3 oz	285	31	3
Honey Dijon Fat-Free, 1.5 oz	60	0	13

Papa John's® (Oct '08)

	C	F	Cb
Original Crust: Per ⅛ Slice of 14" Pizza			
The Meats w. Beef	350	16	38
BBQ Chicken & Bacon	340	11	44
Cheese	300	11	39
Garden Fresh	280	9	39
Hawaiian BBQ Chicken	340	11	46
Pepperoni	310	13	38
Sausage	330	15	37
Spinach Alfredo/Chicken	300	11	37
The Works	330	11	38
Tuscan Six Cheese	320	13	38
Thin Crust: Per ⅛ Slice of 14" Pizza			
BBQ Chicken & Bacon	290	14	29
Cheese	240	13	22
Garden Fresh	210	11	23
Hawaiian BBQ Chicken	290	14	31
Pepperoni	260	15	21
Sausage	280	17	22
Spicy Italian	320	14	24
Spinach Alfredo/Chicken	230	13	21
The Works	280	14	24
Tuscan Six Cheese	250	14	21
Side Orders: Bread Stick (2), 4 oz	290	4.5	53
Cheese Sticks, 4 sticks	370	16	42
Papa's Chickenstrips, 2 strips	160	8	10
Cinna Swirl Pie, 2 slices, 3¾ oz	420	21	53
Sauces: Garlic, 1 oz	150	17	0
Honey Mustard, 1 oz	150	15	5
Pizza, 1 oz	20	0	3

Papa Murphy's® (Oct '08)

Pizzas: Per Slice of Family Size	C	F	Cb
Gourmet: Chicken Garlic, ⅒₂ pizza	320	14	30
Classic Italian, ⅒₂ pizza	350	18	31
Veggie, ⅒₂ pizza	300	13	31
Papa's: BBQ Chicken, ⅒₂ pizza	335	12	36
Cheese, ⅒₂ pizza	260	10	29
All Meat; Cowboy, ⅒₂ pizza, avg.	350	17	30
Hawaiian, ⅒₂ pizza	285	11	33
Murphy's Combo, ⅒₂ pizza	355	18	31
Pepperoni, ⅒₂ pizza	310	15	29
Specialty; Perfect, ⅒₂ pizza, avg.	310	14	31
Rancher, ⅒₂ pizza	325	15	30
Veggie Combo, ⅒₂ pizza	285	12	32
Stuffed: Big Murphy, ⅒₆ pizza	360	16	40
Chicago Style, ⅒₆ pizza	365	16	38
Chicken and Bacon, ⅒₆ pizza	375	15	38
Five Meat, ⅒₆ pizza	365	16	38

Papa Murphy's® cont... (Oct '08)

Pizzas Cont:	C	F	Cb
Thin Crust deLITEs: Cheese, ⅒₀	140	7	13
Hawaiian, ⅒₀ pizza	150	7	15
Meat, ⅒₀ pizza	190	11	13
Pepperoni, ⅒₀ pizza	165	9	13
Veggie, ⅒₀ pizza	150	8	13
Salads: Club, w/o dressing	290	18	12
Garden, w/o dressing	200	12	16
Italian, w/o dressing	270	20	14

Pei Wei Asian Diner (Oct '08)

First Tastes: Per Serving	C	F	Cb
Crab Wontons (4)	190	13	9
Crispy Potstickers (4)	130	7	10
Edamame	310	16	24
Minced Chicken w. Lettuce Wraps	250	4	31
Spring Rolls (2)	90	5	11
Rice & Noodle Bowls: Per Bowl			
Dan Dan Noodle, Chicken	780	14	108
Fried Rice: Beef	1260	42	136
Chicken	1050	22	136
Japanese Udon Noodles: Beef	1200	52	114
Chicken	980	32	114
Lo Mein Noodles: Chicken	920	22	122
Beef	1140	42	122
Pad Thai: Beef	1340	60	126
Chicken	1120	40	122
Soba Miso Bowls: Shrimp	720	12	102
Beef	1060	36	106
Chicken	840	16	106
Teriyaki Bowl:			
with Brown Rice: Beef	1160	34	132
Chicken	920	14	128
with White Rice: Beef	1120	32	124
Chicken	880	12	120
Shrimp	980	34	120
Thai Blazing Noodles: Beef	1260	64	110
Chicken	1040	44	110
Shrimp	960	44	110
Salads: Per Dish, w/o Dressing			
Asian Chopped Chicken	400	16	20
Spicy Chicken	420	5	46
Salad Dressings: Per Serving			
Lime Vinaigrette, 2 oz	230	20	13
Sesame Ginger, 2 oz	170	16	5
Sauces: Lettuce Wrap, 2 oz	70	4.5	2
Sweet Chile, 2 oz	140	0	34
Thai Peanut, 2 oz	170	11	15
Soup, Hot & Sour, 1 bowl	500	28	37
Cookies: Chocolate Chip (1)	340	14	53
Fortune Cookie (1)	30	0	7

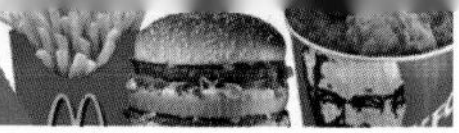

Fast - Foods & *Restaurants*

Penn Station® (Oct '08)

Subs (6")

	C	F	Cb
Artichoke: w. mayo	360	18	37
No mayo	260	7	37
Cheese Bread	250	5.5	42
Chicken Salad	360	15	41
Chicken Teriyaki	435	13	48
Grilled Vegetarian	245	4	46
Ham Dagwood, no cheese	260	6.5	35
Philadelphia Cheesesteak	500	25	45
Philadelphia Cheesesteak, no mayo	395	14	45
Reuben	500	21	40
Reuben, w/o Dressing	390	12	37
Tuna Salad	365	15	41
Turkey Dagwood	420	18	36
Turkey Dagwood, no Cheese/Mayo	240	4	34

Pepe's Mexican® (Oct '08)

	C	F	Cb
Burritos: Beef & Bean	510	24	52
Beef & Bean Suizo	640	34	55
Chicken & Bean	480	21	51
Chicken & Bean Suizo	610	31	54
Pork & Bean	470	19	51
Pork & Bean Suizo	600	29	54
Flauta: Beef, plain	160	9	10
Beef w. cheese & sauce	190	12	11
Chicken, plain	190	10	16
Chicken w. cheese & sauce	230	13	17
Taco Salad: (Includes Taco Shell)			
Beef w. 4 oz salsa	550	26	52
Chicken w. 4 oz salsa	520	23	51
Pork w. 4 oz salsa	500	20	52
Without Taco Shell, deduct	290	13	19
Tacos: Beef Crisp	210	11	16
Beef Soft Corn	250	10	28
Beef Soft Flour	250	11	24
Chicken Crisp	190	9	15
Chicken Soft Corn	230	8	27
Chicken Soft Flour	230	9	23
Pork Crisp	170	6	16
Pork Soft Corn	220	6	27
Pork Soft Flour	220	7	24
Tostada			
Beef & Bean	380	23	26
Beef & Bean Suiza	440	29	26
Chicken & Bean	360	21	21
Chicken & Bean Suiza	410	26	25
Pork & Bean	350	20	26
Pork & Bean Suiza	410	25	26

Perkin's® Family Restaurant (Oct '08)

	C	F	Cb
Entrees			
Chicken Dinner	620	13	60
Fish Dinner	470	7	60
'Lite & Healthy'	105	2	15
Omelettes: Country Club	930	79	6
Deli Ham & Cheese	960	79	8
'Everything' Omelette	695	54	9
Granny's Country Omelette	940	82	7
w. 9 oz Hash Browns	1245	90	57
Salads: Chef's, Mini	215	11	7
Muffins: Banana	650	33	78
Blueberry; Pumpkin	550	26	78
Bran Muffin	550	16	94
Carrot	455	26	55
Chocolate Chips	620	26	81
Cranberry Nut	585	29	75
Lemon Poppyseed	685	33	88
Oat Bran	455	15	68
Peaches & Cream; Apple, avg.	520	23	72
Raspberry & Cream	585	26	81
Pancakes: Buttermilk (1), no syrup	140	4.5	20
Short Stack (3), no syrup	425	14	60
Regular Stack (5), no syrup	705	24	100
Pies (Per Slice): Apple Pie, ⅙ pie	375	15	56
Wildberry, ⅙ pie	390	16	66
Bundt Cake, w. Icing (sugar free)	385	17	70
Fruit Cup	50	0.5	12

For Complete Nutritional Data ~ See CalorieKing.com

Peter Piper® Pizza (Oct '08)

Pizza: Per Slice	C	F	Cb
Original Crust: *Per ⅛ of 14" Pizza*			
Cheese	300	9	37
Ham & Pineapple	280	7	38
Pepperoni	300	10	36
Hand-Tossed Crust: *Per ⅛ of 14" Pizza*			
Cheese	290	9	38
Ham & Pineapple	280	7	39
Pepperoni	290	10	37
Pan Crust: *Per ⅛ of 14" Pizza*			
Cheese	290	9	38
Ham & Pineapple	310	7	46
Pepperoni	330	10	44
Specialty			
Original Crust: *Per ⅛ of 14" Pizza*			
5 Meat Supreme	350	13	38
Chicago Classic	300	10	38
New York 3 Cheese w. Pepperoni	380	16	38
Smokehouse	370	15	38
The Werx	320	11	38

P.F. Chang's® (Oct '08)

Appetizers: Per Whole Dish	C	F	Cb
Crab Wontons w. Plum Sauce	550	26	60
Harvest Spring Rolls (4) no sauce	285	15	30
Lettuce Wraps: w. Rice Sticks, no sauce			
Chicken	510	13	68
Vegetarian	415	4	70
Spare Ribs: w. Barbecue Sauce	1355	89	43
Northern Style	720	54	6
Peking Dumplings: Pan-Fried	425	24	21
Steamed	385	19	21
Shrimp Dumplings: Pan-Fried	330	13	26
Steamed w. Ginger Sauce	290	8	26
Vegetable Dumplings: Pan-Fried	365	12	43
Steamed	325	8	43
Meals: Per Whole Dish			
Beef: A La Sichuan	1170	64	56
Mongolian	1180	73	29
Orange Peel	1570	85	115
Chicken: w. Black Bean Sauce	680	23	33
Chang's Spicy	925	37	88
Kung Pao, regular	1230	79	58
Mu Shu	715	38	49
Orange Peel	1150	46	125
Philip's Better Lemon	1050	42	113
Spicy Ground w. Eggplant	790	40	73
Sweet & Sour	765	20	107
Lamb, Wok Seared	1080	80	29
Seafood: Cantonese Scallops	410	16	26
Cantonese Shrimp	330	12	21
Chang's Lemon Scallops	950	28	100
Crispy Honey Shrimp	1060	44	118
Kung Pao Scallops	1135	57	66
Kung Pao Shrimp	975	58	58
Lemon Pepper Shrimp	700	36	59
Scallops	1030	36	98
Shrimp	730	37	55
Traditions: Beef w. Broc.	1120	65	38
Almond Cashew Chicken	815	30	63
Crispy Honey Chicken	865	11	121
Lo Mein Beef	1375	80	94
Lo Mein Chkn	1200	67	97
Moo Goo Gai Pan	660	34	32
Shrimp w. Lobster Sauce	480	22	24
Vegetarian Plate: Buddha's Feast	135	1	29
Coconut Curry Vegetables	685	46	48
Ma Po Tofu	535	19	51
Sides: Large			
Garlic Snap Peas	205	10	23
Shanghai Cucumbers	125	6	8
Sichuan Asparagus	205	6	34
Spicy Green Beans	600	40	48
Spinach Stir-Fried w. Garlic	140	6	16
Soups: Hot & Sour, 1 bowl	650	18	82
Egg Drop Soup, 1 bowl	365	14	51
Wonton, 1 bowl	355	10	45
Desserts: Banana Spring Rolls	815	37	130
Great Wall of Chocolate Cake	2235	90	376
Tiramisu Mini Dessert	200	14	15

Piccadilly Cafeteria® (Oct '08)

Meals: No Sides Included	C	F	Cb
Beef: Chopped Steak Fried, 4.5 oz	415	33	6
Roast Leg, small, 4 oz	350	22	2
Steak: Filet Mignon, 6 oz	340	20	1
New York Strip, 10 oz	875	71	1
Ribeye, 10 oz	1040	91	2
Chicken: Breast, Mesquite Smoked	210	8	1
Baked Cajun, Boneless Breast	430	27	9
Fish: Catfish Cajun Baked	405	28	6
Catfish Filet Stuffed	550	40	9
Tilapia Baked	210	11	10
Trout Almondine Baked, large	490	22	11
Trout Cajun Baked	520	27	7
Trout Filets Baked	465	19	10
Pork Loin: Bone in Roast, 5 oz	375	13	10
Shrimp, Fried	460	19	34
Turkey Breast, Carved, 5.5 oz	265	10	5
Salads			
Caesar Salad, 3 oz	145	11	7
Chef's Salad, Small, 6 oz	145	9	4
Italian Coleslaw, 3.7 oz	165	16	5
Louisianne Bowl	45	3	2
Mexican	60	3	8
Piccadilly Bowl	25	0	6
Shrimp Remoulade	515	28	33
Dressings			
Au Jus, 3 fl.oz	5	0	1
Blue Cheese, 2 Tbsp	160	18	1
Cheese Sauce, 2 fl.oz	35	1	5
French, 2 Tbsp	130	13	5
Italian, 2 Tbsp	160	17	1
Ranch, 2 Tbsp	150	17	1
Ranch Fat-Free, 2 Tbsp	35	0	7
Thousand Island, 2 Tbsp	170	18	2
Soups: Per 9.5 oz (No Rice)			
Gumbo: Chicken	100	2	11
Chicken & Sausage	225	15	10
Extras			
Broccoli w. Cheese Sauce	105	7	9
Cabbage: Buttered, Steamed	70	5	6
Bacon Seasoned	105	8	6
Cauliflower, Buttered	90	6	8
Fried Okra	240	13	26
Greens: Collard Mustard & Turnip	135	10	3
Turnip w. Diced Turnips, 3.2 oz	150	12	4

Pita Pit (Oct '08)

Breakfast Pitas: *Includes meat, pita, eggs, hashbrowns, green peppers & onions*

	C	F	Cb
Awakin' with Bacon	510	33	17
Chicken Classic	710	26	73
Ham n' Eggs	745	26	72
Meat the Day	590	39	21
Morning Glory	350	21	15
Sausage Sunrise	510	33	21

Meat Pitas: *Only includes meat and pita bread. Add extra for toppings and sauces*

	C	F	Cb
Black Forest Ham	400	5.5	56
B.L.T.	515	19	57
Chicken Breast	370	5	57
Chicken Caesar	550	19	57
Chicken Crave	440	7.5	58
Chicken Souvlaki	430	10	54
Dagwood	435	6	59
Gyro	550	26	61
Philly Steak	360	3	59
Roast Beef	365	3.5	56
Tuna	375	1	57
Turkey	365	3	60

Veggie Pitas: *Add extra for toppings and sauces*

	C	F	Cb
Babaganoush	330	3.5	58
Cheddar	415	13	54
Falafel	515	14	91
Feta	340	7	55
Garden	260	0.5	54
Hummus	310	2.5	58
Pita Bread (1)	260	0.5	54

Toppings:

	C	F	Cb
Avocado	90	9	3
Babaganoush	70	3	4
Hummus	50	2	4
Pineapple	50	0	12
Salad Veggies, average	5	0	1

Sauces:

	C	F	Cb
BBQ	20	0	3.5
Caesar	140	15	1
Hot Sauce	0	0	0
Mayo	100	11	0.5
Ranch	70	7	1
Sour Cream	60	5	2
Teriyaki	45	0	10
Tzatziki	40	3.5	2
Cheeses: American Swiss	100	8	1
Cheddar	150	13	0

For Extra Listings ~ see CalorieKing.com

234

Pizza Hut® (Oct '08)

Thin 'n Crispy (12"): *Per ⅛ Pizza*

	C	F	Cb
Cheese Only	200	8	22
Italian Sausage & Red Onion	230	11	23
Meat Lovers	310	18	22
Pepperoni	210	10	21
Quartered Ham & Pineapple	190	7	23
Supreme	240	11	23
Super Supreme	260	13	23

Pan (12"): *Per ⅛ Pizza*

	C	F	Cb
Cheese Only	270	13	27
Italian Sausage & Red Onion	300	15	28
Meat Lover's	380	22	28
Pepperoni	280	15	27
Pepperoni & Mushroom	270	13	27
Quartered Ham & Pineapple	250	11	28
Supreme	310	16	28
Veggie Lover's	250	11	28

Hand-Tossed Style (12"): *Per ⅛ Pizza*

	C	F	Cb
Cheese Only	230	10	25
Pepperoni	240	11	26
Pepperoni & Mushroom	230	9	25
Pepperoni Lover's	290	15	25
Quartered Ham & Pineapple	210	7	28
Super Supreme	290	14	26
Supreme	270	13	26
Veggie Lover's	210	8	26

Fit n' Delicious (12"): *Per ⅛ Pizza*

	C	F	Cb
Diced Chicken Mushr. & Jalapeno	160	4.5	22
Diced Chkn Red On. & Pepper	170	4.5	23
Diced Tomato Mushr. & Jalapeno	150	4	23
Green Pepper Red On. & Tomato	160	4	24
Ham Pineapple & Diced Tomato	170	4.5	24
Ham Red Onion & Mushroom	160	4.5	23

Pizza Mia: *Per ⅛ Pizza*

	C	F	Cb
Cheese Only	210	8	26
Pepperoni	210	8	26

Stuffed Crust (14"): *Per ⅛ Pizza*

	C	F	Cb
Italian Sausage & Red Onion	410	19	41
Pepperoni Lover's	450	24	38
Quartered ham & Pineapple	350	13	41
Super Supreme	450	23	39

Pizza Hut® cont... (Oct '08)

Personal Pan (6")	C	F	Cb
Cheese Only	610	25	69
Italian Sausage & Red Onion	690	33	71
Meat Lover's	890	49	70
Supreme	720	34	70
Super Supreme	750	37	71

P'Zone: Per ½ P'Zone			
Classic	620	23	78
Meaty	700	29	77
Pepperoni	640	25	76

Sandwiches & Burgers

Toasted Sandwiches:			
Black Forest Ham & Cheese	710	27	79
Roasted Turkey & Provolone	680	23	80
Steak & Chse Hoagie	690	25	67
Supremo	790	39	67

Appertizers

Wings: Hot (2)	120	7	1
Mild (2)	110	7	1
Breadsticks: Plain (1)	160	7	18
Cheese (1)	190	9	19
Dipping Sauce: Wing Ranch, 1.5 oz	220	23	3
Wing Blue Cheese, 1.5 oz	220	23	3
Breadstick Dipping Sauce, 3 oz	40	0	8

Pastas

3-Cheese Penne Bake	980	61	62
Bistro Chicken Alfredo Bake	900	51	61
Spaghetti w. Meat Sauce	920	42	97
The Meaty Ziti Bake	990	59	64

Tuscani Pasta: *Per ¼ Order*			
Bacon Mac N Cheese	520	22	54
Chicken Alfredo	630	33	56
Meaty Marinara	510	24	48

Soups: 1 Cup, 8 fl.oz			
Broccoli Cheddar	200	13	9
Tomato & Basil	180	14	13

Desserts

Cinnamon Sticks, 2 pieces	170	5	27
Hershey's Chocolate Dunders (4)	410	20	51
Hershey's Chocolate Sauce, 1.5 oz	120	2.5	24
White Icing Dipping Cup, 2 oz	190	0	47

Pizza Ranch® (Oct '08)

Pizzas, 12 ": Per Slice (⅛ Pizza)	C	F	Cb
Original: BBQ Beef	220	8	28
BBQ Chicken	210	6	27
Bacon Cheeseburger	220	9	26
Beef; Canadian Bacon, avg.	210	7	25
California Chicken	250	12	26
Cheese; Chicken Broccoli, avg.	220	8	26
Garlic Cheese	230	11	25
Italian Sausage; Pepperoni	220	9	25
Prairie; Sweet Swine, avg.	210	7	26
Roundup; Tabasco Pepperoni	230	10	26
Stampede	250	10	27
Texan	240	9	31
Skillet: BBQ Beef	230	8	30
BBQ Chicken	220	6	29
Bacon Cheeseburger	230	9	28
Beef; Canadian Bacon, avg.	220	7	27
Bronco; California Chicken, avg.	270	12	28
Cheese; Chicken Broccoli, avg.	230	8	28
Garlic Cheese	240	11	27
Italian Sausage; Pepperoni, avg.	230	9	27
Prairie; Sweet Swine	220	7	27
Roundup; Tabasco Pepperoni	240	10	28
Stampede	260	11	29
Texan	250	9	33
Thin: BBQ Beef	170	7	17
BBQ Chicken	150	6	16
Bacon Cheeseburger	170	8	15
Beef; Canadian Bacon, avg.	150	7	14
California Chicken; Bronco, avg.	200	11	15
Cheese; Chicken Broccoli, avg.	160	8	14
Garlic Cheese	170	10	14
Italian Sausage; Pepperoni, avg.	160	8	14
Prairie; Sweet Swine, avg.	150	7	15
Roundup; Tabasco Pepperoni	180	9	15
Stampede	190	10	16
Texan	190	9	20
Broasted Chicken: Breast, 1 pce	440	23	4
Leg, 1 piece	190	12	2
Thigh, 1 piece	370	26	4
Wing, 1 piece	190	13	2
Sides: Potato Wedges (1)	60	0	13

For Complete Nutritional Data ~ see CalorieKing.com

Planet Smoothie® (Oct '08)

	C	F	Cb
Cool Blended Smoothies			
Per 22 fl.oz Unless Otherwise Stated			
Captain Kid, 12 fl oz	195	1.5	47
PBJ	560	11	97
Shag-a-delic	430	1	104
The Last Mango	355	3.5	82
Twig & Berries	300	0.5	74
Vinnie del Rocco	385	3.5	92
Energy Smoothies: Per 22 fl.oz			
Berry Bada-Bing	360	0.5	88
Chocolate Elvis	520	9	109
Frozen Goat	360	1	85
Grape Ape	305	0.5	78
Road Runner	280	0.5	72
Spazz	265	0.5	68
Workout Smoothies: Per 22 fl.oz			
Big Bang	350	0.5	80
Chocolate Chimp	400	1	94
Merlin's Pineapple LB	415	1.5	57
Strawberry LB	485	1.5	78

Pollo Tropical® (Oct '08)

	C	F	Cb
Chicken			
Boneless Breast, 2 pieces	230	4	0
¼ Chicken: Dark Meat with skin	270	17	0
without skin	180	9	0
White Meat with skin	350	17	0
w/o skin, serving	230	7	0
Sandwiches & Burgers			
Chicken Caesar Sandwich	740	33	45
Grilled Chicken Sandwich	740	34	51
Roast Pork Sandwich	710	27	57
Menu Items			
TropiChop: Regular			
Chicken w. Rice & Beans	530	10	90
Chicken with Rice & Vegetables	330	5	51
Grilled Chicken Deluxe	410	7	53
Picadillo with Rice	680	22	96
Pork with Rice & Black Beans	680	22	92
Pork with Rice & Vegetables	490	18	54
Ropa Vieja	600	16	98
Shrimp Creole	505	11	77
TropiChop Max: Ropa Vieja	1120	38	159
Chicken with Rice & Beans	1090	27	142
Chicken with Rice & Veggies	840	22	93
Grilled Chicken Deluxe	740	12	94
Picadillo with rice	1280	51	156
Pork with Rice & Black Beans	1260	49	145
Pork with Rice & Vegetables	1000	44	97
Shrimp Creole	1000	29	129
Vegetarian	950	21	178

For Complete Nutritional Data ~ see CalorieKing.com

Popeye's® (Oct '08)

	C	F	Cb
Chicken: Chkn Breast, Mild/Spicy avg.	355	21	8
Chicken Leg, Mild/Spic, avg.	105	6	3
Chicken Thigh, Mild/Spicy, avg.	290	22	7
Chicken Wing, Mild/Spicy, avg.	145	10	5
Sides: Biscuit, 2.1 oz	240	13	26
Cajun Rice, regular, 4.1 oz	170	6	22
Cinnamon Apple Turnover, 3 oz	250	12	34
Coleslaw, regular, 5 oz	260	23	14
Corn on the Cob (1), 7.8 oz	190	2	37
French Fries, 3 oz	310	17	35
Mashed Potatoes: no Gravy, reg.	100	3	17
w. Gravy, regular, 5 oz	120	4	18
Red Beans & Rice, regular, 6 oz	320	19	31

Port of Subs® (Oct '08)

	C	F	Cb
Light Submarine: Per 5" Sub (Five Grams of Fat or Less)			
#2 Ham Turkey	330	5	46
#5 Smoked Ham & Turkey	320	5	46
#6 Vegetarian, no Cheese	240	2	44
#7 Roast Beef	315	4	43
#8 Turkey	315	4	47
#9 Peppered Pastrami	295	4	44
#10 Roasted Chicken Breast	305	3	44
#14 Smoked Ham	300	4	44
#18 Roast Beef & Turkey	315	4	45
Cold Submarine Sandwiches: Per 5" Sub (No Mayo.)			
#1 Ham, Salami, Capicolla & Pepperoni w. Provolone	530	26	45
#2 Ham & Turkey w. Provolone	435	15	46
#3 Salami & Turkey w. Provolone	465	20	46
#4 Ham & Salami w. Provolone	470	21	45
#5 Smkd Ham & Turkey w. Cheddar	430	15	47
#6 Vegetarian w. Avocado & Olives	600	33	49
#7 Roast Beef w. Provolone,	420	14	43
#8 Turkey w. Provolone	420	14	47
#9 Peppered Pastrami w. Swiss	440	17	44
#10 Rstd Chicken Brst w. Provolone	410	13	45
#11 Ham w. American	380	20	45
#12 Salami w. Provolone	480	25	45
#13 Combination of Cheeses	510	26	44
#14 Smoked Ham w. Swiss	445	17	45
#15 Salami & Pepperoni w. Prov.	510	27	45
#16 BLT Sandwich	520	30	43
#17 Tuna no Cheese	420	18	45
#18 Rst Beef & Turkey w. Provolone	420	14	45

Updated Nutrition Data ~ www.CalorieKing.com
Persons with Diabetes ~ See Disclaimer (Page 24)

Port of Subs® cont... (Oct '08)

	C	F	Cb
Hot Subs: Per 8" Sub			
Grilled Chicken	565	11	68
Hot Pastrami	760	17	62
Meatball	655	25	76
Tortilla Wrap: Per Wrap, 12" Tortilla			
Chicken Caesar	760	35	63
Hot Grilled Chkn & Smokey Cheddar	660	23	63
Turkey & Bacon Ranch	785	44	190
Tortilla (1)	330	8	55
Sauces & Dressings: Per 2 Tablespoons			
Mayo & Mustard Mix	110	12	0
Mayonnaise	130	14	0
Mustard	0	0	0
Soups: Medium 6 oz Bowl			
Campbell's: Boston Clam Chowder	105	4	13
Broccoli Cheese	120	6	13
Minestrone	55	1	8
Roasted Chicken Noodle	85	2	9

Pret A Manger® (Oct '08)

	C	F	Cb
Bakery: Banana Cake	420	24	48
Carrot Cake	460	29	47
Chocolate Brownie	390	20	51
Pecan Pie	390	21	50
Raspberry Bar	390	18	55
Salads: Per Pack			
Cobb & Greens	430	24	30
Grilled Chicken Caesar	400	16	24
Salmon Sushi	350	15	37
Tuna Sushi	430	20	36
Chicken & Avocado	430	28	41
Sandwiches			
Chicken & Bacon Sandwich	460	13	58
Chicken Avocado Sandwich	500	20	64
Natural Turkey	520	21	59
Tuna Roast Red Pepper	550	19	58
Baguettes:			
Rst Beef Arugula & Parm.	670	13	65
Chicken & Mozzarella	510	14	77
Ham & Swiss	620	16	68
Wraps: Avocado Salad	460	30	36
Chicken Jalapeno	500	21	46
Spicy Falafel Hot	540	24	61
Swedish Meatball Ragu	710	37	49

For Complete Menu ~ See CalorieKing.com

Pretzelmaker® (Oct '08)

	C	F	Cb
Pretzels			
Bites: Small, 5.3 oz	450	11	80
Medium, 7½ oz	640	16	112
Large, 11½ oz	1020	26	176
Cinnamon Sugar, 6 oz	520	12	95
Pretzels: Caramel Crunch	300	4	58
Caramel Nut	390	7	74
Cinnamon Sugar	370	8	68
Garlic	350	7	64
Original	340	7	61
Parmesan	360	9	61
Plain	290	2	61
Pretzel Dog	440	27	34
Ranch	240	7	63
Sauces: Per Container			
Caramel, 1½ oz	140	0	35
Cheddar Cheese, 1½ oz	70	5	6
Cream Cheese, 1½ oz	200	20	4
Cream Cheese Icing, 1½ oz	180	9	22
Ketchup	10	0	2
Mustard	5	0	0.5
Nacho Cheese, 1½ oz	80	5	7
Pizza, 1½ oz	30	0.5	6
Beverages: Per 20 fl.oz			
Breezer: Coffee	640	21	107
Mocha	620	20	106
Peach	650	20	117
Raspberry	650	20	117
Strawberry Banana	650	20	115
Lemonade: MCF	160	0	92
MCF	270	0	147

Pretzel Time® (Oct '08)

	C	F	Cb
Pretzels			
Bites: Plain, small, 5.3 oz	450	11	80
Medium, 7½ oz	640	16	112
Large, ½ order, 5.8 oz	510	13	88
Cinnamon Sugar (1), 4.3 oz	370	8	68
Garlic (1), 4.15 oz	350	7	64
Parmesan (1), 4.2 oz	360	9	61
Plain (1), 3.8 oz	290	2	61
Original (1), 4 oz	340	7	61
Ranch (1), 4.2 oz	240	7	63
Sauces & Dressings: Per Container			
Caramel Sauce	140	0	35
Cream Cheese Icing	180	9	22
Cheddar/ Nacho Cheese Sauce	75	5	7
Cream Cheese Sauce	200	20	4
Ketchup	20	0	4
Mustard	5	0	1
Pizza Sauce	30	1	6

Qdoba (Oct '08)

Burritos: With 13" Flour Tortilla

	C	F	Cb
Ancho Chile BBQ Burrito	950	21	145
Grilled Vegetable Burrito	930	32	126
Fajita Ranchero Burrito			
Chicken/Steak	790	24	101
Queso Burrito with fajita veggies	810	26	125
Poblano Pest Burrito	930	29	121
Shredded Beef Burrito	1070	36	126

Tacos: With cheese, lettuce, pico de gallo, lite sour cream

Chicken, Crispy Shell	170	10	18
Grilled Veggie, Crispy Shell	130	8	10
Ground Sirloin, Crispy Shell	190	13	8
Pork, Crispy Shell	160	8	11
Shredded Beef, Crispy Shell	170	10	10

Taco Salads: With lettuce, black bean & corn salsa, cheese, picante ranch dressing, lite sour cream

Ground Beef, Crispy Shell	910	50	64
Chicken with Shell	850	43	64

Quesadillas: With13" flour tortilla, 4 oz. cheese, pico de gallo

Plain	780	44	56
Chicken	970	54	57
Shredded Beef	970	52	61
Chicken/Shredded Beef	970	53	59

3-Cheese Nachos: With Chips, 3-cheese queso, beans, lite sour cream, salsa verde

Regular	970	47	111
with Ground Beef	1210	64	112
with Chicken	1150	57	112
with Pork	1130	52	121

Breakfast Items: With 10" Flour Tortilla

Breakfast Burrito:

with 3-Cheese Queso Sauce	540	26	54
with Fajita Ranchero Sauce	480	20	53
Breakfast Quesadilla, w/ Chorizo	650	34	52

Sides: 3-Cheese Queso, 4 oz | 190 | 16 | 6

Black Bean & Corn Salsa, 2 oz	70	0	9
Chile Corn Salsa, 2 oz	60	0.5	11
Chips, 4 oz	560	26	75
Cilantro Lime Dressing, 1.5 oz	90	8	5
Guacamole, 3 oz	130	4	7
Lite Sour Cream, 2 oz	60	4	3
Mango Salsa, 4 oz	60	0	14
Picante Ranch Dressing, 1.5 oz	45	0	10
Poblano Pesto Salsa, 2 oz	60	5	3
Salsa Verde/Roja/Habanero, 2 oz	15	0	4

Quizno's Subs® (Oct '08)

Subs Regular:

	C	F	Cb
With Cheese & Dressing Unless Indicated			
Signature Classic Subs:			
Classic Italian	920	50	69
Classic w. Bacon	890	50	67
The Traditional	690	30	68
Premium Steak Subs:			
Prime Rib Sub: w. Peppercorn	980	55	72
w. Cheesesteak	1090	64	71
Black Angus Steak	850	26	86
Delectable Chicken Subs: Baja	780	34	70
Honey Bourbon, w/o Cheese	550	8.5	72
Honey Mustard	860	41	72
Carbonara w. Bacon	840	40	66
Mesquite w. Bacon	790	36	68
Deli Favorite Subs:			
Honey-Cured Ham & Swiss	810	45	67
Oven Roasted Turkey	770	41	66
Roast Beef & Cheddar	760	41	66
Tuna Melt	1270	101	64
The 5 Meat Stack	850	49	65
Primo Meatball	760	36	75
Inspired Turkey Subs:			
Turkey & Swiss	650	26	68
Tuscan Turkey	660	25	75
Turkey, Bacon & Guacamole	800	38	74

Flatbread Sammies:
With Cheese & Dressing Unless Indicated

Alpine Chicken	285	14	25
Bistro Steak Melt	280	13	26
Cantina Chicken, w/o Cheese	205	4	29
Italiano	305	17	24
Roadhouse Steak, w/o Cheese	205	4	29
Sonoma Turkey	270	14	26

Breakfast Sandwiches:

Black Angus, Steak & Cheddar	390	17	36
Egg & Cheddar	350	20	36
Bacon, Egg & Cheddar	440	26	36
Ham, Egg & Cheddar	350	17	37
Garden Vegetable w. Cheddar	310	16	38

Soups: Per Bowl with 2 Crackers

Broccoli Cheese, Bowl	360	22	28
Chili, Bowl	360	15	36
Bread Bowls: Chili	760	22	107
Country Fresh Chicken	760	26	103

Flatbread Salads: With Cheese & Dressing

Black & Bleu	720	24	84
Chicken Caesar	1000	64	63
Classic Cobb w Ranch Dressing	960	62	62
Rstd Chicken w. Honey Mustard	1110	74	70
Raspberry Chipotle Chicken	820	32	95

Rally's Hamburgers® (Oct '07)

Burgers/Sandwiches

	C	F	Cb
Rallyburger	435	22	35
with Cheese	490	27	35
Big Buford	745	48	35
Chicken Fillet Sandwich	400	15	43
Chili w. Cheese & Onion: 7 oz	360	22	20
13 oz size	670	41	37
Super Barbecue Bacon	595	31	49
Super Double Cheeseburger	760	48	37
French Fries: Regular	210	11	26
Large	320	16	39
X-Large	425	21	52

Ranch 1® (Oct '08)

	C	F	Cb
Sandwiches: American Rancher	390	10	51
Club Sandwich	470	16	53
Grilled Chicken Philly	450	15	53
Ranch Classic	370	5	53
Spicy Grilled Chicken	420	11	58
Specialities			
Grilled Chicken & Vegetable Platter	790	7	129
Grilled Chicken Fajita	330	16	25
Chicken Tenders	370	15	7
Grilled Chicken Hot Pasta	590	10	86
Baked Potato: with Broccoli	510	0.5	117
with Chicken	610	4	114
with Cheese	790	25	118
Salads			
Chicken on Gourmet Greens	350	11	31
Gourmet Greens Salad	220	7	31
Zesty Caesar	180	3	31
Zesty Chicken Caesar Salad	290	6	31
Side Kicks			
Ranch Fries: Regular	350	14	51
Large	420	17	62
Fruit Cup	90	0.5	18

Red Hot & Blue® (Oct '08)

BBQ Platters

	C	F	Cb
Five Meat Treat	1160	85	15
Memphis Half Chicken	1510	103	11
Pulled Chicken	365	24	7
Pulled Pork	485	34	7
Smoked Sausage	950	67	36
BBQ Sandwiches: Regular			
Carolina Chopped Pork	460	23	34
Pulled Chicken	390	17	36
Pulled Pork	470	23	37
Ribs, Half Slab: Dry	1350	100	32
Sweet	1320	95	40
Wet	1260	95	26

Red Hot & Blue cont... (Oct '08)

Salads

	C	F	Cb
Grilled Chicken Caesar	755	45	45
RH & B Chopped Salad	935	55	54
Smokehouse Salad	770	45	44
Southern Fried Chicken	690	31	58
Soup: Corn Chowder, 1 bowl	320	18	22
Kids: Chicken Tenders Meal	305	14	20

Red Lobster® (Oct '08)

	C	F	Cb
Fresh Fish:			
Broiled Flounder, lunch portion	240	5	0
Atlantic Salmon, full portion	580	33	0
Atlantic Salmon, half portion	260	12	0
Broiled Flounder, dinner portion	240	5	0
Rainbow Trout, full portion	510	25	6
Rainbow Trout, half portion	275	14	2
Tilapia, full portion	345	10	0
Tilapia, half portion	185	6	0
Meals:			
Grilled Chicken Breast	315	8	0
Signature Shellfish:			
Garlic Chili Jumbo Shrimp	140	3	1
Garlic Grilled Jumbo Shrimp	140	3	1
Chilled Jumbo Shrimp Cocktail	140	1	2
Live Maine Lobster, 1¼lb	145	1	2
Lobster Chops	320	8.5	0
North Pacific King Crab Legs	490	9	0
Rock Lobster Tail	260	3	0
Snow Crab Legs	260	4.5	0
Sides:			
100% Pure Melted Butter, 1 oz	190	21	0
Baked Potato w. Pico de Gallo	185	2	37
Baked Potato, no topping	180	2	36
Cheddar Bay Biscuit (1)	160	9	17
Cocktail Sauce, large	85	2	17
Garden Salad, no dressing	50	2	9
Jumbo Shrimp Cocktail	140	2	1
King Crab Legs	165	3	0
Lemon Wedge (1)	5	0	1
Petite Shrimp Topping	30	1	1
Red Wine Vinaigrette Dressing	50	3	5
Seasonal Vegetables w. butter	145	11	9
Seasoned Broccoli	55	0	10
Snow Crab Legs	130	2	0
Wild Rice Pilaf	205	5	36

For Complete Nutritional Data ~ see CalorieKing.com

Red Robin® (Oct '08)

Entrees	C	F	Cb
Artic Cod Fish & Chips	990	60	76
Carnitas Fajitas	1160	63	81
Chicken Parmigiano Pasta	1570	74	155
Clucks & Fries	1260	80	90
Buffalo Style	1485	106	91
Ensenada Chicken Platter	590	30	14
Jumbo Shrimp & Slaw Platter	1235	58	120
Red's Rice Bowl,	1010	29	64
Shrimp & Cod Duo	1405	83	107
Southwest Chicken Pasta	1540	89	121
Sandwiches & Burgers			
Chicken Burger: Blackened	790	48	50
California	980	62	50
Crispy	930	56	71
Jamaican Jerk'd	680	34	53
Teriyak	900	47	65
Whiskey River BBQ,	955	51	72
Classic Gourmet Burgers:			
5 Alarm	905	58	50
Blackened Bayou	860	57	44
Bleu Ribbon	1060	63	71
Cheeseburger	1030	70	47
Gourmet Cheeseburger	850	49	57
Guacamole Bacon	1150	76	52
Monster	1150	69	57
Royal	1180	82	48
Santa Fe	1035	63	63
Sauteed 'Shroom	970	60	52
Sicilian	1070	66	46
The Banzai	1055	63	69
Whiskey River BBQ	1130	69	72
Insanely Delicious Burgers			
Bruschetta Chicken	875	54	54
Chili Chili Cheeseburger	405	57	58
Honky Tonk BBQ Pork	680	24	78
Prime Rib Dip	990	56	57
Lighten Up Burgers: Crispy Fish	565	27	58
Grilled Salmon	745	38	52
Grilled Turkey	705	43	51
Lettuce-Wrapped Protein	440	27	10
The Garden, 1 burger, 10.4 oz	515	18	63
Wraps: Caesar's Chicken	1245	60	122
Whiskey River BBQ Chicken	1525	81	138
Meals			
Cheeseburger Con Queso	455	25	55
Chili Chili Nachos	1185	80	66
Chili Chili Nachos w. Chicken	1380	89	67
Creamy Artichoke & Spinach Dip	1200	73	101
Fresh-Fried Cheese Sticks	1180	70	86
Guacamole, Salsa & Chips	800	47	88
Just-in-Quesadilla	1075	55	72
RR's Buzzard Wings	1025	81	4
Towering Onion Rings	1835	124	160

Rita's® (Oct '08)

	C	F	Cb
Italian Ice: Kids, 7.5 oz	175	0	54
Regular, 12 oz	285	0	86
Large, 19 oz	445	0	136
Cream Ice: Kids, 7.5 oz	210	3	48
Regular, 12 oz	340	4.5	76
Large, 19 oz	535	7	120
Custard: Kids, 4 oz	270	15	145
Regular, 5.75 oz	385	21	43
Large, 7.5 oz	505	28	56
Gelati with Custard:			
Vanilla: Regular, 10 oz	375	12	63
Chocolate: Regular, 10 oz	365	11	64
Misto w. Custard:			
Vanilla: Reguar 15 oz	445	7	95
Large, 23 oz	670	11	143
Chocolate: Regular, 15 oz	440	6	96
Large, 23 oz	665	9	144
Blendini: *Per 11 oz*			
Banana Cream Pie; Berry Ban. Crunch	570	24	82
Chunky Chocolate Brownie	610	27	84
Coconut Cream Pie	580	25	82
Cookie Lover's Delight	620	27	87
Crazy Banana Split	570	25	83
Green Apple Pie A La Mode	560	24	81
Orange Cream Dream	560	27	74
Oreo Blitz	550	24	96
Pineapple Upside Down Cake	570	24	81
Strawb. Shortcake; Twisted Float	560	24	81
Vanilla Mango Crunch	580	24	84

For Complete Nutritional Data ~ see CalorieKing.com

Robeks (Oct '08)

Smoothies: Per 12 fl.oz	C	F	Cb
Acai Energizer	165	1	36
Big Wednesday	170	1	40
Cardio Cooler	215	1	44
Cranberry Quest	175	0	40
Dr. Robeks	180	1	40
Green Tea Sensation	220	1	42
Guava Lava	180	1	42
Hummingbird	185	1	44
Mahalo Mango	175	1	42
Malibu Peach	155	0	36
Outrageous Raspberry	175	1	39
Passionfruit Cove	170	1	38
Pomegranate Passion	195	0	48
Pomegranate Power	210	0	50
Raspberry Romance	170	0	42
Robeks Rejuvenator	195	1	43
Robeks MuscleMax	200	1	38
Strawnana Berry	180	0	44
Venice Burner	230	1	46
Zen Berry	190	1	45

Rocky Rococo® (Oct '08)

Pastas: Per Serving

	C	F	Cb
Can't Decide, 14 oz	465	9	77
Fettuccine w. Alfredo Sauce:			
Regular, 14 oz	460	14	66
Light, 7 oz	230	7	33
Spaghetti with Meat Sauce: Reg.	500	7	87
Light, 7 oz	250	3	44
Spaghetti w. Meatballs: Reg., 15 oz	630	16	89
Light, 7.5 oz	315	8	45
Spaghetti w. Tomato Sauce: Reg.	470	4	87
Light, 7 oz	235	2	44

Pizzas: Per Slice, ⅛ Pizza

	C	F	Cb
Cheese	380	9	54
Garden	390	10	56
Pepperoni	425	13	54
Sausage	495	19	54
Sausage Mushroom	500	19	55

Sides

	C	F	Cb
Breadsticks: w. Marinara Sce (6)	420	7	72
w. Jalapeno Cheese Sauce (6)	530	18	72
Wheat Muffin (1)	200	4	38

Roly Poly® (Oct '08)

Tortilla Wraps: Per Whole Wrap

	C	F	Cb
Baked Ham & Roast Pork:			
BarBQ Pork Melt	600	20	52
Italian Classic	660	24	56
Key West Cuban Mix	640	24	54
Peachtree Melt	650	22	56
Porky's Nightmare	620	24	52
Chicken: Basil Cashew Chicken	580	22	54
Catalina Chicken Salad	610	24	54
Chicken Caesar	620	24	56
Chicken Cordon Bleu	610	22	54
Chicken Fajita	620	25	54
Chicken Popper	560	18	58
Cobb Salad	640	28	56
Delhi Chicken	640	24	64
Hickory Chicken	670	22	54
Oriental Chicken	520	12	62
Santa Fe Chicken	610	24	54
Seafood: Popeye's Tuna	620	9	60
Classic Tuna Melt	670	36	54
Texas Tuna Melt	620	26	52
Thai Hot Tuna	650	26	54
Tuna Luau	650	30	58

Round Table® Pizza (Oct '08)

Appetizers

	C	F	Cb
Buffalo Wings, 6 pieces	420	28	2
Garlic Bread	470	21	59
with Cheese	630	33	59
Garlic Parmesan Twists, 3 pieces	500	14	73
Honey BBQ Wings 6 pieces	390	25	8

Pizzas (Large 14"): Per Slice, ½₂ Pizza

	C	F	Cb
Original Crust: Cheese	230	8	25
Chicken & Garlic Gourmet	240	9	25
Chicken Smokehouse	260	10	26
Gourmet Veggie	230	9	26
Guinevere's Garden Delight	210	7	26
Hawaiian	220	7	27
Italian Garlic Supreme	270	13	25
King Arthur Supreme	270	12	26
Maui Zaui with Polynesian Sce	260	9	29
Milano Roastano	280	14	25
Montague's All Meat Marvel	290	14	25
Pepperoni	240	10	24
Primo Supremo	390	18	35
Pan Crust: Cheese	300	9	38
Chicken & Garlic Gourmet	330	11	39
Chicken Smokehouse	350	12	39
Gourmet Veggie	320	11	40
Guinevere's Garden Delight	300	8	39
Hawaiian	310	8	40
Italian Garlic Supreme	360	15	39
King Arthur Supreme	340	12	39
Maui Zaui with Polynesian Sce	340	11	43
Milano Roastano,	350	14	39
Montague's All Meat Marvel	360	14	38
Pepperoni	320	11	38
Skinny Crust: Cheese	190	8	18
Chicken & Garlic Gourmet	210	9	19
Chicken Smokehouse	230	10	20
Gourmet Veggie	200	9	19
Guinevere's Garden Delight	180	7	20
Hawaiian	190	7	20
Italian Garlic Supreme	240	13	18
King Arthur Supreme	240	12	19
Maui Zaui with Polynesian Sce	220	9	22
Montague's All Meat Marvel	260	14	18
Pepperoni	210	10	18

Sandwiches:

	C	F	Cb
Chicken Club	760	34	67
Ham Club	810	37	76
RT Pizza	690	34	65
Turkey Club,	800	37	75
Turkey Sante Fe	850	44	74

For Complete Nutritional Data ~ see CalorieKing.com

Roy Rogers® (Oct '08)

Breakfast Itrems

	C	F	Cb
Big Country Breakfast: w. Bacon	740	43	61
w. Sausage	920	60	61
w. Ham	710	39	67
Burgers: Hamburger	260	9	33
Cheeseburger	300	13	34
¼ lb Hamburger	430	18	41
¼ lb Cheeseburger	470	22	42
Sourdough Grilled Chicken	500	21	46
Sandwiches: Roast Beef	260	4	30
Chicken Fillet	500	24	49
Grilled Chicken	340	11	32
Fries: Regular	350	15	49
Large	430	18	59
Desserts: Hot Fudge Sundae	320	10	50

Rubio's Mexican Grill®

(Oct '08)

	C	F	Cb
Burritos: Served with Chips			
Chicken	600	24	58
Steak	640	30	58
Big Burrito Especial: Chicken	820	30	115
Steak	870	36	103
Fish Burrito	800	45	73
Grilled Mesquite Shrimp Burrito	740	32	78
Mahi Mahi Burrito	730	37	56
Grilled Veggie Burrito	690	46	77
Health Mex: Chicken Burrito	540	13	73
Mahi Mahi Burrito	530	13	72
Tacos: Carnitas Rajas	260	17	28
Grilled Chicken	300	15	24
Fish, Especial	390	23	30
Health Mex: Chicken	190	4.5	23
Mahi Mahi	220	5	22
Grilled Mesquite Shrimp	280	14	26
Grilled Steak	250	11	23
Street: Chicken	110	3	9
Steak	110	3	9
World Famous Fish	330	18	29
Quesadillas: Cheese	890	59	55
Chicken; Steak	1000	61	57
Salads: Chicken Tropical	230	6	19
Chicken Chopped	400	17	31
Chicken Fiesta	340	18	11
Chipotle Chicken Ranch	460	20	40
Grande Bowl Chicken	550	18	60

Ruby Tuesday® (Oct '08)

	C	F	Cb
Appetizers: Per ¼ Order without Sides or Sauce			
Asian Dumplings	110	5	12
Cheddar Fries	300	17	27
Classic Sampler	340	19	27
Fire Wing	195	12	1
Grand Sampler	325	18	19
Jumbo Lump Crab Cake	110	8	4
Quesadillas: Chicken	230	14	13
Fresh Avocado	185	15	14
Southwestern Spring Rolls	175	10	15
Thai Phoon Shrimp	195	13	12
Beef: Without Sides or Sauce			
Baby Back Ribs,Asian Glazed, ½ Rack	655	46	18
Ribs: & Asian Chicken	1115	68	34
& Fire Wings	875	56	16
& Louisiana Fried Shrimp	1410	82	69
& Steak	700	37	16
Steaks: Bayou Sirloin	440	21	5
Peppercorn Mushroom Sirloin	605	36	16
Rib Eye	590	35	6
Sirloin & Bistro Chicken	740	34	21
Sirloin & Louisiana Fried Shrimp	630	22	42
Chicken: Without Sides			
Bistro Barbecue Chicken	845	45	25
Chicken Bella	625	36	14
Chicken Fresco	465	23	7
Chicken Oscar	470	22	4
Gourmet Chicken Pot Pie	1550	121	53
Sandwiches & Burgers: Per Burger without Sides			
Handcrafted Burgers			
Bacon Cheeseburger	1195	85	52
Bison Bacon Cheeseburge	1070	71	53
Buffalo Chicken	1040	71	67
Chicken BLT	980	63	64
Classic Cheeseburger	1105	78	52
Ruby Minis, 4 ruby minis	1310	90	74
Ruby's Classic	1015	71	52
Smokehouse	1390	96	77
Turkey	810	45	53
Veggie	955	52	75
Premium Burgers:			
Blackened Fish	795	44	49
Jumbo Lump Crab	755	45	63
The Ultimate Chkn Burge	1085	61	50
Triple Prime	885	56	53
Triple Prime Cheddar	1065	70	53

Updated Nutrition Data ~ www.CalorieKing.com
Persons with Diabetes ~ See Disclaimer (Page 24)

Ruby Tuesday® cont... (Oct '08)

Seafood: *Without Sides*

	C	F	Cb
Asian Glazed Salmon	425	27	7
Creole Catch	310	16	0
Lemon Grilled Salmon	505	37	2
Louisiana Fried Shrimp	425	17	40
New Orleans Seafood	495	31	2
Parmesan Shrimp Pasta	1220	64	108

Sides

	C	F	Cb
Baked Potato: w. Butter & Sour Crm	460	19	62
w. Cheese, Bacon, Sour Cream	615	32	63
Brown Rice Pilaf w. Cheese & Tom.	220	6	35
Creamy Mashed Cauliflower	155	10	14
Fries	360	13	57
Mashed Potatoes	255	15	33

Salads: *Without Dressing*

	C	F	Cb
Signature House	440	34	28
Tomato & Mozarella	110	7	7
Tossed Caesar	175	15	7
Sauteed Baby Portobella Mushr.	175	14	9

Salads: *Without Dressing*

	C	F	Cb
Carolina Chicken	975	68	40
Club House	655	45	16
Signature House, ¼ Order	440	34	28

Salad Dressings & Condiments: *Per 1 oz Serving*

	C	F	Cb
Balsamic Vinaigrette	35	2	4
Blue Cheese	175	19	1
Caesar	95	10	2
Creamy Parmesan	95	10	2
Ranch: Regular	100	11	1
Fresh Avocado	60	5	3
Light	55	5	1
Sour Cream	30	2	2

Sauces

	C	F	Cb
Asian Barbecue	60	3	7
Barbecue	50	0	13
Chocolate	100	1	24
Lemon Butter	95	9	1
Marinara	15	1	2
Parmesan Cream	95	9	2
Peanut	65	3	8
Sweet & Spicy Chile	170	17	2

Desserts

	C	F	Cb
Blondie	675	31	93
Cookie: Chocolate Chip	320	15	42
White Choc. Macadamia Nut	340	20	39
Double Chocolate Cake	955	48	118
Gourmet Cookie & Ice Cream	750	37	94
Strawberries & Ice Cream	915	50	98
Strawberry Cream Puff	840	40	103

For Complete Menu ~ see CalorieKing.com

Runza® (Oct '08)

Sandwiches

	C	F	Cb
Original Overstuffed Sandwich	495	17	65
Cheese Overstuffed Sandwich	555	21	66
BBQ Chicken Sandwich, grilled	390	9	46
Fish Sandwich	490	24	50
Polish Dog	425	26	30
Smothered Chicken, grilled	380	10	41
Special Deluxe Chicken, crispy	485	19	51

Burgers

	C	F	Cb
Junior: Cheeseburger	325	17	28
Cheeseburger Runza	305	14	30
Swiss Mushroom	380	21	26
Legendary: ¼ lb Cheeseburger	430	21	32
½ lb Double Cheeseburger	640	32	37
¼ lb Bacon Cheeseburger	515	29	36
¼ lb Legend Supreme	765	37	62
¼ lb Swiss Cheese Mushroom	450	25	36

Sides

	C	F	Cb
French Fries: Small, 3.1 oz	280	15	31
Medium	410	23	46
Large	625	35	70
Frings, 6.3 oz	540	28	64
Onion Rings: Medium, 4 oz	370	20	41
Large, 6.5 oz	590	32	66
Onion Ring Dip, 2.1 oz	90	6	4

Salads: *No Dressing*

	C	F	Cb
Tossed Salad w. Crispy Chicken	435	27	29
Tossed Salad w. Grilled Chicken	275	13	13
Dressing: Ranch, 2.4 oz	300	32	5
Reduced Calorie Ranch, 2.5 oz	170	11	17
Lite Italian, 2.6 oz	85	5	10
Raspberry Vinaigrette	25	0	6

Soups: *Per Bowl*

	C	F	Cb
Boston Clam Chowder	320	23	33
Broccoli Cheese	360	27	35
Cauliflower Cheese	335	26	32
Chicken Noodle	170	5	21
Homemade Chili	310	10	26
Potato w. Bacon	305	20	40
Vegetable Cheese	330	22	28
Wisconsin Cheese	425	35	36
Kids-Size: Mini Corn Dogs (5)	275	17	25
Chicken Strips (2)	185	10	11

Desserts & Drinks

	C	F	Cb
Chocolate Chip Cookie (1)	310	16	34
Vanilla Shake, regular, 12 fl.oz	465	16	69
Oreo Shake, regular, 12 fl.oz	605	24	84
Pepsi Slushie, medium, 18 fl.oz	225	0	60

243

Ryan's® Family Steakhouse (Oct '08)

Main Courses: Sides Not Included	C	F	Cb
BBQ Beef, 6 oz	225	12	9
BBQ Chicken, ¼, 5 oz	230	15	5
Carved Turkey Breast, 6 oz	280	12	0
Chkn Fried Beef Steak (1), no gravy	180	9	16
Chkn Fried Beef Steak (1), w. gravy	220	11	24
Chicken Pot Pie, 8 oz	350	16	48
Grilled Chicken Breast, plain, 6 oz	280	18	0
Grilled Pork Chop: Plain, 1 chop	240	14	1
BBQ; Teriyaki, avg., 1 chop	160	8	8
Grilled Salmon, 7 oz entree	240	9	0
Grilled Sliced Sausage: BBQ Sce, 6 oz	555	48	8
in Peppers and Onions, 8 oz	450	42	6.5
Grilled Teriyaki Chicken Thighs, 6 oz	215	6	6
Macaroni and Cheese, 8 oz	350	16	40
Meat Lasagne, 8 oz	370	16	30
Meat Loaf, 4 oz	220	12	9
Mexican Casserole, 8 oz	415	16	46
Pizza: Cheese, 1 slice, 3½ oz	200	10	11
Pepperoni, 1 slice, 3½ oz	230	13	10
Rotisserie Chicken, ¼, 5 oz	250	15	0
Salisbury Steak w. gravy, 1 patty	200	11	11
Sirloin Steak: 8 oz	485	33	0
10½ oz	640	44	0
16 oz	970	67	0
Sirloin Tips, 5.5 oz	330	23	0
Stuffed Alaskan Pollock Fillet, 6 oz	360	30	18
Taco Beef, 4 oz	180	10	8
Vegetable Lasagne, 8 oz	355	16	30
White Turkey w. gravy, 6 oz	140	3	6.5
Sides: Baked Potato, plain, 8 oz	250	0	57
Bowtie Pasta and Veges, 8 oz	210	0	38
Chicken Salad, Low-Fat, 8 oz	245	4	24
Coleslaw, 4 oz	180	12	12
Corn Cobbet (1) 4 oz	90	6	11
Garlic Mashed Potatoes, 4 oz	120	4	16
Glazed Baby Carrots w. Sauce, 4 oz	125	8	12
Low Carb Grilled Veggies, 8 oz	40	0	8
Marinated 7-Bean Salad, 6 oz	300	0	66
Pinto Beans, 4 oz	105	2	16
Potato Salad, 6 oz	280	12	33
Sweet Pot. w. M'mallows, 4 oz	240	18	16
Yellow Squash w. Onions, 4 oz	50	2	7
Desserts: Cheesecake, 1 sl.	190	15	11
Ice Cream Cone (flat bottom)	20	0	4
Key Lime Pie, 1 slice	410	17	58
Lemon Creme Cake, 1 slice	170	15	9
Cookies: Oatmeal Raisin (1)	110	3.5	18
Sugar Cookie (1)	120	5	18

7-Eleven® (Oct '08)

Breakfast Sandwiches	C	F	Cb
Big Bite Breakfast Sandwich	430	27	29
Croissant: w. Bacon, Egg & Chse	400	33	34
w. Ham, Egg & Chse	390	22	34
Engl. Muffin w. Saus., Egg, Chse	450	24	37
Sausage, Egg & Cheese Biscuit	500	31	34
Sausage, Egg & Twister Roll	430	27	29
Hot Dogs (Big Bite)			
¼ Pound Hot Dog, no bun	360	34	6
⅓ Pound Hot Dog, no bun	480	45	3
Spicy Bite, 1 link, 4 oz	425	38	2
Bacon Cheeseburger Bite, no bun	270	12	1
Reynaldo's Jumbo Burritos (10 oz)			
Beef & Bean; Beef & Potato	590	20	82
Red Hot Burrito	640	20	88
Green Burrito	710	26	93
Sandwiches (7-Eleven)			
Black Forest Ham	380	6	59
Chicken Salad, 7.3 oz	500	28	44
Chicken w. Ancho Lime Spread	500	26	47
Classic Chicken Caesar, 8.3 oz	590	27	45
Classic Sub on Roll, 7.6 oz	380	6	49
Combo Sub w. Turkey, 5.5 oz	270	7	33
Ham & Swiss, 4.9 oz	330	11	39
Hearty Ham, 8.3 oz	570	30	48
Pastrami & Swiss on Wheat	480	21	48
Smoked Turkey w. Chse/Mayo	550	27	46
Turkey & Ham on Tom. Basil Brd	490	23	42
Turkey & Ham on White Bread	350	6	53
Tuna Salad, 7.5 oz	540	27	45
Bakery Stix™ Treats: *Per Stick (3.5 oz)*			
Grilled Cheese	270	11	30
Ham & Cheese	280	12	32
Pepperoni & Cheese	340	18	30
Sushi: California Rolls, 3 pieces	155	2	39
Imperial Rolls, 3 pieces	210	11	22
Salads			
Tuna Macaroni Salad, 8 oz	270	8	29
Reser's Coleslaw, 3½ oz	130	7	17
Reser's Macaroni Salad, 3½ oz	220	15	20
Reser's Potato Salad, 3½ oz	200	10	19
Go-Go Taquitos			
Beef Taco & Cheese, 3 oz (1)	250	11	30
Fiesta Chicken, 3 oz (1)	220	12	23
Jalapeno & Cream Cheese, 3 oz	240	13	27
Monterey Jack Chkn, 3 oz (1)	280	14	30
Go-Go French Toast Sticks, 3 oz	270	16	23

Updated Nutrition Data ~ www.CalorieKing.com
Persons with Diabetes ~ See Disclaimer (Page 24)

7-Eleven® cont... (Oct '07)

Donuts & Muffins (World Ovens) C F Cb

	C	F	Cb
Donuts: Blueberry Cake (1)	330	22	31
Chocolate Iced (1)	250	11	35
Glazed (1)	250	16	24
Jelly (1)	420	16	66
Sour Cream Donut (1)	450	19	65
Muffins: Banana Nut, 7 oz	660	26	97
Blueberry, 5.6 oz	310	8	54
Brownies: Original, 5 oz	570	28	83
Peanut Butter Cup Brownie, 4.4 oz	560	20	55
Walnut Brownie, 5 oz	600	31	78

Fountain Drinks (Figures Assume ⅓ Ice)

Coca-Cola/Pepsi/Dr.Pepper/7Up:

	C	F	Cb
Gulp, 20 oz	195	0	51
Big Gulp, 32 oz	310	0	82
Super Gulp, 44 oz	430	0	112
Double Gulp, 64 oz	625	0	163
Diet Coke/Diet Pepsi, 16 oz	1	0	0
Slurpees: Average All Flavors,			
12 oz size	95	0	24
22 oz size	175	0	44
28 oz size	220	0	56
40 oz size	315	0	80
Crystal Light, 12 fl.oz	45	0	9
Hawaiian Punch; Dr Pepper, avg.,			
12 oz size	180	0	48
22 oz size	330	0	88
28 oz size	420	0	112
40 oz size	600	0	160
Cafe Select Coffee: 12 fl.oz	8	0	2
16 fl.oz size	10	0	2
20 fl.oz size	14	0	3
24 fl.oz size	16	0	4
Hot Drinks: Hot Chocolate, 8 fl.oz	180	3	36
French Vanilla Cappuccino, 8 fl.oz	160	6	26

Sammy's®
Woodfired Pizza (Oct '08)

Healthy Dining Meals C F Cb

	C	F	Cb
Pasta, Tomato Angel Hair Pasta	700	18	115
Individual Salad: Chinese Chicken	450	12	47
Chopped Chicken	425	11	30
Oak Roasted Salmon on Ponzu	470	19	21
Fresh Tomato Basil Soup	110	5	10
Roast Chicken Pesto Wrap	480	20	22

Samurai Sam's® (Oct '08)

Bowls: With White Rice C F Cb

	C	F	Cb
Low-Carb, regular	230	4	16
Spicy Beef 'n Broccoli: Regular	620	13	97
Large	930	16	152
Sweet & Sour White Chicken: Reg.	580	4.5	96
Large	820	6	136
Teriyaki Dark Chicken, regular	540	10	79
Teriyaki Steak: Regular	530	8	86
Large	750	11	123
Teriyaki Veggie: Regular	365	1	81
Large	525	1	117
Yakisoba Bowls: Shrimp	680	10	110
Steak	810	20	112
White Chicken	795	14	114
Veggie	510	8	110

Wraps: With White Rice

	C	F	Cb
Teriyaki White Chicken	640	11	96
Teriyaki Steak	650	14	101
Teriyaki Veggie	510	8	94

Sandella's Flatbread Cafe (Oct '08)

Wraps C F Cb

	C	F	Cb
Chicken Fajita	465	15	54
Classic BLT	670	28	54
Pacific Chicken	530	21	59
Pesto Turkey	460	16	57
Spicy Roast Beef	590	14	56
Paninis			
Chicken Delicato	515	21	51
Spinach, Ham & Swis	480	14	55
Tuscan Chicken	560	24	55
Turkey & Mozzarella	515	22	54
Quesadillas			
California	525	24	52
Chicken Fajita	435	12	52
Mediterranean	325	10	50
Grilled Flatbread			
Aloha	635	21	71
Brazilian Chicken	550	13	72
Pesto Chicken	560	23	53
Spinach & Bacon	685	39	50
Vegetarian	420	11	62
Salads			
Chef's Salad	550	25	55
Greek Salad	320	8	53
Rice Bowls			
Cheddar Chicken & Broccoli	795	9	146
Chicken Fajita	700	9	124

For Extra Menu Items ~ see CalorieKing.com

Sbarro's® (Oct '08)

Entrees	C	F	Cb
Baked Ziti w. Sauce	700	41	43
Chicken Parmigiana	520	22	16
Meat Lasagna	650	37	36
Spaghetti w. Sauce	820	28	120
Pizza: Per Slice (Thin Crust)			
Cheese	460	13	60
Pepperoni	730	37	61
Sausage	670	31	60
Supreme	630	27	63
Stuffed Pizza: Per Slice			
Spinach & Broccoli	790	34	89
Pepperoni	960	42	89

Schlotzsky's® (Oct '08)

	C	F	Cb
Oven-Toasted Sandwiches: Per Medium Sandwich			
Angus: Beef & Provolone	755	29	80
Corned Beef Reuben	920	41	78
Corned Beef	580	13	77
Pastrami Reuben	920	40	78
Pastrami & Swiss	905	36	82
Roast, Beef & Cheese	785	33	73
BLT	545	18	74
Chicken & Pesto	565	14	72
Chicken Breast	510	6	77
Chipotle Chicken	550	14	68
Dijon Chicken	575	11	79
Homestyle Tuna	565	16	73
Mediterranean Tuna	505	7	76
Santa Fe Chicken	620	15	76
Smoked Turkey Breast	515	9	76
Smoked Turkey Reuben	905	39	83
Texas Schlotzsky's	755	31	73
Turkey & Guacamole	565	13	80
Turkey Bacon Club	785	31	76
Original Style: The Original	770	34	76
Deluxe	955	46	78
Ham & Cheese	730	27	78
Turkey	830	35	78
Panini: Classic Swiss & Tomato	625	26	63
Grilled Chicken Romano	570	16	62
Italiano	735	32	67
Mozzarella & Portobello	485	15	63
Smoked Ham Crostini	645	23	67
Smoked Turkey & Guacamole	605	21	68
Wraps: Asian Chicken	535	11	80
Feta & Portobello	620	39	55
Grilled Chicken & Guacamole	695	36	59
Homestyle Tuna	455	17	55
Mediterranean Tuna	420	12	57
Parmesan Chicken Caesar	650	33	56

Schlotzsky's® cont... (Oct '08)

8" Pizzas: Per Pizza	C	F	Cb
BBQ Chicken & Jalapeno	715	16	99
Baby Spinach Salad	470	8	83
Bacon, Tomato & Portobello	615	22	76
Combination Special	640	25	76
Double Cheese	600	21	74
8" Pizzas (Cont): Per Pizza			
Fresh Tomato & Pesto	555	19	73
Grilled Chicken & Pesto	685	22	85
Mediterranean	560	20	74
Pepperoni & Double Cheese	685	30	74
Smoked Turkey & Jalapeno	640	19	78
Thai Chicken	725	23	85
Vegetarian Special	540	17	74
Salads: without Dressing/Croutons Unless Indicated			
Baby Spinach & Feta	195	15	10
Caesar Salad	105	5	10
Chicken Salad	290	15	12
Fruit Salad	100	0	25
Garden Salad	50	1	12
Greek Salad	135	8	13
Grilled Chicken Caesar w. Croutons	220	8	12
Ham & Turkey Chef Salad	255	13	14
Pasta Salad	70	3	12
Potato Salad	240	13	29
Side Salad	25	1	7
Turkey Chef Salad	305	16	15
Kid's Meals: Without Cookie or Drink			
Cheese Pizza	480	13	73
Cheese Sandwich	395	15	48
Ham & Cheese Sandwich	425	16	49
Pepperoni Pizza	525	17	73
Turkey Sandwich	305	5	49
Desserts			
Brownie	415	24	47
Carrot Cake	715	42	80
Cheesecake	350	23	30
Cookies: Chocolate Chip	160	7	24
Fudge Chocolate Chip	160	7	23
Oatmeal Raisin	145	5	24
Sugar	150	6	23
White Choc Macadamia	165	8	23

Second Cup® ~ *see CalorieKing.com*

Updated Nutrition Data ~ www.CalorieKing.com
Persons with Diabetes ~ See Disclaimer (Page 24)

Shakey's® (Oct '08)

Pizzas (12"): Per Slice (1/10 Pizza)

	C	F	Cb
Cheese only:			
Thin Crust	135	5	13
Thick Crust	170	5	22
Homestyle Pan	305	14	31
Onion/Olives/Mushrooms:			
Thin Crust	125	5	14
Thick Crust	160	4	22
Homestyle Pan	320	15	32
Sausage Pepperoni:			
Thin Crust	165	8	13
Thick Crust	205	8	22
Homestyle Pan	375	20	31
Sausage Mushroom			
Thin Crust	140	6	13
Thick Crust	180	6	22
Homestyle Pan	340	17	31
Pepperoni:			
Thin Crust	150	7	13
Thick Crust	185	6	22
Homestyle Pan	345	15	31
Shakey's Special:			
Thin Crust	170	9	13
Thick Crust	210	8	22
Homestyle Pan	385	21	32
Other Items			
3-Piece Chicken & Potato	945	56	51
5-Piece Fried Chicken & Potato	1700	90	130
Hot Ham & Cheese Sandwich	550	21	56
Potato Wedges, 15 pieces	950	36	120
Shakey's Super Hot Hero	810	44	67
Spagh. w. Meat Sce/Garlic Bread	940	33	134

Sheetz® (Oct '08)

	C	F	Cb
M.T.O Breakfast: Includes Cheese			
Shmagels: Bacon & Egg	575	28	53
Egg	425	16	51
Ham & Egg	490	17	54
Shmiscuits: Bacon & Egg	595	37	40
Egg	445	28	38
Ham & Egg	510	26	41
Sausage & Egg	620	42	38
Shmuffins: Bacon & Egg	465	27	30
Egg	315	15	28
Ham & Egg	380	16	31
Sausage & Egg	490	32	28
Steak & Egg	505	25	29

Sheetz® (Oct '08)

	C	F	Cb
Coffeez™: Per 16 fl.oz			
Hot Chocolate, medium	250	4	52
Cupo'ccino®: Per Medium (16 fl.oz)			
Cupo'ccino: Almond Amaretto	275	8	52
Fat-Free French Vanilla	140	0	34
M.T.O Cold Subs: Per 6" Sub (No Cheese Unless Indicated)			
BLT Sub	405	13	53
Cheese	255	1	51
Chicken Salad	505	22	60
Club	375	4	56
Deli	370	10	54
Ham	330	3	54
Italian	450	12	53
Roast Beef	295	3	52
Tuna Salad	470	17	60
Turkey	310	3	53
M.T.O Hot Subs: Per 6" Sub			
Chicken	375	5	51
Meatball w. Marinara Sauce	395	12	55
Pepperoni	455	19	51
Steak	445	11	52
M.T.O Deli Bagel: No Cheese Unless Indicated			
Chicken Salad	490	23	57
Deli	355	11	51
Ham & Cheese	125	1	15
Italian	430	13	50
Roast Beef	310	4	48
Tuna Salad	455	18	57
Turkey	290	4	50
M.T.O Hot Dogz: No Cheese			
Deli Dogz,	610	32	53
Hot Dogz	265	15	24
M.T.O Nachos: Per Serving, No Topping			
Nachos Bueno w. Nacho cheese	505	23	65
M.T.O Salads: No Dressing Unless Indicated			
Chef Salad	145	3	12
Crispy Chicken	270	8	30
Garden Salad	25	0	7
Grilled Chicken	145	4	7
Grilled Chicken Caesar w. Dressing	405	27	19
Steak Salad	215	10	8
Taco Salad	255	10	38
Sides			
Fryz: Bag, 3.2 oz	160	6.5	23
Cup, 5.1 oz	260	11	37
Cheese, 14.3 oz	650	30	81
Smokehouse, 15.3 oz	975	52	103

Shoney's® (Oct '08)

Breakfast	C	F	Cb
All Star, no Sides	190	15	1.5
Big Eater Steak, no Sides	630	41	1.5
Country Fried Steak	995	66	49
Biscuits, biscuit	310	14	41
Biscuits & Gravy, serving	685	32	88
Biscuits, Sausage, biscuit	540	34	42
Black/Blueberries, ¼ cup, 1.3 oz	20	0	5
Half Stack Pancake Platter	930	14	187
Sunrise Breakfast	975	60	88
Burgers: All American	690	32	44
A A Bacon Cheeseburger	890	49	45
Famous Patty Melt	945	60	40
Half-O-Pound Burger	1350	53	130
Mushroom Swiss	970	58	49
Sandwiches: Blackened Chicken	885	21	122
Charbroiled Chicken, sandwich	895	22	122
Chicken Parmesan, sandwich	750	30	80
Corned Beef Reuben, sandwich	795	53	37
Fish, sandwich	825	17	127
Fried Chicken, sandwich	560	15	77
Hot Roast Beef w. Potatoes & Gravy	770	24	95
Hot Turkey w. Potatoes & Gravy	840	30	94
Original Slim Jim	1005	34	123
Raymond's French Dip	500	15	54
Turkey Club	950	53	47
Ultimate Grilled Cheese	895	47	77
Beef: BBQ Ribs	1520	78	125
Choice Sirloin	1225	51	128
Half-O-Pound: w. Mushrooms	1315	53	128
with Grilled Onions	1335	52	133
Southwest	1305	69	83
Ribeye	1480	75	128
T-Bone	1810	100	128
Rib Combos:			
¼ Rack & BBQ Chicken w. Fries	1230	54	104
¼ Rack & Fried Shrimp w. Frie	1145	51	114
¼ Rack & Gr. Shrimp w. Fries	1125	53	103
¼ Rack & Tenderloins w. Fries	1370	70	121
Surf & Turf: Ribeye & 5 Fried Shrimp	1640	82	139
Ribeye & 6 Grilled Shrimp	1590	81	128
Sirloin & 5 Fried Shrimp	1380	58	139
Sirloin & 6 Grilled Shrimp	1330	57	128
T-Bone & 5 Fried Shrimp	1965	107	139
T-Bone & 6 Grilled Shrimp	1920	106	128

Shoney's® cont... (Oct '08)

Blue Plate Specials	C	F	Cb
Baked Whitefish	505	8.5	58
Cajun Whitefish	480	11	56
Grandma's Meatloaf w. Glaze	1090	47	93
Grandma's Meatloaf w. Gravy	1090	49	88
Grilled Liver & Onions	710	22	80
Ham Steak Dinner	665	26	60
Original Country Fried Steak	1150	62	103
Roast Beef Platter	880	30	96
Chicken: Chicken Stir-Fry	1200	35	172
Charbroiled Blackened Chicken	830	26	100
Charbroiled Chicken Breast	795	23	99
Fried Chicken Tenderloins	1155	61	121
Monterey Chicken	910	40	84
Smothered Chicken	890	35	90
Seafood: Fried Fish Platter	1050	39	123
Grilled Salmon	750	19	95
Grilled Shrimp	720	20	96
Lite: Grilled Cod, serving	200	4	1
Grilled Salmon	180	4	0
Grilled Shrimp	320	9	30
Shrimp Stir-Fry	875	19	131
Shrimper's Feast	1030	40	128
Pastas: Chicken Alfredo	1705	78	171
Italian Feast	1435	46	204
Pasta Ya Ya	1845	81	176
Shrimp Alfredo	1780	85	172
Kids Menu: Junior Chicken	190	10	12
Junior Fish & Chips	310	12	30
Sides: Baked Potato, Plain,	345	6.5	68
French Fries, 4 oz	215	11	26
Macaroni & Cheese, ½ cup	240	15	18
Mashed Potatoes & Gravy	225	10	30
Onion Rings (7)	500	15	83
Sweet Potato Casserole, 4 oz	245	6	44
Turnip Greens, 4 oz	45	3.5	4
Desserts			
Cheesecake, 1 slice, 4 oz	365	26	23
Pies: Apple a la Mode	1205	53	174
Cherry Nutrasweet	465	18	66
Original Strawberry	330	17	45
Peach Nutrasweet	480	21	68
Sundaes: Caramel	620	27	83
Hot Fudge	600	30	75
Strawberry	610	28	86
Ultimate Hot Fudge Cake	875	37	127
Walnut Brownie a la Mode	575	34	61
Milk Shakes: Chocolate	1080	52	142
Strawberry	1115	50	151
Vanilla	1075	50	139.5

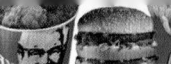

Sizzler® (Oct '08)

Hot Entrees: *(No Sides)*	C	F	Cb
Hamburger	625	33	36
Dakota Ranch Steak: 6 oz	315	20	0
8 oz	420	27	0
9½ oz	500	32	0
Hibachi Chicken Breast,			
w. Pineapple	195	3	13
Lemon-Herb Chicken Breast	140	3	0
Malibu Chicken Patty, each	310	19	11
Salmon	250	12	0
Santa Fe Chicken Breast	150	3	0
Shrimp: Broiled	150	6	0
Fried, 4 only	225	2	35
Mini	150	1	24
Shrimp Scampi	145	3	0
Swordfish	315	14	0

Low Carb Grill Menu

	C	F	Cb
Grilled Salmon w. Broccoli	405	19	14
Hibachi Chicken w. Broccoli	295	6	15
Petite Sizzler Steak w. Broccoli	520	26	11

Hot Bar

	C	F	Cb
Broccoli Chse Soup, 4 oz	140	9	10
Chicken Noodle Soup, 4 oz	30	1	4
Chicken Wings, 1 oz	75	4	4
Clam Chowder, 4 oz	120	6	11
Focaccia Bread, 2 pces	110	7	9
Meatballs, 4 balls	155	11	5
Minestrone Soup, 4 oz	35	0	7
Pasta: Fettucine, 2 oz	80	1	15
Spaghetti, 2 oz	80	0	16
Potato Skins, 2 oz	160	8	22
Refried Beans, ¼ cup	60	1	11
Saltine Crackers, 2 crackers	25	1	4
Taco Filling, 2 oz	105	9	3
Taco Shells, each	50	2	7
Dessert Bar: Chocolate Syrup, 1 oz	90	0	21
Choc/Vanilla Soft Serve, 4 oz	135	4	24
Strawberry Topping, 1 oz	70	0	18
Whipped Topping, 1 Tbsp	10	1	1

Salads & Toppings

Prepared Salads: *Per 2 oz*	C	F	Cb
Carrot & Raisin	130	10	10
Chinese Chicken; Teriyaki Beef	55	2	6
Mediterranean Minted Fruit	30	0	7
Mexican Fiesta	55	1	10
Old Fashioned Potato	85	5	10
Red Herb Potato	120	9	9

Sizzler® cont... (Oct '08)

Salads & Toppings (Cont	C	F	Cb
Seafood	55	3	4
Seafood Louis Pasta	65	2	9
Spicy Jicama	15	0	4
Tuna Pasta	135	10	6

Sides

	C	F	Cb
Baked Potato, plain	220	0	50
Cottage Cheese, 2 oz	50	1	2
Eggs, 1 oz	45	3	0
Garbanzo Beans, ¼ cup	65	1	11
Kidney Beans, ¼ cup	50	0	10
Olives, 1 oz	60	6	1
Peaches, ¼ cup	35	0	9
Peas, ¼ cup	30	0	6
Real Bacon Bits, 1 Tbsp	30	2	1
Turkey Ham, 1 oz	60	5	0

Dressings: *Per 2 Tbsp (1 oz)*	C	F	Cb
Blue Cheese	110	12	1
Honey Mustard	160	16	4
Italian, Lite	15	0	2
Japanese Rice Vinegar, Fat-Free	10	0	2
Parmesan Italian	100	10	2
Ranch	120	12	2
Ranch, Reduced-Calorie	90	8	4
Thousand Island	145	15	3

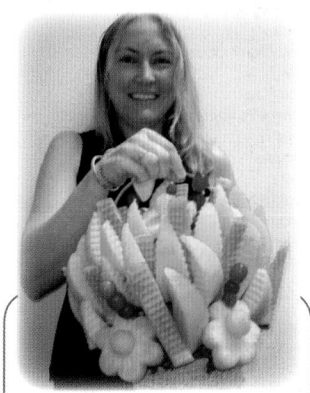

Balance eating out with fruit and veggies
(EdibleArrangements.com)

Skyline Chili® (Oct '08)

Burritos	C	F	Cb
All Chili Burrito	560	30	37
All Chili Deluxe Burrito	650	35	45
Salads: *Without Dressing*			
Buffalo Chicken Salad	150	7	7
Classic Chicken Salad	150	7	8
Garden Salad	80	5	6
Greek Chicken Salad	170	8	9
Greek Salad	60	3.5	5
Southwestern Chkn w. Tortilla Chips	760	44	66
Meals: *Per Regular Serving*			
Coney w. Cheese	340	22	17
Coney, no Cheese	220	12	17
Black Bean & Rice, 3-Way	800	40	74
Black Bean & Rice, 4-Way	810	40	77
Black Bean & Rice, 5-Way	880	40	89
Black Bean & Rice, Spaghetti	490	12	79
Bowls:			
Chili	270	16	6
Chili Bean	270	12	17
Chili Cheese	440	30	6
Coney	870	69	9
Loaded Chili	580	40	18
Vegetarian Black Beans & Rice	320	9	46
Chili Spaghetti:			
Regular	450	18	43
w. Bean & Onion	530	17	64
w. Bean	520	17	61
w. Onion	470	17	51
Steamed Potatoes:			
Plain	310	0	72
Cheddar	740	41	72
Chili	440	8	74
Sour Cream	570	27	72
Wraps			
Buffalo Chicken	520	21	55
Classic Chicken	510	21	55
Greek Chicken	510	21	54
Southwest Chicken	670	30	85
Sides:			
Cheese	230	19	1
Chili	130	8	3
Crackers	100	3	20
French Fries	630	33	79

Smoothie King® (Oct '08)

Fruit Smoothies (Low-Fat): Per 20 fl.oz Cup
Figures Include Turbinado. Without Turbinado,
deduct 100 calories and 23 carbs.

	C	F	Cb
Angel Food	355	0	84
Blackberry Dream	365	1	88
Cranberry Cooler	495	0	120
Cranberry Supreme	555	1	130
Grape Expectations	400	0	95
Mangofest	285	0	72
Muscle Punch	365	1	75
Orange Ka-BAM	465	0	117
Peach Slice	315	0	72
Pineapple Pleasure	280	0	66
Raspberry Sunrise	390	0	95
Strawberry Kiwi Breeze	375	0	90
Youth Fountain	255	0	61
Slim-N-Trim: Chocolate	300	2	57
Orange Vanilla	215	1	46
Strawberry	375	1	84
Vanilla	255	1	53
High Protein Smoothies: Per 20 fl.oz			
Almond Mocha	365	9	42
Banana	320	9	32
Chocolate	365	9	42
Lemon	370	9	44
Pineapple	320	9	29
Shredder: Chocolate	310	3	36
Strawberry	355	1	56
The Activator: Chocolate	405	1	83
Strawberry	555	1	121

32 fl.oz Cup: Multiply 20 fl.oz figures by 1.5
40 fl.oz Cup: Multiply 20 fl.oz figures by 2

Exotic Smoothies: Per 20 fl.oz Cup

Acai Adventure	435	5	92
Go Goji	435	0	104
Green Tea Tango	305	4	54
Mangosteen Madness	385	0	94
Passion Passport	395	0	96
Sorbet Smoothies: Per 20 fl.oz Cup			
Banana Berry Treat	370	0	88
Berry Punch	365	0	93
Fruit Fusion	360	10	84
Island Impact	310	0	73
Raspberry Collider	345	0	88

32 fl.oz Cup: Multiply 20 fl.oz figures by 1.5
40 fl.oz Cup: Multiply 20 fl.oz figures by 2

For Complete Nutritional Data ~ see CalorieKing.com

Smoothie King® cont...(Oct '08)

Kids Kup Smoothies

	C	F	Cb
Berry Interesting	275	0	69
Choc-A-Laka	250	3	45
Gimme-Grape	265	0	64
Smarti Tarti	200	0	49

Snappy Tomato (Oct '08)

Pizza: Per Slice (⅛ Pizza)

	C	F	Cb
Buffalo Grilled Chicken	250	8	32
Cheese Pizza	220	7	30
Hawaiian Pizza	370	18	33
Pepperoni Pizza	340	17	31
Ranch Pizza	370	21	31
Snapperoni Pizza	390	22	31
Meat Topper	430	23	31
Supreme Pizza	340	17	32
Veggie Pizza	240	8	33

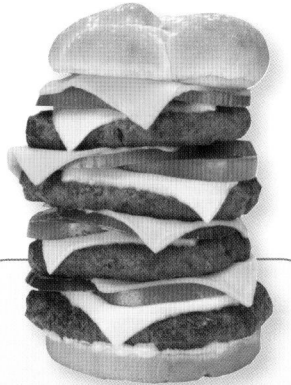

*This **Quadruple Bypass Burger**® is offered by Heart Attack Grill in Chandler, Arizona.*

With some 5000 calories, it contains 2 lbs beef, 4 fried eggs, 8 slices cheese, mayo and garnish – all in a large bun dipped in pure lard.

Definitely not for anyone with a heart!
(Photo: Ken Epstein)

Sonic Drive-In® (Oct '08)

Burgers

	C	F	Cb
Sonic Burger w. Mayonnaise	650	37	55
Sonic Burger w. Mustard	560	26	54
Sonic Cheeseburger w. Mayo	720	42	56
Sonic Cheeseburger w. Mustard	620	31	55
Sonic Bacon Cheeseburger	780	48	57
Super Sonic Chseburger: w. Mayo	980	64	58
w. Mustard	890	53	57
Jr. Burger	310	15	30
Jr. Cheeseburger	380	20	31

Sandwiches/Coneys/Wraps

	C	F	Cb
Coney: Extra-Long Cheese (1)	600	33	54
Corn Dog (1)	210	11	32
Sandwiches: Breaded Chicken	580	33	496
Grilled Chicken	340	12	32
Toaster Sandwiches: Chkn Club	740	46	55
Bacon Cheeseburger	670	39	52
Wraps: Chicken Strip	470	20	54
Fritos Chili Cheese	670	38	66
Grilled Chicken	380	11	44

Chicken

	C	F	Cb
Chicken Strip Dinner	930	43	100
Jumbo Popcorn Chicken:			
Snack, no Sauce, 4 oz	380	22	27
Large, no Sauce, 6 oz	560	32	41

Fresh Tastes Salads: No Dressing

	C	F	Cb
Grilled Chicken	310	13	19
Jumbo Popcorn Chicken	480	27	39
Santa Fe Grilled Chicken	380	15	29

Salad Dressings & Sauce: Per Serving (2 oz)

	C	F	Cb
Golden Italian Fat-Free	50	0	13
Honey Mustard	240	21	14
Original Ranch	260	28	0
Original Ranch Light	120	7	14
Popcorn Chicken Sauces: BBQ	45	0	11
Honey Mustard	90	7	7
Ranch	150	16	1

Sides

	C	F	Cb
French Fries: Plain, regular, 2.6 oz	220	9	32
w. Cheese, regular, 3.3 oz	280	14	33
w. Chili & Cheese, regular, 4.3 oz	310	16	35
Mozzarella Sticks (5), no Sauce	440	22	40
Onion Rings, regular, 5½ oz	440	21	55
Tater Tots: Plain, regular, 3 oz	220	9	32
w. Cheese, regular, 3.6 oz	310	21	26
w. Chili & Cheese, regular, 4.6 oz	340	23	27

Sonic Drive-In®cont... (Oct '08)

Breakfast	C	F	Cb
Burritos: Bacon Egg & Cheese	450	26	38
Ham Egg & Cheese	440	23	37
Sausage Egg & Cheese	470	30	38
SuperSonic	550	35	47
French Toast Sticks: w. Syrup (4)	580	31	70
no Syrup (4)	500	31	49
Breakfast Sandwiches			
Bistro: Bacon Egg & Cheese	510	30	37
Ham Egg & Cheese	460	24	36
Sausage Egg & Cheese	590	40	37
Toaster: Bacon Egg & Cheese	530	32	40
Ham Egg & Cheese	490	26	40
Sausage Egg & Cheese	620	42	40
Desserts: Per Regular			
Banana Split	420	9	80
Vanilla Cone	180	6	30
Vanilla Dish	240	9	36
Cream Pie Shakes: Reg., Banana	590	19	98
Chocolate	660	19	114
Coconut	580	20	93
Strawberry	620	19	106
CreamSlush;			
Lemon-Berry; Strawb., avg.	450	12	81
Other varieties, average	440	13	77
Floats: Diet Coke; Diet Dr Pepper	220	8	33
Coca-Cola	290	8	54
Shakes: Chocolate	540	16	89
Banana; Vanilla, avg.	470	17	34
Pineapple; Strawberry, avg	505	16	82
Sonic Blast: Butterfinger	580	31	91
M&M's	600	24	88
Reese's Peanut Butter Cups	560	19	89
Single Topping Sundaes: Choc.	410	13	67
Hot Fudge	440	18	63
Pineapple; Strawberry	375	13	60
Drinks: Barq's Root Beer, 20 fl.oz	190	0	52
Cranberry Juice, regular	170	0	46
Limeade Cranberry, medium	200	0	53
Fruit Smoothie: Strawberry, reg.	500	0	124
Strawberry-Banana, regular	460	0	113

For Complete Nutritional Data ~ see CalorieKing.com

Souper Salad® (Oct '08)

Soups: Per 5 oz Serving	C	F	Cb
Adobe Rice & Chicken	100	5	10
Black Bean	85	2	2
Cherokee Joe's Cornbread	70	1.5	13
Chicken Noodle	80	3	9
Chicken Tortilla	60	2	7
Holiday Harvest	90	6	5
Mama Mia Chicken	80	3	8
Minestrone	70	1	13
Mr. B's Hot & Sour Chicken	60	1.5	8
Pasta Tortellini	100	3.5	14
Red French Onion, no Crouton	40	1	6
Seafood Bisque	120	8	8
Spicy Meatballs with Rice	100	4.5	10
Vegetable Lentil	70	0	16
Vegetarian Vegetable	50	0.5	11
Bread			
Blueberry Bread, piece	150	2.5	29
Cheese Drop Biscuit, piece	70	3	8
Cornbread, piece	170	4.5	30
Garlic Breadstick, piece	130	4.5	18
Gingerbread, piece	180	6	30

For Complete Nutritional Data ~ see CalorieKing.com

Souplantation® (Oct '08)

Soups: Per Cup	C	F	Cb
Low Fat: Chicken Tortilla	100	3	5
Classical Minestrone	120	2	20
Vegetable Medley	90	1	14
Regular Soup: *Per Cup*			
Chesapeake Corn Chowder	280	16	30
Cream of Mushroom	290	21	15
Irish Potato Leek	260	16	23
Manhattan Clam Chowder	130	4	16
Minestrone w. Italian Sausage	210	11	14
Navy Bean w. Ham	340	10	30
Vegetarian Harvest	190	8	23
Chili: Low-Fat Kettle House, 1 cup	230	3	26
Breads: Sourdough	150	0.5	27
Buttermilk Cornbread, 1 pce	140	2	27
Focaccia: Garlic Asiago	140	5	19
Tomatillo	140	6	16
Fresh Tossed Salads: Per Cup			
Antipasto Salad; BBQ, average	140	10	6
Caesar Salad Asiago	190	14	10
Won Ton Chicken Happiness	150	8	12

Souplantation® cont... (Oct '08)

Prepared Salads: *Per ½ Cup*	C	F	Cb
Aunt Doris' Red Pepper Slaw	70	0	18
Baja Bean & Cilantro	180	3	29
BBQ Potato	160	8	20
Carrot Raisin	90	3	17
Dijon Potato w. Garlic Dill Vinegar	150	12	9
Greek Couscous w. Feta Cheese	170	9	19
Oriental Ginger Slaw w. Krab	70	3	8
Southern Dill Potato	120	3	20
Thai Noodle w. Peanut Sauce	170	8	17
Zesty Tortellini	190	15	18
Dressing & Croutons: *Per 2 Tbsp*			
Balsamic Vinaigrette	180	19	1
Blue Cheese Dressing	140	14	3
Italian Dressing, creamy	120	13	1
Fat Free	20	0	5
Honey Mustard Dressing	150	13	8
Fat Free	45	0	10
Ranch Dressing	130	13	1
Fat Free	50	0	2
Thousand Island Dressing	110	11	3
Croutons, Garlic Parmesan, 5 pcs	40	3	2
Hot Tossed Pastas: *Per Cup*			
Bruschetta	260	4	41
Creamy Bruschetta	360	16	43
Garden Vegetable: w. Meatballs	270	7	42
w. Italian Sausage	300	10	42
Italian Vegetable Beef	270	6	43
Vegetarian Marinara w. Basil	260	4	44
Muffins: *Chocolate Brownie*	170	8	22
Georgia Peach Poppyseed	150	6	20
Tangy Lemon	140	4	24
Wildly Blue Blueberry, small	140	5	22
Fruit Medley Bran	80	0.5	17
Desserts			
Apple Cobbler, ½ Cup	350	10	64
Apple Medley (fat-free), ½ cup	70	0	18
Banana Royale (fat-free), ½ cup	80	0	20
Chocolate Chip Cookie, small	70	3	10
Chocolate Lava Cake, ½ cup	295	8	55
Jello, flavored, ½ cup	85	0	20
Rice Pudding, ½ cup	110	2	20
Vanilla Pudding, ½ cup	140	4	24
Chocolate Syrup, 2 Tbsp	70	0	18
Granola Topping, 2 Tbsp	110	4	16
Soft Serve: *Chocolate, ½ cup*	95	0	21
Vanilla Soft Serve (reduced fat)	140	4	22

For Complete Nutritional Data ~ see CalorieKing.com

Southern Tsunami® (Oct '08)

Sushi: *Per Pack*	C	F	Cb
California Roll, 12 pieces	360	6	66
California Roll & Inari, 9 pieces	505	11	87
California Roll Plus	495	10	88
Cream Cheese Roll w. Salmon (12)	515	20	59
Crunchy Shrimp Roll, 12 pieces	510	21	64
Dragon Roll, 12 pieces	505	18	66
Eel Roll (Freshwater Eel), 12 pieces	495	16	65
Eel Roll (Sea Eel), 12 pieces	435	12	66
Futomaki	505	6	96
Inari, 4 pieces	420	9	73
Inari & Maki	560	9	102
M&M Roll: *Shrimp & Avocado (16)*	330	5	59
Tuna & Cucumber, 16 pieces	305	1	57
Nigiri: *Cuttlefish, 1 piece*	40	0	8.5
Egg Cake, 1 piece	75	1	13
Fish Roe, 1 piece	60	0.5	9
Fresh Salmon, 1 piece	70	1	9
Fresh Water Eel, 1 piece	110	5	11
Octopus, 1 piece	55	1	9
Sea Eel, 1 piece	90	3	11
Shrimp, 1 piece	45	0	8
Smoked Salmon, 1 piece	70	1	9
Tilapia, 1 piece	50	0.5	8
Tuna, 1 piece	60	0	8
Yellowtail, 1 piece	55	0.5	8
Ocean Crab Roll, 12 pieces	390	7	60
Orange Roll, 12 pieces	385	5	67
Rainbow Roll, 12 pieces	490	9	66
Snack Pack: *Cucumber, 16 pieces*	265	0	57
Imitation Crab & Cucumber (16)	290	1	61
Spicy Roll: *Salmon, 12 pieces*	485	16	59
Shrimp, 12 pieces	395	11	64
Tuna, 12 pieces	450	11	57
Tempura Roll, 12 pieces	530	11	82
Tofu Roll, 12 pieces	320	3	62
Tsunami Roll, 12 pieces	470	13	71
Vegetable Combo: 12 pieces	350	7	65
24 pieces	445	4	92
Combinations: *Fullmoon, 12 pcs*	425	13	64
Marina Plate, 6 pcs	380	8	52
Meteor Special, 14 pieces	385	3	69
Seaside, Tuna & Salmon, 16 pcs	360	3	58
Seaside, Tuna, Salmon, Shrimp, Eel	355	4	59
Shoreline, 12 pieces	480	8	78
Stardust, 16 pieces	540	12	94

Spaghetti Warehouse® (Oct '08)

Lunch	C	F	Cb
Minestrone Soup	80	1.5	12
Grilled Chicken Marinara	530	8	65
Seafood Marinara	385	5	65
Spaghetti: w. Tomato Sauce	425	5	82
w. Marinara Sauce #12	440	5	84
Spicy Marinara Sce Spaghetti	280	4	52
Vegetable Primavera	340	4	65
Dinner			
Minestrone, 1 bowl	110	2	18
Grilled Chicken Marinara	640	10	85
Grilled Halibut Dinner	880	14	106
Grilled Marinated Chicken Breast	910	17	116
Marinara Sauce #12	520	6	99
Seafood Marinara	520	8	86
Spaghetti w. Tomato Sauce	525	6	101
Spicy Marinara Sce Spaghetti	330	6	60
Vegetable Primavera	610	8	116

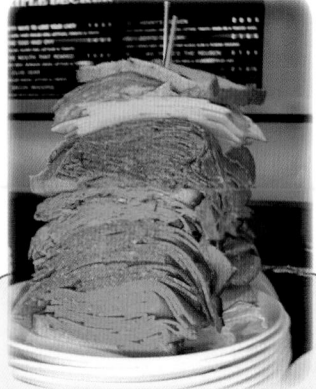

This Triple Decker (Carnegie Deli, New York) contains up to 3 lb meat and 8 oz cheese ~ approx. 4000 calories and 300 grams fat.

Note: Only half the sandwich is shown – the other half is hidden behind!

Carnegie's Challenge: Eat one Triple Decker . . . get the second one free!

Starbuck's® (Oct '08)
Figures Based on Grande (16 fl.oz) Without Whip Unless Indicated

Classic Favorites	C	F	Cb
Apple Juice	240	0	60
Apple Juice, Steamed	230	0	58
Brewed Coffee			
Caffe Misto: w. Whole Milk	130	7	10
w. Nonfat Milk	70	0	10
w. Soy Milk	95	3	13
Espresso Hot			
Caffe Americano	20	0	3
Caffe Latte: w. Whole Milk	230	12	18
w. Nonfat Milk	135	0	20
w. Soy Milk	175	5	24
Caffe Mocha: w. Whole Milk	305	12	41
w. Nonfat Milk	225	2.5	42
w. Soy Milk	255	6.5	46
Cappuccino: w. Whole Milk	145	7	1
w. Nonfat Milk	90	0	13
w. Soy Milk	110	3	15
Caramel Macchiato: w. Whole Milk	270	10	34
w. Nonfat Milk	190	1	35
w. Soy Milk	225	5	38
Con Panna: 1 doppio, 2 fl.oz	35	2.5	3
1 solo, 1 fl.oz	20	1.5	1.5
Dulce de Leche Latte: w. Whole Milk	390	10	63
w. Nonfat Milk	310	0	64
w. Soy Milk	345	4	67
Espresso: 1 doppio, 2 fl.oz	10	0	2
1 solo, 1 fl.oz	5	0	1
Macchiato, w. Whole Milk: 1 doppio	15	0	2
1 solo, 1 fl.oz	10	0	1
White Choc. Mocha: w. Whole Milk	440	16	61
w. Nonfat Milk	360	5.5	62
w. Soy Milk	390	9.5	66
Espresso Iced			
Caffe Americano	15	0	2.5
Caffe Latte: w. Whole Milk	140	6.5	11
w. Nonfat Milk	85	0	13
w. Soy Milk	115	3	15
Caffe Mocha: w. Whole Milk	205	7.5	34
w. Nonfat Milk	165	2.5	35
w. Soy Milk	195	4.5	37
Dulce de Leche Latte: w. Whole Milk	300	5.5	56
w. Nonfat Milk	260	0	57
w. Soy Milk	280	2.5	59
White Choc. Mocha: w. Whole Milk	345	11	54
w. Nonfat Milk	305	6	55
w. Soy Milk	325	8	57
Espresso: 1 doppio, 2 fl.oz	10	0	2
1 solo, 1 fl.oz	5	0	1

Continued Next Page...

Updated Nutrition Data ~ www.CalorieKing.com
Persons with Diabetes ~ See Disclaimer (Page 24)

Starbuck's® cont... (Oct '08)

Figures Based on Grande (16 fl.oz)
Without Whip Unless Indicated

Frappuccino Blended Coffee	C	F	Cb
Caffe Vanilla	295	3	63
Caramel	255	3.5	51
Cinnamon Dolce	245	3	51
Coffee	225	3	45
Dulce de Leche	280	3	59
Espresso	195	2.5	38
Java Chip	325	7.5	61
Mocha	255	3.5	52
White Chocolate Mocha	295	4.5	57
Frappuccino Blended Creme			
Double Chocolate Chip	365	7.5	69
Dulce de Leche	365	2	76
Strawberries & Creme	415	2	89
Tazo Chai	315	2	64
Tazo Green Tea	360	2.5	74
Vanilla Bean	325	2.5	67
White Chocolate	420	6	79
Frappuccino Light Blended Coffee			
Caffe Vanilla	185	0.5	39
Caramel	145	1	29
Coffee	120	0.5	23
Dulce de Leche	165	0.5	35
Espresso	100	0.5	19
Java Chip	200	4.5	37
Mocha	140	1.5	29
White Chocolate Mocha	185	2.5	35
Frappuccino Juice Blend			
Pomegranate	215	0	52
Tangerine	155	0	37
Vivanno Blends: Per 16 fl.oz			
Banana Chocolate	270	5	44
with Espresso shot	260	4.5	42
Orange Mango Banana	250	2	47
with Matcha	290	2	57
Drink Extras			
Flavored Syrup: 1 pump, 0.35 oz	20	0	5
Sugar-Free, 1 pump, 0.35 oz	0	0	0
Mocha Syrup, 1 pump, 0.6 oz	25	0.5	6
Topping: Caramel, 0.53 oz	15	0.5	2
Chocolate, 1 serving, 0.14 oz	5	0	1
Sprinkles, 1 serving	0	0	0.5
Whipped Cream Topping:			
Cold Beverage, 1 venti, 1.2 oz	110	11	3
Hot Beverage, 1 venti, 0.78 oz	70	7	2

Starbuck's® cont... (Oct '08)

Breakfast Items	C	F	Cb
Apple Bran Muffin	330	8	61
Chewy Fruit & Nut Bar	250	10	38
Baked Berry Stella	280	9	45
Perfect Oatmeal: 1.3 oz	140	2.5	25
Brown Sugar Topping, 0.5 oz	50	0	13
Dried Fruit Topping, 1 oz	100	0	24
Nut Medley Topping, 0.5 oz	100	9	2
Protein Plate w/ P'nut Butter, 6.6 oz	330	16	35
Baked Items:			
Apple Fritter, Top Pot	480	22	64
Bagels: Cinnamon Raisin	310	2	65
Plain	310	1	62
Bars: Crispy Marshmallow Square	370	10	71
Toffee Almond	450	20	61
Oat: Cranberry	440	17	69
Organic Blueberries	380	16	55
Brownies, Espresso	340	19	40
Cakes: Marble Pound	370	27	55
Old-Fashioned Crumb	500	22	68
Coffee Cakes: Banana Walnut	470	27	63
Reduced-Fat: Blueberry	310	10	58
Banana Chocolate Chip	390	8	76
Cinnamon Swirl	300	8	59
Orange Creme	320	8	56
Cookies: Chocolate Chip	400	21	53
Oatmeal Raisin	350	12	56
Croissants: Butter	300	15	36
Pain Au Chocalat	450	24	56
Cupcakes: Vanilla	330	16	44
Chocolate Chocolate	350	19	44
Danish, Cheese	370	18	42
Doughnut, Old Fashioned	450	21	59
Loaves: Banana Walnut	410	17	60
Cinnamon Sour Cream	460	22	61
Lemon	430	21	59
Zucchini Walnut	460	27	50
Muffins: Blueberry	430	16	65
Low-Fat Blueberry Apricot	360	5	74
Mini: Bran	150	5	26
Zucchini Walnut	380	24	39
Roll, Cinnamon	470	16	76
Sandie, Dulce de Leche	150	8	18
Scones: Blueberry	400	18	55
Cherry Almond Multigrain	430	20	56
Cranberry Orange	420	16	66
Maple Oat Nut	440	21	57
Raspberry Thumbprint	370	16	51
Twist, Cinnamon	480	21	68

Ice Cream & Ice Cream Bars ~ See Page 35, 38
For Bottled Drinks ~ See Page 164

Steak Escape® (Oct '08)

Sandwiches & Burgers

	C	F	Cb
Lighter Side: Chicken Philly	425	5	64
Philly Cheesesteak	430	6	64
Ragin Cajun Chicken	420	5	63
Turkey Club	390	2	67
Wild West BBQ	470	6	72
7" Sandwiches: Chicken Philly	410	6	60
Classic Italian Sub	470	11	60
Meatball Sub	630	26	69
Philly Cheesesteak	420	6	60
Portabello Vegetarian	310	1	65
Ragin' Cajun Chicken	410	5	58
Turkey Club	380	2	67
Turkey Philly	365	2	63
Wild West BBQ	455	6	60
12" Sandwiches: Chicken Philly	640	10	84
Classic Italian Sub	760	22	85
Meatball Sub	1120	52	102
Philly Cheesesteak	660	12	84
Portabello Vegetarian	440	2	93
Ragin' Cajun Chicken	630	10	80
Turkey Club	580	3	88
Turkey Philly	550	3	90
Wild West BBQ	730	12	84

Salads

	C	F	Cb
Grilled Side: Salad	40	0.5	8
w. Chicken	175	5	11
w. Ham/Turkey	130	2	8
w. Meatball	560	24	58
w. Portabello	290	1	63
w. Steak	185	6	11

Sides

	C	F	Cb
Fresh Cut Fries: Small, 6 oz	500	26	67
Medium, 8 oz	650	34	87
Large, 11 oz	920	48	123
Loaded French Fries:			
Bacon & Cheddar, 16½ oz	635	26	91
Ranch & Bacon, 16½ oz	690	34	87
Smashed Potatoes: Plain, 14 oz	245	0	53
w. Chicken, 20 oz	385	4	56
w. Ham, 20 oz	340	2	59
w. Meatball, 19 oz	560	24	58
w. Portabello, 18½ oz	290	1	63
w. Steak, 20 oz	395	5	56
w. Turkey, 20 oz	340	2	59

For Complete Nutritional Data ~ see CalorieKing.com

Steak 'n Shake® (Oct '08)

Meals

	C	F	Cb
Chicken Fingers, without fries	260	18	14
Chili 3-Way	825	45	65
Chili 5-Way	1120	69	74
Chili Deluxe, 6 oz cup	540	32	21
Fish Fillet Sandwich w. Cheese	340	22	20
Frisco Melt Sandwich	980	72	42
Grilled Cheese & Bacon Sandwich	650	47	40
Grilled Chicken Breast Sandwich	240	7	29
Original Dbl Steakburger w. Cheese	410	21	26
Original Single w. Cheese	310	15	26
Philadelphia Sandwich	595	32	34
Triple Steakburger	490	22	36
Turkey Melt Sandwich	915	65	47
Fries: French, reg., 5 oz	450	23	57
French, large, 7.25 oz	645	34	82
Cheddar Cheese, reg., 9 oz	615	36	64
Salads: Beef Taco w. Lt Rnch	1160	85	68
Grilled Chicken no dressing	465	25	23
Fried Chicken w. Caesar	765	62	20
Soups: Per 6 fl.oz Cup			
Chicken Gumbo	80	2	14
Chicken Noodle	80	1.5	10
Broccoli & Cheese	90	4.5	10
Vegetable Beef	60	1.5	12
Breakfast: Sausage Bagel	575	30	51
Biscuits, Gravy 'n Hash Browns	1565	91	143
Buttermilk Pancakes (2)	160	2	31
Country Scrambler	790	52	42
Cinnamon Swirl French Tst, 3 sl.	255	7	40
Egg & Saus. S'wch w/ Hash Browns	680	43	54
Desserts: Berry Berry Cobbler	670	18	72
Brownie Fudge Sundae	865	44	112
Hot Fudge Sundae	770	37	106
Outrageous Parfait, no cream	715	34	97
Strawberry Sundae	280	14	36
Beverages: Per Regular			
Root Beer	195	0	53
Orange Freeze	615	19	101
Shake: Chocolate, no Cream	650	15	116
Banana, with cream	720	22	116
Vanilla, with cream	715	22	115

Updated Nutrition Data ~ www.CalorieKing.com
Persons with Diabetes ~ See Disclaimer (Page 24)

Fast - Foods & Restaurants

Subway® (Oct '08)

6" Subs (6g Fat or Less) | C | F | Cb

Figures based on wheat bread and toppings: lettuce, tomato, onion, green peppers, olives and pickles. **Cheese, oil or mayo not included.**

	C	F	Cb
Ham	285	5	47
Ham w. American Cheese	330	8	47
Oven Roasted Chicken Breast	315	5.5	47
Roast Beef	290	5	45
Subway Club	320	6	47
Sweet Onion Chicken Teriyaki	375	5	59
Tuna	530	31	44
Turkey Breast	280	4.5	46
Turkey Breast & Ham	290	5	47
Veggie Delite	225	3	44

6" Double Meat Subs: *Figures based on wheat bread*

	C	F	Cb
Chicken Bacon Ranch with Cheese	710	35	48
Ham	350	7	49
Italian BMT with Cheese	630	35	49
Meatball Marinara with Cheese	860	42	82
Oven Roasted Chicken	400	8	51
Roast Beef	360	7	46
Steak & Cheese	540	18	52
Subway Club	420	8	50
Subway Melt	490	17	51
Sweet Onion Chicken Teriyaki	480	7	65
Turkey Breast	330	5	48

Wraps:

	C	F	Cb
Chicken Breast	410	10	56
Ham	390	10	58
Roast Beef,	400	10	56
Subway Club	430	11	58
Sweet Onion Chicken Teriyaki	480	10	70
Turkey Breast	380	9	57
Turkey Breast & Ham	400	10	58

4" Mini Subs: *Figures based on wheat bread*

	C	F	Cb
Ham	180	3	30
Roast Beef	190	3.5	30
Tuna with Cheese	320	18	30
Turkey Breast	190	3	30

8" Pizzas

	C	F	Cb
Cheese & Veggies	740	25	100
Cheese	680	22	96
Pepperoni	790	32	96
Sausage	820	34	97

Subway® cont... (Oct '08)

6" Breakfast Sandwiches | C | F | Cb

Omelet Sandwiches: Cheese	420	18	44
Chipotle Steak & Cheese	600	32	49
Dble Bacon & Cheese	510	25	45
Honey Mustard Ham & Chse	470	19	52
Western with Cheese	450	19	46
Wraps: Cheese	520	23	55
Chipotle Steak & Cheese	700	37	60
Dble Bacon & Cheese	610	30	56
Honey Mustard Ham & Cheese	580	25	64
Western with Cheese	550	24	58

Salads (6g Fat or Less)
Includes lettuce, tomato, onions, green peppers, olives, carrot, cucumber. **Dressing and croutons are not included in figures.**

	C	F	Cb
Ham	120	3	14
Oven Roasted Chicken Breast	140	2.5	11
Roast Beef	120	3	12
Subway Club	150	4	14
Sweet Onion Chicken Teriyaki,	210	3	26
Turkey Breast & Ham	120	3	14
Turkey Breast	110	2.5	13
Veggie Delite	60	1	11

Sandwich Components: *For 6" Sub, Wrap or Salad*

	C	F	Cb
Bacon, 2 strips	45	3.5	0
Cheese: American	40	3.5	1
Monterey Cheddar	50	4.5	1
Natural Cheddar	60	5	0
Pepperjack	50	4	0
Provolone	50	4	0
Swiss	50	4.5	0
Meats: Chicken Strips	80	1.5	0
Cold Cut Combo	140	11	2
Ham	60	2	3
Italian BMT	180	14	2
Meatballs	300	18	19
Roast Beef	70	2	1
Seafood Sensation	190	16	7
Steak w. Peppers & Onions	140	6	4
Subway Club	100	3	3
Tuna	260	24	0
Turkey Breast	50	1	2
Veggie Patty	160	5	12

Sauces & Dressings:

	C	F	Cb
Chipotle Southwest, 1¼ Tbsp	95	10	1
Honey Mustard, Fat-Free, 1¼ Tbsp	30	0	7
Mayonnaise: 1 Tbsp, ½ oz	110	12	0
Light, 1 Tbsp, ½ oz	50	5	0.5
Mustard, Yellow or Deli Brown, 2 tsp	5	0	0.5
Olive Oil Blend,1 tsp	45	5	0
Ranch Dressing, 1¼ Tbsp	120	13	1
Sweet Onion, Fat-Free, 1¼ Tbsp	40	0	9

257

Fast - Foods & *Restaurants*

Subway® cont... (Oct '08)

Soups: Per Bowl

	C	F	Cb
Chicken & Dumpling	170	5	23
Chili Con Carne	290	8	35
Cream of Broccoli	160	7	18
Cream of Potato with Bacon	240	13	26
Golden Broccoli & Cheese	200	12	17
Minestrone	80	1	15
New England Style Clam Chowder	150	5	20
Roasted Chicken Noodle	80	2	11
Spanish Style Chicken with Rice	110	2	17
Tomato Garden Vegetable w. Rotini	90	0	20
Vegetable Beef	100	2	15
Wild Rice with Chicken	210	11	21
Apple Pie, 1 pie, 2.5 oz	250	10	37
Fresh Fit: Apple Slices, 2.5 oz	35	0	9
Backed Lay, 1.1 oz	130	1.5	23
Dannon Strawberry Yogurt, 4 oz	110	1	20
Raisins, 1.5 oz	140	0	33

Beverages: Per Small Container

Fresh Fit

	C	F	Cb
MM Fruit Punch (100% Juice)	100	0	24
1% Low-Fat Milk	190	3.5	24

Fruizle Express

	C	F	Cb
Berry Lishus	110	0	28
w. Banana, 1 small, 14 oz	140	0	35
Peach Pizzazz	100	0	26
Pineapple Delight	130	0	33

For Complete Nutritional Data ~ see CalorieKing.com

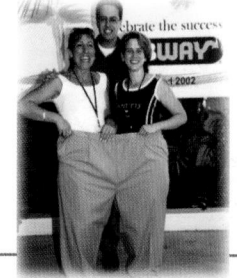

Jared Fogle lost over 200 lbs with low-fat Subway® Sandwiches and lots of walking

Sub Station® (Oct '08)

Sandwiches
Per ½ Sub (Incl. Oil, Vinegar, Salad)

	C	F	Cb
Ham & Cheese	580	36	48
Ham, Turkey & Cheese	605	37	49
Turkey & Cheese	600	37	48
Roast Beef & Cheese	630	40	44
Ham, Salami, Pepperoni, Cappicola, Bologna, Turkey & Cheese	825	57	43

Sweet Tomatoes®
~ *Same Menu & Data as Souplantation* (See Page 253) ~

Swiss Chalet® (Oct '08)

Burgers: Includes Garnishes

	C	F	Cb
Bacon Cheese Burger	870	46	45
Hamburger	730	49	44
Veggie Burger	430	13	51

Rotisserie Chicken: Meat Only

	C	F	Cb
Double Leg w. Skin	630	38	4
Half Chicken, w. Skin	610	31	5
Quarter Chicken: Leg, no Skin	230	11	1
Leg meat w. Skin	310	19	2
Breast meat, no Skin	210	7	0
Breast meat w. Skin	300	11	3
Chicken Pot Pie, 1 pie	580	33	42

Appetizers

	C	F	Cb
Baked Garlic Cheese Loaf, 9 oz	910	57	78
Chalet Chicken Wings, 8 wings	640	44	16
Pierogies w. Cajun Sauce, 6.5 oz	420	10	69
Soup: Chalet Chicken, 1 cup	160	4	17
Side Salads: Greek	130	11	5
Caesar Salad	210	19	9

Meals:

From The Grill: No Flatbread

	C	F	Cb
BBQ Ribs: Half Rack	630	38	4
Full Rack	1270	77	9
⅓ Rack	420	26	3

Lighter Favorites: Includes Salad & Vegetables

	C	F	Cb
Quarter Chicken Breast Dinner	360	11	14
Santa Fe Grilled Chicken Salad	300	4	35
Spinach Chicken Salad, no dress.	370	10	19
Vegetable Stir-Fry, no rice	270	2.5	54
w. Grilled Chkn Breast, no rice	400	4	55

258

Updated Nutrition Data ~ www.CalorieKing.com
Persons with Diabetes ~ See Disclaimer (Page 24)

Swiss Chalet®cont... (Oct '08)

Sides	C	F	Cb
Baked Potato	220	0	48
Flatbread, 1.6 oz	140	3.5	22
Butter, ½ oz	70	8	0
Coleslaw Ramekin	70	5	5
Corn Chips, 1 oz	140	7	19
French Fries, 6 oz	470	25	56
Gravy, 4 oz	40	1.5	7
Mashed Potatoes	100	3.5	17
Mushrooms, 6 oz	220	16	11
Seasoned Rice	240	3	48
Sour Cream & Chives, 1½ oz	70	5	3
Sandwiches: No Sides			
Chicken Club Wrap	840	40	61
Chicken on Kaiser, white meat	440	8	31
Salad Dressings: Light Italian, ½ oz	35	4	7
Famous Chalet Sauce, 4 oz	30	0.5	5
Light Mayonnaise, ½ oz	45	4.5	1
Dipping Sauce: Blue Cheese, ½ oz	70	7	1
Cajun Sauce, 2 oz	100	9	3
Salsa, 1½ oz	20	0	4
Tangy Plum Sauce, 1 oz	50	0	24
Desserts: Apple Blossom	470	28	52
Apple Pie	440	19	65
Carrot Cake	740	48	70
Chocolate Eruption Cheesecake	820	55	72
Coconut Cream Pie	540	33	57
Colossal Caramel Fudge Chsecake	700	39	78
Cranberry, Raspberry Yogurt	110	2	22
Lemon Meringue Pie	400	11	73
Pecan Pie	590	29	79
Swiss Alps Choc Layer Cake	590	39	55
Ice Cream: Butter Pecan	150	7	21
Chocolate	130	5	19
Vanilla	120	6	17
Sauce: Butterscotch	100	0	24
Chocolate	80	0	20
Strawberry	40	0	10

For Complete Nutritional Data ~ see CalorieKing.com

Taco Bell® (Oct '08)

Burritos	C	F	Cb
½ lb Beef & Potato	530	23	66
½ lb Beef Combo	440	18	51
½ lb Cheesy Bean & Rice	470	20	58
7-Layer	490	18	65
Bean	350	9	54
Cheesy Double Beef	460	20	52
Chilli Cheese	370	16	40
Fiesta: Beef	370	13	49
Chicken	350	10	47
Steak	340	11	47
Fresco Style: Bean	330	7	54
Cheesy Dble Beef	410	16	50
Fiesta, Chicken	330	8	48
Supreme, Chicken; Steak	330	8	49
Grilled Stuft: Beef	680	30	76
Chicken	640	23	73
Steak	630	25	72
Spicy Chicken	400	17	48
Supreme, Beef	420	17	51
Menu Items			
Chalupas			
Baja: Beef	410	27	30
Chicken; Steak	390	24	28
Nacho Cheese: Beef	370	22	32
Chicken; Steak	340	19	30
Supreme: Beef	380	23	30
Chicken; Steak	360	21	28
Gorditas			
Baja: Beef	340	19	29
Chicken; Steak	320	17	27
Fresco Style:			
Baja: Beef	250	10	29
Chicken; Steak	230	8	28
Nacho Cheese			
Beef	300	14	31
Chicken; Steak	280	11	29
Supreme			
Beef	310	16	29
Chicken; Steak	290	13	28
Caramel Apple Empanada (1)	290	15	38
Cheese Roll-Up (1)	200	10	19
Nachos			
Regular	330	21	31
BellGrande	770	44	77
Fresco Style, Triple Layer	220	10	28
Pinto & Cheese	120	2	19
Supreme	440	26	40

259

Taco Bell® cont... (Oct '08)

Specialties	C	F	Cb
Border Bowls:			
Southwest Steak	600	24	68
Zesty Chicken with dressing	640	35	60
Crunchwrap Supreme	560	24	68
Enchirito, Chicken; Steak	340	13	33
Fresco Style			
Enchirito, Beef	260	8	34
Chicken; Steak	240	6	32
Mexican Pizza	535	30	47
MexiMelt	280	14	22
Quesadillas, Chicken; Steak	520	28	39
Taco Salads: Express with Chips	610	32	56
Fiesta with Shell	840	45	80
Tacos			
Big Taste	420	22	43
Crunchy	170	10	13
Crunchy Supreme	210	13	15
Double Decker	320	13	38
Double Decker Supreme	370	17	40
Fresco Style: Big Taste	330	12	43
Crunchy	150	8	13
Soft: Beef; Spicy Chicken	180	7	21
Grilled Steak	160	4.5	20
Ranchero Chicken	170	4	21

Taco Cabana® (Oct '08)

Grilled Chicken: Per Serving			
¼ Chicken White, 5 oz	295	14	1
No Skin, 4 oz	170	3	0
¼ Chicken Dark, 4.5 oz	300	18	0.5
No Skin, 3.5 oz	170	7	1
Fajitas: Beef, 4 oz	245	12	4
Chicken White, 4 oz	190	6	3
Chicken Dark, 4 oz	235	11	2
Sides: Black Beans, 4 oz	110	0.5	21
Borracho Beans, 4 oz	110	2.5	17
Chips, 2 oz	290	14	36
Guacamole, 1 oz; Sour Crm, 1 oz	50	4	2
Queso, 3 oz	185	12	7
Refried Beans, 4 oz	170	6	21
Salsa, all types, 1 oz	10	0	2
Spanish Rice, 4 oz	180	5	30
Tortillas: 6" Flour	130	3.5	22
6" Table Corn	60	1	11
Tortilla Soup: Small, 8.5 oz	250	8.5	26
Large, 19 oz	375	13	32
Tacos: Bean & Cheese	290	12	35
Black Bean	215	5	37
Carne Guisada	200	8	20
Crispy Beef	150	7	13
Soft Chicken	220	9	21

Taco Cabana® cont... (Oct '08)

Burritos	C	F	Cb
Bean & Cheese	710	27	85
Beef/Chicken, average	660	25	75
Black Bean	560	11	95
Breakfast Tacos: Barbacoa	305	15	2
Chorizo & Egg	250	12	22

Taco John's® (Oct '08)

Burritos: Bean Burrito	380	9	58
Beefy Burrito	440	20	45
Chicken & Potato Burrito	470	19	56
Combination Burrito	400	14	50
Crunchy Chicken & Potato Burrito	600	28	65
Meat & Potato	500	23	58
Super Burrito	450	18	54
Grilled Burrito: Steak	610	34	49
Beef; Chicken, avg.	595	31	51
Tacos: Bravo	340	13	40
Crispy Taco	180	10	13
Softshell Taco: Regular	220	11	21
Cilantro Lime Steak	240	14	19
Chicken	190	6	19
Taco Burger w. Cheese	270	12	28
Burrito: Ranch Beef	440	22	45
Ranch Chicken	400	17	44
Smothered	510	20	60
Chili Enchilada	310	16	24
Mexi Rolls w. Nacho Cheese (6)	470	21	47
Potato Oles, Chili Cheese	590	36	55
Specialties: Cheese Quesadilla	450	23	43
Chicken Taco Salad, no dressing	480	27	35
Crunchy Chicken Taco, no dress.	660	40	47
Potato Oles Super	1030	65	87
Super Nachos	810	48	74
Taco Salad, no Dressing	520	33	37
Sides: Mexican Rice	250	6	45
Nachos	380	23	38
Potato Oles, medium	600	36	62
Refried Beans	320	6	47
Desserts: Apple Grande	270	12	39
Choco Taco	390	20	48
Churro	190	7	15

For Complete Nutritional Data ~ see CalorieKing.com

Taco Mayo® (Oct '08)

Burritos	C	F	Cb
Bean	495	16	71
Beef	490	23	41
Super Chicken	405	16	39
Combo	495	20	56
Super Burrito, Beef	540	24	58
Quesadillas			
Cheese	590	35	45
Chicken	670	37	46
Fajita Chicken	700	39	47
Fajita Steak	725	40	47
Tacos			
Crispy Taco, Beef	160	10	10
Soft: Beef Taco	230	11	17
Chicken Taco	185	6	16
Tamale Melt	615	34	50
Tostada Melt	525	32	35
Salads			
Acapulco Chicken Salad	760	55	39
Taco Salad, Beef	705	38	57
Taco Chicken Salad	440	23	30
Sides			
Mexicali Rice	160	1	36
Refried Beans	295	9	43
Potatos Locos, Small	380	24	36

Target Food Court (Oct '08)

	C	F	Cb
Breakfast: Pancakes (3) + Syrup	490	4	104
Breakfast Sandwich w. Bacon	380	20	29
Cinnamon Swirl French Toast, 2 slices	230	5	36
Pretzels (Cinnabon): Cinnamon, 5¾ oz	550	9	105
Mega Cinnamon, 6½ oz	650	15	115
Salted Pretzel, 5½ oz	435	3.5	89
Meals: Bowl of Chili, 9 oz cup	300	10	32
Chicken Breast Sandwich, 4 oz	280	9	31
Chicken Tenders, 5 strips, 3 oz	280	19	14
Hot Dog Meal: w. Chips & Soda	570	22	84
w. Applesauce & Soda	520	12	93
Hot Dog: Plain, 3½oz	260	12	28
All Beef Meat, 5 oz	350	20	30
Cheddar, 4 oz	310	16	38
Macaroni & Cheese: 8 oz	340	13	45
w. Apple Sauce & Soda Meal	600	13	106
w. Chips & Soda, Meal	650	23	97
Mini Pizza (6"), 5½ oz	360	14	42
Nachos w. Cheese, 40 chips, 4 oz	1100	59	132
Spaghetti O's Meal: w. Chips & Soda	490	11	93
w. Apple Sauce & Soda	440	1	102

For Complete Nutritional Data ~ see CalorieKing.com

Taco Time® (Oct '08)

Burritos	C	F	Cb
Beef, Bean & Cheese	615	23	66
Big Juan: Chicken	620	24	69
Ground Beef	640	25	71
Shredded Beef	790	27	113
Casita: Chicken	545	26	50
Ground Beef	650	31	54
Shredded Beef	725	23	93
Crisp Burrito: Bean	425	18	53
Meat	550	30	39
Chicken	420	25	32
Soft Bean Burrito	380	10	58
Soft Meat Burrito	490	21	48
Veggie Burrito	490	16	70
Tacos: ¼ lb Crisp Taco	295	17	16
½ lb Soft Tacos: Chicken	380	14	42
Ground Beef	525	24	47
Shredded Beef	580	14	84
Jr Soft Taco	315	15	23
Super Soft Taco	510	23	50
Specialties: Cheddar Melt	200	11	17
Nachos: Regular	680	38	61
Deluxe	1050	57	91
Taco Cheeseburger	635	36	48
Sides: Cheddar Fries, med. 7 oz	665	44	47
Mexi Fries®, medium, 6 oz	415	24	48
Mexi-Rice, 4 oz	160	2	30
Stuffed Fries, medium, 6.2 oz	495	26	47
Refritos, 7 oz	325	10	44
Salads: Chicken Fiesta, 13 oz	540	17	67
Chicken Taco Salad, regular	370	21	27
Taco Salad, regular	480	28	30
Tostada Salad	630	33	48
Salsas, Sauces & Dressings: Per 1 oz			
Green Sauce; Original Hot	10	0	2
Guacamole	30	2	2
Salsa Fresca	5	0.5	1.5
1000 Island Dressing	160	16	4
Desserts: Cinnamon Crustos, 4 oz	580	38	51
Fruit Filled Empanadas, 4 oz	270	7	46

Tacone® (Aug '08)

Gourmet Wrapped Sandwiches	C	F	Cb
Campfire, ½ wrap	340	12	41
Malibu Melt, ½ wrap	360	17	25
Pilgrim, ½ wrap	260	14	21
Thai Cone, ½ wrap	300	9	35

For Complete Nutritional Data ~ see CalorieKing.com

TCBY® (Oct '08)

	C	F	Cb
Soft Serve Frozen Yogurt: Average all Flavors			
96% Fat-Free: Kids Cup	110	2	18
Small Cup	280	6	46
Regular Cup	360	8	60
Large Cup	460	10	76
Non-Fat: Small Cup	220	0	48
Regular Cup	290	0	64
Large Cup	360	0	79
No Sugar Added/Non-Fat: Small	190	0	50
Regular Cup	230	0	62
Large Cup	300	0	79
Hand Scooped Frozen Yogurt: Average all Flavors			
Kids Cup	90	3	14
Small Cup	180	6	28
Regular Cup	280	10	44
Large Cup	370	13	58
No Added Sugar: Chocolate Swirl			
Small Cup	130	0.5	32
Regular Cup	200	1	49
Large Cup	270	1.5	65
Sorbet: Average all Flavors			
Kids Cup	80	0	21
Small Cup	205	0	49
Regular Cup	265	0	64
Large Cup	345	0	82
Frappe Chillers: Per 16 fl.oz Cup			
Caramel de Leche	240	9	32
Coffee	190	7	25
French Vanilla, no sugar added	200	9	23
Frozen Hot chocolate	230	0	32
Mocha	240	9	31
Cappuccino Chillers: Per 16 fl.oz Cup			
Mocha	560	21	82
Oreo-Joe	780	29	115
Toffee Coffee	640	28	8
Shakes: Regular			
Chocolate	640	20	103
Moussed	1000	49	127
Oreo	970	33	152
Peanut Butter	1130	66	112
Strawberry	580	15	101
Desserts			
Banana Split: Dulche Delight	1120	35	195
Fruit Grove	800	27	135
Mississippi Mud	750	19	14
Monkey's Uncle	990	45	139

Teriyaki Stix® (Oct '08)

	C	F	Cb
Bowls: Beef Bowl	620	7	102
Chicken Bowl; Hot & Spicy	730	15	101
Chicken Curry	680	17	92
Teriyaki Chicken Salad	360	13	26
Teriyaki Special	740	13	111
Veggie Bowl	440	1	99
Yakisoba	360	4.5	56

The Taco Maker® (Oct '08)

	C	F	Cb
Burritos			
Bean	295	9	43
Beef	445	16	44
Chicken	375	12	44
Crisp Bean; Crisp Beef, avg.	420	27	30
Enchiladas: Beef	375	20	22
Cheese	595	38	25
Chicken	320	13	21
Nachos: Cheese	605	35	49
Chips 'n Beans	290	16	32
Macho Nacho w. Beef	815	50	57
Macho Nacho w. Guacamole	845	55	62
Salad: Chicken Fiesta	625	35	38
Taco	685	42	39
Tacos: Crisp	185	9	16
Crisp Super	310	15	24
Soft	180	6.5	20
Soft Super	390	15	43
Tater Gem Fries, Regular	485	30	48

ThunderCloud Subs® (Oct '08)

	C	F	Cb
Classic Subs: Cheese/Mayo/Sauce not included			
BLT, small	400	17	40
Roast Beef, small	315	4	40
Smoked Chicken, small	295	4	40
Turkey, small	280	4	40
Hot Subs: Meatball, small	650	32	56
Hot Pastrami, small	515	15	49
Signature Subs: Club, small	480	19	43
California Club, small	510	23	45
N.Y. Italian, small	570	30	42
Office Favorite, small	850	40	81
Texas Tuna, small	700	45	44
Veggie Delite, w/ Hummus, small	360	10	53

Updated Nutrition Data ~ www.CalorieKing.com
Persons with Diabetes ~ See Disclaimer (Page 24)

Tim Hortons® (Oct '08)

Sandwiches	C	F	Cb
Tim's Own: Chicken Salad	380	9	55
Deli Trio	390	9	54
Egg Salad with lettuce	390	13	52
Ham & Swiss w. Tim's Own Dress.	440	12	56
Turkey Bacon Club w. Mustard	440	8	63

Soup: Per Bowl (10 oz)			
Beef Stew	235	8	25
Chili	300	16	18
Cream of Broccoli	160	9	16
Creamy Field Mushroom	150	3	28
Hearty Vegetable	70	0	14
Minestrone	120	3	24
Split Pea with Ham	150	2.5	27
Tim's Own, Chicken Noodle	120	2	18
Turkey Rice	120	1.5	21

Cookies			
Caramel Chocolate Pecan	230	11	32
Oatmeal Raisin	220	8	35
Peanut Butter	280	16	27
Chocolate Chunk	230	9	35
Triple Chocolate	250	13	31

Donuts: Per Donut			
Cake: Chocolate Glazed	260	10	39
Old Fashion Plain	260	19	20
Sour Cream Plain	270	17	27
Filled: Blueberry	230	8	36
Boston Cream	250	9	38
Canadian Maple	260	9	41
Strawberry	230	8	36
Honey Cruller	320	19	37
Yeast: Apple Fritter	300	11	49
Other varieties, avg.	210	8	30

Baked Goods: Per Serving			
Croissant: Plain	200	11	21
Cheese	230	14	19
Tea Biscuit: Plain, 3 oz	250	9	35
Raisin, 3 oz	290	10	45
Cinnamon Roll: Frosted	470	25	57
Glazed	420	23	50
Danish: Cherry Cheese	330	13	46
Chocolate	430	24	51
Maple Pecan	380	20	46
Bagels: Plain	260	1.5	52
Blueberry Cinnamon Raisin	270	1	55
Everything	280	2	53
Onion	260	1.5	53
Sun Dried Tomato	310	3.5	59

Tim Hortons® Cont... (Oct '08)

Muffins: Per Muffin	C	F	Cb
Blueberry Bran	340	10	56
Cranberry Fruit	360	11	60
Chocolate Chip Plain	430	14	71
Fruit Explosion	350	10	61
Raisin Bran	380	9	67
Strawberry Sensation	370	11	62
Wheat Carrot	400	19	55
Low-Fat varieties	290	2.5	62

Timbits: Low-Fat			
Cake: Chocolate Glazed	70	2.5	10
Old Fashion Plain	70	5	5
Filled, all varieties	60	2	10
Yeast: Apple Fritter	50	1.5	9
Honey Dip	60	5	9

Desserts			
Yogurt: Strawberry w. Berries	150	2.5	28
Creamy Vanilla w. Berries	160	2.5	32

Beverages: Per Serving			
Cafe Mocha, 10 fl.oz	160	7	27
Cappuccino: Eng. Toffee, 10 fl.oz	220	6	40
French Vanilla, 10 fl.oz	240	7	39
Iced w. Milk, 12 fl.oz	180	1.5	39
Iced, 12 oz	300	15	41
Coffee w. sugar/cream, 10 fl.oz	75	3.5	9
Hot Chocolate, 10 fl.oz	240	6	45
Iced Tea, 12 fl.oz	50	1	10

T.J. Cinnamons® (Oct '08)

Bakery	C	F	Cb
Chocolate Twist, 2½ oz	250	12	34
Cinnamon Twist, 1 roll, 2½ oz	260	14	33
T.J. Icing, 1 oz	120	5	18
Original Roll: no icing, 5.3 oz	505	10	73
w. Cream Cheese Icing	625	16	91
Pecan Sticky Bun, 1 bun, 6½ oz	690	22	91

Beverages: Per Serving (12 fl.oz)			
Coffee	0	0	0
Mocha Chill: no Whipped Cream	265	4	46
w. Whipped Cream	305	7	47

**For Extra Menu Items
+ Full Nutritional Data**
~ See Author's Website
www.CalorieKing.com

Fast - Foods & Restaurants

Togo's Eatery® (Oct '08)

Sandwiches: Regular 6" Roll

	C	F	Cb
Albacore Tuna	450	10	69
Avocado & Cucumber	590	26	79
Avocado & Turkey	670	27	78
Black Forest Ham & Cheese	630	24	67
Cheese Sandwich	660	30	70
Chunky Chicken & Almond Salad	750	43	64
Cold Roast Beef	680	22	68
Egg Salad & Cheese	650	28	69
Hummus	790	31	104
Salami & Cheese	760	37	70
The Italian	740	37	68
Turkey & Bacon Club	600	21	65
Turkey & Cheese	600	18	71
Turkey Ham & Cheese	600	19	70
Turkey Roast Beef & Cheese	670	23	70
BBQ Beef	530	13	64
California Roasted Chicken	620	15	68
French Onion Dip	640	16	66
Hot Pastrami	810	42	72
Meatballs in Zesty Tomato Sauce	690	23	80
Pastrami Reuben	650	25	68
Roast Beef	680	22	68
Savory BBQ Chicken	520	6	79
Sicilian Chicken	670	22	73

Large Size: Add 50% to Regular Size

Topz® (Oct '08)

Sandwiches & Burgers

	C	F	Cb
½ lb Black Angus Burger: w. sauce	735	40	40
no sauce	670	34	37
¼ lb Black Angus Chili Burger	490	21	42
¼ lb Black Angus Burger: w. sauce	505	25	40
no sauce	445	19	37
Gardenburger	355	12	46
Grilled Chicken Breast Burger	400	10	39
Turkey Burger	450	19	40
Sandwiches: Classic Grilled Cheese	415	18	47
Ginger Grilled Ahi	385	11	37
Grilled Cheese & Tomato	420	18	48

Sides

	C	F	Cb
Aero Fries, 5.6 oz	380	14	58
Aero Onion Rings, 5.8 oz	300	11	46
Chili Cheese Fries 10.6 oz	590	27	66
Signature Chili, 10.2 oz	330	17	17

Tropical Smoothie Cafe (Oct '08)

Sandwiches

	C	F	Cb
American Albacore	725	30	85
Cheese BLT	715	37	72
Chicken Caesar	625	25	66
Chipotle Chicken	660	27	71
Club Sandwich	705	26	77
Ham & Cheese	605	19	78
Roast Beef, Pepper Jack	680	30	63
The Italian	750	39	71
Turkey Bacon Ranch	670	23	69
Tuscan Turkey	440	13	67
Wraps: Breakfast Wrap (Bacon)	535	23	55
Breakfast Wrap (Ham)	525	18	57
Buffalo Chicken	565	21	61
Cool Tuna Wrap	645	27	71
Jamaican Jerk	580	13	79
King Caesar	555	27	55
Sesame Chicken	755	24	103
Totally Turkey	655	27	58

Salads: No Cheese or Dressing

	C	F	Cb
Chef Salad	170	2	11
Garden Classic Salad	60	0.5	10
Sesame Chicken Salad	415	10	53
Thai Chicken Salad	355	4	54

Low Fat Smoothies: With Turbinado

	C	F	Cb
Blimey Limey; Cool Breeze, avg.	410	0	102
Blue Lagoon	330	1	80
Hawaiian Breeze	360	0	88
Island Fever; Orange Passion, avg.	455	0.5	111
Rockin Raspberry	515	0.5	125
Strawberry Beach	450	0	109
Sunrise Sunset	390	0.5	96
Fat Buster	375	0.5	91
Health Nut	620	10	104
Lean Machine; Paradise Point, avg.	475	0.5	115
Muscle Blaster	595	3	119
Peanut Paradise	810	22	119

Dessert Smoothies: With Turbinado

	C	F	Cb
Beach Bum	560	5	125
Chocolate Chiller	555	7	118
Coconut Royale	730	11	155
Mocha Madness	645	12	127
Peanut Butter Cup	840	24	142

With Splenda: Deduct 200 calories & 50g carbs

Fast - Foods & *Restaurants*

Tubby's® (Oct '08)

Subs: Per Regular Sandwich

	C	F	Cb
Burger Subs: Big Tub	670	56	55
Burger Special	900	59	59
Cheeseburger	910	60	59
Pizza Burger	930	60	62
Taco Burger	825	47	67
Deli Style Subs: Ham & Cheese	570	30	54
Club Sub	700	41	53
Tubby's Famous	665	39	55
Turkey & Cheese	600	32	51
Turkey Club Sub	680	38	52
Specialty Subs: BLT	635	42	50
Cold Veggie	460	14	66
Italian Sausage	730	45	56
Tuna Salad	415	18	47
Veggie Stir Fry	650	27	90
Chicken Subs: Per Regular Sandwich			
Chicken & Broccoli	550	23	56
Chicken & Cheddar	545	23	54
Chicken Club Sub	705	41	53
Chicken Fajita Sub	445	12	57
Grilled Chicken	345	5	52
Steak Subs: Per Regular Sandwich			
Mushroom Steak	835	26	52
Pepper Steak	710	46	52
Pizza Steak	985	57	85
Steak & Cheese	825	56	51
Steak Special	745	46	58

Uno Chicago Grill® (Oct '08)

Fab Firsts: Per ⅓ Order

	C	F	Cb
Beer Battered Vidalia Onion Ring	410	24	46
Buffalo Bites	330	19	21
Buffalo Chicken Quesadillas	310	13	34
Crispy Cheese Dippers	280	15	27
Muchos Nachos	480	22	55
Pizza Skins	480	31	38
Rhode Island Style Calamari	350	31	26
Roasted Vegetable Quesadillas	24	9	30
Shrimp & Crab Fondue	210	14	14
The Chi-Town Tasting Plate	510	34	32
Flatbread Pizzas: Per ⅓ Pizza			
BBQ Chicken	270	10	28
Cheese and Tomato	270	11	31
Four Cheese	310	18	22
Mediterranean	230	12	22
Pepperoni	300	16	24
Sausage	290	15	22
Spicy Chicken	300	14	26
Spinach, Mushroom & Gorgonzola	270	11	31

For Complete Nutritional Data ~ see CalorieKing.com

Villa Pizza® (Oct '08)

Pizza (18"): Per Slice (⅙ Pizza)

	C	F	Cb
Neapolitan: Cheese	525	19	60
Sausage and Cheese	675	32	61
Pepperoni and Cheese	635	29	60
Stuffed: Meat	880	42	83
Spinach and Mushroom	790	35	87
Sicilian: Deluxe	945	39	105
Stromboli:			
Sausage and Cheese	880	44	83
Pepperoni and Cheese	745	33	83
Steamtable:			
Baked Ziti	680	35	63
Meat Lasagna	1235	81	86
Spinach and Cheese Lasagna	1065	60	88
Spaghetti	2710	122	349
Chicken Francais	225	11	4
Chicken Cacciatore	780	68	11
Italian Sausage and Peppers	645	64	3
Sauteed Fresh Vegetables	465	43	19
Salads:			
Caesar	110	8	7
Fresh Mozzarella	310	22	10
Greek	155	11	9

Vocelli Pizza® (Oct '08)

Pizze: Per Slice (⅛ Pizza)

	C	F	Cb
Grand Cheese	260	6	38
Grand Pepperoni	410	20	38
Gourmet: Per Slice (⅛ Pizza)			
Deluxe	390	16	40
Meat Magnifico	490	25	38
Philly Steak	360	13	38
Panini: Per Sandwich			
Chicken	900	38	81
Italian	910	42	77
Vegetarian	750	31	83
Insalata: Per Plate			
Chicken Caesar	220	4.5	4
Mediterranean	270	18	20
Tuscany Chicken	350	16	15
Antipasta	630	50	16
Pepperoni Sticks, 2½ slices	470	26	36
Croutons, 1 Package,	30	1	5
Bruschetta, 1 slice	150	8	14
Buffalo Wings (10)	560	39	3
BBQ Wings (10)	610	33	31
Dressings: Per 2 oz Packet			
Italian	200	21	4
Ranch	260	28	2
Bleu Cheese	230	25	2

Wahoo's Fish Taco® (Oct '08)

Bowls

Carne Asada, Steak	760	22	90
Chicken, Skinless Breast	750	18	90
Fish of the Day	705	16	90

Classic Burrito (A la Carte)

Fish, average	455	14	51
Chicken, average	545	17	50
Carne Asada	515	20	49
Carnitas	595	26	49
Shrimp	470	14	51
Veggie	600	14	98
Mushroom	415	17	57

Tacos: Carne Asada, Steak

	195	7	18
Carnitas, Pork	230	10	18
Chicken, Skinless Breast	210	6	18
Fish of the Day	175	4	19
Veggie	200	4	33

Sides: Beans

	445	2	80
Rice	475	6	94

Salads: Chips Not Included

Carne Asada, Steak	555	33	13
Chicken, average	560	28	15
Fish, average	420	23	15

For Complete Nutritional Data ~ see CalorieKing.com

WAWA® (Oct '08)

Breakfast & Baked Goods

	C	F	Cb
Bagel: Plain	285	1	60
w. Butter	505	23	64
w. Cream Cheese	430	13	67
Bagel Melts: Ham & Cheese	485	13	67
Pepperoni & Cheese	660	33	59
Pork Roll & Cheese	655	26	77
Breakfast Bowls: Per Bowl			
Creamed Chipped Beef on a Bisc.	475	23	56
Sausage Gravy on a Biscuit	505	27	56
Hash Brown (1), 2.5 oz	130	8	15
Muffins: Banana Walnut, 6 oz	670	34	83
Blueberry, 6.2 oz	620	33	76
Chocolate Chip, 4 oz	680	36	84
Corn, 6 oz	640	29	87
Sizzli Bagels: Bacon Egg & Chse	410	19	48
Sausage Egg & Cheese	515	28	49
Sizzli Biscuits: Bacon Egg & Chse	535	33	52
Sausage Egg & Cheese	635	42	53
Sizzli Muffins:			
Sausage, Egg & Cheese	460	29	35
Hot Sandwiches: No Cheese Unless Indicated			
Chicken Caesar w. Cheese	455	12	49
Cheese Steak	450	17	36
Classics: Roasted Pork w. Cheese	760	33	66
Cheese Steak	700	25	62
Meatball w. Cheese	700	31	74
Roast Beef Homestyle w. Cheese	740	24	71

WAWA® cont... (Oct '08)

	C	F	Cb
Cold Sandwiches: No Cheese Unless Indicated			
Chicken and Salad	540	30	41
Corned Beef	400	9	35
Egg Salad	540	33	41
Ham	335	7	38
Classics: BLT	780	42	62
Roast Beef Classic	600	10	62
Turkey Carolina Honey Smoked	470	6	70
Turkey	470	6	70
Tuna Salad	900	53	97
Veggie	330	3	62
Cold Shortis: American	685	20	97
BLT; Cheese, average	500	28	37
Chicken Salad	540	29	49
Egg Salad w. Cheese	640	40	49
Turkey	560	7	94
Hot Shortis: Chicken Steak	325	6	42
Meatball w. Cheese	685	21	103
Roast Beef w. Cheese	410	13	46
Wraps: Buffalo Blue Chicken	260	4	37
Chipotle Ranch Roast Beef	350	5	37
Ham, Turkey & Cheddar	370	7	39
Roast Beef & Pepper Jack	410	16	38
Roasted Chicken Caesar	300	5	39
Hot Dogs: ¼ lb Beef Frank	385	28	23
All Beef Hot Dog	250	15	22
Big Bacon Cheese Dog	720	49	45
Hot Sausage	310	20	21
Kielbasa	290	17	21
Bowls: Beef Stew	470	29	45
Chili	390	11	57
Homestyle Roast Beef	500	29	41
Meatballs	475	18	61
Sides: Per Medium Serve			
Beef Stew, 11 oz	265	12	22
Chili, 11 oz	220	8	28
Homestyle Chkn & Noodles, 11 oz	325	16	25
Macaroni & Beef, 11 oz	335	12	41
Macaroni & Cheese, 11 oz	460	22	50
Mashed Potatoes, 11 oz	470	31	47
Meatballs in a Cup, 4 oz	160	11	9
Soups: Per 11 oz Medium Bowl			
Boston Clam Chowder	275	14	25
Chicken Corn Chowder	350	23	29
Cream of Broccoli	215	13	20
Vegetable Beef & Barley	150	5	21
Drinks: Per 12 fl.oz			
Cappuccino	210	8	30
Low-Fat	180	1	39
French Vanilla Cappuccino	210	7	33
Mocha Wakeup, 12 fl.oz	195	7	34

Wendy's® (Oct '08)

Sandwiches	C	F	Cb
¼ lb. Deluxe Double Stack	410	22	29
¼ lb. Double Stack	360	18	28
¼ lb. Single	430	20	39
Baconator Burger	840	51	38
Jr. Bacon Cheeseburger	320	16	26
Chicken Temptations: Homestyle	430	16	48
Spicy Chicken Fillet	440	16	46
Ultimate Chicken Grill Fillet	320	7	36
French Fries: Kid's, 2.5 oz	210	10	28
Small, 4 oz	340	16	45
Medium, 5 oz	425	20	56
Large, 6.5 oz	550	26	73
Chicken: Crispy Nuggets, 5 pce	230	15	12
Sauce: Barbecue	45	0	11
Sweet & Spicy Hawaiian	70	0	17
Kids Meal: Cheeseburger only	270	11	26
Hamburger only	220	8	26
Garden Sensations Salads			
Chicken BLT Salad no dress./topping	340	19	10
with Croutons/Dressings	780	53	42
Caesar Chicken no dress./topping	180	6	8
with Croutons & Dressings	490	33	20
Mandarin Chicken w. Noodles	540	25	50
Southwest Taco no dress./topping	430	22	30
Caesar Side Salad no dress./topping	70	4	7
Side Salad no Dressing	35	0	8
Baked Patatoes: Plain 10 oz	270	0	61
Plain w. Buttery Spread	320	6	61
Bacon & Cheese	450	13	67
Broccoli & Cheese	320	2	69
Sour Cream & Chives	320	4	63
Sides: Chili Large, 12 oz	280	9	29
Cheddar Cheese, shredded, 2 Tbsp	70	6	1
Hot Chili Seasoning, 1 pkg	5	0	4
Saltine Crackers, (2)	25	0.5	4
Chocolate Chip Cookie	270	12	37
Mandarin Orange Cup, 5 oz	80	0	19
Yogurt, w. Granola Cup, 5.7 oz	250	6	42
Frosty: Original Chocolate, 4 oz	160	4	26

For Complete Nutritional Data ~ see CalorieKing.com

Western Sizzlin® (Oct '08)

Steaks (Meat Only, Raw Wts)	C	F	Cb
New York Strip, 14 oz	900	60	0
Ribeye, 10 oz	520	28	0
Sirloin: 8 oz Steak	540	33	0
16 oz Steak	1080	66	0
T-Bone, 20 oz	1230	99	0
Baked Potato, plain, 8 oz	245	0	58

Wienerschnitzel® (Oct '08)

Breakfast	C	F	Cb
Biscuit: w. Bacon	330	17	35
Egg & Bacon	390	21	36
Egg, Bacon & Cheese	440	25	36
Egg, Sausage & Cheese	540	34	40
Burrito: Egg, Bacon & Cheese	490	25	39
Chili Cheese	470	21	43
Country Breakfast	640	40	47
French Toast Sticks	490	29	49
Hash Browns, 2.8 oz	290	16	14
Platter w. Bacon	600	40	40
Burgers: Chili Cheeseburger	350	13	32
Deluxe Cheeseburger	450	23	33
Deluxe Hamburger	400	19	33
Double Chili Cheeseburger	560	24	35
Fries: Regular, 4.5 oz	340	25	28
Large, 6.5 oz	470	34	39
Chili Cheese, 8 oz	540	38	39
Hot Dogs: Chili Dog	290	13	31
Chili Cheese Dog	340	17	31
Deluxe; Kraut; Mustard; Relish, avg.	270	12	30
All Beef: Chili Dog	380	21	33
Chili Cheese Dog	430	25	33
Other varieties, avg.	365	20	31
Turkey: Chili Dog	270	11	31
Chili Cheese Dog	320	15	31
Other varieties, average	250	10	28
For Pretzel Bun add extra	145	3	26
Sandwiches: Bacon Ranch Chkn	430	21	37
Italian Sausage	350	17	31
Pastrami	580	35	38
Polish Sausage	490	29	39
Sides: Onion Straws, 3.4 oz	430	35	25
Ranch Dressing, 1.2 oz	120	12	2
Desserts: Freezee, average	630	25	100
Banana Split	820	24	149
Chocolate Dipped Cone	490	29	57
Plain Cone	300	11	49

Whataburger® (Oct '08)

Burgers/Sandwiches	C	F	Cb
Justaburger	290	15	53
Whataburger: Burger	620	30	58
No Bun	290	20	8
w. Bacon & Cheese	780	43	59
w. Bacon & Cheese, no bun	450	32	9
w. Cheese, no bun	380	27	9
Whataburger Jr.	300	15	28
Double Meat Whataburger	870	49	58
Triple Meat Whataburger	1120	68	58
Grilled Chicken: Sandwich	470	19	49
no bun	250	12	13
Whatacatch Sandwich	460	29	38
Whatachick'n Sandwich	550	20	65
French Fries: Small, 3 oz	260	13	31
Medium, 4½ oz	400	20	47
Large, 6 oz	530	27	63
Onion Rings: Medium, 4.3 oz	420	28	36
Large, 6.4 oz	630	42	55
Chicken Strips (2)	380	45	22
Salads: Chicken Strips Salad	570	38	34
w. Cheddar Cheese, no Bacon	740	51	35
Garden Salad	60	0	12
w. Cheddar Cheese, no Bacon	230	13	13
Grilled Chicken Salad	230	7	19
w. Cheddar Cheese, no Bacon	400	20	20
Dressings: Per 2 oz Package			
Buttermilk Ranch	310	33	3
Caesar	190	19	3
Thousand Island	150	13	10
Reduced-Fat Ranch	230	22	6
Low-Fat Vinaigrette	40	1.5	5
Shakes			
Chocolate; Strawb.: Med., 27 fl.oz	995	26	171
Small, 17 fl.oz	630	16	111
Vanilla: Medium, 27 fl.oz	890	28	139
Small, 17 fl.oz	560	17	87
Breakfast: Cinnamon Roll	400	7	80
Hash Brown Sticks (4)	200	12	20
Texas Toast, 1 slice	150	7	20
Biscuit: Plain	300	17	32
w. Bacon	350	20	32
w. Gravy	530	36	52
w. Sausage	540	37	32
Honey Butter Chicken	610	38	51
Biscuit Sandwich: w. Egg & Chse	450	28	33
w. Bacon, Egg & Cheese	500	32	33
w. Sausage, Egg & Cheese	690	49	33

Whataburger® cont... (Oct '08)

Breakfast (Cont)	C	F	Cb
Breakfast On A Bun: w. Bacon	360	21	25
w. Sausage	550	38	25
Breakfast Platter (Biscuit/Eggs/Hash Brown)			
w. Bacon	740	45	53
w. Sausage	930	62	53
Pancakes: Plain (3)	580	8	112
w. Bacon	630	12	112
w. Sausage	820	29	112
Taquito: w. Bacon & Egg	380	21	27
w. Bacon, Egg & Cheese	420	24	27
w. Potato & Egg	430	23	37
w. Potato, Egg & Cheese	470	27	37
w. Sausage & Egg	410	24	27
w. Sausage, Egg & Cheese	450	28	27
Desserts: Hot Apple Pie	230	11	29
Chocolate Chunk Cookie	230	11	33
White Choc. Macadamia Cookie	250	14	30

White Castle® (Oct '08)

Sandwiches & Burgers	C	F	Cb
Cheeseburger	170	9	15
Double	300	17	23
Hamburger	140	7	14
Double	250	13	22
Sandwiches: Chicken Ring	170	8	17
Chicken Breast w. Cheese	200	7	21
Chicken Supreme	230	10	21
Fish w/ Cheese on Golden Bun	190	8	20
Surf & Turf	390	22	28
Sides			
Chicken Rings: 6 rings, 3.9 oz	340	23	15
9 rings, 5.8 oz	510	34	22
Clam Strips, 4 oz	250	22	4.5
Fish Nibblers, 4.1 oz	315	16	24
French Fries, 3.8 oz	310	15	39
Mozzarella Cheese Sticks, 3 sticks	250	14	22
Onion Chips, 4 oz	490	23	62
Onion Rings Homestyle, 3.4 oz	405	21	49
Sauces & Condiments: Per Packet			
Ranch Dressing, 1 oz	150	17	0
Ketchup, 0.3 oz	10	0	2.5
Lemon Juice, 0.1 oz	0	0	0
Mayonnaise, 0.3 oz	60	7	0
Sauce: BBQ, 0.3 oz	10	0	2.5
Cheese, 1.5 oz	130	10	6
Seafood, 1 oz	30	0	7
White Castle Zesty Zing, 1 oz	110	11	3

Winchell's® (Oct '08)

Baked Products	C	F	Cb
Croissant	260	17	28
Cake Donuts: Chocolate Iced	230	15	28
Traditional Cake	215	14	26
Yeast Raised Donuts: *Per Donut*			
Chocolate Bar	240	16	29
Chocolate Round/Twist	240	16	29
Glazed Round/Twist	230	15	27

WingStreet (Oct '08)

Chicken	C	F	Cb
Crispy Bone In Wings: *Per 2 Pieces*			
All American, 1.7 oz	170	13	7
Buffalo, Mild./Hot, 2.3 oz	210	13	14
Cajun, 2.3 oz	210	13	15
Garlic Parmesan, 2 oz	210	16	8
Bone Out Wings: *Per 2 Pieces*			
All American, 2.2 oz	190	10	11
Buffalo, Mild/Med./Hot, 2.8 oz	220	11	18
Cajun, 2.8 oz	220	10	19
Garlic Parmesean, 2.4 oz	220	14	12
Traditional Wings: *Per 2 Pieces*			
All American, 1.4 oz	80	5	0
Buffalo, Mild./Med./Hot, 2 oz	110	6	7
Cajun, 2 oz	120	6	8
Garlic Parm., 1.7 oz	120	9	1
Sides: Apple Pies, 2 pies, 3.7 oz	360	18	47
Fried Cheese Sticks, 3.4 oz	310	19	25
Taters, 8 oz	790	52	74

Woody's Bar-B-Q (Oct '08)

Entrees	C	F	Cb
½ Chicken	840	56	0
Baby Back Ribs, ½ Rack	520	40	2
Beef Prime Rib	230	19	1
Chicken Breast: 1 piece	250	14	4
Spicy Breaded, 1 piece	200	8	14
Chicken Tenders, 2 pieces	190	7	18
Chicken Wings, 2 pieces	210	13	4
Homestyle Meat Loaf, 4 oz	340	26	10
Hot Dog	330	28	8
Pulled Pork, 5 oz	500	38	8
Sausage, 5 pieces	260	16	20
Shrimp, 6 shrimp	180	1	33
Spare Ribs, ½ slab, 8 oz	540	42	0
Wrap: BBQ Beef	380	13	31
BBQ Pork	440	21	31
BBQ Turkey	320	10	32

For Complete Nutritional Data ~ see CalorieKing.com

Yoshinoya® (Oct '08)

Bowls: Without sauce unless indicated	C	F	Cb
Beef Bowl®: Regular	760	30	92
Large	1090	41	137
Beef Bowl® w/ Beef Soup, regular	800	30	98
Beef Bowl® w/ Vegetables, regular	680	22	95
Beef & Chicken Combo, large	1120	33	151
Chicken Bowl: Regular	660	12	104
Large	1110	22	180
Chicken Bowl w/ Teriyaki Sce, reg.	790	12	135
Shrimp Bowl: Regular	550	4	106
with Seafood Sauce	680	4	136
Spicy Chicken Bowl: Regular	640	12	99
w/ Spicy Teriyaki Sauce	730	12	119
Vegetable Bowl, regular	440	3	95
Kids: Beef w/ Vegetables	350	11	48
Chicken w/ Vegetables	360	7	53
Soups: Chicken Vegetable	70	1.5	7
Clam Chowder	210	7	34
Miso Soup	60	1.5	8
Salad, Chicken	290	14	2
Sesame Wings, 6 pieces	420	27	2

Z Pizza® (Oct '08)

Pizzas: Small 10", Per ⅙ Slice	C	F	Cb
American	240	13	19
Berkeley Soy Cheese Veggie	180	8	19
California	150	6	19
Casablanca	190	9	18
Greek	150	6	17
Italian	180	8	17
Mediterranean	160	7	21
Mexican	180	7	19
Moroccan	190	10	17
Napoli	180	8	18
Provence	160	7	20
Santa Fe	180	7	20
Thai	170	6	19
Tuscan Mushroom	160	7	18
ZBQ	170	5	21
Salads: Salad Dressing is not included in figures			
Antipasto	230	17	6
Arugula	260	20	14
Caesar	100	6	7
California	100	6	10
Greek	120	6	12
Pear and Gorgonzola Salad	220	5	22
Spinach Salad	45	2	7
ZBQ Salad	200	2	19
Sandwiches: Hot Meatball Sub	670	34	45
Pollo Latino Sandwich	350	11	38
Supersub	460	23	34
Turkey Breast Sandwich	400	14	35
Yuppie Veggie Sandwich	460	24	46
Calzones: Classic Calzone	890	49	73
Veggie Calzone	590	16	89

Zaxby's (Oct '08)

Zappetizers	C	F	Cb
Onion Rings, w/o Sce	625	41	55
Spicy Fried Mushroom w/o Sce	505	33	43
Tater Chips, 5.6 oz	800	53	76
Chicken: With Sides, w/o Sauce			
Buffalo Fingerz, 5-pieces	430	20	8
Buffalo Wings, 5-pieces	370	23	0
Chicken Fingerz, 5 fingers, 6 oz	425	20	8.5
Meal Dealz: Without Sauce			
Big Zax Snax	765	34	78
Buffalo Wings	740	39	53
Chicken Finger Plate: Regular	1055	50	91
Large	1585	73	147
Chicken Finger Sandwich	1265	69	116
Grilled Chicken Sandwich	1070	49	107
Kickin Chicken Sandwich	1190	68	107
Nibbler	1235	69	127
Wings & Things: Regular	1140	57	80
Large	1675	80	134
Sandwich Baskets: Includes Fries & Pickles			
Cajun Club	1180	57	107
Chicken Salad	1245	66	118
Zaxby's Club	1220	69	102
Zax Kidz: Kiddie Cheese	435	20	46
Kiddie Finger	390	17	34
Zalads: With Texas Toast, w/o Dressing			
Blue Zalad: w. Blackened Fillet	590	27	37
w. Buffalo Fingerz	750	39	46
Caesar Zalad: with Chicken Fingerz	665	34	31
with Grilled Fillet	515	23	24
House Zalad: with Grilled Fillet	605	30	36
with Chicken Fingerz	755	41	43
Zensation, w. Chicken Fingers	835	39	77
Salad Dressings: Per 1.5 oz Packet			
Blue Cheese	220	23	2
Caesar Salad with Croutons	200	21	2
Honey French	185	15	11
Honey Mustard	180	16	8
Lite Vinaigrette	55	3	8
Mediterranean	170	17	5
Ranch	190	20	2
Thousand Island	270	29	3
Sides: Celery Sticks, 2.6 oz	5	0	2
Cole Slaw, 2.8 oz	115	8	10
Crinkle Fries, 8 oz	590	25	84
Onion Rings, 2.5 oz	310	21	28
Texas Toast, 3 wedges, 1.4 oz	145	6	20

Zero's Subs® (Oct '08)

Oven Baked 6" Subs:	C	F	Cb
Includes cheese, lettuce, tomato, onions, oil & vinegar			
BLT	410	19	48
BLT, no Mayo	330	12	43
Cosmo Vegetarian	470	23	46
Cosmo Vegetarian Deluxe	490	25	48
Grinder	550	31	48
Grinder, Multigrain	560	32	50
Ham & Cheese	440	19	44
Meatball & Cheese	565	30	50
without Cheese	465	22	50
Pepperoni & Cheese	545	31	42
without Cheese	345	15	41
Roast Beef & Cheese	460	19	45
The Club	515	23	44
Tuna & Cheese	520	26	47
Turkey & Cheese	455	17	44
6" Subs From The Grill			
Grilled Veggie	395	14	52
Hot Italian Sausage & Cheese	665	37	45
Philly Chicken & Cheese	400	10	48
w. Mushrooms/Green Peppers	410	10	49
without Cheese	330	4	47
12" Size Subs: Double the figures for 6" size			

Zoup!® (Oct '08)

Soups: Per 8 fl.oz Cup	C	F	Cb
Chicken Potpie	200	8	21
Cream of Broccoli	160	11	12
Fire Roasted Tomato Bisque	290	22	28
Ginger Butternut Squash	240	15	28
Jamaican Bay Gumbo	140	2.5	20
New England Clam Chowder	200	5	22
Seafood Bisque	150	6	12
Tomato Spinach & Brown Rice	100	3	19
Vegetable Bounty	90	1.5	33
Vegetarian Split Pea	140	1.5	25
White Chicken Chili	160	3	23
Other varieties, average	140	7	17
SandwichZ: on Ciabatta, half			
Chicken Greek w. Feta	430	12	5
Southwest Turkey	475	18	52
BLT w. Avocado	340	11	51
Bread: Per Piece			
French, 2 oz	150	2.5	21
Multigrain, 2.4 oz	185	2.5	35
Artisan Ciabatta, 2.8 oz	215	1	35

Notes on Cholesterol

- **Cholesterol** is a white waxy substance produced mainly by our liver. It is also found in animal food products. Plant foods have no cholesterol.

- **Cholesterol is essential to life.** It is a structural part of every body cell wall and is the building block for vitamin D, sex hormones, and bile acids which help in the digestion of dietary fats.

- **The body makes sufficient cholesterol** for its needs and does not rely on cholesterol in the diet. Dietary fats have a major influence on blood cholesterol levels - more so than dietary cholesterol.

- **A high blood cholesterol level increases** the risk of atherosclerosis - the thickening of arteries that can reduce or block blood flow to the heart, brain, eyes, kidneys, sex organs and other body parts.

  This in turn increases the risk of heart attack, stroke, blindness, kidney failure, impotence and other blood circulatory problems.

  Other risk factors which increase the risk of atherosclerosis include high blood pressure, smoking, obesity and uncontrolled diabetes.

BLOOD CHOLESTEROL

CHECK YOUR RISK!

Total Cholesterol Level (mg/dl)		Risk of Heart Attack
240 and above	~	High Risk
200 - 239	~	Borderline/High
Below 200	~	Desirable

♥ **Know your cholesterol level, particularly if there is a family history of heart disease or stroke. If level is high, see your doctor.**

♥ **All adults should have their cholesterol, HDL and triglycerides tested at least every 5 years.**

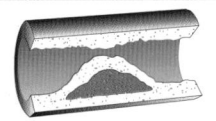

▲ **Atherosclerosis can clog arteries and impede blood flow to the heart or other body organs.**

▼ **A thrombus (blood clot) can form on unstable, festering athero-sclerotic plaque and rapidly block blood flow. A heart attack or stroke can result.**

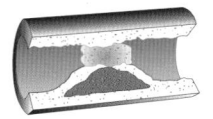

HEART ATTACK WARNING SIGNALS

Many victims die before reaching the hospital by ignoring warning signals and delaying medical help.

Symptoms vary and commonly include:

- **Chest pain,** vice-like squeezing or burning sensation in center of the chest or between the shoulder blades, or in the mid-back. Pain may even feel like severe indigestion.

- **Pain** may be felt in the arms, shoulders, neck or jaw.

- **Shortness of breath** often occurs with or before chest discomfort.

- **Other signs,** with or without pain, include a cold sweat, nausea or light-headedness.

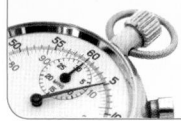

If you experience any of the above symptoms call IMMEDIATELY for medical help. Every minute counts.

Call 9-1-1 *or your emergency number*

The amount and type of dietary fat has the greatest influence on blood cholesterol levels.

Fats in food are a mixture of 3 basic types: saturated, monounsaturated, and polyunsaturated. Animal fats are mainly saturated while plant oils and fish oils are mainly mono- and polyunsaturated.

Saturated fats have subgroups known as long-chain, medium-chain, and short-chain fats. Most of the long chain fats raise blood cholesterol, and increase the risk of blood clots and thrombosis leading to artery blockage.

Long-chain saturated fats are found mainly in full-cream milk, cheese, butter, cream, fatty meats and sausages, and processed foods.

Monounsaturated fats tend to more selectively lower 'bad' LDL cholesterol and maintain the protective 'good' HDL cholesterol in the bloodstream – but only if they replace saturated fats in the diet.

Foods rich in monounsaturates include canola and olive oils, canola margarine, peanuts, and avocados.

Polyunsaturated fats consist of two main classes. **Omega-6** polyunsaturates tend to lower blood cholesterol. Rich sources include safflower, sunflower and corn oils.

Omega-3 polyunsaturated fats can lower blood cholesterol; significantly lower blood triglycerides; and reduce the rise of thrombosis, heart arrythmmia, and artery spasm.

Best practical omega-3 sources include canola oil and margarine, soybean oil and fish.

A balanced intake of the two omega classes is important for optimal health. For most Americans, slightly increasing omega-3 intake would help attain a more ideal balance.

Trans fats from hydrogenated vegetable oils and shortenings should also be avoided. They are common in commercial baked and fried food products such as cakes, muffins, pastries, doughnuts, fried snacks and french fries.

Note: All fats are high in calories and need to be limited for weight control.

DIETARY FATS COMPARISON

■ Saturated Fat   ■ Monounsaturated Fat

Polyunsaturated Fats:
☐ Linoleic (Omega-6)   ■ Alpha-Linolenic (Omega-3)

OILS — PERCENTAGE CONTENT

Oil	Saturated Fat	Monounsaturated Fat	Linoleic (Omega-6)	Alpha-Linolenic (Omega-3)
CANOLA OIL	7	63	20	10
LINSEED/FLAX OIL	9	19	17	55
SAFFLOWER OIL	9	14	77	
GRAPESEED OIL	10	22	68	
SUNFLOWER OIL	11	23	66	
CORN OIL	14	32	52	2
OLIVE OIL	14	76	10	
SOYBEAN OIL	15	23	54	8
PEANUT OIL	19	45	34	2
COTTONSEED OIL	26	16	58	
PALM OIL	51	39	10	

SPREADS & FATS

Saturated Fat includes 'Trans Fats'   ☐ WATER CONTENT

Spread/Fat	Saturated Fat	Monounsaturated Fat	Linoleic (Omega-6)	Alpha-Linolenic (Omega-3)	Water Content
LIGHT MARGARINE	14	14	21		51
CANOLA MARGARINE	18	45	12	6	19
POLYUNSATURATED MARG	24	20	36		20
BUTTER	57	18	2		24
LARD	41	47			12
BEEF FAT	44	37	4		15

GOOD SOURCES OF OMEGA-3 FATS

Plant Sources	Omega-3 Fats (Grams)
Canola Oil, 1 Tbsp, ½ fl.oz	1.5g
Flaxseed Oil, 1 Tbsp	8g
Soybean Oil, 1 Tbsp	1.2g
Canola Margarine, 1 Tbsp, ½ oz	1g
Soybeans, cooked, ½ cup, 4 oz	0.5g
Walnuts, ½ oz	0.5g

FISH - *Per 4 oz Serving*

High Content: Salmon (Chinook), Tuna, Trout (Lake), Sardines, Herring, Mackerel — 3g / 3g

Medium Content:
Salmon, (Pink/Red/Coho), 4 oz — 2g

Fair Content: *Per 4 oz Serving*
Bass, Catfish, Cod, Grouper, Hake, Halibut, Kingfish, Perch, Pollock, Shark, Trout (Rainbow), Tuna, Crab, Oysters, Blue Mussels, Shrimp, Squid — 0.5-1g

How Much Is Needed?

As little as 1-2 grams daily of omega-3 fats may benefit general health. High doses of fish-oil supplements should only be taken as directed by your doctor.

Dietary Cholesterol

Cholesterol in food varies in its effect on blood cholesterol level (BCL) from person to person. Much depends on the amount and type of fat and fiber eaten at the same meal.

Any elevating effect of dietary cholesterol on BCL is more likely to occur when the diet is high in saturated fat. Little elevation, if any, generally occurs when dietary fats are balanced in favor of monounsaturated and polyunsaturated fats (including omega-3 fats).

For example, while fish does contain cholesterol, the omega-3 fats can prevent any increase in BCL. Conversely, a meal containing no cholesterol but rich in saturated fat may result in a significant increase in BCL.

Consequently, the need to be overly-concerned about dietary cholesterol is being de-emphasized in favor of the approach of limiting total fat, saturated fat, and trans fat in particular – and substituting unsaturated fats.

The liver usually cuts back its own cholesterol production in response to cholesterol in the diet. Many people can consume normal amounts of high-cholesterol foods without concern.

However, it is difficult to identify just who is at risk - the so-called 'hyper-responders'. Because over 50% of Americans have a BCL above ideal levels, the **American Heart Association** advises all Americans to be prudent and limit their cholesterol intake to less than 300mg daily, as well as to adopt a heart-healthy diet.

This limitation still allows the inclusion of most foods that are regularly eaten – even the overly-maligned egg.

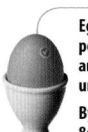

Eggs contain a modest 5 grams of fat per large egg, barely 2 grams of which are saturated, the rest being mono-unsaturated and polyunsaturated.

By comparison, a cup of whole milk has 8g fat of which almost 5g is saturated.

CHOLESTEROL COUNTER

Cholesterol is found only in foods of animal origin. Plant foods contain no cholesterol.
AHA recommends limiting dietary cholesterol to less than 300mg/day.

	Chol mg
Meat - Average all types:	
Lean Meat, cooked, 4 oz	70
Fatty Meat, cooked, 4 oz	105
Fat, thick strip, 2 oz	35

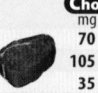

Note: While lean meat and fat have similar amounts of cholesterol, choose lean meat to limit fat intake.

Chicken/Turkey, average, 4 oz	90
Organ Meats: Liver, fried, 4 oz	500
Brains, beef, pan fried, 3 oz	1700
Sausages: Frankfurter, 1.5 oz	25
Salami, 2 slices, 2 oz	40
Bacon: 3 slices, cooked, 1 oz	20
Fish: Fish fillets, average, ckd, 4 oz	70
Tuna/Salmon, canned, 3 oz	30
Scallops, 9 medium, 3 oz	30
Shrimp, 12 large, raw, 3 oz	130
Oysters, raw, 6 medium, 3 oz	45
Lobster, Crab, raw, 3 oz	80
Eggs (Chicken), 1 large	210
1 medium	180
Egg White, *Egg Beaters*	0
Milk/Yogurt: Whole, 1 cup, 8 fl.oz	35
1% Milk, 1 cup	10
Skim/Non-fat, 1 cup	5
Soy Milk, Tofu, Tempeh	0
Cheese: Natural/Hard/Cream, 1 oz	30
Cottage, lowfat, 4 oz	5
Ricotta, part skim, 4 oz	25
Fats: Butter, 2 Tbsp, 1 oz	60
Margarine, Oils (vegetable)	0
Mayonnaise, 1 Tbsp	10
Cream: Heavy, whipping, 2 T, 1 oz	40
Half & Half/Sour, 2 Tbsp, 1 oz	10
Ice Cream: Regular, ½ cup, 4 fl.oz	30
Fruit, Vegetables, Avocados	0
Nuts, Seeds, Grains	0
Coffee, Tea, Soda, Beer, Wine	0

For Comprehensive Food Listings ~ see CalorieKing.com

Blood Cholesterol ~ Diet Hints

DIETARY HINTS TO LOWER BLOOD CHOLESTEROL

1. **Maintain a healthy weight.**
   If overweight, lose weight with a low-fat meal plan and daily exercise.

2. **Reduce saturated fat intake by:**
   (a) eating less dairy fat. Choose low-fat or fat-reduced varieties of milk, yogurt, soy drinks, cheese, and ice cream.
   (b) replacing saturated fats with fats and oils rich in monounsaturated and polyunsaturated fats. Choose vegetable oils such as canola, olive, sunflower and soybean. Avoid solid frying fats.

   Take Control and *Benecol* (spreads) contain plant stanol esters which can lower total and LDL cholesterol.

   (c) eating less fat from meat and poultry. Choose lean cuts of meat and skinless chicken. Go easy on lunch meats, salami and fatty sausages. Enjoy fish.

   (d) eating less saturated and trans fats from baked and fried fast-foods. Avoid deep-fried foods. Avoid donuts, cakes, pastries and cookies unless made with healthier fats and oils.

3. **Increase your soluble fiber intake.**
   Foods rich in soluble fiber include beans, lentils, chick peas, hummus, nuts, seeds, psyllium-seed husks and psyllium-fiber supplements. Oat bran, rice bran and barley are also good sources, as are fruit, veggies and avocados. (*See Fiber Guide - Page 276-281*).

4. **Eat more soy bean products** such as: soy drinks, tofu, tempeh (cultured soy beans), soy flour and soy vegetarian foods. Soy protein in place of animal protein can significantly decrease high blood cholesterol levels as well as 'bad' LDL cholesterol and blood triglycerides while 'good' HDL cholesterol is maintained. For best results, eat at least 25g of soy protein per day (from 3-4 servings).

5. **Eat more fruit, vegetables, and whole grains** in place of high-fat foods. Aim for 2 fruits and 5 servings of vegetables per day. They also contain valuable antioxidants. The fat of avocados (and most nuts) is mainly unsaturated and can lower blood cholesterol levels.

6. **Limit cholesterol to 300mg per day.** (Extra Notes ~ See Previous Page)

7. **Avoid brewed unfiltered coffee** (espresso; plunger-style). Several cups per day may raise blood cholesterol. Filtered coffee is fine.

8. **Spread your food intake over the day.** Have 5-6 small meals per day rather than just 2-3 large meals. Nibbling, versus gorging, favors lower blood cholesterol.

ALCOHOL - WINE

Alcohol is a mixed bag. Moderate amounts of 1-2 drinks daily appear to reduce the risk of heart attack and ischemic stroke in older persons.

However, larger amounts increase the risk of high blood pressure, obesity, heart failure and hemorrhagic stroke, and can aggravate hypertriglyceridemia: as well as many other health hazards. (*See Alcohol Guide – Page 25*)

The speculative benefits of moderate alcohol intake have been overstated in the media. The overriding harmful effects of excess alcohol do not allow its recommendation for any aspects of health promotion.

Fruit, Vegetables & Tea Also Protect:
Red wine and red grapes (more so than white) contain antioxidants which may help protect cholesterol in the blood from becoming oxidized.

Many fruits, vegetables, grains, nuts and tea also contain protective antioxidants.

Fats in the diet affect more than blood cholesterol levels. They can also strongly influence blood clot formation and thrombosis, as well as blood flow and ultimate oxygen delivery to body parts and organs.

While advanced atherosclerosis can impede blood flow to the heart and other organs, it is thrombosis (complete blockage by blood clots) or arterial spasm which commonly results in a heart attack or stroke.

Plant and fish oils rich in omega-3 fats lessen the risk of blood clots, thrombus formation, and artery spasm by reducing platelet stickiness and adhesion to artery walls. This reduces the risk of atherosclerotic plaque becoming unstable and reactive.

Omega-3 fats also improve blood flow by reducing blood viscosity and increasing the flexibility of red blood cells (RBC) that need to flex and twist on themselves in order to squeeze through tiny narrow capillaries often half their diameter.

A diet high in saturated fats has the opposite effect by stiffening RBC membranes and increasing blood viscosity, thereby hindering blood flow. The stiffening of the RBC membrane also reduces its ability to release vital oxygen to body cells and take up carbon dioxide.

Stiff red blood cells may also form aggregates that resemble coin stacks. In narrow blood vessels, this further impedes blood flow and impairs oxygen release through the much-lessened surface area of red blood cell membranes exposed to blood. (Smoking, lack of exercise, and stress can have similar adverse effects on thrombosis, red blood cell flexibility, and blood flow.)

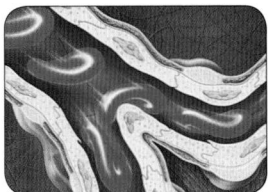

▲ Picture of Healthy Blood Flow

Flexible red blood cells twist and slide through tiny capillaries - often half the diameter of red blood cells.

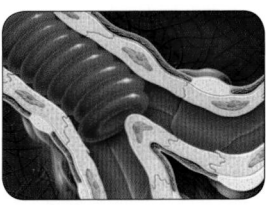

▲ A Not-So-Healthy Picture!

Red blood cells have lost their flexibility and ability to twist and slip through capillaries. They are stacked up, thereby impeding blood flow.

A diet high in saturated fats can contribute to this picture - as can smoking, lack of exercise, and stress.

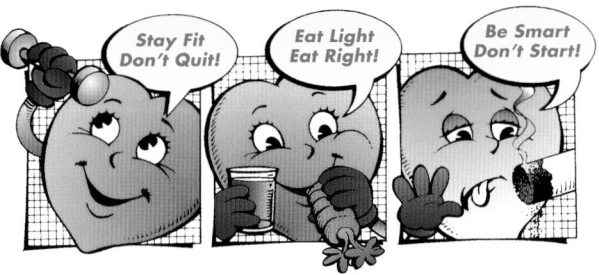

Stay Fit Don't Quit!

Eat Light Eat Right!

Be Smart Don't Start!

Fiber Guide

Introduction

Fiber is the general term for those parts of **plant** food that we cannot digest (although bacteria in the large bowel partly digests fiber through fermentation). It is not found in foods of animal origin (meats, dairy products).

Fiber promotes intestinal health, bowel regularity, can benefit diabetes and blood cholesterol levels, and may help prevent colon cancer. High-fiber foods also assist weight control.

Most Americans don't eat enough fiber - less than 20 grams/day - instead of a healthier **25 to 35 grams/day.**

Types of Fiber

Plant foods contain a mixture of different fibers in varying proportions. Insoluble and soluble fiber categories are based on their solubility in water. All types of fiber are beneficial to the body.

◆ **Insoluble fibers** (cellulose, hemi-celluloses, lignin) make up the structural parts of plant cell walls.

   Best food sources are wheat bran, corn bran, rice bran, whole-grain cereals and breads, beans and peas, nuts, seeds, and the skins of fruits and vegetables.

These fibers absorb many times their own weight in water. They create a soft bulk and hasten the passage of waste products through the intestines.

They promote bowel regularity, and aid in the prevention and treatment of uncomplicated forms of **constipation, diverticulosis and hemorrhoids.**

The risk of colon cancer may also be reduced by fiber's diluting effect on potentially harmful substances.

◆ **Soluble fibers** (pectin, gums, mucilages) are found mainly within plant cells, soy milk (whole bean) and products.

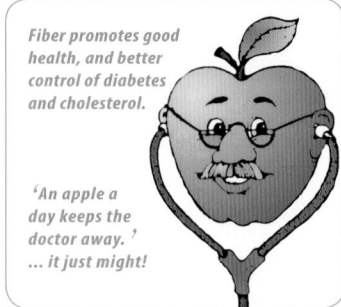

Fiber promotes good health, and better control of diabetes and cholesterol.

'An apple a day keeps the doctor away.'
... it just might!

Types of Fiber (Cont)

Best Sources of Soluble Fiber: Fruits and vegetables, oat bran, barley, beans and peas, prunes, psyllium and flax seed.

These fibers form a gel which slows both stomach emptying and the absorption of sugars from the intestines. **This helps to control blood sugar levels.**

Weight control is also aided by the slower emptying of the stomach and the feeling of **fullness provided by soluble fiber.**

Some soluble fibers can lower **blood cholesterol** by binding bile acids and excreting them. More body cholesterol must then be broken down to supply bile acids for emulsification of dietary fats. **Rice bran, while not high in soluble fiber, can also lower blood cholesterol.**

◆ **Resistant starch** is that part of starchy foods (approx. 10%) which is tightly bound by fiber and resists normal digestion. Friendly bacteria in the large bowel ferment and change the resistant starch into short-chain fatty acids, which are important to bowel health and may protect against colon cancer.

Starchy foods include bread, cereals, rice, pasta, potatoes and legumes.

Fiber & Weight Control

Fiber can assist weight control in several ways. Fiber-rich foods such as fresh fruit and vegetables, potatoes and whole-grain bread contain few calories for their large volume (due to their low-fat, high-water content).

Their bulk fills the stomach and satisfies the appetite much sooner than fiber-depleted foods. The extra chewing time also contributes to satiety, and gives the stomach time to register a feeling of fullness. Excessive calories are less likely to be consumed.

Fiber-depleted foods and drinks are more concentrated in calories; e.g. fats, sugar, candy, soft drinks, fruit juices, alcohol. They require little or no chewing. Large amounts with excessive calories can be consumed before the appetite is satisfied.

Example: Whereas one fresh apple might satisfy the appetite, an apple juice drink with the equivalent sugars and calories of 2-3 apples only minimally satisfies the appetite. (See illustration below.)

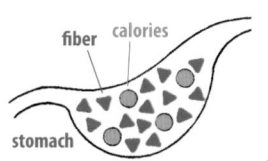

High-fiber foods fill the stomach. Fewer calories are consumed.

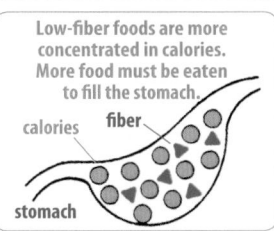

Low-fiber foods are more concentrated in calories. More food must be eaten to fill the stomach.

EFFECTS OF REMOVING FIBER FROM FOOD

2-3 pieces of fresh fruit produces 1 glass of fruit juice. The removal of fiber concentrates the sugar and calories.

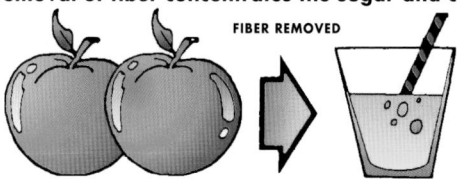

FIBER REMOVED

Fresh Fruit		Fruit Juice
High Fiber	←	Negligible Fiber
Low Calorie Density	←	High Calorie Density
Long Eating Time	←	No Eating Time (Drink)
Satisfies Hunger	←	Does Not Satisfy Hunger
Sugar Slowly Absorbed	←	Sugar More Quickly Absorbed
Less Insulin Required	←	More Insulin Required

Constipation

Constipation can reasonably be defined as a failure to have a bowel movement at least every second day – and just as importantly, without straining or pain.

Typically, constipated stools are too hard, too narrow and too small.

The **main cause** is simply a lack of dietary fiber. Other contributing factors include insufficient fluids, too little exercise, emotional stress, gastrointestinal disease, lack of proper dentition to chew high-fiber foods, and some medications (e.g. some antacids, antidepressants, pain medications).

Note: Check with your doctor to rule out any underlying medical problem – especially if you have a change in bowel habits in middle-age or later years.

DESIRABLE FIBER INTAKE

Adults: 25-35gm per day
Children (under 18): Age + 5gm
Example: 6-year old (6 + 5)= 11gm

SAMPLE FOOD QUANTITIES
For 35 Grams of Fiber/Day

	Fiber
Breakfast Cereal (higher-fiber)	5g
plus 4 slices whole-grain Bread	6g
plus 3 servings fresh Fruit	9g
plus 1 medium Potato (w. skin)	
or 1 cup Brown Rice	4g
or ½ cup whole-grain Pasta	
plus 3-4 servings Veggies/Salad	6g
plus 1 cup Bean Soup	
or ¼ cup Baked/Soy Beans	
or ½ cup Corn/Peas/Lentils	5g
or 1¼ oz Almonds (natural)	
or 3 medium Figs	

HINTS TO INCREASE FIBER AND AVOID CONSTIPATION

❶ **Breakfast is an important** contributor to daily fiber intake. Eat high-fiber breakfast cereals (bran-based cereals, oatmeal etc.). Add 1-2 tablespoons of unprocessed bran.

Dried fruits, chopped nuts, soy grits, and seeds are also excellent additions to cereals.

Note: A gradual increase in fiber will prevent bloating, gas or pain. People intolerant to bran may benefit from psyllium-based fiber supplements and cereals.

❷ **Drink adequate water daily.** Fiber works by absorbing many times its own weight in water.

❸ **Eat whole-grain breads,** or fiber-enriched breads. They have over double the fiber of regular white bread.

❹ **Enjoy fruit as fresh fruit** with skin rather than as fruit juice. Enjoy whole-grain pasta, barley, brown rice, nuts and seeds.

❺ **Eat more vegetables,** salads and legumes – especially cooked beans, lentils, potatoes with skins, avocado, broccoli, brussels sprouts, cabbage, carrots, celery, and peas.

❻ **Add bran** (barley/rice/wheat) or soy grits to soups, casseroles, yogurt, desserts, cookies, cakes. Also use whole-meal flour or soy flour in place of white flour. Use nuts, seeds, and ground linseed.

❼ **Snack** on fresh or dried fruits, carrot or celery sticks, popcorn, nuts or seeds, whole-grain crackers, high-fiber bars (low-fat). Limit amounts if overweight.

❽ **Exercise regularly** to strengthen abdominal muscles and stimulate the gut. Keep up water intake, especially in warm weather.

❾ **Avoid** indiscriminate and regular use of harsh laxatives. They can overstimulate the intestinal muscles and may make normal bowel activity impossible. It may take several weeks to restore normal bowel function.

Fiber Guide

FOODS WITH ZERO FIBER

- **Dairy Products (Milk, Cheese, etc)**
- **Meats, Poultry, Fish, Eggs**
- **Fats/Oils, Sugar/Syrups**
  (Only foods of plant origin contain fiber.)

Breakfast Cereals   **Fiber**

General Mills:

Food	Fiber
Basic 4, 1 cup, 2 oz	3
Cheerios (Honey Nut; Multigrain), 1 c., 1 oz	3
Multi-Bran Chex, 1 cup, 2 oz	7
Oatmeal Crisp Almond, 1 cup, 2 oz	4
Raisin Nut Bran, 1¼ cup, 2 oz	5
Total, average all types, ¾ cup, 1 oz	5
Wheat Chex, 1 cup, 2 oz	5
Wheaties ¾ cup, 1 oz	3

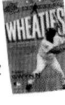

Health Valley:

Food	Fiber
Amaranth Flakes, ¾ cup, 1 oz	4
Crunches & Flakes, ¾ cup, 1.9 oz	4
Fiber 7 Flakes, ¾ cup, 1 oz	4
Golden Flax, ¾ cup, 1.9 oz	6
Granola (Low-Fat), ⅔ cup, 2 oz	6
Healthy Fiber Flakes, ¾ cup, 1.1 oz	4
Oat Bran Flakes, all types, ¾ cup, 1 oz	3
Oat Bran O's, ¾ cup, 1 oz	3
Real Oat Bran, ½ cup, 1.7 oz	5

Kellogg's:

Food	Fiber
All-Bran, ½ cup, 1.1 oz	10
All-Bran w. Extra Fiber, ½ cup, 1 oz	13
All-Bran Bran Buds, ⅓ cup, 1.1 oz	13
Corn Flakes, Fruit Loops, Smacks 1 cup, 1 oz	1
Cocoa/Rice Krispies Treats, 1¼ cup, 1 oz	0
Complete: Wheat Bran Flakes, ¾ c., 1 oz	5
Oat Bran Flakes, ¾ cup, 1.1 oz	4
Corn Pops, 1 cup, 1.1 oz	0.5
Cracklin' Oat Bran, ¾ cup, 1.7oz	6
Frosted Mini Wheats, 24 bisc., 2 oz	5
Granola w. Raisins, ⅔ cup, 2.1 oz	3
Nutri-Grain Cereal Bars, 1 bar, 1.3 oz	1
Raisin Bran, 1 cup, 2.1 oz	7
Smart Start, Healthy Heart, 1¼ cups, 2 oz	5
Product 19, 1 cup, 1.1 oz	1
Special K, 1 cup, 1.1 oz	0.5

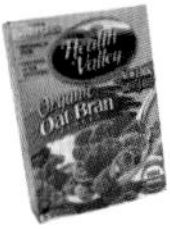

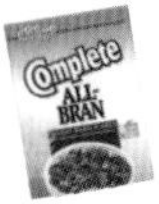

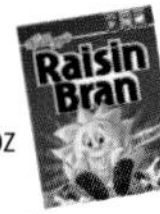

Fiber ~ Fiber (grams)

Breakfast Cereals (Cont)   **Fiber**

Kashi:

Food	Fiber
GoLEAN Cereal, 1 cup, 1.8 oz	10
GoLEAN Crunch!, 1 cup, 1.9 oz	8
GoLEAN Bars, avg. (1)	4
Good Friends: Original, 1 cup, 1.9 oz	12
Cinna-Raisin Crunch, 1 cup, 1.8 oz	8
Heart to Heart, ¾ cup, 1.2 oz	5
7 Whole Grain Pilaf, ½ cup, cooked, 5 oz	6
7 Whole Grain Puffs, 1 cup, 0.7 oz	1

Quaker:

Food	Fiber
Cap'n Crunch, ¾ cup, 1 oz	1
100% Natural Granola, avg., ½ cup, 1.8 oz	3
Crunchy Corn Bran, 1 cup, 1 oz	5
Life Cereal, ¾ cup, 1.1 oz	2
Oat Bran, ½ cup, 1.4 oz	6
Oatmeal, average, 1 packet	3

Post:

Food	Fiber
100% Bran, ⅓ cup, 1 oz	9
Alpha Bits, 1 cup, 1 oz	3
Blueberry Morning, 1 cup, 1.9 oz	2
Cocoa/Fruity Pebbles, 1 cup, 1 oz	3
Cranberry Almond Crunch, 1 cup, 1.8 oz	3
Fruit & Bran, 1 cup, 1.9 oz	6
Grape-Nuts, ½ cup, 2 oz	6
Great Grains, ⅔ cup, 1.9 oz	4
Honey Bunches of Oats, ¾ cup, 1.1 oz	2
Shredded Wheat & Bran, ½ cup, 2 oz	6

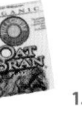

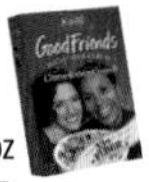

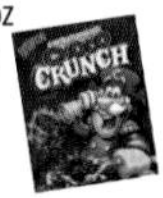

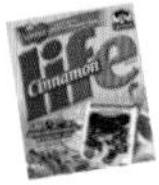

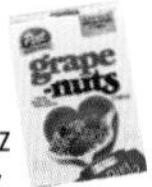

Brans & Supplements

Food	Fiber
Oat Bran: 1 Tbsp (level)	1
⅓ cup, (5⅓ Tbsp), 1 oz	5
Rice Bran, raw. ¼ cup, 1 oz	6
Wheat Bran (unprocessed):	
Raw, 1 Tbsp	1.5
2 Tbsp (level), ¼ oz	3
¼ cup, (4 Tbsp), ½ oz	6
½ cup, 1 oz	12
Corn Germ: Toasted, ¼ cup, 1 oz	1
Wheat Germ: Raw, ¼ cup, 1 oz	4
Psyllium Seed Husks, 2 Tbsp	8
Metamucil, 1 dose	3.5

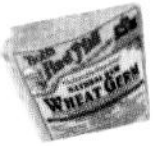

Hot Cereals, Oatmeal

Food	Fiber
Bulgur (cracked Wheat), ckd, 1 cup	8
Corn/Hominy Grits, dry, 3 Tbsp, 1 oz	0.5
Cream of Wheat, cooked, ¾ cup	1
Oatmeal (uncooked ⅓ cup), ckd, ⅔ cup	3

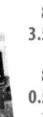

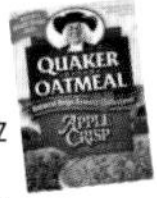

Fiber Guide

Breads & Crackers | Fiber

Bread: White, 1 slice, 1 oz	0.6
Whole-wheat, 1 slice, 1 oz	1.5
Whole-grain, 1 slice, 1 oz	2
Rye, Pumpernickel, 1 oz	1.5
Bagel/Roll/Bun, 1 medium, 2 oz	1.5
Pita, whole wheat, 6½" pocket	4.5
Crackers: Graham, average, 2	0.4
Saltine, 4 crackers	0.4
Crispbreads (Rye), average, 2	4
Matzo 1 board, 1 oz	1
Rice Cakes, average, 1 cake	0.3
Tortilla: Regular, 6"	0.5
Whole-wheat, 6"	1.3

Barley, Pasta, Rice & Flours

Barley, pearled, raw, ¼ cup, 1.7 oz	8
Rice: White, cooked, 1 cup	0.6
Brown, cooked, 1 cup	3.5
Rice-A-Roni, average, 1 cup, prepared	1.5
Spaghetti/Noodles: Cooked, 1 cup	2
Whole-Wheat, cooked, 1 cup	4
Flour: Wheat, All-purpose, 1 cup, 4½ oz	3.5
Whole-Wheat, 1 cup, 4½ oz	15
Cornmeal, stone ground, 1 cup, 4½ oz	13
Carob Flour, 1 cup, 3½ oz	41
Rye Flour, 1 cup, 3½ oz	15
Soy Flour: Defatted, 1 cup, 3½ oz	17
Full-fat, raw, 1 cup, 3 oz	8
Soy Meal, defatted, 1 cup, 4½ oz	14

Frozen Entrees & Dinners

Average All Brands: Per Serving

Beans/Chili base, average	6-10
Potato/Pasta base, average	4-6
Vegetable base, average	3
Meat/Chicken base, average	2-3
Pizzas, ¼ large, average	3
Vegetarian Soy Burgers, 1 pattie	4

Soups

Chicken Noodle, 1 cup	0.5
Tomato Soup, average, 1 cup	0.5
Vegetable Soup, average, 1 cup	3

Health Valley: Per 1 Cup Serving

Black Bean; Minestrone	8
Tomato	
5-Bean Vegetable; Lentil & Carrots	10
Mushroom Barley; Vegetable	4
Split Pea	8

Fast Foods & Restaurants | Fiber

Hamburgers: Small, average	1.5
Large/Whopper, average	2.5
Hot Dog, Regular	1.5
French Fries: Small serving, 2½ oz	2.5
Regular/Medium, 3½ oz	3.5
Chicken Nuggets, 6 pack	0.5
Chicken Sandwich, average	2
Taco, average	4
Sundaes, Shakes, Soft Drinks	0
Arby's: Baked Potato w. Broc. & Cheese	8
Roast Beef Sandwich, regular	2
Denny's: Grilled Chicken Salad, no bread	4
Classic Burger, no fries	4
Club Sandwich, no fries	2
Grilled Chicken Sandwich, no fries	4
Domino's (Classic): Vegi Feast, 1 sl. (12")	2
Hawaiian Feast, 1 slice, (12")	2
Pepperoni Feast, 1 slice (12")	2
McDonald's: Big Mac	3
Hamburger; Quarter Pounder	1
Egg McMuffin	2
Grilled Chicken Caesar Salad	3
McVeggie Burger on Wheat Bun	8
Pizza Hut: Per 1 Slice, Medium	
Pan Pizza: Cheese, Pepperoni	1
Supreme	2
Thin 'n Crispy, Supreme	2
Hand-Tossed, average all varieties	2
Subway: Sandwich, white roll, avg.	4
w. Honey Wheat Roll, average	3.2
Footlong w. Wheat Roll, average	8
Salads, average	4

Cakes, Cookies, Snack Bars

Apple/Fruit Pie, 1 serving, 4 oz	2
Cake: w. plain flour, 1 serving, 3.4 oz	1.5
w. whole-wheat flour, 1 serving	3
Carrot Cake, 1 serving, 1.2 oz	2
Cookies, oatmeal, (3 small/1 large)	1
Donuts, Medium, 1.7 oz	0.7
Fruit Cake, 1 serving, 1½ oz	2
Fig Bars, 1 cookie, ½ oz	0.7
Muffins, Oat Bran (2 small, 1 large), 4 oz	5
Granola Bars, average, 1 bar	2
Atkins Advantage Bars, average	7
Clif Bars, 2.5 oz	5
Curves, Chocolate Peanut Bar, 25g	5
Fi-Bar Chewy & Nutty 1 bar	1
Health Valley: Fruit/Granola Bars	3
Cereal Bars	1
Luna Bars, avg., 1.7 oz	3

Fiber Guide

Chocolate, Chips, Popcorn — Fiber

	Fiber
Cheese Balls/Curls/Twists	1
Chocolate, Hard Candy, 1 oz	0
Chocolate with nuts/fruit, 2 oz bar	1.5
Mars Bar, 1.8 oz	1
Potato Chips, corn chips, 1 oz	1
Popcorn, 3 cups	3
Pretzels, Twists (6)	1

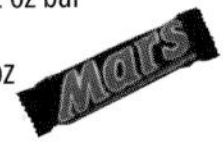

Nuts, Seeds

	Fiber
Almonds: Natural, 25 nuts, 1 oz	3.5
Blanched (skins removed), 1 oz	3
Cashews, Filberts, Pecans, 1 oz	1.7
Peanuts, Mixed Nuts, Coconut, 1 oz	2.5
Peanut Butter, 2 Tbsp, 1 oz	2
Pistachio Nuts, dried, shelled, 1 oz	3
Walnuts, Black/English, dried, 1 oz	2
Seeds: Amaranth, 2½ Tbsp, 1 oz	3.5
Flax Seeds, 3 Tbsp, 1 oz	7
Psyllium Seed Husks, 5 Tbsp, 1 oz	20
Quinoa Seeds, 3 Tbsp, 1 oz	1.7
Sesame Seeds, whole, 1 oz	3.4
Sesame Butter/Tahini, 2 Tbsp, 1.1 oz	1.4
Sunflower kernels, ¼ cup, 1 oz	3.8
Teff Seeds, 1 oz	3.8

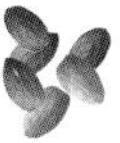

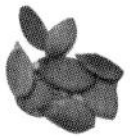

Fruit – Fresh

	Fiber
Apples: 1 medium, 5½ oz (whole)	
with skin + core	3.7
with skin, no core	3.2
without skin, no core	1.7
Apricots, 2 medium, 4 oz	1.5
Avocado, average, ½ medium	6.7
Banana, 1 medium, 6 oz (w. skin)	3
Blueberries, raw, ½ cup, 2½ oz	1.7
Cherries, sweet, raw, 8 fruits, 1.6 oz	1
Grapefruit, average, ½ fruit, 10 oz	1.4
Grapes, 1 medium bunch, seedless, 7 oz	2
Kiwifruit, 1 medium, 2.7 oz	2.3
Mango, 1 medium, 11 oz (whole)	1.6
Melons, Cantaloupe, 4 oz (edible)	1
Nectarine, 1 medium, 4 oz	1.5
Olives, average all types, 7 jumbo, 2 oz	1
Oranges, 1 medium (7-8 oz w. skin)	
5½ oz (peeled)	3.8
Passionfruit, 2 medium, 2½ oz	5
Peaches, 1 large, 6 oz	2
Pears, raw, 1 medium, 6 oz	4.5
Pineapple, 1 slice, 3 oz	1.2
Plums, 2 medium, 6 oz	1.8
Strawberries, 6 medium/3 large, 2 oz	1
Watermelon, 4 oz (edible)	0.5

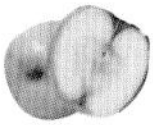

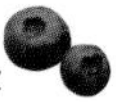

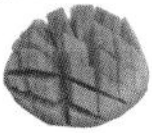

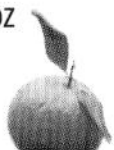

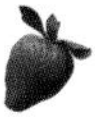

Fruit – Dried, Juice — Fiber

	Fiber
Dried Fruit: Apricots, 8 halves, 1 oz	2.2
Dates (3 med); Raisins (2 Tbsp), 1 oz	1.5
Figs, 3 medium, 1½ oz	5
Prunes, 4 medium, 1 oz	2
Fruit Juice: Orange/Apple etc, 1 glass	<0.5
Prune Juice, 5 oz	1.4
Carrot Juice, 8 oz	1.8

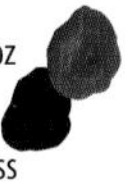

Vegetables

	Fiber
Asparagus, 4 medium spears	1.3
Bean Sprouts, ½ cup, 2 oz	1
Beans: Snap/Green, ½ cup, 2 oz	2
Baked Beans in Tom Sce, ½ c, 4½ oz	5
Dried Beans, ckd, average, ½ cup	7
Beets, ckd, slices, ½ cup, 3 oz	1.7
Broccoli, cooked, ½ cup, 3 oz	2.4
Brussels Sprouts, ckd, ½ cup, 3 oz	3.5
Cabbage: White, ckd, ½ cup, 2½ oz	1
Red, ckd, ½ cup, 2½ oz	2
Carrots, 1 medium (7½"), ½ cup, 3 oz	2.5
Cauliflower, cooked, 3 flowerets, 2 oz	1.5
Celery, raw, diced, 1 cup, 3½ oz	1.6
Chick Peas (Garbanzos), ckd, ½ c., 3 oz	6.5
Corn, kernels, ckd, ½ cup, 2½ oz	2.5
Cream-style, ½ cup, 4½ oz	2
Cucumber/Lettuce/Mushrooms, 2 oz	0.5
Eggplant, raw, sliced, ½ cup , 1½ oz	2
Lentils, cooked, ½ cup, 3½ oz	8
Mixed Vegetables, frozen, cooked, ½ cup	3
Onions, Raw, 1 medium, 4 oz	1.5
Spring Onions, chop., ¼ cup, 1 oz	0.7
Peas: Green, Raw, 2½ oz	3.7
Cowpeas (Black-eyed), ckd, ½ cup	10
Split Peas, ckd, ½ cup, 3½ oz	8
Peppers, sweet, raw, 1 large, 6 oz	3
Potatoes: 1 medium, with skin, 5 oz	4
without skin	2.5
½ cup mashed, 3½ oz	1.5
French Fries, small, 2.6 oz	3
Spinach, cooked, ½ cup, 3 oz	2.5
Squash: Summer, cooked, ½ cup, 3 oz	2.5
Winter, cooked, ½ cup, 3½ oz	2.4
Tomatoes: 1 medium, 4½ oz	1.5
Tomato Sauce, 1 cup	0.3
Soybean Products: Miso, ½ c., 5 oz	7.4
Tempeh, cooked, 1 piece, 3 oz	3
Tofu, ½ cup, 4.4 oz	0.4

Salads: Side Salad, average

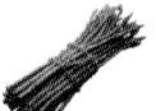

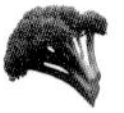

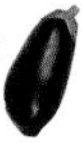

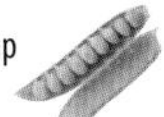

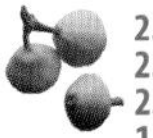

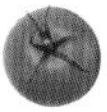

	Fiber
Side Salad, average	1
Bean Salad, ½ cup	5
Coleslaw, ½ cup	1
Potato Salad, ½ cup	2

Protein Guide

General Notes

- **Protein has many important body functions.** It builds and repairs muscle, and is the basis of our body's organs, hormones, enzymes, and antibodies to fight infection.

- **Protein is also an emergency fuel** in the absence of sufficient carbohydrate and fats. For this reason, weight loss should be gradual so as to preserve protein levels in muscle, the heart and other body organs.

- **It is easy to obtain sufficient protein,** even if vegetarian. **Plant proteins are not inferior to animal proteins.** In fact, eating more soy and other plant proteins, and less animal protein, may help to build stronger bones and prevent osteoporosis, and may help to control blood cholesterol levels.

- **When changing to a vegetarian diet,** include soybeans, and other beans, soy milk drinks (calcium-enriched), lentils, tofu, tempeh, nuts and whole-grain breads and cereals. Milk, yogurt, cheese and eggs can enhance nutrient intake.

Protein & Muscle

- Although muscles are built of protein, protein is not a special fuel for working muscle cells – carbohydrates and fats are.

- In fact, a diet high in protein (and fat) and low in carbohydrate can significantly reduce the performance of endurance sports athletes. **Carbohydrates** are the best fuel for muscles exercised for long periods.

- Any **extra protein** required by athletes and body-builders can easily be obtained from the extra food eaten to satisfy hunger and energy needs.

- Remember, **excessive protein** intake will not build bigger muscles. Any excess is converted and stored as fat. Excess protein can also strain the kidneys, which excrete the waste products of protein metabolism.

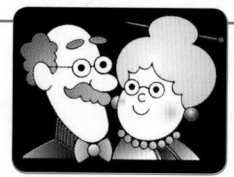

Elderly people (and dieters) must eat sufficient food to ensure adequate protein intake.

Inadequate protein leads to a drop in immune response with greater susceptibility to illness and infections. Muscle strength and muscle mass also drop.

Protein needs are easily met with sensible eating. Athletes who eat enough food for their energy needs can obtain sufficient protein.

RECOMMENDED DAILY PROTEIN INTAKE ~ HEALTHY RANGE ~
(Lower figure is RDA)

		PROTEIN
Children:	1-3 yrs	13g-26g
	4-8 yrs	19g-38g
	9-13 yrs	34g-64g
Males:	14-18 yrs	52g-120g
	19+	56g-120g
Females:	14+	46g-110g
Pregnancy:		71g-120g
Breastfeeding:		71g-120g

Note: On lower-calorie diets, aim for higher amounts of protein within the Healthy Range.

Iron & Anemia Guide

- **Iron deficiency** is one of the most common nutritional deficiencies in women. The risk is increased in dieters who do not eat well-balanced meals. Chronic shortage of iron leads to anemia.

- **Women** between 11 and 50 years of age are at greater risk because of the monthly loss of menstrual blood. Pregnancy, growth, and endurance sports also demand extra iron.

- **In red blood cells**, iron combines with protein to form **hemoglobin** – the red pigment which carries oxygen in the blood. A lack of iron limits the production of hemoglobin and consequently the amount of vital oxygen delivered to body cells.

Note: A blood test will tell you if your Hb and Iron stores (ferritin) are adequate. (Iron stores can be low even when Hb is normal.)

- **Vitamin C** (in fruits/veggies/salads) enhances absorption of 'non-heme' iron in bread, cereals, milk, vegetables, nuts, eggs and iron supplements. Small amounts of meat, fish or poultry also help. (They contain 'heme' iron).

- **Iron absorption is lessened** by up to 60% when high calcium foods are consumed with iron-rich main meals. Tea, coffee, phytates (in bran) and oxalates lessen absorption of non-heme iron.

- **For infants to 1 year,** use iron-fortified milk/soy formula if not breast-feeding. Introduce iron-fortified baby cereals at 4-6 months.

Note: Iron deficiency in children (even without anemia), can result in lethargy, irritability, repeated infections, and developmental problems.

Iron Supplements

- **Most people** can obtain adequate iron from their diet. **A wide variety** of animal and plant foods contain iron. (See Iron Counter)

- **Iron supplements** are only recommended for women with heavy menstrual blood losses or during pregnancy (if tests show a low-iron status), endurance athletes with low blood ferritin (iron stores) and for persons with diagnosed anemia. Check with your doctor.

- While the 5 mg of iron in multi-vitamin/mineral supplements is safe for most people, large amounts can be toxic, (especially for persons with hemochromatosis iron-overload condition).

ANEMIA SYMPTOMS

Anemia reduces the amount of oxygen carried in the blood. The body tissues become starved of oxygen. Symptoms include:

- **Pale skin; brittle fingernails (may turn up into spoon shape)**
- **Excessive tiredness or fatigue**
- **Breathlessness**
- **Feeling of malaise and irritability**
- **Always feel cold**
- **Decrease in attention span**

Note: Other medical conditions may also cause similar symptoms. Check with your doctor.

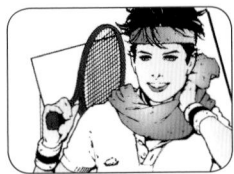

A nutritious diet with adequate iron is important - particularly for women and athletes.

RECOMMENDED DAILY IRON INTAKE (mg)

			Iron
Infants (0-6 mths):			
	Breast-fed	~	0.5mg
	Bottle-fed	~	3mg
	6-12 mths	~	11mg
Children:	1-11 yrs	~	7-10mg
Males:	12-18 yrs	~	11mg
	19+ yrs	~	8mg
Females:	12-18 yrs	~	15mg
	19-50 yrs	~	18mg
	51+ yrs	~	8mg
	Pregnancy	~	27mg
	Breast-feeding	~	12-16mg

Protein & Iron Counter

Pro ~ Protein (grams)

Iron ~ Iron (mg)

Meat

	Pro	Iron
Steak: Average all cuts, lean (no fat)		
Small (4 oz raw/3 oz ckd)	23	2.3
Medium (6 oz raw/4¼ oz ckd)	34	3.4
Large (10 oz raw/7¼ oz ckd)	57	5.7
Roast Beef, lean, 2 slices, 3 oz	24	2.5
Ground Beef patty, lean, ckd, 3 oz	21	2
Lamb chop, broiled, 3 oz	22	1.5
Liver, cooked, 3 oz	23	5.5
Veal cutlet, 1 medium	23	1
Pork, cooked, lean, 3 oz	24	1
Bacon, 3 medium slices	6	0.3
Ham, roasted, 2 pieces, 3 oz	18	1
Ham, luncheon, 2 slices, 1½ oz	7	0.3
Pastrami (Oscar Mayer), 3 sl., 1¾ oz	10	1.3
Sausages: Bologna, 2 sl., 2 oz	7	1
Braunschweiger, 2 sl., 2 oz	8	5.3
Pork link, thick, 2 oz	6	0.5
Frankfurter, 1⅓ oz	5	0.5
Salami, hard, 3 slices, 1 oz	7	0.5
Vegetarian (Boca Burger), 1 pattie	13	2

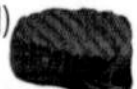

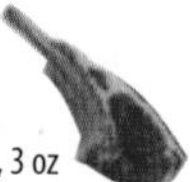

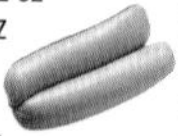

Chicken/Turkey (Without Skin)

	Pro	Iron
Chicken, ckd: Breast, Roasted, 4 oz	36	1.5
Leg/Thigh, Roasted, 2 oz	14	0.5
½ Whole Chicken	60	2.5
Drumstick, Rstd, 1 med., 3 oz	13	0.5
Turkey, cooked: Light meat, 3 oz	28	2
Dark meat, lean, 3 oz	24	2

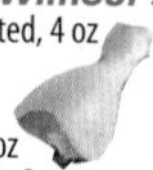

Fish

	Pro	Iron
Fresh Fish: Per 4 oz, cooked		
Cod, Flounder/Sole, Pollock	28	0.5
Catfish, Haddock, Halibut, M/Mahi	28	1.3
Ocean Perch, Swordf., Orange Roughy	28	1.3
Canned Fish: Tuna, Light, 3 oz	25	1.5
White, 3 oz	23	0.5
Salmon, pink, 3 oz	17	0.7
Salmon, red, 3 oz	17	1
Sardines, 3 whole (3"), 1¼ oz	9	1
Anchovies, 1 can, 1½ oz	13	2
Shellfish: Crabmeat, 3 oz	17.5	0.7
Clams, raw, 4 large/9 sml, 3 oz	11	12
Crayfish, cooked, 3 oz	20	2.7
Lobster, cooked, 3 oz	17	0.5
Oysters, raw, 6 medium, 3 oz	7	5
Scallops, 2 lge/5 small, 1 oz	5	0
Shrimp, raw, 6 large, 1½ oz	8.5	1
Fish Products: Fish Sticks, 4 sticks	10	0.5
Fish Portions, in batter, 4 oz	13	0.6
Gefilte Fish, 1 medium ball, 2 oz	8	1

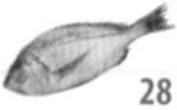

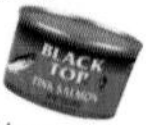

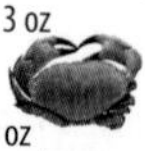

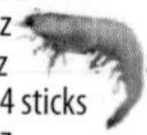

Eggs

	Pro	Iron
1 Large Egg, whole	6	0.7
Egg Yolk	3	0.7
Egg White	3	0
Omelet: Plain, 2 eggs	13	1.7
Ham & cheese	17	3
Egg Substitutes (liquid):		
Egg Beaters, ¼ cup, 2 oz	4.5	1
Better 'n Eggs/Scramblers, ¼ cup, 2 oz	6	0.7

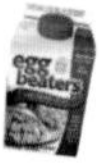

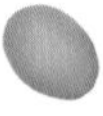

Milk, Yogurt, Ice Cream

	Pro	Iron
Milk: Whole: 2%, 1 cup	8	0
Low-Fat (1%); Fat-Free, 1 cup	8.5	0
Chocolate Milk, 1 cup	8	0.6
Thick Shake, Chocolate, 10 oz	9	1
Vanilla, 10 oz	11	0.3
Soymilk (fortified), average, 1 cup	7	1
Soy Dream Enriched, shelf-stable, 1 cup	7	8
Yogurt: Plain, 6 oz	10	0
Fruit flavors: 6 oz	8	0.3
8 oz	11	0.5
Ice Cream: Rich, ½ cup	2	0
Regular, Vanilla, ½ cup	2.5	0
Sherbet, ½ cup	1	0
Custard, baked, ½ cup	7	0.5

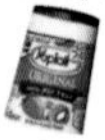

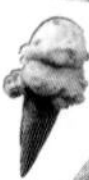

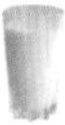

Cheese

	Pro	Iron
Hard Cheeses, average, 1 oz	7	0.2
Cottage Cheese, ½ cup	13	0.3
Cream Cheese, avg., 1 oz	2	0.3
Ricotta, part skim, ½ cup	14	1

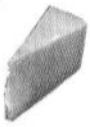

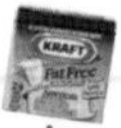

Bread, Bagels, Biscuits

	Pro	Iron
Bread (w. enriched flour): 1 slice, 1 oz	2	1
4 thin slices, 4 oz	8	4
4 thick slices, 6 oz	1.2	6
Bagel, plain 2 oz	6	1.5
Biscuits, 1 oz	2	0.7
Pita Bread, 1 pita, 1½ oz	4	1
Pumpernickel, 1 slice, 1 oz	3	1

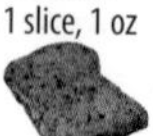

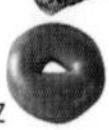

Infant/Baby Foods

	Pro	Iron
Infant Formula Milk:		
Enfamil/Gerber/Similac, 5 fl.oz		
Regular/Low Iron	2.2	0.2
With Iron	2.2	1.8
Isomil/Nursoy/ProSobee	3	1.8
Baby Cereals: Average All Brands		
Dry, 4 Tbsp, ½ oz	1	7
Jars (w. fruit), 4½ oz	1	7

Breakfast Cereals   **Pro** **Iron**

	Pro	Iron
Hot Cereals, cooked:		
Bulgur, cooked, 1 cup, 5 oz	9	2
Oatmeal: Reg., non-fortified, 1 cup	6	1.5
Instant, fortified, avg., 1 pkt	4	8
Quaker, all flavors, ½ cup	5	18
Corn/Hominy Grits: Reg., 1 cup	3	1.5
Quaker: Reg., 3 Tbsp, 1 oz	2	0.8
Instant White, 1 packet	2	8
Cream of Wheat, 1 cup	4	10
Brands ~ Ready-To-Eat		
Arrowhead: Average all varieties, 1 oz	3	1
General Mills: Basic 4, 1 cup, 2 oz	4	4.5
Cheerios, Original, 1 cup, 1 oz	3	8
Cocoa Puffs, 1 cup, 1 oz	1	4.5
Kix, 1⅓ cups, 1 oz	2	8
Multi-Bran Chex, 1 cup, 2 oz	4	16
Country Corn Flakes, 1cup, 1.2 oz	2	8
Total Raisin Bran, 1 cup, 2 oz	3	18
Wheaties ¾ cup, 1 oz	3	8
Health Valley: Oat Bran O's, ¾ cup, 1 oz	3	0.7
Amaranth Flakes, ¾ cup, 1 oz	3	0.7
Bran Flakes w. Raisins, ¾ cup, 1.1 oz	5	1.5
Low-Fat Granola, ⅔ cup, 2 oz	5	1.4
Real Oat Bran Alm. Crunch, ½ cup, 1.7 oz	6	0.7
Golden Flax, ¾ cup, 1 oz	6	1
Kashi: Friends, 1 cup, 1.9 oz	5	1.8
GoLean Crunch!, 1 cup, 1.9 oz	9	1.8
7 Whole Grain Flakes, 1 c., 1.8 oz	5	1.4
Kellogg's: All-Bran: ½ cup, 1 oz	4	4.5
Complete Oat Flakes, ¾ cup, 1.1 oz	3	18
Cocoa Krispies, ¾ cup, 1 oz	1	4.5
Corn Flakes, 1 cup, 1 oz	2	8
Low-fat Granola w. Raisins ⅔ c., 2.1 oz	4	2
Product 19, 1 cup, 1 oz	2	18
Raisin Bran, 1 cup, 2 oz	7	4.5
Rice Krispies, 1¼ cup, 1.2 oz	2	9
Smart-Start Healthy Heart, 1 c., 1.8 oz	6	4.5
Special K: Regular, 1 c., 1 oz	6	8
Protein Plus, ¾ cup, 1 oz	10	8
Post: Raisin Bran, ⅔ cup, 2 oz	4	11
Grape Nuts, ½ cup, 2 oz	6	16
Quaker: Crunchy Corn Bran, 1 cup, 1 oz	2	8
100% Natural Granola, ½ cup, 1.7 oz	5	1.4
Life, ¾ cup, 1.1 oz	3	8
Cap'n Crunch, ¾ cup, 1 oz	1	4.5
Oat Bran, ½ cup, 1.4 oz	7	2.7

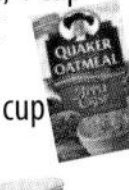

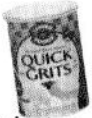

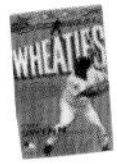

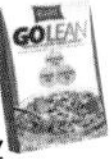

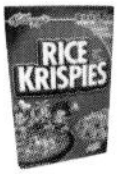

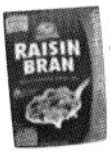

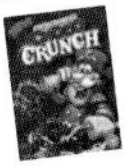

Brans & Wheatgerm   **Pro** **Iron**

	Pro	Iron
Oat Bran, raw, 1 Tbsp	2	0.5
Rice Bran, raw, 2 Tbsp	1	1
Wheat Bran, unprocessed, 2 T.	1	1
Wheat Germ, 2 Tbsp, ½ oz	4	1.3

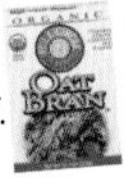

Grains & Flours, Yeast

	Pro	Iron
Amaranth, ½ cup, 3.4 oz	14	7
Barley, ½ cup, 3.2 oz	12	2
Buckwheat Flour: Whole-groat, 1 cup	15	2.7
Carob Flour, 1 cup, 3.6 oz	5	3
Corn Flour, 1 cup, 4 oz	11	2
Corn Meal, 1 cup, 4½ oz	8	3.5
Flour: White, 1 cup, 5.6 oz	9	6
Whole-grain, 1 cup, 4¼ oz	16	5
Millet, whole-grain, 1 cup, 3½ oz	12	7
Rye Flour: Dark, 1 cup, 4½ oz	18	6
Light, 1 cup, 3½ oz	9	1
Soy Flour, full fat, 1 cup, 3 oz	29	5.5
Yeast: Brewers, 2 Tbsp, ½ oz	8	1.5
Nutritional Yeast Flakes *(Red Star),* 1 heaping Tbsp, ½ oz	8	0.8

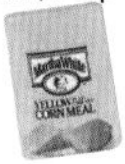

Rice, Spaghetti, Macaroni

	Pro	Iron
Rice: Brown/White, average 1 cup cooked, 6½ oz	5	1
Spaghetti/Macaroni/Noodles (enriched):		
Cooked, 1 cup, 4½ oz	7	2
Canned: in Tomato Sauce, ½ cup	2	0.5
w. Meatballs, 1 cup, 8 oz	10	2
Macaroni & Cheese, 1 cup, 9 oz	8	1

Soups

	Pro	Iron
With Noodles/Vegetables, 1 c.	3	0.5
With Meat/Beans/Peas, 1 c.	8	1.5

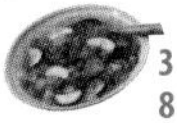

Fruit

	Pro	Iron
Fresh/Canned:		
Average, all types 1 medium/2 small fruit	1	0.5
Avocado, ½ medium	2	1
Dried Fruit: Apricots, 8 halves, 1 oz	1	1.3
Dates, 6 dates, 2 oz	1.5	0.7
Figs, 4 medium figs, 2 oz	2	1.7
Prunes, 5 medium, 1½ oz	2	1
Raisins, 1 oz	1	0.7
Fruit Juice: Average, 1 cup	0.5	0.5
Prune Juice, 6 fl.oz	1	2.5
Tomato Juice, 1 cup, 8 fl.oz	1.5	1

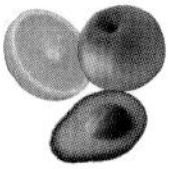

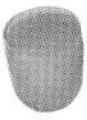

Protein & Iron Counter

Vegetables	Pro	Iron
Beans: Snap/green, ½ cup, 2 oz	1	0.8
Dried: Average all types, cooked, ½ cup	7	2.5
Baked Beans, ½ cup 4½ oz	5	2
Bean Sprouts, mung, 1 c., 4 oz	3	1
Broccoli, 3 raw, ½ cup, 1½ oz	1.5	0.7
Cabbage; Cauliflower, raw, 1 c. 3 oz	1.5	0.6
Corn, raw, ½ cup kernels, 3 oz	2.5	0.3
1 ear trimmed to 3½"	2	0.4
Lentils, cooked, ½ cup, 3½ oz	9	3.3
Mushrooms, raw, ½ c., sliced	1	0.3
Peas: Green, raw, ½ c., 2½ oz	4	1.2
Split Peas, cooked, 1 cup, 7 oz	16	2.5
Potatoes, cooked:		
1 medium, with skin, 5 oz	3.3	2
without skin, 4 oz	2.3	1
French Fries, small, 2.6 oz	2	1
Potato Salad, ½ cup, 4 oz	3.5	2.5
Pumpkin, ½ cup mashed, 4.3 oz	1	1
Seaweed, kelp, 1 oz	<1	2.5
Spinach, cooked, ½ cup, 3 oz	2.7	3.5
Squash, ckd, all types, ½ cup	1	0.3
Tomatoes, 1 medium, 4½ oz	1	0.6
Vegetables, mixed, ckd, 1 cup	2.5	0.7
Soybeans, cooked, ½ cup, 3 oz	14	4.4

Tofu, Tempeh, Miso		
Tofu, raw, firm, ½ cup, 4½ oz	10	1.5
Tempeh, ½ cup, 3 oz	16	2
Miso, ½ cup, 5 oz	16	4
Miso Soup, 1 cup	3	0.4
Soybean Protein (TVP), 1 oz	18	3

Cakes, Pastries, Pies		
(Made with enriched flour)		
Carrot w. cream cheese frosting, 4 oz	4	1.3
Cheesecake, 1 piece, 4 oz	6	0.5
Chocolate, 1 piece, 2 oz	2	2
Fruitcake, 1 piece, 3 oz	4	2
Plain, 1 piece, 3 oz	4	1.2
Croissant, plain, 2 oz	5	2
Danish Pastry, 1 pastry, 2¼ oz	4	1.3
Donuts, average, 2 oz	4	1.2
Muffins, average, 1 med., 1½ oz	3	1
Pancakes, 4" diam., two, 2 oz	4	1
Pies: Fruit, 1 piece, 5½ oz	4	1.5
Pecan, 1 piece, 5 oz	7	4.5
Puddings, average, ½ cup, 4½ oz	4	0.3
Waffles, 1 large, 2½ oz	7	1.5

Peanut Butter	Pro	Iron
Regular: 2 Tbsp, 1.1 oz	8	0.5
Peter Pan Plus, 2 Tbsp, 1.1 oz	8	4.5

Sugar, Honey, Jam		
Sugar: White	0	0
Brown, 1 Tbsp	0	0.3
Molasses: Light/Med., 1 Tbsp	0	1
Blackstrap, 1 Tbsp	0	3
Corn Syrup, 1 Tbsp, ¾ oz	0	1
Honey, Jams, Jelly	0	0.2

Candy, Chocolate, Carob		
Candy, sugar-based	0	0
Chocolate: Plain, 2 oz bar	4	0.8
with nuts, 2 oz bar	6	0.8
Carob, plain, 2 oz	6	0.7

Cookies, Crackers, Chips		
Cookies, average, 4 cookies	2	1
Crackers, Graham, 2½" sq., (2)	1	0
Rice Cakes, average, one	1	0
Corn/Potato Chips, 1 oz	2	0.3
Nuts: Almonds, shelled, 20-25 nuts	6	1
Brazil Nuts, 7-8 medium nuts, 1 oz	4	1
Cashews, 12-16 nuts, 1 oz	5	1.5
Macadamias, 1 oz	2	0.5
Peanuts, dry rsted, 40 nuts, 1 oz	6	0.6
Pecans, 24 halves, 1 oz	2	0.5
Walnuts, 15 halves, 1 oz	4	0.7
Seeds: Sesame Seeds, dry, 1 Tbsp	2	0.6
Pumpkin Kernels, dry, hulled, 1 oz	7	4.2
Sunflower Seeds, dried, hulled, 1 oz	6	2
Tahini, 1 Tbsp, ½ oz	2.5	1.4

Granola & Food/Protein Bars		
Granola Bars, average, 1 bar, 2 oz	2	0.5
Atkins Advantage Bar, avg., 2.1 oz	20	1.8
Balance Bars, Original, 1.76 oz	14	4.5
Bariatrix Proti-Bars (1), 1.4 oz	15	0.7
Dr Soy Protein Bars, 1.76 oz	11	18
GeniSoy Bar, 1.5 oz	14	4.5
Jenny Craig Bars, 1.8 oz	4	3.6
Met-Rx "Big 100", 3.5 oz	27	7.2
Myoplex Carb Sense Bar, 2.5 oz	26	2
Planters Carb Well Bar, 1.2 oz	6	1
PowerBar: Harvest	10	4.5
Performance Bar, 2.3 oz	10	6.3
ProteinPlus, 1 bar, avg., 2.75 oz	24	8
Slim-Fast Optima Diet Bar, 1 oz	2	1.4
Special K:		
Protein Meal Bar, 1.6 oz	10	1.8
Protein Snack Bar, 0.9 oz	4	0.7

Nutritional & High Protein Drinks

	Pro	Iron
Atkins Shakes, 11 fl.oz	18	2.7
Boost Ready To Drink, 8 oz can	10	3.5
Carnation Instant Breakfast, 10 oz	13	4.5
Curves Protein Drink, 2 scoops, dry	15	18
Ensure Plus, 8 oz can	13	2.3
GeniSoy Shake, 1 scoop, 1.2 oz	14	3.6
Kashi GoLean Shake, 2 sc., 2.1 oz	21	2.7
Lightfull, Chocolate, 8.25 oz	5	2.7
Other flavors, avg. 8.25 oz	5	0.4
Met-Rx RTD 40	40	4.5
Myoplex, Original Nutrition Shake, 1 pkt	42	5.4
Optifast 800, made-up, 8 oz	14	3.6
Resource (Novartis) Standard, 8 fl.oz	15	4.5
Revival Soy, Plain, 58g pkt	20	3
Slim-Fast Shakes, 325 ml can	10	3.6
High Protein, 1 can	15	6.3
Special K₂0 Protein Water, 16 fl.oz	5	0
Usana Soyamax, 2 scoops, 1 oz	24	6
Walgreens Slim For Less, 11 oz can	10	2.7
Weider Mass 1000, 4 scoops, 7 oz	34	6

Coffee, Tea, Soda

	Pro	Iron
Coffee, Coffee Substitutes, 1 cup, 8 fl.oz	0	0
Coffee w. 2 oz milk, 1 cup, 8 fl.oz	2	0
Caffe latte, large, 16 fl.oz	12	0
Cappuccino, large, 16 fl.oz	8	0
Frappuccino, avg., 16 fl.oz	6	0
Hot Chocolate:		
(all milk), 1 c., 8 oz	8	1.2
Soft Drinks/Soda	0	0
Tea (all types)	0	0

Beer, Wine, Spirits

	Pro	Iron
Beer, 12 fl.oz	1	0
Wines, red/white, 1 glass	0	0.4
Spirits/Liquor	0	0

Fast-Foods/Burgers

For extra listings ~ see CalorieKing.com

	Pro	Iron
Pancakes: Average all outlets, 3	8	2
Shakes, Chocolate, 16 fl.oz	12	0.4
Sundaes: Average all outlets	7	0.3
Arby's: Roast Beef Sandwich, reg.	20	4.6
Chicken Club Salad	32	3.8
Roast Beef Sandwich, Super	21	3.8
Burger King: Whopper S/wich	29	5.4
Bacon Double Cheeseburger	32	4.5
BK Big Fish Sandwich	24	4.5
Carl's Jr: Famous Star Hamburger	24	2
Bacon Swiss Crispy Chicken	35	2
Charbroiled Chicken Club Sandwich	40	3
Super Star Hamburger	41	3

Fast Foods/Burgers (Cont)

	Pro	Iron
Domino's Pizza: Deep Dish (12")		
Beef, 2 slices	4	0.7
Cheese, 2 slices	13	3.6
Pepperoni, Sausage, 1 sl.	10	1.8
KFC: Original, Breast	37	1
Crispy Strips, 3 strips	29	1.8
Snacker, Regular	15	2.7
McDonald's: Big Mac	25	4.5
Cheeseburger	15	2.7
Chicken McNuggets (6)	14	0.7
Crispy Chicken Classic Burger	28	3.6
Filet-O-Fish	15	1.8
Grilled Chicken Caesar Salad	30	1.8
Hamburger	12	2.7
Quarter Pounder w. Cheese	29	4.5
French Fries: Small, 2.5 oz	3	0.7
Large, 5.4 oz	6	1.5
Salads w. Chicken, average	29	3
Thick Shake, average, 16 fl.oz	13	0.7
Breakfast: Egg McMuffin	18	3.6
Bacon, Egg & Cheese McGriddles	16	2.7
Sausage Burrito	12	2.7
Sausage McMuffin w. Egg	21	3.6
Pizza Hut: Per Medium, 1 slice, ⅛ Pizza		
Thin 'n Crispy, Supreme	11	1
Pan Pizzas, Supreme	10	2
Hand Tossed, Pepperoni	11	1.5
Fit n' Delicious, Ham/Pineapple	8	1
Subway (6" Subs): Roast Beef	19	6.3
Meatball Marinara	24	7.2
Roast Chicken Breast	24	4.5
Subway Club	24	5.4
Sweet Onion Chicken Teriyaki	26	4.6
Taco Bell: Bean Burrito	13	2.7
Chicken Quesadilla	28	1.8
Chicken/Steak Enchirito	21	1.8
Gordita Baja Beef	13	2.7
Steak Burrito Supreme	18	2.7
Taco Supreme	9	1
Tostado	11	1.5
Wendy's: Old Fashioned Single Burger	25	4.5
Chicken Club	34	2.7
Hamburger (Kid's Meal)	15	2.7

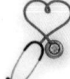
High Blood Pressure

High Blood Pressure

Many American adults have hypertension (high blood pressure), and are unaware of it. It is generally symptomless, so **have your blood pressure checked annually** – particularly if it runs in the family.

Untreated hypertension overworks the heart, damages arteries and promotes atherosclerosis. This in turn greatly increases the risk of heart disease, stroke, blindness, kidney disease and impotence. The earlier hypertension is detected, the sooner it can be brought under control.

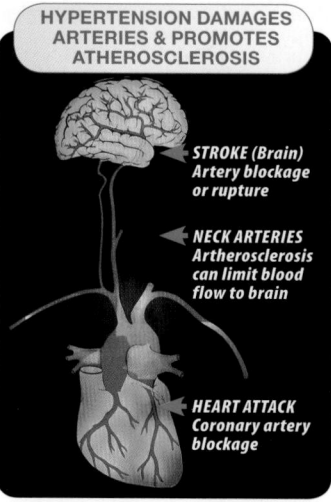

HYPERTENSION DAMAGES ARTERIES & PROMOTES ATHEROSCLEROSIS

STROKE (Brain)
Artery blockage or rupture

NECK ARTERIES
Artherosclerosis can limit blood flow to brain

HEART ATTACK
Coronary artery blockage

BLOOD PRESSURE CLASSIFICATION

For Adults Age 18 & Older ~ Not Acutely Ill or on Medication (American Heart Association)

	DIASTOLIC		SYSTOLIC
Normal ➤	Below 80	and	Below 120
Prehypertension ➤	80-89	or	120-139
Hypertension:			
Stage 1 ➤	90-99	or	140-159
Stage 2 ➤	100 or more	or	160 or more

Treating Hypertension

Prehypertension (in the chart above) means you don't have high blood pressure now but are likely to develop it in the future.

You can take steps to lessen the risk by adopting healthy lifestyle habits such as:
- reducing sodium intake
- eating adequate fruit and vegetables
- losing weight if overweight
- limiting alcohol to 2 drinks or less daily
- quitting smoking
- exercising regularly, managing stress.

Stage 1 hypertension can often be treated with the above lifestyle changes.

Stage 2 hypertension usually requires drug therapy. However, salt restriction, abstaining from alcohol, and the above lifestyle changes will improve the success of drug therapy, and enable smaller drug doses to be prescribed.

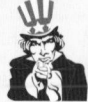

STROKE
KNOW THE WARNING SIGNS

Stroke is a medical emergency!
If you notice one or more of these signs, call 9-1-1 or your doctor immediately.

These signs may be signalling a possible stroke or transient ischemic attack:

- **Sudden weakness** or numbness in your face, arm, or leg on one side of your body
- **Sudden confusion,** trouble speaking or understanding
- **Sudden trouble seeing,** in one or both eyes
- **Sudden trouble walking,** dizziness, loss of balance or coordination
- **Sudden severe headache** - 'a bolt out of the blue' – with no apparent cause

Salt & Sodium

- **Sodium is a mineral element** most commonly found in salt (sodium chloride). It also occurs naturally in much smaller amounts in animal and plant foods, and water – normally sufficient for our needs without having to add salt to our diet.

- **Sodium is required** for nerve and muscle function, as well as to balance the amount of fluid in our tissues and blood.

  Sodium acts like a sponge to attract and hold fluids in body tissues.

- **Excess sodium** can cause water retention, and increase the risk of developing hypertension. Very high salt intake may also increase the risk of stomach cancer.

- **Too little sodium** may cause low blood pressure (hypotension), and decrease blood flow to the heart, brain and kidneys - especially during exercise. (A certain blood volume is required to sustain the blood pressure needed for adequate blood flow in the capillaries).

Salt-Sensitive Persons

- **Normally, our kidneys** excrete excess dietary sodium. The thirst we feel after a salty meal is the body calling for water to dilute the sodium, and enable the kidneys to flush out excess sodium.

- **However, 'salt - sensitive'** persons (up to 50% of adults) tend to retain excess sodium (above approximately 3000mg daily) instead of excreting it. Such persons are more likely to develop hypertension and would benefit most from sodium restriction. Assume you are susceptible if there is a family history of hypertension.

- **Although not everyone will benefit, all Americans are being asked to moderate their salt and sodium intake** as a public health measure – particularly because so many do not know whether or not they have hypertension, and also because we do not know just who is salt-sensitive.

SAFE SODIUM LEVELS

The American Heart Association recommends a **maximum sodium intake of 2300mg per day** for adults with normal blood pressure. However, people who consume **less than 1500mg sodium** have the lowest blood pressure levels.

Persons with hypertension and kidney ailments are usually restricted to as little as **1000mg sodium per day**. Your doctor will discuss the correct sodium level for you.

Persons with Menière's Disease (chronic attacks of vertigo, dizziness, hearing loss, imbalance), often benefit from lower sodium intake of less than 2000mg/day, as well as even distribution of food and fluids over the day (to prevent fluctuations in body fluids and pressure in the inner ear). Also avoid caffeine and MSG. Limit sugar and alcohol.

further info: www.CalorieKing.com

FINDING HIDDEN SODIUM

On average, **less than one third of our sodium intake comes from the salt shaker.** The rest is hidden in processed foods that have salt added during manufacture.

Sodium compounds added to food or medicinals can also contribute significant sodium.

Sodium bicarbonate in particular is widely used in antacid tablets (such as Alka Seltzer) and powders. Sodium bicarbonate contains 27% sodium by weight. Each gram contributes 270mg sodium. Large amounts of sodium can be unwittingly consumed – up to 600mg per tablet. (See Antacids ~ Page 293)

Example: 2 Alka-Seltzer Tablets = 1000mg sodium

Other sodium compounds include monosodium glutamate (MSG), sodium ascorbate, sodium nitrite, and sodium citrate.

ALCOHOL DANGER

Excessive alcohol intake contributes to hypertension. Susceptible persons should limit alcohol intake to 1-2 drinks per day.

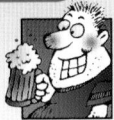

Salt Sodium Guide

Sodium accounts for only 40% of the weight of salt (sodium chloride). Examples:
1 gram (1000mg) Salt has 400mg Sodium
1 teaspoon (5g) Salt has 2000mg Sodium

HINTS TO REDUCE SODIUM

- **Cut down use of the salt shaker.** Start with an easy 50% cut in sodium by using Lite Salt (*Morton*) or *Cardia* Salt. Then gradually cut back until you can leave the salt shaker off the table. Sea salt is still high in sodium.

- **Use fresh herbs,** and salt-free seasonings to add flavor to food.

- **Choose low-sodium,** sodium-free, and reduced-sodium products in place of regular, salted products.

- **Check food labels for sodium levels.** FDA Guidelines for sodium descriptors are:
  - **Reduced Sodium:** At least 25% less sodium than the original product
  - **Low Sodium:** 140 mg or less/serving
  - **Very Low Sodium:** 35mg or less/serving
  - **Sodium Free:** Less than 5mg/serving
  - **No Salt Added:** Made without the salt normally added, but still contains the sodium that is a natural part of the food

- **Use reduced-sodium breads,** butter and margarine. Regular varieties contain up to 2% salt. This is considered high in view of their significant contribution to our diet.

- **Go easy on salty condiments and sauces** such as ketchup, mustard, soy sauce, spaghetti sauces, and salad dressings. Use low-sodium varieties.

- **Limit pizzas and salty fast-foods.** Check *CalorieKing.com* food database.

- **Avoid salty snack foods** such as potato chips, corn chips, salted nuts, pretzels and cheesy-flavored snacks. **Choose unsalted** popcorn, nuts or seeds. Eat more fruit.

- **Don't salt children's food** to your taste.

- **Avoid antacids with** sodium bicarbonate (such as *Alka-Seltzer*). They are high in sodium. Look for low-sodium alternatives.

FOODS HIGH IN SODIUM

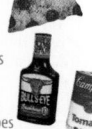

- Cheese, Butter, Margarine
- Pickles, Sauerkraut, Olives
- Condiments, Sauces
- Salad Dressings
- Canned vegetables/salads/beans
- Deli Salads (with dressing)
- Frozen/Packaged Meals/Entrees
- Soups: Canned/dry; bouillon cubes
- Meats: Ham, bacon, sausage, luncheon meats, smoked meats
- Canned Fish (in brine/salt)
- Sea Salt, Garlic/Celery Salt
- Snack Foods (potato chips, pretzels)
- Tomato Juice (Canned), V8 Vegetable Juice
- Fast Foods: Pizza, Burgers, Chicken
- *Alka-Seltzer* Antacid

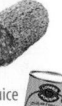

MODERATE SODIUM

- Bread (Reduced Salt)
- Meat, Fish, Poultry - Unprocessed
- Milk, Yogurt, Soy Drinks, Eggs
- Peanut Butter
- Breakfast Cereals (less than 200mg/serving)
- Chocolate Candy, Fruit/Nut Bars
- *Reduced Sodium & Low Sodium Products*

FOODS LOW IN SODIUM

- Products labelled *Very Low Sodium*, or *Sodium Free*
- Fresh fruits and vegetables
- Canned and Dried Fruits
- Potatoes, Rice, Pasta
- Dried Beans & Lentils, Tofu
- Nuts & Seeds (unsalted)
- Corn & Popcorn (unsalted)
- Pepper, Spices, Herbs
- Jam, Honey, Syrup
- Candy, Gum
- Hard & Jelly Candy
- Coffee, Tea, Alcohol
- Fresh Fruit Juices, Water

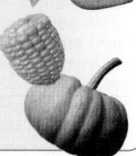

The American Heart Association recommends a sodium intake of **less than 2300mg/day**

Milk & Dairy Products

	Sodium
Milk: Whole/lowfat/skim, average	
1 cup, 8 fl.oz	120
Whole, low sodium, 1 cup	5
Choc Milk *(Hershey's)*, 1 cup	130
Soy Milk, 8 fl.oz	30
Buttermilk, cultured, 8 fl.oz	250
Dry/Powder, skim, ¼ cup, 1 oz	110
Yogurt, with fruit average, 8 oz	130
Cheese: Bleu, 1 oz	330
Parmesan, 1 oz	450
Kraft Cheddar, 2% milk, 1 oz	230
Philadelphia Cream Cheese, 1 oz	90
Process Cheese., average, 1 oz	430
Swiss, 1 oz	40
Cottage Cheese, ½ cup, 4 oz	450
Ricotta Cheese, ½ cup, 4 oz	150

Ice Cream, Frozen Yogurt

Icecream, average, ½ cup	50
Frozen Yogurt, ½ cup	50

Fats/Oils

Butter/Margarine:	
Regular, 2 Tbsp, 1 oz	230
Unsalted, reg., 2 Tbsp, 1 oz	5
Mayonnaise, aver., 2 Tbsp, 1 oz	160
Oils/Lard/Drippings	0
Cream, average, 1 Tbsp	5
Coffee-Mate: Powdered, 1 tsp	2
Liquid, 1 Tbsp	5

Eggs

Whole, 1 large	70
Omelet, 2 egg, plain	220
w. cheese	400
Egg Beaters: Original, ¼ cup	115
Flavors, average, ¼ cup	230

Meats

Meat, average all types, cooked	
(Beef/Lamb/Veal/Pork), 4 oz	80
Corned Beef, cooked, 3 oz	800
Bacon, cooked, 2 sl., ½ oz	270
Ham, 3 oz	1100

Chicken & Turkey

Chicken/Turkey, cooked, unsalted, 4 oz	80
Stuffing Mixes, average., ½ cup	500

Sodium ~ Sodium (mg)

Sausages & Meats

	Sodium
Bologna, 1 oz	280
Frankfurter, 2 oz	640
Ham, chopped, ¾ oz slice	290
Liverwurst (Braunschweiger), 1 oz	320
Pepperoni, 5 slices, 1 oz	570
Salami, cooked, 1 oz	350
dry/hard, 1 oz	600
Sausage, 1 oz link	220
Pork, 2 oz patty	260
Spam: Classic, 2 oz	790
25% Less Sodium, 2 oz	580
Turkey Roll, 1 oz	160

Fish:

Fish: Fresh Fish, average, plain	
Cooked, 4 oz (no bone)	60
Broiled w. butter, 4 oz	150
Breaded & fried, 4 oz	320
Fish fillets, batter-dipped 3 oz	350
Fish sticks, 1 oz stick	160
Gefilte Fish (w. broth), 1 pce, 1½ oz	220
Herring, pickled, 2 pces, 1 oz	260
Lobster, meat only, 4 oz	180
Oysters, fresh, 6 med., 3 oz	95
Salmon: Canned, 3 oz	460
No Salt Added, 3 oz	65
Smoked fish, average, 3 oz	650
Tuna: Canned, regular, 3 oz	330
No Added Salt, 3 oz	40
Spicy Flavored, 5 oz can	550

Entrees & Meals

Frozen Meals, average	600-900
Lean Cuisine, average	700
Stouffer's, average	580
Dinners, average	900-1200
Side Dishes, average	400-600
Pizza, frozen, ¼ large, 6 oz	800-1200
Microwave Cup Meals	900-1200
Cup O'Noodles, average	1500

Fast-Foods & Restaurants

Cheeseburger	750
Chicken Dinner (3 piece)	2200
Chicken Nuggets w. Sauce	800
Fish/Chicken Sandwich	1000
French Fries, small, 2½ oz	150
Hamburger: Regular	500
Large with cheese	1100
Hot Dog (Frankfurter)	800
Pizza, 2 medium slices	1200
Shake, chocolate	250
Taco	400

Extra Listings ~ see CalorieKing.com

Sodium Counter

Sodium ~ Sodium (mg)	Sodium
Soups: Condensed, 1 c., 8 oz	800-1000
Low Sodium	70
Chicken Noodle, 1 cup	900
Bouillon Cube, average	950
Cup-A-Soup: Average	850
Lite, average	450
Soup Mixes, average, 1 cup	900

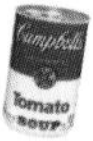

Condiments, Sauces, Dressings

A-1 Sauce, 1 Tbsp	280
Barbecue Sauce, 1 Tbsp	130
Bragg Liquid Aminos, 1 tsp	220
Chili Sauce, 1 Tbsp	230
Ketchup: Tomato, 1 Tbsp	180
Low Sodium, 1 Tbsp	20
Mayonnaise, 1 Tbsp	80
Mustard, 1 tsp	70
Pizza Sauce, ½ cup	700
Salad Dressings, 2 Tbsp, 1 oz	160-400
Spaghetti Sauce, ½ cup	500
Soy Sauce: 1 Tbsp	900
Lite *(Kikkoman),* 1 Tbsp	600
Sweet & Sour, ½ cup	250
Tabasco, 1 tsp	25
Vinegar, Lemon Juice	0
Worcestershire, 1 Tbsp	200
Tomato: Sauce, 1 cup	1200
Paste/Puree (salted), ½ cup	1000
No Salt Added, ½ cup	25

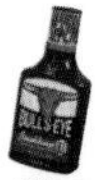

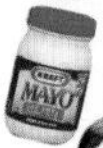

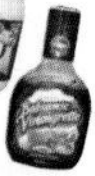

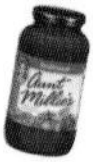

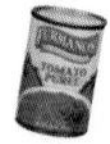

Salt & Salt Substitutes

Table Salt: 1 teaspoon, 6g	2400
Single Serve package, 1 g	400
Cardia Salt, 1 teaspoon	1080
Lite Salt *(Morton),* 1 teaspoon, 6g	1200
Morton Salt Substitute	5
No Salt Salt Substitute, 1 teaspoon	5
Garlic/Seasoned Salt 1 teaspoon, 4g	1300
Sea Salt, 1 teaspoon, 5g	2250

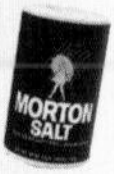

Seasonings, Herbs & Spices

Baking Powder, 1 tsp, 3g	340
Baking Soda (Sodium bicarb), 1 tsp, 3g	810
Accent (Flavor Enhancer), 1 tsp	600
Chili Powder, 1 tsp, 3g	25
Curry Powder	0
Lemon Pepper *(Lawry's),* 1 tsp	340
Meat Tenderizer, 1 tsp, 5g	1750
MSG (Monosodium glutamate), 5g	500
Mrs Dash Blends/Marinades	0
Pepper, Mustard (dry), 1 tsp	1
Yeast, Nutritional, 1 Tbsp	10

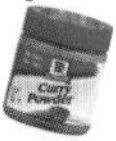

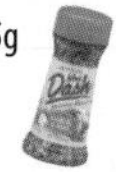

Breakfast Cereals

Kellogg's:	Sodium
All-Bran, ½ cup, 1 oz	80
Special K, 1 cup, 1.1 oz	220
Corn Flakes, 1 cup, 1 oz	200
Just Right, ¾ cup, 2 oz	240
Mini Wheats Frosted, 24 bisc., 1.8 oz	5
Health Valley Cereals, 1 serving	5
Quaker: Cap'n Crunch, ¾ cup, 1 oz	200
Crunchy Corn Bran, ¾ cup, 1 oz	230
100% Natural Granola, ½ cup, 1 oz	15
Puffed Rice/Wheat, 2 cups, 1 oz	1
General Mills: Total, ¾ cup, 1 oz	190
Oatmeal: Regular, ¾ cup	1
Instant *(Quaker),* ⅔ cup (1 pkt)	270

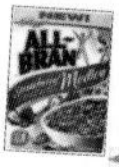

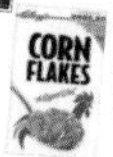

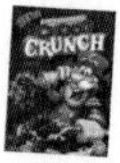

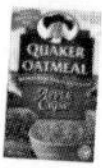

Breads, Bagels, Crackers

Bread: Average all types, 1 oz	140
Low Sodium, 1 oz	10
Bagels: Plain, 2 oz	200
Sara Lee, 3 oz	500
Biscuits, average, 1 oz	180
Bun/Roll, 1 medium, 1½ oz	200
Crackers: Saltine, 2 crackers	70
Low Salt *(Premium),* 2	25
Graham, 2 regular	50
Croissant, average, 2 oz	280
Rice Cakes, average	25
Ry-Krisp Crispbread, Sesame, 1	100

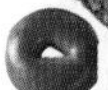

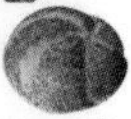

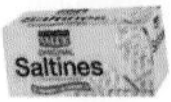

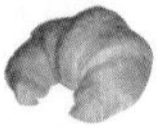

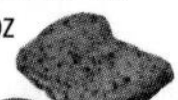

Cookies, Cakes, Desserts

Cookies: Average, 2-3 cookies, 1 oz	100
Mrs Fields', average, 2½ oz	180
Baked Custard, ½ cup	100
Brownie, ¼ oz piece	75
Cake, average, 3 oz piece	250
Cinnamon Sweet Roll, 2 oz	250
Danish, Apple	250
Donut, average	150
Muffins: 1 medium, 2 oz	150
Pancakes, 3 x 4"	360
Pie, average ⅙ of 9" pie	300
Pudding: Average, ½ cup	160
Jell-O (Mix), Instant, ½ cup	400
Waffles:	
Home-made, 7", 2½ oz	350
Frozen: Average, 1¼ oz	260
Aunt Jemima, avg, 2½ oz	565

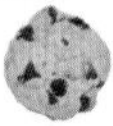

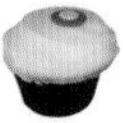

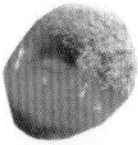

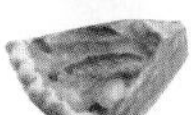

Sodium Counter

Fruit & Juices
	Sodium
Fresh Fruit, average all types, 1 serving	1
Dried/Canned Fruit, ½ cup	1
Fruit Juice: Fresh, sqz'd, 6 fl.oz	1
Commercial, aver., 6 fl.oz	20
Carrot Juice (Ferraro's), 8 fl.oz	230
Tomato Juice (Campbell's), 6 fl.oz	570
Low Sodium (No Salt Added)	20
V8 Vegetable (Campbell's), 6 fl.oz	600
(No Salt Added), 6 fl.oz	45

Vegetables
Fresh/Frozen (No Salt Added): Per ½ Cup	
Asparagus, Bean Sprouts, Corn	3
Beets, Carrots, Celery, ½ cup	40
Broccoli, Cabbage, Cauliflower	10
Cucumber, Green Beans, Mushroom, Okra	3
Onions, Peas, Potato, Pumpkin, Squash	3
Peppers, Hot Chili, raw, each	3
Spinach, Turnips, ½ cup, ckd	40
Tomato, 1 medium, 5 oz	10
Canned: Asparagus, 4 spears	300
Beans, baked in tomato sauce	450
Beets, ½ cup, 3 oz	240
Corn Kernels, ½ cup, 3 oz	190
Creamed, ½ cup, 4½ oz	330
Mushrooms w. butter sce, 2oz	550
Peas, ½ cup, 3 oz	250
Sauerkraut, ½ cup, 4 oz	750

Pickles, Olives
Olives, pickled: Green, 1 large	90
Ripe/black, 1 large	40
Pickles: Bread & Butter, 4 sl., 1 oz	200
Dill, 1 pickle, 2½ oz	900
Sweet, 1 gherkin, ½ oz	130

Soybean Products
Miso (Soy Paste), ¼ c., 2½ oz	2500
Soybean Protein Isolate, 1 oz	280
Tempeh, ½ cup, 3 oz	5
Tofu, average, ½ cup, 4 oz	5

Jam, Honey, Syrups
Jam/Jelly, 1 Tbsp	2
Honey/Maple Syrup, 1 Tbsp	1
Log Cabin Syrup, 1 fl.oz	35
Lite, 1 fl.oz	90

Peanut Butter
Peanut Butter: Regular, 2 Tbsp, ½ oz	190
Low Sodium (Jif), 2 Tbsp	65
Unsalted (Trader Joe's), 2 Tbsp	5

Snacks, Nuts
	Sodium
Cheese Balls/Curls, 1 oz	280
Corn/Tortilla Chips, average, 1 oz	220
Granola bars, average, 1 bar	80
Nuts: Plain, unsalted, 1 oz	1
Lightly salted, 1 oz	80
Salted or Honey Roasted, 1 oz	160
Popcorn: Plain (unsalted), 1 cup	1
Flavored, average, 1 cup	60
Salt added, 1 cup	180
Potato Chips: Plain, 1 oz	160
Flavored, average, 1 oz	250
Pretzels, regular, 3, 1 oz	450

Candy, Chocolate
Chocolate, milk, 1 oz	30
Fudge, chocolate, 1 oz	55
Candy Bars, average, 1½ oz	60
Hard Candy, Jelly Beans, 1 oz	10
Licorice, 1 oz	30

Beverages, Alcohol
Coffee (& Substitutes), Tea, 1 cup	1
Cocoa, dry, plain, 1 Tbsp	1
Mix, average, 1 envelope	120
Quik (Nestle), 2 tsp	35
Soft Drinks, average, 8 fl.oz	20
Mineral Water, Perrier, 8 fl.oz	5
Gatorade Thirst Quencher, 8 fl.oz	110
Water: Average, 1 cup, 8 fl.oz	5
Drier regions, 1 cup	20+
Alcohol: Beer, average, 12 fl.oz	15
Wines, average, 4 fl.oz	10
Spirits (distilled), 1½ fl.oz	1

Antacids – Alka-Seltzer
	Sodium
Alka-Seltzer (Per Tablet):	
Alka-Seltzer P.M., 1 tablet	500
Original (Light Blue Box)	570
Extra Strength (Dark Blue Box)	590
Flavored Lemon/Lime & Cherry	500
Antacid (yellow Box)	310
Gelatine Capsule, 1	0
Alka-Mints, chewable	0
Bromo Seltzer, ¾ capful	760
Rolaids, All types	0
Tums, Regular/Extra Strength	0
Sodium Bicarbonate (27% sodium), 1g	270

Index A - B

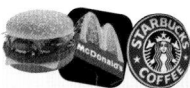

FAST-FOOD RESTAURANTS INDEX
~ SEE PAGE 183 ~

Index C - F

Index K - M

Index P - S

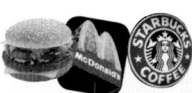

FAST-FOOD RESTAURANTS INDEX
~ SEE PAGE 183 ~

Index T - Z

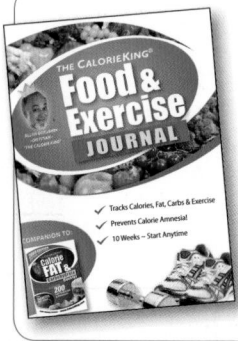
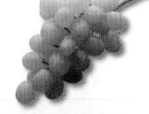

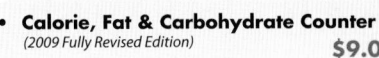
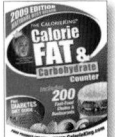
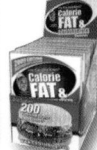
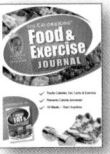
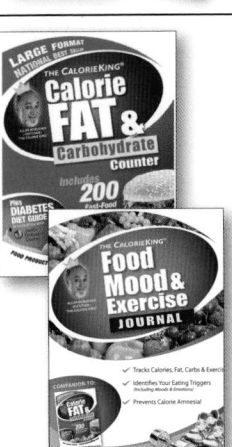
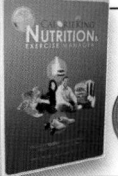
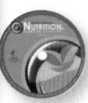

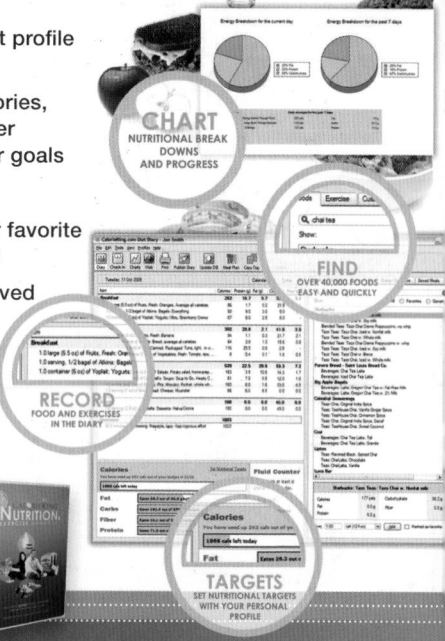